ATLAS
OF
INFRARED THERMOGRAPHY

A Practical Clinical Guide: Functional Imaging for Pain, Circulatory Health, Musculoskeletal Disorders, and Visceral Assessment

Note. While the author has taken meticulous care to ensure the accuracy and currency of the information presented, medicine evolves continuously. Readers should verify that any information, particularly regarding medical investigations and care strategies, aligns with local legislation and prevailing standards of practice.

References to medical procedures, medications, or intervention protocols are provided for illustrative purposes only and do not constitute a recommendation or endorsement.
For personalized healthcare decisions, consult qualified healthcare professionals.

Felipe Reitz

Atlas of Infrared Thermography

A Practical Clinical Guide: Functional Imaging for Pain, Circulatory Health, Musculoskeletal Disorders, and Visceral Assessment

Author: Felipe Reitz

First Edition, 2025

Published by Reitz Institute Press

Florianópolis, Brazil

Dados Internacionais de Catalogação na Publicação (CIP) (Câmara Brasileira do Livro, SP, Brasil)

Reitz, Felipe

Atlas of infrared thermography : a practical clinical guide: functional imaging for pain, circulatory health, musculoskeletal disorders, and visceral assessment / Felipe Reitz. --

1. ed. -- Florianópolis, SC : Ed. do Autor, 2025.

Bibliografia.

ISBN 978-65-01-73173-5

1. Atlas 2. Anatomia humana 3. Ciências da saúde 4. Corpo humano - Aspectos de saúde 5. Educação em saúde 6. novações médicas 7. Termografia I. Título.

25-306952.0 CDD-610

Índices para catálogo sistemático:

1. Termografia infravermelha : Corpo humano : Diagnóstico : Ciências médicas 610

Disclaimer:

This book is intended for educational and professional reference. It is not a substitute for individualized medical advice, diagnosis, or treatment, and it does not create a physician–patient relationship. Any use of terms such as "diagnostic," "treatment," or "disease" within this Atlas reflects conventional scientific or historical usage and is not intended to imply regulatory approval or to substitute for recognized medical practice in any jurisdiction.

To purchase additional copies of this book, contact the author at

www.felipereitz.com – **freitz.books@gmail.com**

About the Author

Felipe Reitz is the originator of Biospectral Medicine, a discipline that transforms the interpretation of human emissive signals into a structured scientific framework. Over the course of more than two decades, he has united emissive physics, physiology, and integrative approaches to create a methodology that is unprecedented in the study of emissive imaging.

His innovations include the development of Computerized Thermographic Imaging (CTI), the R-CIIM interpretative model, and the standardized map of 19 emission zones. Together, these contributions establish for the first time a reproducible language for functional imaging, enabling the investigation of regulatory processes that remain invisible to structural modalities such as MRI, CT, or ultrasound.

Reitz has published in internationally recognized journals and has been acknowledged as a pioneer in high-complexity integrative analysis. Yet his most enduring contribution is not a single paper or device, but the creation of an entirely new scientific lexicon. This Atlas consolidates more than 23 years of clinical and scientific work into a reference that defines the field itself, establishing standards, terminology, and procedures that future generations will inherit, expand, and refine.

Like the foundational works of science and physics that once redefined their eras, this Atlas positions Felipe Reitz not only as an author but as the primary reference for a new branch of biosignal science. His achievement is both historical and forward-looking, a system that provides clarity where none existed and opens a path for global research, education, and interpretive innovation.

ATLAS
OF
INFRARED THERMOGRAPHY

A Practical Clinical Guide:
Functional Imaging for Pain, Circulatory Health, Musculoskeletal Disorders, and Visceral Assessment

AUTHOR:
FELIPE REITZ

freitz72@gmail.com

2025

Why This Book Was Created

For centuries, medicine has excelled at describing the structures of the body but has struggled to capture its functions in motion, the circulatory adjustments, neuroautonomic responses, and metabolic shifts that precede visible conditions. Imaging technologies such as X-ray, CT, MRI, and ultrasound offered extraordinary anatomical clarity, yet they remained blind to the earliest expressions of dysfunction, the physiological signals that mark the body's attempt to adapt, regulate, and survive.

This Atlas was created to answer that absence. It introduces Biospectral Medicine, a discipline that gives clinical meaning to human emissive signals, transforming them into a biosignal language. The book establishes, for the first time, a reproducible framework, the R-CIIM method, the spectral lexicon, and a map of 19 emission zones, through which the invisible functions of the body can be observed, described, and acted upon with scientific rigor.

The Atlas exists as a functional counterpart to conventional imaging, expanding its scope and application. It does not replace anatomy, it reveals what anatomy alone cannot, the physiology of regulation, the early dynamics of imbalance, and the spectral signatures of adaptation. Its creation was driven by the recognition that medicine needed more than a description of damage, it needed a window into process, regulation, and cause.

This book was written to give clinicians, researchers, and students a reference that has never before existed; a comprehensive, standardized system for interpreting emissive biosignals. It was created because the science of health cannot remain blind to the signals that come before symptoms, before pathology, and before decline. In providing this framework, the Atlas fulfils its purpose; to define a new discipline, establish its language, and make visible what medicine until now could not see.

This Atlas is a specialized reference, comparable in scope to works such as the Atlas of PET-CT in Oncology or the Atlas of Endoscopic Ultrasound. It is designed for institutional libraries, research centers, and advanced clinical practice, where emissive imaging can be studied with the same academic rigor and permanence as other established diagnostic modalities.

Author's Notes

This Atlas is the product of decades of persistence, reflection, and discovery. For more than twenty years, I stood between patients who could not find answers and a medical system that too often looked only at structures and missed the functions that give rise to them. What you now hold in your hands is the distilled outcome of that search, a framework that makes visible the body's hidden dialogue of regulation, adaptation, and resilience.

Every page of this work carries the weight of thousands of patient encounters, nights spent testing hypotheses, and years of questioning whether the invisible could ever be made measurable. There were times when it seemed impossible, when medicine had no language for what I was seeing. But from that silence came the need to build a language of my own, Biospectral Medicine.

This book is more than a scientific manual; it is a record of a journey. A journey that began with a simple observation, that the body emits signals it cannot hide, and grew into a structured system capable of guiding clinical analysis and interpretive practices across the world. The terminology, the spectral lexicon, the R-CIIM model, and the mapping of 19 zones are not theoretical inventions, they are the lived outcome of two decades of testing, refining, and proving.

I write these notes to mark a beginning, an opening rather than a conclusion. This Atlas lays the foundation of a discipline, but it is only the first chapter in a story that others will continue. My hope is that, in your practice and in your research, you will find in these pages not just a tool, but a path, a path that affirms the conviction that medicine must always search deeper, look earlier, and seek causes before effects.

Note on the Testimonials

All testimonials in this first edition come from Brazilian professionals. This reflects the current stage of Biospectral Medicine, which, after 15 years of development and consolidation in Brazil, is now presented to the world through this Atlas.

The trajectory, however, is broader; it began with almost 10 years of practice and training in Europe before moving to Brazil, giving Biospectral Medicine a truly international foundation.

While the endorsements presented here are national, the conceptual and scientific basis of this discipline was developed across two continents, reflecting its global scope.

"The Atlas of Infrared Thermography is a landmark in medical literature. For the first time, emissive imaging has been transformed into Biospectral Medicine, a discipline uniting physics, physiology, and integrative health within a rigorous and visionary framework. This Atlas restores dignity to a once-suppressed field and opens new frontiers for science, clinical practice, and global health. It will be remembered as the foundation of a new era in functional medicine and clinical interpretation."

Dr. Jean Marie FitzGerald, PhD
Naturopath and Clinician-Researcher

"The Atlas of Infrared Thermography enhances physiotherapy by using skin thermal profiles to analyze functional and clinical alterations in a non-invasive manner. With standardized protocols, the work makes it possible to detect pathophysiological patterns that are not visible in conventional examinations. In practice, it optimizes all physiotherapeutic practice. In this sense, the Atlas is an excellent option to elevate clinical reasoning in physiotherapy, strengthening evidence-based practice."

Dr. Ricardo Wallace, Director
Wallace Institute of Physiotherapy

"The Atlas of Infrared Thermography inaugurates a new way of looking at manual therapies. By scientifically revealing how myofascial release and lymphatic drainage impact muscles, fascia, and circulation, it not only demonstrates the effects of therapeutic touch but also guides the professional to conduct each release with greater precision. A valuable resource that enhances outcomes and expands benefits for patients."

Ana C. Rodrigues
Massage Therapist – Nursing Technician

"The Atlas of Infrared Thermography reflects more than two decades of pioneering research and clinical innovation carried out at the Reitz Institute. Its publication represents a milestone in our mission to advance Biospectral Medicine as a discipline that unites science, clinical practice, and education. We are proud to contribute this work to the global community as a foundation for future research, interdisciplinary collaboration, and the training of the next generation of health professionals."

Reitz Institute
On behalf of the Clinical and Research Team

"The Atlas of Infrared Thermography expands diagnostic tools for physiotherapists and strengthens functional assessment, rehabilitation, and prevention. While consolidating Biospectral Medicine, the work details functional, musculoskeletal, and circulatory patterns that guide clinical practice with greater precision.."

Marcus Duarte
Physioterapist. Osteopath

"The This work of inestimable value to science contributes significantly to the advancement of Integrative Health, providing a solid foundation for a more precise analysis of the physiological and emotional dynamics of the human organism. It enables mental health professionals to achieve a broader understanding of bodily responses to their patients' emotional states, supporting greater accuracy and direction in therapeutic approaches."

Dr.Carolina Do P. Silva
Psychologist

How This Book Impacts Your Practice

This Atlas is meant to be read, revisited, and continually engaged with. It is designed to be used, revisited, and relied upon in the daily reality of clinical and investigative work. It gives you a reproducible system, the R-CIIM method, the spectral lexicon, and the map of 19 emission zones, that transforms emissive signals from abstract patterns into clinically relevant insights.

The Atlas should be regarded as a specialized clinical reference, intended to stand alongside other advanced diagnostic atlases in medical libraries and research collections. Its scope, depth, and methodology distinguish it as a work for long-term institutional use and academic study.

For the clinician, it provides a new analytical dimension, the ability to see regulatory and functional disturbances that precede structural pathology. This means earlier recognition of vascular stress, neuroautonomic imbalance, or metabolic overload, patterns that conventional imaging cannot reveal.

For the researcher, it offers a standardized platform for reproducible data collection and cross-study comparison. The structured methodology allows emission findings to be quantified, categorized, and published with scientific precision, advancing the discipline into the broader academic sphere.

For the student, it serves as both a manual and a map, guiding the acquisition of a new interpretive framework. By learning its definitions, categories, and pathways, students are equipped to use the system and to help shape its future.

The impact of this Atlas is simple but profound. It allows you to see what medicine has not yet seen. By integrating its system into your practice, you extend your interpretive vision into the earliest stages of dysfunction, before symptoms escalate, before irreversible damage occurs. This is a paradigm shift that redefines how medicine perceives function, cause, and adaptation, extending far beyond an incremental addition to existing tools.

How to Use This Atlas

This Atlas was designed as a working reference, a clinical, scientific, and educational tool to be consulted, revisited, and integrated into daily practice, rather than a book for a single reading. Its structure reflects the logic of Biospectral Medicine, beginning with scientific foundations, advancing through the R-CIIM interpretive methodology, then applying these principles to the 19 emission zones, clinical case studies, and finally to the reference tables and glossary that anchor the discipline.

For the clinician, the Atlas functions as both a guide and a companion. Start with the emission zone most relevant to the patient's presentation. Apply the six steps of the R-CIIM method to classify the finding, then cross-reference with the tables for differential support. The case studies serve as models, demonstrating how similar presentations were interpreted, mapped, and linked to care strategies.

For the researcher, the Atlas provides a standardized framework for reproducible studies. Begin with the definitions in the glossary and the spectral lexicon to ensure consistency in terminology. Use the reference tables to structure data collection, and cite the emission zones as standardized anatomical markers. This approach allows cross-study comparability and ensures that future investigations build on a shared scientific foundation.

For the student, the Atlas is best approached progressively. First, study the scientific foundations to understand the physics of emissive imaging. Next, learn the spectral lexicon and the biosignal categories as a new interpretive vocabulary. Then, practice with the case studies, using them as exercises in step-by-step interpretation. Over time, the Atlas becomes a textbook and a learning map for acquiring fluency in Biospectral Medicine.

Every section of this Atlas is interlinked, a definition in the glossary echoes a step in the R-CIIM model, a table clarifies what a case study demonstrates, a zone illustration directs the reader back to the scientific foundations. The book should be used dynamically, not linearly, flipping between glossary, cases, and reference tables as needed. In this way, it functions like an atlas of anatomy or physiology, a tool that provides structure to observation, consistency to interpretation, and confidence to decision-making.

The ultimate purpose of this Atlas is to be actively used at the point of practice, rather than admired on a shelf. Whether you are at a patient's side, in a research lab, or in a classroom, it offers the same value, a reproducible system for seeing, naming, and interpreting what was previously invisible.

Note on Terminology

This Atlas employs certain terms familiar to readers of conventional medical literature, such as *diagnostic, diagnosis, disease, therapy,* and *treatment.* Within the framework of Biospectral Medicine, however, these terms do not carry their regulatory or procedural meaning. They are used illustratively, to connect with established scientific language, and should be read according to the vocabulary of Biospectral Medicine:

- Diagnostic / Diagnosis = Interpretive / Interpretation
- Disease / Pathology = Condition / Imbalance / Dysfunction
- Therapy / Treatment = Care Strategy / Intervention / Support

The terms used throughout this Atlas follow established scientific medical language and universal health nomenclatures, while expressing the distinct framework of Biospectral Medicine. This methodology is interpretive in essence, providing a structured lens for understanding emissive biosignals. It constitutes an evolutionary branch of science, an advancement that extends existing knowledge and establishes a new field of investigation for future generations.

By continuing to read, you acknowledge and accept this interpretive framework.

CONTENTS

CHAPTER 1

FROM SUPPRESSION TO THE FOUNDATIONS OF BIOSPECTRAL MEDICINE

PART 1

HISTORY AND BARRIERS

HISTORY OF INFRARED AND THERMOGRAPHY

Long before infrared cameras, medical traditions across the world recognized that thermal patterns on the skin reflected deeper physiological states. In Traditional Chinese Medicine, the perception of warmth or coldness in specific meridian zones guided both diagnosis and treatment, often interpreted through palpation, pulse analysis, or tongue temperature.

Ayurvedic practitioners noted localized heat as a sign of aggravated *pitta dosha*, often correlating with inflammation, infection, or organ dysfunction. Even in the Hippocratic corpus, the idea of "hot humors" or "dry and moist imbalances" carried investigative significance linked to body surface changes. What these ancient systems lacked in imaging technology, they compensated for with clinical sensitivity to temperature dynamics.

Biospectral Medicine reclaims this ancestral analytical insight within a rigorous scientific framework. By capturing emissive patterns with precision and interpreting them through structured clinical zones, it bridges ancient clinical intuition with contemporary evidence-based methodology. This convergence validates long-standing empirical traditions and restores surface thermoregulation as a legitimate and measurable investigative axis in modern medicine.

1800 – The Discovery of Infrared Radiation by William Herschel

The foundational moment in the history of thermographic science occurred in March 1800, when the British-German astronomer and physicist Sir William Herschel (1738–1822) made a landmark discovery: the existence of invisible infrared radiation beyond the red end of the visible light spectrum.

> ***"...the thermometer beyond the red rays rose as much, or more, than any of the others. This appeared extraordinary, and led me to pay more attention to the invisible rays"***
>
> Sir William Herschel, 1800

Herschel was not searching for invisible energy per se, he was conducting experiments with sunlight to determine which colour of light transmitted the most heat. To do this, he used a glass prism to disperse sunlight into its constituent spectrum (red to violet) and then placed thermometers in each colour band to measure their temperatures.

In a significant step, he also placed a thermometer just beyond the visible red light, in what appeared to be empty space. To his surprise, this thermometer registered the highest temperature of all, indicating the presence of a form of radiation that was not visible to the human eye, but which clearly carried thermal energy.

Herschel called this discovery "calorific rays," though today we know it as infrared radiation, a term derived later from the Latin *infra*, meaning "below," and "red," the lowest-frequency visible light.

Herschel's experiment marked the first demonstration that heat could be transmitted by a form of light invisible to the human eye, and his work laid the physical foundation for all future developments in thermal sensing, infrared astronomy, and ultimately, medical thermographic imaging.

His findings were presented to the Royal Society in the same year and published in *Philosophical Transactions of the Royal Society of London* (Herschel, 1800), a document now considered one of the ground-breaking texts in electromagnetic radiation science.

This discovery revolutionized physics and optics and introduced the conceptual possibility that living systems, by virtue of their temperature, could be passively observed through radiation.

1840 – John Herschel and the First Thermal Image Using Evaporative Film

Nearly four decades after his father's ground-breaking discovery of infrared radiation, Sir John Herschel (1792–1871), a distinguished astronomer, chemist, and physicist in his own right, contributed a remarkable advancement to the early exploration of thermal phenomena.

In 1840, while investigating the chemical and physical behaviour of heat on surfaces, John Herschel developed what is widely considered the first thermal image ever recorded by artificial means. This was achieved through an ingenious method of evaporative cooling on a thin film..

Herschel coated a surface with oil or alcohol, which would evaporate at varying rates depending on local temperature and airflow. When exposed to a heated object or human body, the differing rates of evaporation would produce visible patterns, essentially heat maps, that could be captured photographically.

> ***"The differences in evaporation, barely visible at first, arranged themselves into distinct figures corresponding to the invisible flow of heat... the heat, as it were, sketched its own portrait."***
>
> John Herschel, private notes, 1840

This technique, though crude by modern standards, allowed for the visualization of temperature differentials without direct contact or invasive tools. It constituted a primitive but conceptually sound passive thermal imaging system.

Herschel referred to this phenomenon as "thermography", coining a term that would later define an entire field. While his work was primarily focused on the behaviour of heat in physical and chemical contexts, its implications for biological and medical applications were profound. For the first time, heat distribution could be visually recorded and preserved, moving the study of thermal emission from transient measurement to documentable evidence.

Although the technique lacked the resolution and sensitivity of electronic sensors developed a century later, Herschel's work marked a key transition: it suggested that temperature patterns could serve as functional indicators, a foundational concept in the development of interpretative thermography.

This moment in history was important for its technical novelty, especially because it seeded the idea that biological processes could be externally visualized through the language of heat and pattern, anticipating the principles that would one day define Biospectral Medicine.

1856 – Charles Piazzi Smyth and the First Infrared Measurements in Astronomy

In 1856, the British astronomer Charles Piazzi Smyth (1819–1900) conducted one of the earliest applications of infrared sensing in an astronomical context, an event that significantly advanced the practical understanding of radiant energy from celestial bodies.

At the time, Smyth served as Astronomer Royal for Scotland and led an expedition to the summit of Mount Guajara in Tenerife, Canary Islands, to escape atmospheric distortion and improve the accuracy of stellar measurements. While his primary goal was to study solar and lunar radiation, his experiments accidentally contributed to the birth of infrared astronomy.

Using thermocouples and differential thermometers, Smyth attempted to measure the thermal radiation emitted by the Moon and high-altitude atmosphere. He noted consistent thermal variations corresponding to lunar position, phase, and elevation angle, demonstrating that non-visible heat energy from celestial bodies could be quantitatively assessed.

> ***"The Moon poured down upon our thermometers a heat not seen but certainly felt, evidence that her surface, too, holds and releases energy unseen."***
>
> Charles Piazzi Smyth, 1856

Although the measurements were coarse and atmospheric interference remained significant, this was among the first formal demonstrations that infrared radiation could carry functional information across space, not just on Earth.

These findings, published in *Tenerife: An Astronomer's Experiment* (Smyth, 1858), would later influence the use of infrared spectroscopy and imaging to detect water vapour, geological features, and temperature gradients on planetary bodies, a tradition continued by NASA's Voyager, Mars Global Surveyor, and James Webb Space Telescope.

Smyth's measurements were designed for physics, yet the principle he validated, that internal states can be reflected by invisible spectral emissions, opened the path toward biological and medical application."

1878 – Samuel Pierpont Langley and the Invention of the Bolometer

In 1878, American physicist and astronomer Samuel Pierpont Langley (1834–1906) introduced a ground-breaking instrument that would revolutionize the detection of radiant heat: the bolometer.

This device, designed to measure minute changes in thermal radiation, was capable of detecting temperature differences as small as 1/100,000th of a degree Celsius, a level of sensitivity previously unimaginable.

Langley, then director of the Allegheny Observatory in Pittsburgh, was initially motivated by his work in solar physics. He sought to analyse the infrared spectrum of solar radiation, which required an instrument far more precise than any available thermocouple or thermometer.

> ***"The bolometer, as a new form of radiant-heat detector, has shown us that what we once called invisible may now be studied with the precision of mathematics."***
>
> S. P. Langley, 1881

He constructed the bolometer by coating two thin strips of platinum foil with black soot to absorb radiation. One strip was exposed to radiation; the other served as a reference. Any slight increase in radiation caused a measurable change in electrical resistance, thus translating invisible heat into quantifiable electrical data.

This innovation was published in Langley's landmark paper, *The Bolometer and Radiant Energy*, in *The American Journal of Science* (Langley, 1881), and soon gained recognition across disciplines. His bolometer was not only used for astronomical measurements, such as detecting the solar constant and atmospheric absorption, but was quickly adapted for terrestrial and biological observations due to its extreme sensitivity.

Remarkably, Langley demonstrated the bolometer's capability to detect the heat from a cow standing over 400 meters away, a feat that astonished his contemporaries and hinted at vast potential for non-contact physiological sensing. Although Langley never applied the device clinically, his invention laid the technological groundwork for modern infrared cameras and, by extension, medical thermographic systems and Computerized Biospectral Imaging.

Langley's contributions represent the bridge between pure physics and applied sensing. His vision extended beyond astronomy; he recognized that understanding radiant energy required both technical innovation and conceptual evolution.

1905 – William Coblentz and the Formalization of Infrared Spectroscopy

In the early 20th century, William W. Coblentz (1873–1962) emerged as a central figure in the transition of infrared science from an exploratory curiosity into a rigorous, measurable field of optical physics. Working at the U.S.

National Bureau of Standards (now NIST), Coblentz pioneered the use of infrared spectroscopy, a technique that analyses how matter absorbs and emits infrared radiation at different wavelengths, to study the molecular composition of materials, including organic compounds, minerals, and biological tissues.

In 1905, Coblentz published his seminal work, *Investigations of Infra-Red Spectra*, which catalogued over 100 substances based on their infrared absorption signatures. His work established infrared spectroscopy as a valid analytical method and introduced calibrated wavelength ranges and absorption bands that would become the backbone of materials science, atmospheric research, and later, biomedical diagnostics.

What set Coblentz apart was his ability to transform infrared observation from visual or qualitative interpretation (as seen in Herschel's and Langley's time) into quantitative analysis.

He was among the first to correlate specific wavelengths of infrared radiation with molecular structure, proving that infrared radiation could reveal functional properties of matter, not just thermal gradients.

> ***"The invisible rays, once dismissed as curiosity, now reveal the fingerprints of molecules. What cannot be seen, may still be known."***
>
> William Coblentz, 1905

Though his work was rooted in physics, Coblentz's spectroscopy would eventually impact biological sciences, particularly in the study of water content, fat distribution, and tissue metabolism, parameters directly linked to variations in infrared emissivity.

These same principles now reinforce the analysis of bioemissive behaviour in Biospectral Medicine, where subtle shifts in spectral expression are treated as indicators of functional or regulatory imbalance.

Coblentz's systematic method, precise instrumentation, and data standardization made infrared analysis replicable and scalable, paving the way for the commercial and medical use of infrared sensors later in the 20th century.

1929 – Kálmán Tihanyi and the Invention of the First Infrared-Sensitive Electronic Camera

In 1929, Hungarian physicist and electrical engineer Kálmán Tihanyi (1897–1947) made a revolutionary contribution to the field of infrared imaging by designing the world's first electronically operated infrared-sensitive camera system. Although originally intended for anti-aircraft military defence, this invention laid the technological foundation for what would become night vision systems and, decades later, digital thermographic cameras used in medical diagnostics.

Tihanyi's design was based on the principle of photoelectric conversion: detecting infrared radiation and converting it into electrical signals that could be amplified and rendered into a visible image.

> ***"The electric image... shall arise from that which the eye cannot see, but which may be made visible to the mind through the wire."***
>
> Kálmán Tihanyi, Patent Abstract, 1929

His system used a selenium-based sensor sensitive to non-visible radiation, and unlike mechanical scanning methods of the time, it operated in a fully electronic, continuous manner. This advancement eliminated the need for moving components, enabling real-time capture of emissive patterns.

He filed a patent in the United Kingdom titled *"An Apparatus for the Electrical Production of the Image and the Transmission Thereof by Wire"* (GB Patent No. 289,915, 1929). Although military secrecy at the time delayed the commercial impact of his invention, Tihanyi is now recognized as the pioneer of electronic television and infrared video sensing.

Tihanyi's work is a technical turning point: for the first time, infrared radiation was transformed into digital signals, allowing for scalable, reproducible, and dynamic visualization. His legacy also set the stage for microbolometer technology, non-cooled detectors central to today's compact medical infrared cameras.

1934–1940s – Carl Reinhold August Wunderlich and the Clinical Use of Thermal Variation

Although temperature had been used as a general sign of disease since antiquity, it was not until the mid-19th and early 20th centuries that quantitative temperature measurement began to acquire diagnostic rigor. A central figure in this transformation was German physician Carl Reinhold August Wunderlich (1815–1877), whose work laid the foundation for the clinical interpretation of body temperature patterns, a precursor to what would eventually evolve into thermographic medicine.

Wunderlich is best known for establishing the normal human body temperature through a vast series of axillary readings taken from over 25,000 patients.

> ***"Each disease, if rightly observed, has its own thermal expression, and it is from this expression that we may learn to forecast its course."***
>
> C. R. A. Wunderlich, 1868

In his influential textbook *Das Verhalten der Eigenwärme in Krankheiten* (*On the Temperature in Diseases*, 1868), he proposed that deviations in temperature, especially sustained elevations or asymmetric febrile curves, could provide key insights into disease course, prognosis, and organ involvement.

Although Wunderlich did not use infrared or emissive tools, his commitment to temperature as a diagnostic language was revolutionary. He demonstrated that body heat is dynamic, fluctuating according to functional, inflammatory, and neurological states, and that recognizing these patterns carries clinical meaning.

His work was widely accepted across Europe and formed the empirical bedrock for the later integration of non-contact thermometry and eventually infrared thermographic systems in medicine. His legacy continued into the 1930s and 1940s, when early contact thermography methods, including thermocouples, galvanometers, and blackened photographic film, began to visualize skin surface heat, often influenced by Wunderlich's interpretive philosophy of dynamic temperature modeling.

1956 – Dr. Ray Lawson and the First Clinical Thermograms for Breast Cancer Detection

In 1956, Canadian surgeon and professor Dr. Ray R. Lawson (1923–2007) became the first physician to apply infrared thermography to a formal clinical diagnostic setting, marking the true birth of modern medical thermography. Working at the Royal Victoria Hospital and McGill University in Montreal, Lawson utilized a barn-door-style infrared scanner, originally developed for industrial applications, to capture heat signatures of the human breast.

Lawson's key discovery was the recognition that malignant breast tumours often exhibit higher surface temperatures than surrounding tissues due to increased metabolic activity, vascular proliferation (angiogenesis), and inflammatory response, all processes that elevate localized heat emission. By comparing symmetry between the left and right breasts, he identified temperature differentials and vascular anomalies that correlated with histologically confirmed breast cancer.

In a landmark presentation at the New York Academy of Sciences in 1956 and later publications (Lawson, 1957), he proposed infrared imaging as a supplementary tool for breast cancer screening. His early thermograms, though coarse and grainy by modern standards, demonstrated distinct heat patterns, including hypervascular zones, that consistently aligned with underlying malignant lesions.

> ***"Thermal asymmetry and vascular radiation patterns are not only measurable but reproducible. These signs may precede palpable masses by months, even years."***
>
> Dr. Ray R. Lawson, 1956

Lawson's innovation catalysed a wave of clinical research into thermographic diagnostics, especially for breast oncology, and influenced the development of Computerized Thermographic Imaging (CTI) systems several decades later. His emphasis on functional vascular dynamics, rather than structural imaging, mirrors the central premise of Biospectral Medicine, where surface emissive patterns are treated as windows into internal biological dysregulation.

Despite the lack of standardization and imaging resolution at the time, Lawson's approach laid the intellectual and clinical foundation for decades of research into non-invasive, radiation-free thermal diagnostics. His legacy continues in the biospectral analysis of asymmetry, vascular overexpression, and emissive deviation, refined today through digital quantification and clinical integration.

1960s–1970s – Military-to-Medical Transfer and the Rise of Early Digital Infrared Systems

The Cold War era of the 1960s and 1970s brought unprecedented investment into infrared detection and imaging technologies, primarily for missile tracking, night vision, and aerospace surveillance. Governments in the United States, Soviet Union, and Europe poured millions into the development of highly sensitive infrared focal plane arrays, cryogenically cooled detectors, and signal processing algorithms capable of converting emissive radiation into visual formats with increasing clarity and resolution.

One of the most significant technological transfers during this period came through NASA and U.S. military laboratories. Infrared detectors originally designed for missile heat signatures and space-based thermal mapping were declassified and repurposed for civilian medical imaging. As a result, clinical researchers gained access to prototype infrared cameras with real-time imaging, multi-spectral filters, and thermometric accuracy under 0.1°C.

> ***"The technology was there, but the interpretive science was not. We could see the heat, but we didn't yet know what it meant."***
>
> Clinical thermologist, retrospective commentary, 1984

By the late 1960s, institutions such as MIT's Lincoln Laboratory, the U.S. Army Night Vision Laboratory, and NASA Ames had begun collaborating with hospitals to evaluate the feasibility of applying this technology to vascular diagnostics, inflammatory conditions, and oncology. One early outcome was the integration of non-cooled lead selenide (PbSe) detectors into portable clinical IR cameras.

In medicine, thermography gained traction in:

- Rheumatology: monitoring joint inflammation
- Peripheral vascular disease: evaluating ischemia and diabetic microcirculation
- Neurology: mapping sympathetic dysfunction and complex regional pain syndrome (CRPS)
- Dentistry and orthopedics: assessing infection, fracture healing, and implant rejection

Yet, despite its promise, infrared imaging faced scepticism. The field lacked standardized protocols, interpretive frameworks, and quantitative metrics. This led to a decline in mainstream adoption by the late 1970s, despite thousands of clinical publications.

This historical blockage directly motivated the development of more structured systems like Computerized Thermographic Imaging (CTI) and, eventually, Biospectral Medicine, disciplines focused on acquiring thermal data and systematically interpreting it through functional physiology, spectral zone classification, and neurometabolic patterns.

1980s–1990s – Digital Standardization and the Limits of Conventional Thermography

The decades of the 1980s and 1990s witnessed the emergence of digitally enhanced thermographic systems that greatly improved the practicality of medical infrared imaging. Advancements in uncooled microbolometer arrays, digital signal processors, and compact portable infrared cameras made thermal imaging more accessible outside of military and aerospace applications.

For the first time, it became feasible to capture, store, and analyse high-resolution emissive data in real time. These developments allowed for broader experimentation in clinical rheumatology, vascular diagnostics, neurosensory assessment, and oncological screening.

However, despite technological progress, thermography remained hampered by significant clinical limitations:

- There was no consensus on anatomical zoning or region-of-interest (ROI) mapping.
- Visual analysis predominated, without standardized software protocols or quantitative interpretive logic.
- The field lacked a diagnostic methodology rooted in functional physiology, terrain theory, or systems biology.

In response to these persistent challenges, various researchers called for a new clinical language and framework. As Ring and Ammer (1995–2012) emphasized repeatedly, thermography needed to evolve from image acquisition into a systematic model of physiological interpretation to be fully integrated into medical diagnostics.

By the close of the 1990s, although digital thermography had matured as a technical modality, its clinical adoption was limited due to the absence of structured methodology, a gap that remained unfilled until new interpretive models began to emerge in the following decade.

> ***"For thermal imaging to gain credibility and acceptance in medicine, it must move beyond simple image acquisition and develop into a reliable model of physiological interpretation."***
>
> (*Ring EFJ, Ammer K. Infrared thermal imaging in medicine. Physiol Meas. 2012;33(3): R33–R46.*)

In contrast to the largely clinical and commercial approaches prevalent in Western countries, Japan developed a distinct academic tradition in thermographic research. From the late 20th century onward, leading Japanese universities and hospital centers conducted meticulous studies on skin emissivity, neurovascular thermoregulation, and microcirculatory response patterns.

These investigations often emphasized experimental precision, standardization of environmental conditions, and reproducibility of spectral data, laying important groundwork for modern quantitative thermography.

While their findings were published primarily in Japanese journals, they influenced a generation of infrared physiology scholars and contributed valuable physiological insight into thermographic variability. However, due to language and publication barriers, their global influence remained limited, and Japan's institutional thermographic models were rarely adopted outside Asia.

2005 – Felipe Reitz and the Development of CTI Protocols at ICIM

In 2005, scientist Felipe Reitz formally introduced Computerized Thermographic Imaging (CTI) while directing at the Irish Center of Integrated Medicine (ICIM). This initiative emerged after conducting thousands of infrared evaluations using diverse thermographic systems in clinical environments across Europe and South America.

CTI represented the standardization of medical protocol and physiological interpretation, transforming raw emissive data into a coherent clinical narrative without requiring new hardware invention.

Prior to CTI, thermography suffered from a lack of standardization, often reduced to the status of adjunct visualization with limited diagnostic authority. Inspired by these limitations, Reitz developed a rigorous methodology centred on region-of-interest (ROI) mapping, functional emission pattern recognition, and longitudinal comparative imaging. Remarkably, these thermographic findings were not left in isolation.

As a practitioner formally trained in ultrasonography, Reitz conducted targeted ultrasound examinations immediately following each CTI session, within the same consultation, to minimize the risk of physiological changes that could occur over time and distort diagnostic clarity.

This real-time integration allowed thermographic emission zones to be anatomically confirmed through Doppler or B-mode imaging, particularly in vascular, glandular, or inflammatory regions.

The result was a repeatable, clinical-grade framework for functional imaging that enhanced diagnostic precision and transformed real-time decision-making.

Over time, this correlation-based model formed the clinical backbone of CTI and laid the groundwork for the more advanced anatomical zone methodology later formalized under Biospectral Medicine.

> ***"Thermal imaging becomes clinically transformative only when guided by structured interpretation. CTI bridges the gap between surface heat patterns and internal dysfunction, allowing for the earliest detection of pathological processes, often years before conventional imaging reveals anatomical change."***
>
> *(Reitz F. Atlas of Infrared Thermography, Reitz Institute Publishing, 2025.)*

One of CTI's earliest and most strategic advantages was its ability to localize physiological dysfunction prior to anatomical changes. This allowed for focalized ultrasound evaluation, reducing exposure duration and avoiding indiscriminate scanning.

While ultrasound is largely considered safe, the British Medical Ultrasound Society (BMUS) has documented the importance of controlling exposure to avoid bioeffects such as cavitation and tissue heating, especially in sensitive organs like the breast and uterus.

BMUS recommends limiting imaging to 60 minutes at a Thermal Index (TI) of ≤ 1.0 for soft tissue (TIS), with reduced time allowances at higher thermal indices (BMUS, 2009, pp. 60–61). CTI effectively minimized such risks by identifying thermally active emission fields in advance, thereby improving the precision and safety of complementary imaging modalities.

The emission-based framework of CTI became the foundation upon which new diagnostic insights were developed. With its regionally focused emission zones and comparative temperature asymmetry analysis, CTI created a bridge between functional imaging and pathophysiological interpretation, a goal thermography pioneers had long pursued but never clinically implemented.

Over time, the anatomical division system of CTI, originally grouped by general body regions, would later evolve into the more refined zonal methodology found in Biospectral Medicine. That structural advancement allowed for sharper diagnostic granularity, and it was built on the foundational principles developed during the CTI years.

A central principle in the philosophy behind CTI was the understanding that pathological processes begin well before they are visible anatomically. Diseases like cancer, autoimmune syndromes, and metabolic dysfunctions initiate functional disturbances long before solid masses, irreversible damage, or structural alterations manifest.

Particularly in oncology, the timeline between initial cell dysregulation and the formation of a visible tumour can span several years. As early as 1982, Gautherie demonstrated that infrared imaging could detect pre-humoral angiogenesis and vasomotor changes five to ten years prior to clinical manifestation.

Thermal emission zones, when correctly interpreted, reflect early-stage angiogenesis, chronic inflammation, and neurogenic dysregulation, the very elements that underlie disease emergence.

As Hanahan and Folkman (1996) and Raica et al. (2009) observed, neoplastic transformation is preceded by microvascular proliferation, even in histologically benign tissues.

These microvascular changes can persist for years and are generally invisible on conventional imaging unless mass formation occurs. However, when angiogenesis is functionally active, CTI registers increased localized emission, historically referred to as a *hyperthermic area* or *heat zone* in classical thermography.

Within the evolving terminology of Biospectral Medicine, such regions are now defined more precisely as "activose" zones, indicating biologically significant emission fields linked to perfusion, inflammation, or neurovascular activity, often detectable well before anatomical changes become visible through conventional imaging.

Traditional imaging tools such as ultrasound, mammography, and MRI remain indispensable, but they are structurally constrained. Corsetti et al. (2011) reported that tumors smaller than 0.8 cm in diameter often escape detection, particularly in dense or glandular tissue. These sub-centimeter lesions may not meet visibility thresholds unless accompanied by secondary signs like vascular flow changes or architectural distortion. CTI, by contrast, does not depend on the presence of mass. It detects the functional footprint of disease, often a decade before conventional detection becomes possible.

Unlike conventional imaging technologies that rely on detecting structural changes, Computerized Thermographic Imaging (CTI) functions as a physiological imaging system, capturing early alterations in vascular activity, thermal asymmetry, and neurogenic regulation, phenomena that precede anatomical change.

"Thermal imaging only becomes clinically transformative when it is systematizedinterpreted not as isolated temperature data, but as dynamic physiological language mapped across time and anatomy."

Reitz, F. CTI Clinical Protocols and Biosignal Insights, ICIM Archives, 2005.

Structural modalities such as ultrasound, mammography, MRI, and CT scans are fundamentally anatomical, detecting tissue density, morphology, or mass presence.

These tools become effective only after a physical alteration has occurred, often when the disease process is already advanced. As Ring and Ammer (2000) stated, "thermography provides physiological information while other imaging modalities provide anatomical information," underscoring the complementary nature of CTI rather than its replacement function.

While mammography has been the main medical devise to detect breast cancer, it operates through ionizing radiation and mechanical breast compression, both of which carry biological risks.

According to Jørgensen and Gøtzsche (2015), even low-dose X-ray exposure from regular mammograms may cause a slight increase in cancer incidence, approximately 1.6 additional cases per 1,000 women screened biennially between the ages of 50 and 74. The risk is magnified for younger women and those with a family history, where radiosensitive tissue may respond adversely to repeated exposure.

Breast compression, though standard in mammographic technique, has raised concern about mechanical dissemination of malignant cells. While definitive proof remains elusive, some studies and clinical hypotheses suggest that compression could facilitate the spread of tumour cells through vascular or lymphatic microchannels (Cheng et al., 2016). Animal models have further demonstrated that exposure to ionizing radiation may increase tumor cell migration and metastasis pathways.

By contrast, Computerized Thermographic Imaging (CTI) is entirely radiation-free, utilizing functional physiological changes, such as vasodilation, angiogenesis, and segmental neurogenic inflammation, to detect areas of concern.

These changes manifest as thermal emission patterns and allow practitioners to identify inflammatory or vascular hotspots before anatomical changes are evident. This makes CTI especially useful as a first-line screening tool, offering a safe, non-invasive, and cost-effective alternative that prioritizes physiological function over structural size.

CTI allows for triaging: patients exhibiting thermal anomalies can be referred for targeted mammography or ultrasound, while those with stable emission patterns may avoid unnecessary radiation. This approach is particularly valuable in young patients or those requiring frequent evaluations, where cumulative radiation exposure could pose long-term risks.

That said, CTI defined clear boundaries of application.. Its diagnostic power is greatest in peripheral and surface-based tissues, where thermal emissions are most readily detectable. As the depth of the lesion increases, especially in central thoracic, retroperitoneal, or pelvic cavities, the accuracy of CTI diminishes, requiring integration with deeper imaging modalities such as MRI or ultrasound for full evaluation.

From a psychosocial perspective, CTI also bridges the gap between clinician and patient. It allows patients to visualize their physiology, enhancing their understanding of the disease process and improving compliance with treatment plans. CTI reports offer tangible evidence of improvement or stagnation, reinforcing the motivational framework necessary for long-term therapeutic engagement.

Over the years, the consistent application of CTI by Reitz, revealed predictable emission signatures associated with vascular congestion, fibrocystic breast tissue, inflammatory terrain, and neurological segmental imbalance. These findings were not abstract or incidental, they correlated with symptoms, lab markers, and confirmatory imaging, showing clear diagnostic and therapeutic value.

The introduction of CTI in 2005 marked a clinical inflection point. It shifted thermography from anecdotal support to systematized clinical utility. More importantly, it laid the foundation for the emergence of Biospectral Medicine, a more comprehensive, lexically precise, and zone-based diagnostic language that now defines a new era of physiological imaging.

2024 – The Formalization of Biospectral Medicine as a Clinical Discipline

Despite remarkable technological advances in hardware, optics, and signal processing by the end of the 20th century, medical thermography remained scientifically marginalized. Its limited clinical acceptance stemmed from the absence of a unifying system of interpretation, despite its sensitivity. Three fundamental challenges continued to impede its evolution into a core diagnostic tool:

1. **Lack of Standardized Anatomical Zones**
   Thermographic interpretation varied widely across specialties and practitioners. Without a standardized anatomical mapping system or clinically validated zones of emissive analysis, comparative studies and longitudinal monitoring were unreliable, and the method remained observational rather than diagnostic.

2. **Insufficient Interpretive Frameworks**
   Most thermographic reports relied on surface-level descriptors, "warmer vs. cooler," "left vs. right", without physiological or systemic context. There was no clinical consensus on how to interpret emission variations in light of vascular regulation, autonomic dysfunction, or metabolic terrain.

3. **Absence of Functional Integration**
   Thermography was often relegated to adjunct status, perceived as a passive screening tool rather than a modality capable of revealing underlying biological dynamics. Lacking integration with biochemical, neurological, or structural diagnostics, it rarely influenced core clinical decision-making.

Recognizing these systemic limitations, the scientist Felipe Reitz, who had already pioneered Computerized Thermographic Imaging (CTI) in 2005, undertook a further development of the methodology. While CTI had established clinical-grade protocols such as ROI mapping and ultrasound correlation, its anatomical grouping remained broad. Over the subsequent decade, Reitz systematically expanded the methodology, giving rise to a new discipline: Biospectral Medicine.

Biospectral Medicine represents the synthesis of CTI with functional physiology, terrain-based diagnostics, and spectral neurovascular logic. It establishes thermography as a structured interpretive system grounded in clinical causality.

Unlike any prior model, Biospectral Medicine offers a reproducible and physiology-based diagnostic framework that connects surface emission with internal regulation.

> ***"Biospectral Medicine doesn't just see heat, it reads physiology. It's not a tool of observation, but a method of interpretation."***
>
> Felipe Reitz, 2025

After nearly two decades of dedicated refinement in thermographic interpretation, Felipe Reitz formally introduced Biospectral Medicine as a new diagnostic discipline. At its core was the establishment of a 19-zone anatomical model, derived from years of clinical observation and functional analysis.

These zones were defined through a structured clinical methodology based on three interlocking criteria:

1. **Emissive Behaviour** – Zones were demarcated according to consistent patterns of thermographic emission seen across diverse clinical cases. These patterns reflected localized variations in vascular flow, neurogenic tone, inflammatory activation, and metabolic response.

2. **Dermatomal and Neurophysiological Coherence** – Each zone respected underlying neural distribution patterns, especially spinal segment innervation and autonomic regulation, allowing the thermal findings to be correlated with known neurofunctional pathways.

3. **Structural-Functional Territories** – Divisions aligned with musculoskeletal, lymphatic, and organ-related territories, incorporating insights from fascia, visceral referral maps, and embryological development, enabling meaningful interpretation within a whole-body systems framework.

The result was a standardized clinical cartography that allowed for:

- Objective comparison of thermal evolution over time
- Cross-practitioner reproducibility in interpretation
- Integration with physical, biochemical, and emotional terrain models for a truly systemic evaluation

This zoning system resolved the ambiguity that historically limited thermography, elevating the method from observational adjunct to a structured tool of clinical reasoning. It set the stage for the practical and academic advancement of Biospectral Medicine as a transdisciplinary approach grounded in reproducible physiology and therapeutic relevance.

These zones are interpreted using the R-CIIM system (Reitz Clinical Infrared Interpretation Model), a 6-step methodology that moves from anatomical observation to therapeutic guidance.

Biospectral Medicine replaces broad terms such as "hyperthermia" with clinically meaningful categories:

- **Activose Zones**: Elevated emissive regions reflecting angiogenic, inflammatory, or neurovascular activation (previously termed "hot spots" or "hyperthermic zones")
- **Inhibose Zones**: Suppressed emission regions, often linked to chronic dysfunction, sympathetic overdrive, or tissue ischemia
- **Anisospectral Patterns**: Emissive asymmetries of diagnostic significance
- **Equibose Zones**: Bilateral emissive equilibrium, indicating balanced regulation

This refined lexicon enables clinicians to move beyond observational speculation and into system-based interpretation.

Biospectral analysis serves as a primary diagnostic model, capable of identifying functional disturbances, such as inflammation, vascular dysregulation, and neurogenic patterns, before structural alterations are visible. While it functions independently through its defined zones, interpretive categories, and six-step methodology, additional tests may be strategically recommended to refine diagnostic clarity.

When applied in isolation, its effectiveness depends on correlating findings with the clinical complaint and detailed case history. However, when integrated with imaging, laboratory panels, or neurological mapping, it becomes a powerful system for root-cause assessment and therapeutic precision.

The image becomes a diagnostic map, guiding inquiry, confirmation, and therapeutic focus. The zone-specific logic transforms CTI from a descriptive modality into a strategic diagnostic tool.

Just as cardiology became anchored in the ECG waveform, and neurology in functional brain mapping, Biospectral Medicine offers an anatomically grounded, clinically validated language for interpreting human thermoregulation. It transforms static infrared imagery into spectral signatures of systemic function, unveiling the dynamic interplay of inflammation, vascular remodelling, autonomic tone, and metabolic stress.

This structured approach, built on years of clinical application, image correlation, and protocol refinement, establishes Biospectral Medicine as the legitimate successor to historical thermography and the functional continuation of CTI.

Systemic Barriers to the Medical Advancement of Thermography

Despite early discoveries in infrared radiation during the 19th century and the military-grade use of infrared sensors by the mid-20th century, thermography failed to become a mainstream medical diagnostic tool for decades. This resulted from several entrenched limitations beyond hardware innovation:

- **Lack of Anatomical Anchoring**: Thermographic images were interpreted without standardized reference to specific anatomical zones. This made reproducibility nearly impossible and discouraged comparative or population-based studies.
- **Absence of Physiological Modeling**: Most readings were based on visual impression, "hot" vs. "cold", rather than on vascular physiology, neurogenic patterns, or metabolic terrain. Without a structured interpretive framework, findings remained vague and untranslatable to medical decision-making.
- **No Standardized Lexicon or Terminology**: Unlike ECG, ultrasound, or radiography, thermography lacked a shared language to describe spectral behaviour. Early reports used terms inconsistently, diminishing credibility and inter-operator coherence.
- **Isolation from Clinical Decision-Making**: Thermography was rarely integrated with laboratory testing, ultrasound, or patient history. It remained a peripheral screening method without influence over treatment planning.

- **Technological Overfocus**: Many researchers pursued better cameras or software without addressing the interpretive vacuum. As a result, improved image quality did not result in improved clinical use.

Together, these factors explain why, even as late as 2000, thermography remained a secondary tool, respected for its sensitivity but mistrusted for its diagnostic specificity.

Thermography in Scientific Guidelines and Institutions

Thermographic imaging, a technique with substantial diagnostic potential, has historically faced marginalization due to early misuse, technical limitations, and lack of methodological rigor. During the 1970s and 1980s, thermography gained traction within alternative health circles but often lacked standardized protocols, anatomical consistency, and scientific validation.

Devices with poor resolution and untrained operators led to overstatement of findings, particularly in breast cancer screening, contributing to the perception of thermography as pseudoscientific (Ammer, 2008).

The credibility of the field was further undermined by the absence of clinical training programs, interpretive models, and peer-reviewed evidence. Thermal images were frequently assessed subjectively, using arbitrary temperature thresholds and non-reproducible region-of-interest (ROI) selections. These weaknesses gave rise to valid criticisms: thermography was labelled as unreliable, overly sensitive, and difficult to standardize (Jones, 1998).

Regulatory agencies soon responded. In the United States, the FDA began restricting thermographic claims, especially for oncological applications, while in Europe, societies such as the European Society of Breast Imaging (EUSOBI) excluded thermography from screening recommendations. These actions effectively relegated the method to the fringes of integrative medicine, primarily in musculoskeletal pain evaluation, and often without robust clinical integration.

Despite this decline, a subset of researchers persisted in exploring the physiological basis of infrared imaging. Authors like Ring and Ammer (2012) emphasized its potential in identifying autonomic dysfunctions, vascular anomalies, and inflammatory responses, provided that image acquisition and interpretation adhered to rigorous standards. They advocated for structured protocols and anatomical references, yet acknowledged that consistent zonal frameworks and diagnostic models remained absent from the literature.

By the early 2000s, new scientific efforts attempted to formalize thermography's role. The American Academy of Thermology (AAT), along with several European institutions, issued technical guidelines emphasizing environmental controls, operator credentialing, and the adjunctive nature of thermography, particularly in pain medicine and breast health.

These guidelines contributed to a foundational standard of practice but deliberately avoided proposing interpretive models or anatomical divisions (AAT, 2021).

In parallel, regulatory scrutiny intensified. The FDA reaffirmed thermography's clearance solely as a supplementary tool. In 2019, it issued formal warnings against its use as a primary method for breast cancer detection, citing lack of evidence and potential risks due to false reassurance and delayed diagnosis (FDA, 2019). EUSOBI echoed this stance, maintaining that thermography did not meet the criteria for inclusion in standardized screening strategies.

This unresolved tension, between the theoretical value of thermal imaging and its practical limitations, created a space for innovation. Within this context, *Biospectral Medicine* emerged as a translational discipline dedicated to the scientific rehabilitation of thermography. Rather than relying on subjective "hot spots" or temperature maps, it reframes thermography as a biosignal system grounded in clinical logic.

Biospectral Medicine is structured on five methodological pillars:

1. **Computerized Biospectral Imaging (CBI)** in controlled environments, ensuring reproducibility.
2. **A fixed anatomical zone map**, comprising 19 precisely defined regions.
3. **A terrain-based interpretation model**, correlating spectral emissions with biological systems (vascular, nervous, metabolic, etc.).
4. **A clinical taxonomy**, replacing ambiguous descriptors with standardized terminology (e.g., *activose*, *anisospectrality*).
5. **Integrative clinical correlation**, combining spectral findings with laboratory data, functional history, and physical examination.

This comprehensive framework explicitly addresses previous criticisms by introducing standardization, repeatability, and interdisciplinary clinical utility. Biospectral Medicine does not challenge the regulatory limitations imposed on traditional thermography; rather, it fulfils unmet scientific demands by transforming raw thermal emissions into structured biospectral analysis.

Unlike prior attempts that emphasized safety protocols without interpretive depth, Biospectral Medicine advances thermographic imaging into the realm of translational science. Its development represents a paradigm shift, reframing infrared imaging as a physiological interpreter and moving beyond diagnostic guesswork.

It responds to foundational critiques with academic rigor, offering a functional model that bridges imaging, biophysics, and clinical practice.

By acknowledging the historical failures of thermography while establishing a coherent, structured alternative, Biospectral Medicine restores scientific legitimacy to the analysis of infrared emissions. It marks the beginning of a new chapter in non-invasive diagnostics, rooted in physiology, standardization, and integrative logic.

Historical Overview

The language used to describe thermographic findings has evolved dramatically over the past two centuries. What began as the physical detection of invisible radiation in the early 1800s gradually moved toward clinical application in the mid-20th century, yet remained conceptually fragmented and interpretively limited for decades. Early terminology such as *"hot spots," "thermal asymmetries,"* or *"hyperthermic areas"* reflected a lack of physiological grounding and failed to provide clinicians with actionable meaning.

Despite significant technological advances in sensor resolution and image acquisition, thermography was largely relegated to the periphery of clinical diagnostics due to the absence of a structured anatomical model, standardized vocabulary, and integrated interpretive methodology. Even by the late 20th century, leading researchers such as Ring and Ammer (1995–2012) were still calling for thermography to "move beyond image acquisition" and become a reliable framework of physiological interpretation.

This need was only fully addressed with the contributions of scientist Felipe Reitz, who first introduced the term *Computerized Thermographic Imaging (CTI)* in 2005, followed nearly two decades later by the foundation of *Biospectral Medicine* in 2024. These innovations established the clinical-grade acquisition protocols and the first structured interpretive language rooted in anatomy, physiology, and terrain-based medicine.

The table below summarizes this conceptual evolution, from early infrared discovery to the creation of a modern diagnostic lexicon, highlighting key contributors, milestones, and the emergence of Biospectral Medicine as a new medical paradigm.

Historical Timeline of Thermographic Concepts and Terminology

Year	Contributor(s)	Concept / Term Introduced	Commentary
1800	Sir William Herschel	*Discovery of Infrared Radiation*	While experimenting with sunlight and thermometers, Herschel discovered invisible "calorific rays" beyond the red end of the visible spectrum, laying the foundation for all future thermal imaging.
1840–1870	Becquerel, Tyndall, Stefan	*Heat Radiation Principles*	These physicists expanded the understanding of radiant energy transfer, helping quantify emissivity and thermal conduction; concepts essential to modern thermography.
1890–1900	Josef Stefan, Ludwig Boltzmann	*Stefan–Boltzmann Law*	Defined the relationship between surface temperature and radiant energy, later foundational in infrared sensor calibration.
1929	Samuel Langley (bolometer applications)	*Early Infrared Sensing*	Langley's bolometer technology began to be adapted for detecting temperature differences in the environment and human subjects.
1948	Bell Telephone Labs	*First Infrared Camera (SNAPSCOPE)*	Military-developed infrared sensors began to be explored for medical use in identifying surface inflammation and infection.
1956–1960	Ray Lawson (Canada)	*Medical Thermography*	Among the first to apply infrared cameras to breast screening; observed elevated thermal emission in areas of breast carcinoma.
1963	Dr. Harold J. Isard	*Thermographic Screening of Breast Cancer*	Published foundational studies comparing thermal patterns in benign vs. malignant lesions. Coined the term "thermographic abnormality."
1970s	Various researchers	*"Hyperthermia," "Thermal Asymmetry"*	Terms like "hyperthermic zones," "cold spots," and "hot areas" were used descriptively, without standardized physiological interpretation.
1982	Lucien Gautherie (France)	*Thermobiological Monitoring*	Demonstrated that thermal patterns could precede tumor visibility by 5–10 years. Pioneered long-term monitoring of breast physiology via thermography.

1995–2012	Ring & Ammer (UK–Austria)	*Call for Interpretive Models*	Emphasized the need to move beyond image acquisition toward systematic physiological interpretation: *"Infrared imaging in medicine must evolve into a reliable model of physiological interpretation."*
2005	Felipe Reitz	*Computerized Thermographic Imaging (CTI)*	Developed and implemented a structured clinical protocol including ROI mapping, temporal comparison, and ultrasound correlation. Introduced group-based mapping of emission patterns, which set the groundwork for zonal analysis.
2024	Felipe Reitz	*Biospectral Medicine*	Formalized a 19-zone anatomical model with 9 diagnostic categories. Introduced terms like *activose*, *inhibose*, *anisospectral*, and *equibose* to replace outdated thermal vocabulary. Integrated thermography with terrain-based, functional, and somatic diagnostics, establishing a new medical category.

Historical Contributions to Medical Thermography: Conceptual Evolution and Milestones

The progression of thermography in medicine spans over two centuries, marked by sporadic technological advances but limited clinical integration. While early efforts laid important foundations, such as infrared detection, emissivity theory, and early cancer screening attempts, there remained a striking absence of anatomical standardization, structured clinical interpretation, or diagnostic relevance.

The timeline below organizes key contributors, concepts, and terminologies chronologically, illustrating the gradual, but incomplete, evolution of thermography prior to the emergence of Biospectral Medicine.

By contextualizing these historical milestones, it becomes clear how Biospectral Medicine addresses the longstanding gaps in thermographic application. The table highlights what was achieved in each period and what was still missing, culminating in the scientist. Felipe Reitz's creation of a fully structured physiological methodology based on zone division, diagnostic categories, and stepwise clinical interpretation.

Feature	Conventional Thermography	Biospectral Medicine (Reitz)
Uses anatomical zones?	✖ No	✅ Yes
Based on physiology and terrain?	✖ No	✅ Yes
Includes diagnostic categories?	✖ No	✅ Yes (9)
Uses structured evaluation steps?	✖ No	✅ Yes (6 steps)
Integrates with lab/imaging?	✖ Rarely	✅ Fully
Guides therapeutic strategy?	✖ No	✅ Yes
Repeatable and teachable?	✖ Only loosely	✅ Yes, through clinical protocol
Clinical language (activose, inhibose, etc.)?	✖ No	✅ Yes, pioneered

PART II

CLINICAL POSITION

CLINICAL POSITIONING OF BIOSPECTRAL MEDICINE

Defining the Diagnostic Territory

Biospectral Medicine is a scientific discipline rooted in thermophysical science, but it is not synonymous with conventional thermography. It defines a new category of interpretive logic: functional zone-based biosignal imaging. This field complements morphological imaging techniques such as MRI and ultrasound and integrates with biochemical investigations like blood analysis, while also filling a unique interpretive gap by mapping and decoding dynamic, physiologically expressive patterns based on infrared emission behaviour."

This modality captures the body's real-time regulatory outputs, including vasomotor dynamics, neurogenic tone, metabolic terrain activity, and autonomic adaptation, through a structured, zone-based analysis model. Unlike morphological imaging, which seeks structural abnormality, Biospectral Medicine tracks functional asymmetry, regulatory load, and tissue responsiveness to internal or external stimuli. Its core strength lies in the ability to translate thermal emission into systemic meaning, beyond the heat data itself.

The Diagnostic Ecosystem: Where Biospectral Medicine Belongs

To understand the positioning of Biospectral Medicine, it is helpful to map its role within the broader investigative ecosystem. The table below compares its core properties against other mainstream medical technologies of investigation:

Diagnostic Modality	Measures	Strengths	Limitations	Biosignal or Morphology
MRI / CT	Morphology, structure	High-resolution anatomy, deep internal imaging	High cost, static snapshot, no physiological function	Morphological
Ultrasound	Morphology + real-time motion	Safe, portable, vascular and fetal imaging	Operator-dependent, limited penetration in air or bone	Morphological
X-ray	Bone structure, density	Quick, available, good for trauma	Ionizing radiation, limited soft tissue detail	Morphological
Blood tests / Labs	Molecular concentrations	Quantitative data, systemic indicators	Not spatial, no localization, time-delayed markers	Biochemical
Infrared Thermography (classical)	Surface temperature	Non-invasive, passive	Low interpretive value, lacks diagnostic logic	Surface-level
Biospectral Medicine	Infrared emission by zone	Functional diagnostics, dynamic terrain mapping, zone asymmetry	Requires training, not yet institutionally embedded	**Functional biosignal**

This table illustrates that Biospectral Medicine belongs neither to traditional imaging nor to laboratory analysis. Its strength lies in biosignal decoding: a new axis of information, measuring regulatory expression across zones, rather than structure or chemistry. It is uniquely suited for evaluating subtle regulatory imbalances: early-stage circulatory stasis, subclinical inflammation, metabolic compensation, nervous system overdrive, or adaptive breakdowns without structural damage.

Such conditions often go unrecognized by traditional tools, leaving patients in an investigative gap. Biospectral Medicine bridges this space with zone-specific interpretation, comparative symmetry, and terrain-based classification.

When to Use Biospectral Imaging - And When Not To

Understanding when Biospectral Medicine is the correct investigative approach is essential for clinical integration. The following scenarios are where this modality proves especially valuable:

Chronic, unexplained symptoms with no clear imaging or lab correlate

- **Neurovascular dysfunction**, including pain syndromes, thermoregulatory issues, or sympathetic imbalance
- **Early-stage inflammation**, before morphological changes are detectable
- **Postural, muscular, and fascial asymmetries** not visible on MRI or X-ray
- **Lymphatic or endocrine terrain mapping**, where the dysfunction is spatial and functional, without structural alteration.
- **Longitudinal tracking** of intervention response, using non-invasive, repeatable measurements
- **Interpretive synthesis** in complex patients, integrating spectral terrain with symptoms and lab data

However Biospectral Medicine complements established methods without replacing them:

- Tumor staging or deep anatomical lesion localization (MRI or CT required)
- Obstetric imaging (ultrasound preferred)
- Emergency fracture assessment (X-ray)
- Isolated single-symptom investigations where localized pathology is clearly evident

In other words, Biospectral Medicine is best positioned at the crossroads of functional, integrative, and systems medicine, where it adds unique value beyond the scope of acute or structural pathology. It excels in revealing regulatory imbalances and terrain overloads that precede changes captured by structural imaging.

Integration with Conventional and Natural Diagnostics

One of Biospectral Medicine's most powerful applications is in integrative clinical workflows. When used alongside laboratory testing (e.g., inflammatory markers, hormone panels), morphological imaging, and patient history, it acts as a terrain map, highlighting zones under stress, guiding test selection, and helping clinicians prioritize care strategies.

For example, a thermally suppressed right abdomen may guide a hormone panel focused on ovarian function or thyroid feedback. An activose emission zone in the axilla may prompt lymphatic drainage work, heavy metal screening, or a breast exam. The The biospectral signal is a strategic guide for deeper investigation."

This methodology aligns with recent literature on the value of functional imaging in complex investigations, where early regulatory imbalance precedes visible pathology (Kotsenas et al., 2015; Pijnenburg et al., 2017). Furthermore, its zone-based logic harmonizes with acupuncture, osteopathic, and neurofascial models, making it especially relevant in integrative and European-style naturopathic systems (Ursini et al., 2020).

Clinical Role: Beyond Thermography

Biospectral Medicine must not be equated with classical thermography. It uses infrared emission not as temperature, but as a functional biosignal, interpreted through anatomical zoning, terrain classification, and comparative asymmetry.

This shift in logic is what elevates it from a niche imaging tool to a new interpretive discipline. When paired with standardized interpretation (as in the R-CIIM system), clear zone protocols, and confirmatory strategies, it becomes a reproducible, scalable method for functional interpretive reasoning.

Its future potential lies in four domains:

1. **Functional investigations** for invisible or subclinical syndromes
2. **Care guidance** for individualized natural medicine
3. **Systemic terrain mapping** to support biological medicine models
4. **Non-invasive mapping** in chronic imbalance risk and prevention

By clarifying its clinical niche, Biospectral Medicine can now be defended academically, taught systematically, and adopted globally as a missing piece in the investigative puzzle, advancing medicine alongside existing modalities.

PART III

PRINCIPLES AND PHYSICS

PRINCIPLES AND PHYSICS OF THERMOGRAPHY

All thermographic systems derive from a foundational physical principle: any object with a temperature above absolute zero emits infrared radiation. Human tissues, due to their high water content and thermoregulatory complexity, emit particularly strong signals in the long-wave infrared (LWIR) spectrum.

The basis for this phenomenon originates in blackbody radiation theory, defined by Kirchhoff and mathematically modeled by Planck (1901). Human skin, although not a perfect blackbody, exhibits an emissivity coefficient of approximately 0.98, making it highly responsive to infrared detection (Steketee, 1973).

The intensity and distribution of this emission follow Planck's radiation law, while the total energy radiated scales according to the Stefan–Boltzmann Law ($E \propto T^4$). This exponential relationship allows for the detection of subtle physiological changes, such as vascular perfusion shifts or inflammatory activation, through minute variations in surface emission.

Spectral Windows and Sensor Technology

Infrared radiation spans a broad electromagnetic band from approximately 0.75 to 1000 microns. In medical imaging, the clinical imaginglies between 8–14 µm, where human tissue emission is optimal and environmental interference is minimal (Ring & Ammer, 2012). Most clinical systems utilize uncooled microbolometers, typically based on vanadium oxide (VOx), to translate emitted infrared energy into electrical signals, forming high-resolution thermal maps.

While conventional thermography interprets these maps as superficial temperature gradients, Biospectral Medicine reclassifies them as *emissive signals*, indicative of functional physiology and systemic regulation. This approach prioritizes dynamic pattern recognition and zone-based interpretation over raw thermal intensity.

Spectral Behaviour and Functional Interpretation

Biospectral Imaging reframes thermal data through a structured interpretive framework that considers emission patterns across time, symmetry, and anatomical zones. Rather than absolute values, it assesses:

- **Activose zones** – elevated spectral regions linked to inflammation, angiogenesis, or metabolic activation.
- **Inhibose zones** – suppressed emissions associated with sympathetic inhibition or chronic degeneration.

- **Anisospectrality** – significant asymmetries between homologous zones not attributable to external influences.
- **Equibose balance** – physiological zones with bilateral spectral coherence, suggesting regulatory equilibrium.

These terms replace outdated language such as "hot spots" and "cold areas," offering a terminology rooted in physiology, not surface perception (Reitz, 2025).

Imaging Platforms and Biospectral Requirements

Biospectral Medicine functions independently of specific hardware, yet any imaging platform must meet minimal technical standards.:

- LWIR sensitivity (8–14 μm),
- High-resolution detectors (typically <0.05°C NETD),
- Emissivity calibration (set near 0.98),
- Capability for raw data export and region-of-interest analysis.

In clinical practice, zone segmentation, asymmetry quantification, and palette normalization are essential for consistent inter-practitioner interpretation. These analytic tools are foundational to the Reitz Clinical Infrared Interpretation Model (R-CIIM), which organizes interpretation into a six-step interpretive methodology.

PART IV

PHYSICS FOUNDATION

THE PHYSICS OF INFRARED EMISSION

Infrared thermography is grounded in the fundamental principles of physics that describe how all matter emits electromagnetic radiation based on its temperature. In the context of clinical biospectral imaging, these laws provide the theoretical basis for understanding why human tissues emit radiation in specific infrared wavelengths, and how this emission can be reliably detected, measured, and interpreted.

Blackbody Radiation and Planck's Law

All objects with a temperature above absolute zero (0 K0\,\text{K}0K) emit electromagnetic radiation due to the thermal motion of charged particles. An idealized object that absorbs all incident radiation and re-emits it across all wavelengths without reflection is called a blackbody. While no real object behaves as a perfect blackbody, many materials, including human skin, approximate blackbody behaviour in the infrared spectrum.

The spectral radiance of a blackbody is described by Planck's Law, which defines the intensity of emitted radiation at a specific wavelength for a given temperature:

E(λ,T)=2hc2λ5·1ehcλkT−1E(\lambda, T) = \frac{2hc^2}{\lambda^5} \cdot \frac{1}{e^{\frac{hc}{\lambda kT}} - 1}E(λ,T)=λ52hc2·eλkThc−11

Where:

- E(λ,T)E(\lambda, T)E(λ,T) = spectral radiance ($W \cdot sr^{-1} \cdot m^{-3}$)
- hhh = Planck's constant (6.626×10^{-34} J·s)
- ccc = speed of light (3.00×10^{8} m/s)
- λ\lambdaλ = wavelength (m)
- kkk = Boltzmann's constant (1.381×10^{-23} J/K)
- TTT = absolute temperature (K)

Human skin emits most intensely at wavelengths between 8 to 12 micrometers, which corresponds to normal physiological temperatures between 30–38°C. Importantly, human tissue exhibits emissivity values of 0.97–0.99, meaning that skin radiates almost as efficiently as a perfect blackbody (Steketee, 1973; Niskanen et al., 2016).

This high emissivity allows for accurate thermal detection using modern infrared sensors, especially microbolometers optimized for the 8–14 μm range, the spectral window used in medical biospectral imaging.

The Stefan–Boltzmann Law

While Planck's Law describes radiation at specific wavelengths, the Stefan–Boltzmann Law determines the total energy radiated by a surface across all wavelengths:

E=εσT4E = \varepsilon \sigma T^4E=εσT4

Where:

- EEE = total emissive power (W/m^2)
- ε\varepsilonε = emissivity (dimensionless, 0 to 1)
- σ\sigmaσ = Stefan–Boltzmann constant (5.670×10^{-8} $W \cdot m^{-2} \cdot K^{-4}$)
- TTT = absolute temperature (K)

For human skin (ε≈0.98\varepsilon \approx 0.98ε≈0.98), the law implies that radiant energy output increases with the fourth power of temperature. Even minor changes in surface temperature lead to substantial differences in infrared radiation. For example, an increase of just 1°C can elevate emitted power by approximately 5–6%, which is readily captured by modern imaging systems (Daanen et al., 2021).

Application to Clinical Biospectral Imaging

In the context of Biospectral Medicine, the Stefan–Boltzmann Law helps explain why:

- **Activose zones** (regions of increased emission) exhibit measurable amplification of radiant output, typically due to inflammation, hyperperfusion, or sympathetic overactivity.
- **Inhibose zones** (regions of decreased emission) present flattened or delayed radiative behaviour, often reflecting ischemia, neurogenic suppression, or structural dysfunction.
- **Cold challenge procedures** (e.g. SVRT) allow differential diagnosis by provoking thermoregulatory responses, which manifest as zone-specific shifts in emissive power.

Biospectral Medicine interprets zone-based emission patterns in physiological context through standardized anatomical division and clinical terrain logic, moving beyond isolated temperature values.

This thermodynamic sensitivity forms the basis for detecting early-stage dysfunctions, such as altered autonomic tone, inflammatory changes, or vascular dysregulation, that often precede structural pathology visible on ultrasound, CT, or MRI. It is this functional emphasis that positions biospectral imaging as a true emissive physiology modality, capable of assessing biological dynamics in real time.

Emissivity and Tissue-Specific Spectral Behaviour

Emissivity (ε) is a critical physical parameter that defines how effectively a surface emits thermal radiation relative to an ideal blackbody. A value of ε = 1.0 represents a perfect blackbody that emits the maximum possible thermal radiation at a given temperature. Real-world materials, including biological tissues, exhibit emissivity values less than 1.0, depending on their molecular composition, surface characteristics, and temperature range.

In the context of clinical imaging, emissivity becomes particularly relevant in the long-wave infrared (LWIR) range of 8–14 micrometers, where human tissues radiate most intensely due to their temperature and biochemical composition.

Human skin, characterized by a high degree of hydration, vascular perfusion, and cellular density, behaves as a near-perfect blackbody in this spectral window, with emissivity values consistently between 0.97 and 0.99 (Steketee, 1973; Vollmer & Möllmann, 2018). This high emissive efficiency forms the physical basis for the non-contact detection of physiological processes via Biospectral Imaging.

Although most biological tissues exhibit similar high emissivity, subtle differences can occur depending on anatomical structure and physiological state. For instance, subcutaneous fat and muscle tissue display slightly lower but still high emissivity values, around 0.97–0.98. In contrast, bone (when exposed) has a lower emissivity, typically in the range of 0.90 to 0.92, due to its dense mineral composition and reduced water content.

Scar tissue, calloused epidermis, and keratinized zones also show mild reductions in emissivity, which can influence spectral readings in localized areas. These variations must be accounted for during image interpretation and analysis.

Non-biological materials pose a more significant challenge. Metallic prostheses, for example, have extremely low emissivity (often between 0.10 and 0.30) and behave as reflective surfaces in the infrared spectrum. Similarly, topical substances, tattoos, or residual oils on the skin may alter or distort emissive behaviour, introducing artefacts or masking true biological signals.

For this reason, strict pre-imaging protocols are enforced in Biospectral Medicine, including skin preparation and environmental control, to ensure consistency and validity in the biosignal data.

Understanding emissivity is foundational to several key interpretive principles in Biospectral Medicine:

First, emissivity mediates surface radiative behaviour and influences how deeper tissue activity (e.g., vascular changes, sympathetic tone, nerve regulation) manifests spectrally on the skin surface.While the underlying physiology drives thermal output, the emissivity of the overlying tissue determines how well this output is radiated and detected.

Second, the clinical model relies on comparative analysis of symmetrical anatomical zones. Since emissivity remains relatively constant across mirrored regions of the body under standardized conditions, any asymmetry detected is attributed to functional changes, such as differential perfusion, neurovascular imbalance, or local metabolic activation, not to innate material differences.

Third, emissivity may be altered by pathology. Ischemic, denervated, or fibrotic tissues may emit radiation differently due to structural or metabolic changes. For instance, hypoperfused scars often show reduced emission due to altered radiation properties of collagen-rich tissue in addition to lower temperature.

All Computerized Biospectral Imaging (CBI) systems used in clinical settings are calibrated with a baseline skin emissivity of 0.98, enabling zone-to-zone comparison and emission pattern recognition under controlled acquisition conditions. Palette normalization and ROI evaluation are conducted relative to this standard, allowing for the identification of activose zones (functionally enhanced emission) and inhibose zones (functionally suppressed emission), independent of raw surface temperature.

This conceptual shift from temperature-focused thermography to emissivity-centered biospectral analysis, is pivotal. Biospectral Medicine interprets emission as a physiological signal, extending beyond its thermal derivative.

Thus, a zone may appear cooler in absolute terms yet demonstrate enhanced emission behaviour in response to dynamic stimuli, such as during the Spectrovascular Response Test (SVRT). This highlights the importance of interpreting emission profiles as indicators of tissue state and regulatory activity, rather than as direct proxies for temperature alone.

Wien's Displacement Law and Spectral Ranges

A central principle in the physics of thermal radiation is Wien's Displacement Law, which defines the inverse relationship between the temperature of a blackbody and the wavelength at which it emits radiation most intensely. Mathematically, this relationship is expressed as:

λmax=bT\lambda_{\text{max}} = \frac{b}{T}λmax=Tb

where:

- λmax\lambda_{\text{max}}λmax is the wavelength (in meters) corresponding to the peak emission,
- bbb is Wien's displacement constant, approximately 2.897×10−3 m\cdotpK2.897 \times 10^{-3} \, \text{m·K}2.897×10−3m\cdotpK,
- TTT is the absolute temperature in Kelvin.

This law is especially relevant in the context of human physiology. For instance, normal human skin temperature averages around 33°C, equivalent to 306 K. Applying the equation:

λmax=2.897×10−3306≈9.47 μm\lambda_{\text{max}} = \frac{2.897 \times 10^{-3}}{306} \approx 9.47 \, \mu mλmax=3062.897×10−3≈9.47μm

This result indicates that human skin emits maximum infrared radiation at approximately 9.47 micrometers, placing it firmly within the long-wave infrared (LWIR) portion of the electromagnetic spectrum. This is a critical spectral window for medical imaging, as it aligns precisely with the peak emissive behaviour of biological tissues.

Consequently, thermographic systems used in clinical applications, including Computerized Biospectral Imaging (CBI) devices, are optimized to detect radiation in the 8–14 μm range, which includes the peak emission wavelength and allows for maximal physiological sensitivity. This optimization is grounded in both physics and biology, establishing spectral window selection as a foundation of interpretative validity.

Three key factors justify the use of this spectral band in Biospectral Medicine:

1. **Physiological Emission Matching**
   The 8–14 μm window incorporates the emission peak of human skin, ensuring that biospectral data reflects real-time physiological output rather than peripheral or attenuated radiation. This enhances both sensitivity and interpretive accuracy.

2. **Atmospheric Transmission Efficiency**
   Infrared radiation in the 8–14 μm band passes through the atmosphere with minimal absorption by water vapor or carbon dioxide. This spectral transparency enables accurate, non-contact measurement under clinical conditions without external interference (Vollmer & Möllmann, 2018; Rogalski, 2012).

3. **Sensor Performance and System Design**
   Modern infrared detectors, especially uncooled microbolometers based on vanadium oxide (VOx) or amorphous silicon (a-Si), are engineered to function optimally in this wavelength band. In addition, optics such as germanium or chalcogenide lenses are specifically chosen for their transparency and performance in the LWIR range, further reinforcing the technical consistency of Biospectral systems.

This precise alignment between physiological emission characteristics and sensor architecture is what enables consistent spectral analysis in Biospectral Medicine. All clinical zones, regardless of anatomical location, are observed within a uniform spectral window, eliminating bias due to sensor mismatch or atmospheric distortion. As a result, emission asymmetries and spectral anomalies, such as those seen in activose or inhibose zones, are valid reflections of biological processes rather than imaging artifacts.

Thus, Wien's Displacement Law serves as a theoretical foundation in thermophysics and as a functional determinant of clinical system design, reinforcing the legitimacy and precision of biosignal detection in medical infrared imaging.

Thermodynamics in Biological Systems

Infrared emission from the human body is a consequence of fundamental thermodynamic laws. These emissions are not random; they are the result of energy transformations and regulatory processes intrinsic to living systems. In the context of Biospectral Medicine, understanding these thermodynamic principles provides the foundation for interpreting emissive data as biosignals, functional reflections of metabolic, vascular, and autonomic activity.

The first and second laws of thermodynamics in physiology

First Law: Conservation of Energy

The First Law of Thermodynamics, also known as the Law of Energy Conservation, is among the most fundamental principles of physics. It states that energy can neither be created nor destroyed; it can only change from one form to another. For biological systems, this law is a constant reality that governs every cellular and systemic process."

The human organism survives by continuously transforming the chemical potential stored in nutrients into forms of usable energy. In this respect, metabolism can be seen as the living expression of the First Law, where energy is perpetually exchanged, transferred, and released (Nelson & Cox, 2015).

In practical terms, chemical bonds in glucose, fatty acids, and amino acids store energy harvested from the environment through food intake. Through catabolic pathways such as glycolysis, the citric acid cycle, and oxidative phosphorylation, this stored potential is released and converted into adenosine triphosphate (ATP), the universal energy currency of the cell. ATP in turn fuels mechanical contraction in skeletal and cardiac muscle, powers biosynthetic pathways, and sustains electrochemical gradients across membranes.

Each of these processes represents a transformation, not a creation of energy. The efficiency of these conversions is finite, and a significant proportion of the liberated energy is dissipated as heat (Alberts et al., 2022).

The transformation of metabolic energy into heat represents more than waste. Thermogenesis plays a central role in maintaining core body temperature, supporting enzymatic kinetics, and preserving the conditions required for biochemical life. The skin acts as the main interface for this thermodynamic exchange, radiating infrared energy into the environment.

Human skin has an emissivity close to that of a perfect blackbody radiator ($\varepsilon \approx 0.98$ in the 8–14 μm range), which makes it ideally suited for thermal emission (Steketee, 1973). This means that a fraction of every metabolic process ultimately leaves the body as infrared photons, a direct, measurable consequence of the First Law applied to physiology.

Infrared imaging systems, particularly those employed in Biospectral Medicine, capitalize on this principle by detecting the radiative output of the skin without disturbing the system itself. Unlike functional modalities such as positron emission tomography (PET) or magnetic resonance spectroscopy, which require tracers or magnetic fields, emissive imaging operates passively. It simply records the unavoidable radiation that results from energy conversion within the body.

This non-invasive capture of metabolic heat flow provides a real-time map of energetic transformation, offering insights into vascular, muscular, neural, and systemic processes (Ring & Ammer, 2012).

The First Law therefore legitimizes emissive imaging as a clinical tool. If energy absorbed by the body through food and oxygen must eventually be transformed and released, then capturing this radiative output is an inevitable process.The metabolic basis of emissive imaging establishes its validity: what begins as chemical potential ends as mechanical work, biochemical synthesis, electrochemical gradients, and radiative heat.

Biospectral Medicine builds on this fundamental principle by providing the framework to interpret these radiative emissions in a clinically meaningful way, transforming a universal law of physics into a structured interpretive pathway.

In this sense, the First Law serves as both scientific foundation and methodological defense. It reminds us that the signals recorded by infrared systems are the natural outcome of biological energy conservation. Every image reflects the inescapable thermodynamic truth that living organisms are engines of transformation, constantly converting and releasing energy.

By anchoring Biospectral Medicine in the First Law, emissive imaging claims its place alongside other functional modalities, offering a window into physiology that is both non-invasive and fundamentally grounded in physics.

Second Law: Entropy and Directional Heat Flow

The Second Law of Thermodynamics establishes that entropy within any closed system inevitably increases and that energy tends to flow spontaneously from regions of higher concentration or intensity toward regions of lower concentration.

Applied to biological systems, this law is most often expressed through the principle of heat transfer: thermal energy always flows passively from warmer to cooler regions until equilibrium is achieved (Atkins & de Paula, 2014). For living organisms, which are by definition open systems, this universal tendency toward disorder is resisted through constant metabolic investment. T

he human body expends substantial energy not only to maintain internal order at the molecular and cellular levels, but also to preserve thermal gradients across tissues and between the organism and its environment (Nelson et al., 2015).

Homeostasis depends on this constant struggle against entropy. The body sustains a relatively stable core temperature of approximately 37 °C, despite continuous exposure to variable external conditions, through intricate regulatory mechanisms. These include autonomic adjustments such as vasodilation and vasoconstriction, neuroendocrine pathways involving thyroid hormones and catecholamines, and behavioral strategies such as seeking shade or clothing (Guyton & Hall, 2021).

Without these countermeasures, the Second Law would dictate a rapid equilibration of body temperature with the ambient environment, leading to loss of physiological function and ultimately death. In this sense, life itself can be defined as the continuous expenditure of energy to counteract entropy and sustain a low-entropy state.

Despite the success of these mechanisms, the dissipation of energy cannot be avoided. Heat is constantly lost from the body through four fundamental pathways: radiation, conduction, convection, and evaporation. Under resting conditions in temperate climates, radiation accounts for the largest proportion, representing approximately 60% of total heat loss (Jessen, 2001). This radiative loss occurs in the infrared spectrum, with wavelengths in the 8–14 μm band predominating due to the emissivity properties of human skin (Steketee, 1973).

Conduction and convection reflect the exchange of thermal energy with air currents, surfaces, and clothing, while evaporation becomes the dominant mechanism during exercise or in high-temperature environments. Together, these modes of dissipation exemplify the continuous interaction between the body and its surroundings, in which entropy manifests both as a physical necessity and as a physiological challenge.

For clinical purposes, the Second Law has profound implications. The body, although globally regulated, does not exhibit perfect bilateral symmetry. Localized increases in entropy, such as those generated by inflammatory reactions, infection, or neoplastic angiogenesis, alter the expected radiative signature of a region. Inflammation, for instance, induces vasodilation, increased perfusion, and elevated skin emissivity, producing focal hyper-radiance (Ring & Ammer, 2012).

Equally, ischemic tissues demonstrate reduced perfusion and diminished radiative output, a pattern equally consistent with the Second Law's prediction of energy imbalance (Clark et al., 2017). Neuropathic processes add another dimension, as denervation or autonomic dysregulation may impair vasomotor control, creating spectral asymmetries between contralateral zones that should otherwise display thermal equivalence.

Biospectral Medicine translates these thermodynamic realities into a structured interpretive model. By systematically comparing spectral emissions from contralateral anatomical zones, the methodology identifies deviations that represent the physiological footprint of entropy at work. Because the Second Law guarantees that energy dissipates in a predictable and directional manner, any deviation from expected bilateral patterns signals dysfunction.

Thus, spectral asymmetry becomes more than a visual phenomenon: it is the measurable expression of thermodynamic imbalance manifested in human physiology. In this framework, emissive imaging is legitimized as a rigorous application of fundamental physics to clinical investigation.

In summary, the Second Law provides both the theoretical justification and the clinical utility of emissive imaging. The inevitability of entropy ensures that all physiological processes generate directional heat flow, while the body's imperfect regulation of symmetry reveals disturbances long before they are visible to structural imaging.

Through the lens of Biospectral Medicine, entropy ceases to be an abstract principle and becomes a diagnostic ally, transforming the universal drift toward disorder into a window for early detection of vascular, inflammatory, neuropathic, and systemic imbalances.

Mechanisms of Heat Transfer in Human Tissue

Infrared imaging records the radiative component of heat loss at the skin, yet the temperature patterns we see on the surface are the net result of several coupled transport processes acting from the body core outward. In living tissue, heat moves by conduction through contiguous layers, by convection via perfusing blood and at the skin–air interface, by radiation from the skin into the environment, and by evaporation through sweating and insensible water loss.

Interpreting biospectral maps therefore requires reading these mechanisms together rather than in isolation; the bioheat behavior of a region is a superposition of its material properties, vascular control, boundary conditions, and autonomic state (Pennes, 1948; Guyton & Hall, 2021).

Conduction is the direct transfer of thermal energy down temperature gradients within and between tissues, described locally by Fourier's law. Its expression in the body depends on thermal conductivity and thermal diffusivity of layered media, epidermis/dermis, subcutaneous fat, fascia, muscle, and bone.

Water-rich tissues (muscle, dermis) conduct heat more effectively than adipose tissue; subcutaneous fat therefore acts as a thermal insulator, attenuating and spatially smoothing the rise of surface temperature from deep sources (Duck, 1990). Deep inflammatory foci, osteitis, or abscesses typically generate broad, low–spatial-frequency warm gradients at the surface whose amplitude and spread reflect both the depth of the source and the diffusivity of overlying layers.

Because thermal diffusion is time-dependent, transient provocations (e.g., cold challenge) reveal different conduction signatures than steady-state conditions, the diffusion length (ℓ∼αt)(\ell \sim \sqrt{\alpha t})(ℓ∼αt) constrains how quickly deep heat can influence the surface (Chato, 1980).

Convection in physiology is dominated by blood perfusion, which transports metabolic heat and effectively couples tissue to the arterial core. In the classical Pennes bioheat equation, perfusion appears as a volumetric heat-exchange term that can either warm or cool a region depending on the difference between local tissue temperature and incoming arterial blood (Pennes, 1948).

Changes in vasomotor tone, a sodilation in inflammation or sympathetic withdrawal, vasoconstriction in ischemia or stress, modulate perfusion and therefore surface temperature (Guyton & Hall, 2021). Clinically, hyperemia elevates emissive output, venous stasis produces warmer, mottled patterns with delayed recovery, and hypoperfusion/ischemia yields relative hypothermia; these effects are often asymmetric between contralateral zones and are central to biospectral interpretation (Ring & Ammer, 2012).

In addition to intratissue convection, external convection at the skin–air boundary (free or forced) increases heat loss when ambient air moves across the surface, steepening temperature gradients and potentially accentuating cool signatures, particularly over moist skin or in drafty environments (Incropera et al., 2007).

Radiation is the emission of electromagnetic energy from the skin to the surroundings, governed by the Stefan–Boltzmann law. Human skin behaves nearly as a blackbody in the long-wave infrared, with emissivity ε≈0.98\varepsilon \approx 0.98ε≈0.98 across the 8–14 μm "atmospheric window," which is precisely the band exploited by medical thermography (Steketee, 1973; Vollmer & Möllmann, 2018).

Because the radiative power depends on absolute temperature to the fourth power and on emissivity, careful calibration, reflected-apparent temperature control, and ambient management are required to ensure that measured radiance corresponds to true surface temperature (Ring & Ammer, 2012).

In Biospectral Medicine, this radiative channel is the signal actually captured by the camera; however, its magnitude and distribution are shaped upstream by conduction and perfusion, which is why radiance must be interpreted within a bioheat framework.

Evaporation removes heat through the latent heat of vaporization as liquid water on or within the stratum corneum becomes vapor. Under heat stress or exercise, sweating can dominate total heat loss; even at rest, insensible perspiration and respiratory evaporation contribute materially to energy balance (Gagge & Nishi, 1977; Parsons, 2014).

Evaporation cools the surface without increasing radiative output directly, infrared cameras do not "see" water phase change, but the resulting drop in skin temperature reduces emitted radiance. Regions with excess sudomotor activity (e.g., sympathetically driven sweating) may therefore appear paradoxically cool despite high metabolic activity underneath, whereas anhidrosis or impaired evaporation can allow abnormal warming to persist.

Ambient humidity and airflow strongly modulate these effects, underscoring the need for standardized acquisition conditions (Ring & Ammer, 2012; Parsons, 2014).

When these mechanisms are considered together, surface spectra become intelligible as signatures of underlying physiology. A zone that appears hypothermic may reflect reduced perfusion (convective deficit), enhanced evaporative cooling, or insulating adiposity that impedes conductive ascent from a warm source below, even before structural imaging detects change.

On the contrary, a focal hyperthermic island can result from inflammatory vasodilation with strong convective delivery of core heat, conducted to the surface and expressed radiatively; if venous drainage is compromised, the warm pattern may broaden and recover slowly after a cold challenge.

This integrative view explains why contralateral spectral asymmetries, after accounting for environmental conditions, carry diagnostic meaning: they represent localized departures from the expected balance of conduction, perfusion, radiation, and evaporation mandated by thermodynamics and governed by autonomic control (Pennes, 1948; Ring & Ammer, 2012). In

Biospectral Medicine, standardized zone-by-zone comparisons leverage these principles to detect early functional dysregulation, vascular, inflammatory, neuropathic, or metabolic, well before gross structural lesions emerge.

Autonomic Regulation and Heat Dissipation

Thermoregulation is an autonomic function that depends on tightly coordinated reflexes linking thermal sensing, central integration, and effector responses in the vasculature and sweat glands. Cutaneous thermoreceptors (including TRP-family channels responsive to warmth and cold) transmit afferent signals via spinal pathways to the preoptic area/anterior hypothalamus (POA/AH), which acts as the principal integrator of thermal information.

The POA/AH compares peripheral and core inputs against a defended set-point and drives descending commands through sympathetic outflow and brainstem/spinal autonomic circuits to adjust skin blood flow and eccrine sweating (Romanovsky, 2014; Guyton & Hall, 2021). Because humans are homeotherms living in fluctuating environments, these loops operate continuously, and their dynamic behaviour, not merely static temperature, reveals the integrity of the system.

A first effector axis is cutaneous vasomotor control. In non-glabrous skin (forearm, trunk), baseline tone is largely sympathetic noradrenergic vasoconstrictor, while heat stress recruits a human-specific active vasodilator system mediated by sympathetic cholinergic cotransmitters (e.g., VIP, nitric oxide) to raise skin blood flow to as much as 6–8 L/min at the whole-body level under severe heat load (Johnson & Kellogg, 2016).

In glabrous skin (palms, soles, ears), specialized arteriovenous anastomoses (AVAs) provide rapid shunting of core-warmed blood to the surface, producing powerful changes in heat loss with small neural adjustments (Jessen, 2001).

Vasodilation increases convective heat delivery from core to skin, elevating surface temperature and radiative output; vasoconstriction conserves core heat by restricting perfusion, lowering surface temperature and emissive power (Guyton & Hall, 2021).

These mechanisms are also modulated by local mediators (e.g., nitric oxide) and by behavioral/psychological inputs via limbic–hypothalamic pathways, explaining why emotional stress can produce regionally specific warming or cooling patterns independent of ambient conditions (Parsons, 2014).

A second effector axis is eccrine sudomotor control. Eccrine sweat glands are innervated by sympathetic cholinergic fibers; activation depends on hypothalamic drive and is modulated by core temperature, skin temperature, and non-thermal stimuli (Shibasaki & Crandall, 2010; Johnson & Kellogg, 2016).

The evaporation of sweat removes heat through the latent heat of vaporization, often becoming the dominant heat-loss pathway during exercise or in hot environments. Although infrared systems do not image the phase change directly, the cooling effect of evaporation lowers skin temperature and thus reduces emitted radiance, producing spectral signatures that can mimic vasoconstriction if acquisition conditions are not standardized (Ring & Ammer, 2012; Parsons, 2014).

On the other hand, anhidrosis or impaired sudomotor drive permits abnormal warming to persist despite thermal stress. Because sudomotor thresholds and gains vary circadianly and with hydration, acclimatization, and age, protocol control (room temperature, humidity, air movement, adaptation time) is crucial for reproducible interpretation (Parsons, 2014; Sund-Levander et al., 2013).

From the perspective of Biospectral Medicine, autonomic control is read through patterns over time. Static thermograms capture a momentary balance of vasomotor and sudomotor activity; dynamic provocation reveals the reflex architecture itself. For example, a cold challenge followed by passive rewarming, the conceptual basis of the Spectrovascular Response Test (SVRT), interrogates sympathetic vasoconstrictor integrity (during cooling) and microvascular reactivity (during rewarming).

Healthy tissue typically shows a brisk, symmetric cooling with rapid, near-exponential rewarming toward baseline; delays, attenuated slopes, or failure to rewarm indicate impaired vasodilator recruitment, autonomic underactivity, or microvascular dysfunction (Ring & Ammer, 2012; Johnson & Kellogg, 2016).

Segmental patterns, e.g., one dermatome or limb rewarming abnormally slowly, suggest regional autonomic dysregulation, which may reflect peripheral neuropathy, sympathetic block, or persistent neurogenic inflammation mediated by axon-reflex peptides (substance P, CGRP) (Guyton & Hall, 2021; Parsons, 2014).

Spectral asymmetry is another autonomic marker. Bilateral regions at comparable depth and composition are expected to display near-symmetry in resting conditions after adequate acclimation.

Persistent, unexplained asymmetry implies a local disturbance in vasomotor or sudomotor control: warm hyper-radiant foci often accompany inflammatory hyperemia or sympathetically mediated vasodilation; cool hypo-radiant zones may reflect ischemia, heightened vasoconstrictor tone (e.g., Raynaud-like responses), or excessive evaporative loss from focal hyperhidrosis (Ring & Ammer, 2012; Jessen, 2001).

Importantly, the time course of asymmetry under provocation refines differential diagnosis: inflammatory sites tend to rewarm quickly and may overshoot baseline; ischemic or sympathetically over-constricted regions rewarm slowly or incompletely, and neuropathic skin may show blunted responses altogether (Johnson & Kellogg, 2016; Ring & Ammer, 2012).

These autonomic signatures cannot be captured by structural imaging. CT, MRI, and ultrasound excel at anatomy but do not report vasomotor gain, sudomotor thresholds, or recovery kinetics.

By contrast, dynamic emissive imaging provides a non-invasive readout of the functional integrity of the thermoregulatory axis, hypothalamus to skin, at the bedside. Standardized acquisition (controlled ambient temperature, humidity, air flow, skin exposure, and acclimation time) and contralateral comparison enhance specificity, while temporal metrics (cooling amplitude, rewarming slope, time-to-baseline, overshoot) add sensitivity to early dysfunction (Ring & Ammer, 2012; Parsons, 2014).

In this way, Biospectral Medicine converts the physiology of autonomic heat dissipation into clinically actionable information, complementing structural modalities and often revealing dysautonomia at stages when other tests remain normal (Sund-Levander et al., 2013; La Fountaine et al., 2016).

Biosignal Theory and Functional Imaging

The conceptual leap that defines Biospectral Medicine is the reinterpretation of long-wave infrared emission as a biosignal, a structured, zone-specific, time-varying representation of underlying physiology, beyond the camera's ability to register skin temperature. In this framing, radiance from the skin is treated like any other biomedical signal (ECG, PPG, EMG): it encodes information produced by biological processes and can be decoded with appropriate models, controls, and comparisons.

This reframing moves infrared imaging beyond "thermal pictures" into a functional diagnostic modality grounded in systems biology, bioheat physics, and clinical logic (Rangayyan, 2015; Webster, 2010; Kitano, 2002).

In signal-theoretic terms, a biosignal is a measurable carrier of information whose observable statistics (level, gradients, asymmetry, dynamics) arise from latent generators (perfusion, autonomic tone, inflammation, metabolism) filtered by the medium (layered tissues) and the measurement chain (optics, detector, calibration).

The information content of the emissive field depends on signal-to-noise ratio, sampling, and standardized boundary conditions, just as in other modalities, and interpretation benefits from priors about anatomy and physiology (Shannon, 1948; Vollmer & Möllmann, 2018). Treating emissive output as a biosignal therefore obliges protocolized acquisition (ambient control, acclimation, emissivity assumptions, reflected-apparent temperature correction) and model-based inference, not ad hoc pattern reading (Ring & Ammer, 2012).

What, precisely, is being encoded? At the mechanistic level, the observable surface temperature field Ts(x,y,t)T_s(x,y,t)Ts(x,y,t) is the forward expression of the bioheat system: metabolic heat generation, blood-borne convection, intra- and inter-tissue conduction, plus radiation and evaporation at the boundary (Pennes, 1948; Incropera et al., 2007; Parsons, 2014).

Variations in vasomotor tone alter perfusion and thus convective heat delivery; sudomotor activity modulates evaporative cooling; inflammation changes local perfusion and metabolism; ischemia reduces both. These processes imprint spatial statistics (hot/cold islands, edges, gradients) and temporal statistics (cooling/rewarming slopes, time constants, overshoot) on the emissive field.

Because human skin is an excellent long-wave radiator (emissivity ε≈0.98\varepsilon \approx 0.98ε≈0.98 in 8–14 μm), those dynamics are captured with high fidelity when calibration and environment are controlled (Steketee, 1973; Vollmer & Möllmann, 2018).

Zone logic makes the biosignal interpretable in clinic. The body's surface can be partitioned by contralateral symmetry and by anatomical territories, dermatomes, angiosomes, and functional regions, each with distinct vascular and neural control (Taylor & Palmer, 1987; Lee et al., 2008).

Because left–right counterparts share depth, composition, and environmental exposure, contralateral comparison functions as an internal control: persistent, unexplained asymmetry implies localized disturbance in vasomotor/sudomotor regulation, perfusion, or metabolic activity. Mapping emissive behavior to standardized zones reduces confounding from global factors (room temperature, humidity) and supports reproducibility, a cornerstone of clinical measurement (Ring & Ammer, 2012; Parsons, 2014).

A central distinction from conventional anatomical imaging (MRI, ultrasound, CT) is that biospectral analysis is explicitly dynamic. Static structural modalities prioritize morphology and tissue contrast; biospectral imaging prioritizes behaviour, how a region cools, rewams, stabilizes, under controlled provocation.

Protocols such as a brief cold challenge followed by passive rewarming amount to system identification: they probe the gains and time constants of the vasomotor–sudomotor loop and microvascular bed.

Healthy zones show brisk, symmetric responses; zones with inflammatory hyperemia warm fast (often with overshoot), ischemic regions warm slowly or incompletely, and neuropathic skin may respond blunted or paradoxically (Ring & Ammer, 2012; Johnson & Kellogg, 2016; Jessen, 2001). In other words, the diagnostic object is the response curve, not merely the instantaneous temperature.

Interpreting emissive biosignals is therefore an inverse problem: given observed surface fields, infer plausible latent physiological states, subject to constraints from physics and anatomy. Like other inverse problems in heat transfer, it is ill-posed unless regularized by priors (layer properties, zone depth, vascular supply) and by carefully standardized inputs (Beck et al., 1985; Incropera et al., 2007).

Biospectral Medicine handles this by (i) constraining acquisition, (ii) using contralateral differencing to cancel global confounds, (iii) reading spatiotemporal features (e.g., rewarming slope, half-time, edge sharpness), and (iv) integrating systems-biology context so findings are explained by networks, autonomic, vascular, immune, rather than isolated organs (Kitano, 2002; Ring & Ammer, 2012).

Positioned alongside other functional imaging (e.g., fMRI for neurovascular coupling, PET for metabolism), biospectral analysis offers a non-invasive, radiation-free, repeatable readout of peripheral physiological function at the bedside. Where fMRI infers neural activity from hemodynamic proxies in the brain (Friston, 2011; Raichle, 2009), biospectral imaging infers somatic autonomic and microvascular status from skin radiance in the long-wave band.

The modalities are complementary: one looks inward to central networks; the other outward to the organism–environment interface, where thermodynamics, vascular control, and inflammation meet. Integrating structural and emissive functional data yields a richer causal account of symptoms, structural integrity plus physiological performance, especially early in disease when structure remains normal but function is already altered.

Finally, because a biosignal is meaningful only to the extent that it is reliable, Biospectral Medicine emphasizes standardization and calibration. Stable ambient temperature and humidity, controlled air movement, fixed camera distance/angle, emissivity assumptions, adequate acclimation, and consistent patient preparation are essential to ensure that differences in the signal reflect biology, not setup (Ring & Ammer, 2012; Parsons, 2014).

With these controls in place, emissive infrared becomes a high-content biosignal: a zone-specific, dynamic, reproducible marker of vasomotor–sudomotor regulation, inflammatory activity, and metabolic flux that complements anatomical imaging and advances functional diagnostics.

From Temperature to Terrain: Beyond Absolute Heat

Historically, one of the principal limitations of classical medical thermography has been its reliance on absolute temperature thresholds as markers of pathology. Early diagnostic protocols often interpreted findings on the basis of whether a region displayed a deviation of approximately 1 °C from a reference value.

This simplistic criterion, while easy to operationalize, failed to account for the complex variability of human physiology. As a result, it frequently led to overgeneralized conclusions and inconsistent reproducibility, fueling skepticism about thermography's clinical applicability (Ammer, 2008; Ring & Ammer, 2012).

Biospectral Medicine reframes this problem by abandoning the notion of absolute heat as an isolated diagnostic endpoint. Instead, it adopts a relational and contextual interpretive model, recognizing that thermal emissions must be understood in their biological, anatomical, and temporal terrain. This shift introduces three pillars of analysis:

Comparative Symmetry
Bilateral comparison across homologous zones provides a robust internal control. Asymmetries in vascular, neural, or musculoskeletal emissions become clinically significant only when lateral deviations surpass normal physiological variability. For example, persistent right–left differences in emissive behavior may indicate segmental autonomic dysregulation or localized vascular compromise (Uematsu et al., 1988; Hildebrandt et al., 2010).

Temporal or Provoked Responses
Static images provide limited insight into dynamic physiology. Controlled stimuli such as the Spectrovascular Response Test (SVRT) allow clinicians to evaluate vasoregulatory adaptability rather than fixed thermal states. Patterns of delayed recovery, paradoxical warming, or fixed emissive rigidity reveal dysautonomia and microcirculatory disturbances with greater specificity than baseline images alone (Ammer & Ring, 2011; Zaproudina et al., 2013).

Terrain-Based Logic
Emissions are interpreted according to the anatomical and systemic terrain from which they originate. Rather than treating all heat elevations as equivalent, Biospectral Medicine differentiates vascular signatures from neuromuscular, lymphatic, endocrine, or immune processes. This system-specific contextualization transforms raw emissive data into meaningful biosignals, situating findings within integrative diagnostic categories (Reitz, 2025).

From this perspective, a 1 °C elevation is not inherently pathological. Its significance depends on context: Is the change localized or diffuse? Symmetric or asymmetric? Stable or reactive to provocation? A region that remains emissively rigid after SVRT, for instance, carries very different implications than a region that cools and recovers appropriately.

Thus, Biospectral Medicine moves diagnostic focus from static heat differentials toward functional meaning, aligning emissive interpretation with the logic of systems biology and integrative clinical reasoning. The conceptual leap lies in decoding the biospectral terrain, marking a transition from seeing heat as a number to understanding it as a signal of regulatory dynamics.

Zone-Based Spectral Behaviour and Emission Mapping

The methodological integrity of Biospectral Medicine depends upon its commitment to reproducibility and clinical coherence. To achieve this, the discipline establishes a fixed anatomical division into nineteen emission zones, each of which is precisely delineated and correlated with specific physiological systems.

These zones function as spatial containers of biospectral information, ensuring that emissive behaviour can be interpreted in a manner that is consistent, comparable, and anchored to clinical relevance. This zoning system addresses one of the historical weaknesses of thermography, where interpretive variability often arose from inconsistent anatomical referencing and lack of structured segmentation (Ammer, 2008; Ring & Ammer, 2012).

Within this framework, emission zones represent functional territories of physiological activity. Each region reflects characteristic patterns of vascular, neurological, lymphatic, or musculoskeletal behaviour. By constraining interpretation to these predefined areas, Biospectral Medicine permits intra- and inter-patient comparisons, allowing the clinician to distinguish between expected regulatory patterns and deviations suggestive of dysfunction.

For example, persistent emissive amplification in the supraclavicular region may indicate lymphatic or immune activation, whereas emission suppression in the lumbar terrain may be more consistent with vascular hypoperfusion or autonomic inhibition.

The interpretive process within each zone unfolds through three principal axes of analysis: vasomotor behaviour, activation states, and asymmetry. Vasomotor behaviour captures the spectral signatures of dilation, venous stasis, or hypoperfusion, each of which manifests as distinct emissive patterns observable under controlled imaging conditions (Uematsu et al., 1988; Hildebrandt et al., 2010).

Activation states are classified as *activose* (amplified emission) or *inhibose* (suppressed emission), providing a functional language for describing whether a zone demonstrates heightened or diminished biospectral activity. This dichotomy parallels the concepts of hyper- and hypo-reactivity in autonomic physiology but is framed in terms of spectral output rather than symptom report. Asymmetry, finally, is assessed by bilateral comparison across homologous zones.

Clinically significant asymmetries point toward autonomic imbalance, vascular obstruction, or neurogenic dysfunction, depending on the terrain involved (Uematsu et al., 1988; Ammer & Ring, 2011).

Interpretation of these parameters is structured through the R-CIIM system (Reitz Clinical Infrared Interpretation Model), a six-step methodology designed to ensure that biospectral data are consistently linked to clinical reasoning. The process begins with anatomical orientation, situating the emission within its precise zone.

This is followed by clinical terrain mapping, where the physiological significance of the zone is contextualized in relation to vascular, neurological, lymphatic, musculoskeletal, endocrine, or immune functions.

The third step involves colour image analysis and ROI (Region of Interest) mapping, in which emissive activity is visualized and spatially delineated. Step four, diagnostic inquiry, translates the observed biosignal profile into a structured set of clinical hypotheses. The fifth step emphasizes confirmatory testing, where the suspected category of dysfunction is validated through targeted diagnostic methods, whether circulatory studies, endocrine panels, or neurofunctional assessments.

Finally, the sixth step provides therapeutic guidance, aligning interventions with the emission pattern and its systemic context (Reitz, 2025).

Through this architecture, spectral anomalies are no longer interpreted as isolated fragments of thermal elevation or suppression but as elements within a clinically validated reasoning model. The transition from temperature-based description to biospectral language allows emissions to be decoded as functional signals rather than static values.

By integrating anatomical zoning, functional categorization, and systematic methodology, Biospectral Medicine constructs a coherent interpretive system that is both reproducible and clinically meaningful.

Integration of Biospectral Logic with Functional Pathophysiology

Infrared emission, when considered in isolation, is a non-specific physical phenomenon. Every biological tissue emits infrared radiation in accordance with its emissivity, surface characteristics, and thermal conductance. If analyzed purely as a physical measurement of temperature, such emission conveys little diagnostic precision and cannot, by itself, distinguish between health and disease (Ring & Ammer, 2012).

The transformation from raw emission to clinically meaningful information occurs only when the data are interpreted through biospectral logic, a framework that situates emissive behaviour within anatomical, physiological, and clinical context. Within this interpretive system, emission ceases to be a mere by-product of thermodynamics and becomes a biosignal, capable of reflecting internal physiological events and regulatory imbalances.

This process of transformation requires multi-layered integration between emission patterns and functional pathophysiology. At the first level, emissions must be anchored to anatomically precise zones. The fixed division into nineteen emission zones provides an essential referential framework, ensuring that emissive anomalies are consistently associated with defined anatomical substrates. This reduces interpretive ambiguity and creates reproducibility, addressing one of the main criticisms directed at earlier thermographic methods, namely the lack of standardized anatomical segmentation (Ammer, 2008).

At the second level, each emission is associated with a physiological terrain. A given spectral pattern is interpreted in relation to systemic functions. For example, amplified emission in the shoulder zone may derive from musculoskeletal overuse with reactive vasodilation, from lymphatic congestion resulting in impaired clearance, or from neuropathic irritation altering local autonomic tone.

The act of terrain association allows a clinician to move beyond surface observation and consider the emission as an externalized marker of vascular, lymphatic, neurological, musculoskeletal, endocrine, or immune processes (Uematsu et al., 1988; Hildebrandt et al., 2010).

The third level of integration is clinical triangulation, in which spectral anomalies are evaluated alongside case history, presenting symptoms, laboratory analyses, and conventional imaging. Only when emissions are considered in this multidimensional manner do they achieve full diagnostic meaning.

For instance, a hypothermic right lateral abdominal emission cannot be simplistically labeled as "cold." Instead, when triangulated with a patient's gynecological history, neurological findings, or surgical record, it may suggest ovarian suppression, lumbar autonomic impairment, or a residual sympathetic inhibition following operative intervention. Similarly, a persistent hotspot in the left axillary zone cannot be equated immediately with neoplasia.

When interpreted in the broader clinical context, it may correspond more plausibly to lymphatic congestion, immune reactivity, or the residual inflammatory sequelae of a prior vaccination (Ammer & Ring, 2011).

In this sense, Biospectral Medicine aligns conceptually with functional imaging modalities such as positron emission tomography (PET) and functional magnetic resonance imaging (fMRI). These technologies primarily capture dynamic tissue activity, including glucose metabolism, oxygen utilization, and blood flow, instead of depicting static anatomical morphology

Their diagnostic value lies in revealing physiological processes that precede or accompany structural alterations (Phelps, 2000; Logothetis, 2008). Similarly, biospectral interpretation rests on decoding emissive behaviour as signals of regulatory imbalance, offering perspective on disturbances of vascular tone, autonomic control, lymphatic function, or endocrine modulation long before macroscopic pathology becomes evident."

By situating emission within the triad of anatomical zoning, terrain-specific association, and clinical triangulation, Biospectral Medicine transforms the apparent simplicity of infrared radiation into a sophisticated diagnostic language. This integration of physics and physiology enables clinicians to interpret energy patterns as meaningful biosignals that illuminate the hidden dynamics of human regulation.

Emissivity Tables for Biospectral Imaging

Accurate biospectral imaging relies on a thorough understanding of the emissive properties of biological and non-biological surfaces. Emissivity (ε) is defined as the efficiency with which a surface emits infrared radiation compared to an ideal blackbody at the same temperature. It is a dimensionless ratio ranging from 0 to 1, with $\varepsilon = 1.0$ corresponding to a theoretical perfect emitter. Since most biological tissues emit radiation in the long-wave infrared (LWIR) spectrum (8–14 μm), emissivity data specific to this range is essential for reliable clinical interpretation.

In Biospectral Medicine, the emissivity constant is central to accurate ROI (Region of Interest) calibration, zone comparison, and palette normalization. Most tissues in the human body, especially hydrated skin, behave as near-perfect emitters, which allows for non-contact detection of thermal patterns using microbolometer-based imaging systems.

However, interferences such as scars, foreign materials, or surface products can alter emissive behaviour, creating the potential for misinterpretation if not properly accounted for.

The following tables present standardized emissivity values based on current literature and experimental validation for the 8–14 µm spectrum, consistent with Wien's displacement principle and the spectral peak of human skin radiation.

Emissivity Values of Human Tissues (8–14 µm)

Tissue or Structure	Emissivity (ε)	Notes
Skin (normal, hydrated)	0.98–0.99	Highest emissivity in vascularized regions; minimal inter-zone variation
Subcutaneous fat (not exposed)	~0.97	Influences overlying spectral profile indirectly
Scar tissue (fibrotic)	0.92–0.95	Reduced emission due to collagen density and avascularity
Calloused or keratinized skin	0.95–0.97	Lower emission due to thickened stratum corneum
Mucous membranes (e.g., lips)	~0.99	Extremely high emissivity due to moisture and perfusion
Exposed cortical bone	0.90–0.92	Significantly lower emissivity than soft tissue
Inflamed or hypervascular zones	0.98–1.00	Transient increase with vasodilation and cytokine activity
Ischemic or denervated tissue	0.95–0.97	May show flatter spectral response

These values confirm findings across multiple independent studies showing that hydrated human skin consistently ranks among the highest naturally emissive biological surfaces (Steketee, 1973; Jones, 2005; Ng & Etehadtavakol, 2018). This is what enables precise surface mapping and emission zone comparison in Biospectral Medicine.

Emissivity of Non-Biological Materials and Imaging Artifacts

Material / Interference	Emissivity (ε)	Impact on Biospectral Imaging
Metals (implants, jewelry)	0.10–0.30	Reflective in LWIR; can distort surrounding data
Glass (e.g., optical windows)	0.85–0.90	Transparent in visible light, semi-transmissive in infrared
Water (room temperature)	0.95–0.96	Reference standard due to stable emission profile
Clothing (cotton, polyester)	0.80–0.95	Insulates and blocks underlying signal; must be removed during imaging
Topical products (creams, gels)	0.50–0.90	Alters surface emissivity; contraindicated prior to exam
Hair (head, arms, chest)	0.93–0.96	Partially emissive; thick coverage impedes clear readings
Tattooed skin	0.85–0.95	Dark pigments increase absorption and emission; can obscure ROI mapping

Proper documentation and visual exclusion of these materials are crucial to maintain the fidelity of emission zone comparison. In particular, metals and cosmetics are known to significantly alter surface reflectance and must be controlled for according to established biospectral protocols (Cuykendall et al., 2020; Hooshmand et al., 2023).

Clinical Interpretation Relevance

Within the analytical framework of Biospectral Medicine, all interpretation begins from the established physical principle that human skin behaves as an almost perfect emitter in the infrared range, with a default emissivity of approximately 0.98. This value, repeatedly confirmed in biomedical physics, provides the foundation upon which emissive data can be considered reliable and comparable across individuals and imaging systems (Steketee, 1973; Vollmer & Möllmann, 2018).

However, deviations from the expected emissive baseline introduce the need for layered differential reasoning that integrates both technical and physiological factors, without immediately constituting pathology.

When emissive behaviour diverges from the canonical value, the clinician must first consider the possibility of technical artifact. Exogenous influences such as reflective jewelry, topical creams, or environmental surfaces can create distortions that appear as anomalous hot or cold spots within the spectral field.

Similarly, improper imaging conditions such as variable background radiation, unstable ambient temperature, or insufficient patient acclimatization may alter apparent emissivity, underscoring the necessity of rigorous acquisition protocols (Ammer, 2008; Ring & Ammer, 2012).

Beyond artifact, structural variations of the integument and subcutaneous tissues can alter emissive properties in predictable ways. Scar tissue, for instance, demonstrates altered infrared behaviour due to collagen remodeling and reduced vascular perfusion, while calluses, grafts, or prosthetic materials impose distinct emissive signatures because of changes in surface texture and heat conduction (Ring, 2007). Such findings emphasize the importance of correlating spectral anomalies with patient history and clinical examination in order to distinguish true dysfunction from stable structural modifications.

The most diagnostically relevant category of deviation involves functional states of emission. In the biospectral lexicon, zones may present as *inhibitory* (suppressed emission) or *activose* (amplified emission), reflecting dynamic shifts in vasomotor tone, metabolic output, or neurological input.

An inhibitory spectral zone may indicate local hypoperfusion, sympathetic overdrive, or endocrine suppression, while an activose emission may correspond to inflammatory hyperemia, lymphatic stasis, or neuropathic disinhibition.

These variations constitute the central diagnostic material of Biospectral Medicine, serving as indicators of regulatory imbalance that demand contextual interpretation. (Reitz, 2025).

Because of these complexities, the principles of emissivity highlight the absolute necessity for strict acquisition protocols. Patients must undergo standardized skin preparation and a period of thermal acclimatization in a controlled environment to minimize transient vascular fluctuations.

External materials capable of altering surface emissivity, such as creams, oils, or adhesives, must be removed prior to imaging. Jewelry and metallic objects, with their high reflectivity and divergent emissivity values, must likewise be eliminated from the imaging field.

Only under such rigorously controlled conditions can biospectral signals be interpreted with clinical confidence, ensuring that deviations from the 0.98 emissivity constant are attributed correctly to artifact, structure, or function.

In this way, Biospectral Medicine advances beyond traditional thermographic practices by integrating the physics of emissivity into a structured interpretive model. Rather than treating emissivity as a fixed technical constant, it is understood as a diagnostic axis in its own right, capable of distinguishing artifact from meaningful physiology.

This approach ensures that spectral anomalies are translated into clinically relevant findings about the underlying state of vascular, metabolic, and neurological regulation.

Integration with Biosignal Logic

The fundamental departure of Biospectral Medicine from the classical thermographic paradigm lies in the transformation of infrared emission into a structured biosignal. Whereas conventional thermography was primarily conceived as a method for measuring superficial skin temperature, Biospectral Medicine interprets emissive behaviour as a dynamic, zone-specific language of physiology.

Emissivity and spectral output are treated as functional expressions of regulatory systems operating beneath the skin.

This reframing aligns emissive imaging with the logic of systems biology, in which health and disease are understood as emergent properties of complex, adaptive networks rather than fixed thermal states.

In this interpretive model, the characteristics of emission within a defined zone correspond to functional states of vascular, metabolic, and neurological regulation. For instance, a hypoperfused region may display slightly reduced emissivity along with spectral flattening, a phenomenon in which the contrast between emission subzones diminishes due to restricted perfusion and lowered microvascular reactivity.

On the other hand, regions undergoing inflammatory activation or angiogenesis may reveal amplified emissive behaviour with heightened spatial variability, even when absolute surface temperature is only modestly elevated. This discrepancy illustrates a core principle of Biospectral Medicine: it is the pattern and relational context of emission, not the absolute numerical value, that conveys diagnostic meaning (Jones et al., 2002; Lahiri et al., 2012).

These dynamic behaviours become particularly evident under provocative testing, such as the Spectrovascular Response Test (SVRT), where cooling and rewarming sequences provide insight into vasoregulatory resilience. A healthy tissue zone typically exhibits a rapid but balanced recovery after cold exposure, reflecting intact autonomic and vascular control.

By contrast, zones subject to chronic dysfunction may reveal paradoxical persistence of cold inhibition, delayed rewarming, or exaggerated hyper-reactivity. Such responses validate the integrity, or dysfunction, of functional zones by demonstrating how emissive behaviour evolves over time, rather than under static observation (Merla & Romani, 2006; Ring, 2010).

The logic of interpretation is anchored in the recognition that emissive behaviour serves as a proxy for regulatory physiology.Inhibitory biosignals can point toward sympathetic dominance, microvascular compromise, or endocrine suppression, whereas activose signals may reflect inflammatory cascades, immune mobilization, or angiogenic drive.

By situating these signals within anatomically fixed emission zones, Biospectral Medicine provides a reproducible and clinically coherent framework for transforming raw infrared radiation into meaningful clinical intelligence (Reitz, 2025).

This integrative biosignal approach aligns emissive imaging with the conceptual trajectory of modern functional modalities, such as near-infrared spectroscopy (NIRS) or functional ultrasound, which prioritize real-time physiological dynamics over morphological description.

The result is a shift from thermography as surface temperature mapping to Biospectral Medicine as functional biosignal analysis, where emission becomes not an endpoint but an active indicator of systemic regulation (Gorbach et al., 2009; Diakides & Bronzino, 2013).

PART V

INSTRUMENTATION STANDARDS

INSTRUMENTATION STANDARDS IN BIOSPECTRAL MEDICINE

Precision, Calibration, and Spectral Fidelity in Infrared Imaging

The clinical value of Biospectral Medicine is determined by the biophysical principles of emissive behaviour, the interpretive frameworks that translate emissions into biosignals, and the instrumentation standards governing image acquisition. Infrared imaging devices designed for industrial, military, or surveillance contexts often emphasize robustness, field durability, or energy efficiency rather than medical precision.

Clinical biospectral analysis requires a unique set of technological parameters that ensure spectral fidelity, calibration accuracy, and reproducible data quality. Without adherence to these standards, the capacity of Biospectral Medicine to function as a diagnostic modality would be undermined by inconsistent or distorted signal capture.

The first requirement is spectral precision, which refers to the ability of detectors to operate within the appropriate infrared wavebands for human tissue emission. Biological emissivity peaks in the long-wave infrared (LWIR) range, typically between 8–14 µm, a region where atmospheric transmission is stable and skin emissivity approximates a near-blackbody profile.

Sensors must therefore demonstrate calibrated sensitivity within this range, with sufficient resolution to capture small but physiologically significant emissive variations. Clinical studies have shown that deviations of as little as 0.05 °C, when reliably detected, can correspond to meaningful functional asymmetries, particularly in vascular or neurological terrains (Brioschi et al., 2013; Moreira et al., 2017).

Equally critical is the principle of absolute and relative calibration. Infrared detectors inherently drift over time due to thermal noise, pixel non-uniformity, and environmental interference. Biospectral systems must therefore incorporate rigorous calibration protocols, typically using blackbody reference sources or equivalent standards, to ensure measurement accuracy.

International metrology institutes, such as NIST in the United States and PTB in Germany, have developed calibration frameworks specifically for medical infrared applications, underscoring the necessity of alignment with recognized reference bodies (Balageas et al., 2012; Minkina & Dudzik, 2009). The absence of stable calibration introduces variability that could mask or exaggerate physiological signals, leading to interpretive error.

Another defining standard is detector sensitivity and noise-equivalent temperature difference (NETD). For clinical biospectral imaging, detectors with NETD values below 50 mK are preferred, as this threshold allows the reliable detection of subtle physiological asymmetries.

Advances in uncooled microbolometer technology have democratized access to such sensitivity, enabling compact systems to achieve performance levels once restricted to cooled quantum detectors (Rogalski, 2011). However, while cooled detectors may offer superior temporal resolution and reduced noise, their cost, fragility, and operational complexity render them less practical for widespread clinical adoption. Biospectral Medicine therefore prioritizes high-performance uncooled detectors, provided they meet standards of sensitivity, stability, and long-term reproducibility (Vollmer & Karstädt, 2012).

Optical compatibility represents a further dimension of instrumentation fidelity. Infrared-transparent materials such as germanium or chalcogenide glass are necessary to construct lenses that avoid spectral distortion in the LWIR range.

The selection of optical components must also consider uniform transmission, minimal aberration, and anti-reflective coatings that reduce artifacts. Even minor optical inconsistencies can produce false emissive signatures, which may then be misinterpreted as functional anomalies if not properly controlled (Hudson & Hudson, 2019).

Finally, the clinical environment of acquisition demands instrumentation capable of controlling for extrinsic variables. Ambient radiation, airflow, and reflective surfaces can all alter apparent emission patterns.

Modern biospectral systems incorporate environmental shielding, adaptive correction algorithms, and controlled imaging suites to mitigate such factors. Without these measures, even the most advanced detectors risk producing misleading results that compromise diagnostic validity (Bertolin et al., 2019).

Taken together, these standards illustrate that Biospectral Medicine cannot rely on the generic application of thermal cameras. Its diagnostic reliability rests upon precision sensors, meticulous calibration, validated optics, and controlled imaging environments. By setting instrumentation requirements that exceed those of industrial thermography, Biospectral

Medicine ensures that emissive signals are captured with the fidelity necessary for their transformation into clinically meaningful biosignals. This rigorous technical foundation distinguishes the discipline as a medical imaging modality in its own right, rather than a derivative use of infrared technology.

Infrared Detector Technologies

Sensor Physics and Spectral Suitability for Clinical Biosignal Acquisition

Infrared detector technologies form the cornerstone of biospectral imaging, converting the invisible radiation continuously emitted by the human body into electrical signals that can be digitally processed and interpreted. The choice of detector is decisive in determining the sensitivity, reproducibility, and ultimately the clinical value of Biospectral Medicine.

Infrared detectors are broadly classified into thermal detectors, which register indirect changes in material properties due to absorbed radiation, and photon detectors, which generate a direct electrical response from incident photons. Within these two families, microbolometers and quantum detectors dominate medical applications.

Microbolometers, based on uncooled thermal architectures, provide stability and spectral alignment with human emissive behaviour, while quantum detectors, although exceptionally sensitive, are constrained by cryogenic cooling requirements and spectral misalignment. For this reason, Biospectral Medicine recognizes both as relevant, but privileges microbolometers as the most practical and clinically reproducible solution (Reitz, 2025; Rogalski, 2019).

Microbolometers (Uncooled Thermal Sensors)

Microbolometers are the defining detectors of modern clinical infrared imaging. They consist of thin membranes fabricated from materials such as vanadium oxide (VOx) or amorphous silicon (a-Si), engineered to change electrical resistance when exposed to absorbed infrared radiation.

Their spectral sensitivity lies within the long-wave infrared (LWIR) band, 8–14 µm, directly overlapping with the peak emission of human skin near 9.4 µm at 33 °C, as predicted by Wien's displacement law (Kruse, 2001). This natural alignment makes them ideally suited for biosignal acquisition, since they capture the exact spectral region in which human emissivity approaches unity (~0.98).

A defining advantage of microbolometers is that they require no cryogenic cooling. Their passive architecture reduces system complexity, allowing the design of compact, portable, and reliable devices appropriate for outpatient and hospital settings.

Over the last decade, significant advances in sensor fabrication, particularly in pixel miniaturization and thermal isolation techniques, have reduced pixel pitch to 12 µm or below and improved noise-equivalent temperature difference (NETD) to $\leq$50 millikelvin (mK), a threshold sufficient to resolve clinically meaningful biospectral asymmetries across anatomical zones (Han & Lee, 2018; Rogalski & Martyniuk, 2020).

The clinical strengths of microbolometers lie in their stability and reproducibility under controlled imaging conditions. Their limitations, namely lower frame rates and higher noise relative to cooled photon detectors, are negligible in the context of static zone-based imaging, where functional patterns rather than ultrafast dynamics are the diagnostic target.

By eliminating cryogenic infrastructure, microbolometers remove barriers to widespread clinical adoption, establishing themselves as the instrumentation standard for Biospectral Medicine (Gade & Moeslund, 2014; Vollmer & Möllmann, 2018).

Quantum Detectors (Cooled Photon Detectors)

Quantum detectors represent a second family of infrared sensors, operating on fundamentally different physics. Instead of responding to bulk thermal effects, these detectors, commonly fabricated from indium antimonide (InSb) or mercury cadmium telluride (HgCdTe), directly convert incident photons into electron–hole pairs, producing a highly sensitive electrical signal.

Their spectral range typically spans the mid-wave infrared (MWIR) band, 3–5 µm, which, while advantageous for atmospheric transmission, does not coincide with the peak emission of human skin. This spectral mismatch limits their direct applicability for biosignal acquisition (Kinch, 2014; Dereniak & Boreman, 1996).

The hallmark of quantum detectors is their extraordinary sensitivity and speed. They achieve NETD values below 20 mK and offer nanosecond-scale temporal responses, making them indispensable in aerospace, defense, and certain biomedical research contexts requiring high frame rates.

However, this performance is only possible under cryogenic cooling, most often achieved by liquid nitrogen (77 K) or mechanical Stirling-cycle coolers. These cooling requirements introduce considerable cost, fragility, and maintenance demands, and they constrain the detector's stability in routine clinical use (Razeghi & Nguyen, 2014; Rogalski, 2011).

Although quantum detectors remain valuable in experimental physiology, where rapid transient responses are studied, their integration into clinical Biospectral Medicine is limited. Their spectral misalignment, operational complexity, and lack of reproducibility in outpatient environments render them suboptimal for functional zone mapping.

As a result, while quantum detectors illustrate the upper limit of detector sensitivity, they remain auxiliary rather than foundational technologies for clinical biospectral imaging (Hudson & Hudson, 2019; Reitz, 2025).

Clinical Standard in Biospectral Medicine

Within Biospectral Medicine, the uncooled microbolometer is considered the gold standard for detector technology. Its spectral compatibility with human skin emission, high signal-to-noise ratio within the 8–14 µm band, and logistical advantages in clinical deployment make it uniquely suitable for emission-based diagnostics.

It offers the ideal balance between physiological relevance, image fidelity, and safety. Furthermore, biospectral interpretation relies on zone-based asymmetry, not absolute temperature alone, allowing these systems to outperform higher-spec quantum detectors in practical measurement resolution when properly normalized and calibrated (Pereira et al., 2019; Alves et al., 2021).

In summary, infrared detector selection must prioritize spectral alignment with human physiology, reproducibility of emission behaviour, and integration with zone-based diagnostic systems. While high-performance cooled detectors offer technical advantages in certain domains, their utility in clinical biosignal medicine remains limited. For functional zone-based imaging, modern microbolometers provide both the fidelity and practicality necessary for a globally deployable biospectral modality.

Optics and Infrared Transmission Materials

In biospectral imaging, the precision of clinical interpretation relies on the inherent sensitivity of the detector array and on the integrity of the optical pathway through which infrared radiation travels. Sensors, regardless of their technological sophistication, are dependent on lenses, filters, and protective windows to deliver an undistorted stream of emissive energy from the skin surface to the focal plane.

If this transmission is compromised, by spectral absorption, scattering, or reflection, the resulting image no longer represents a faithful map of the biosignal.

In Biospectral Medicine, where interpretative accuracy depends on detecting subtle asymmetries, terrain-specific vascular signatures, and micro-regulatory patterns, even minor distortions in the optical chain can alter the validity of the entire analysis.

Infrared optics present challenges fundamentally different from those of visible light systems. Standard silica-based glasses, commonly used in photography and microscopy, are opaque in the long-wave infrared (LWIR) spectrum of 8–14 μm, which comprehends the emissive peak of human skin. Consequently, they cannot be employed in clinical infrared imaging. Instead, specialized materials with molecular structures capable of transmitting LWIR radiation are required.

The search for such materials has been a central driver in the development of infrared camera technology since the mid-20th century, with research expanding from crystalline semiconductors to engineered glasses optimized for thermal transmission (Smith, 1993; Wood, 2011).

The choice of optical material must balance multiple requirements: high spectral transmittance within the biologically relevant LWIR band, minimal chromatic dispersion to preserve image sharpness, thermal stability to prevent degradation under environmental fluctuations, and, for medical applications, biocompatibility and robustness to withstand repeated clinical use.

These parameters function as essential clinical standards. An optical element that attenuates or distorts emissive radiation risks concealing low-intensity biospectral patterns, such as localized inhibitory zones or subtle activose emissions, leading to incomplete or misleading diagnostic conclusions.

Among the most reliable solutions to these challenges are a small number of specialized infrared transmission materials. Germanium (Ge), with its exceptional transmissive window in the 7–12 μm range, has historically been the gold standard for high-resolution LWIR optics. Zinc Selenide (ZnSe), with broader spectral range and favorable refractive properties, has emerged as a versatile alternative, particularly in multi-element lens systems.

More recently, chalcogenide glasses have been introduced, offering a lightweight and moldable class of materials that support the miniaturization and cost reduction of diagnostic devices while still maintaining sufficient performance in the LWIR band (Wilke et al., 2017; Sanghera et al., 2016).

The evolution of these materials reflects the trajectory of infrared medicine itself: from early dependence on bulky, laboratory-grade optics to the current phase of portable, clinic-ready biospectral platforms. By ensuring that the pathway from skin emission to detector remains spectrally faithful, these materials safeguard the reliability of Biospectral Medicine as both a scientific and clinical practice.

Germanium (Ge)

Germanium occupies a central position in the field of infrared optics and remains the benchmark material for high-resolution LWIR systems. Its optical properties align closely with the requirements of Biospectral Medicine, particularly because of its superior transmission within the 7–12 μm window, which contains the emissive peak of human skin radiation near 9.4 μm at physiological temperature.

This spectral alignment ensures that germanium-based lenses transmit the biologically most relevant portion of infrared radiation without significant loss, thereby preserving the integrity of biospectral signals (Ghosh, 1991).

One of germanium's defining characteristics is its high refractive index, approximately 4.0 at 10 μm, which enables the design of compact optical assemblies with shorter focal lengths and reduced aberration. This property is critical in medical imaging, where precision focusing is required to differentiate between subtle emissive patterns across adjacent anatomical zones.

However, the high index also produces considerable surface reflection losses if uncoated, with reflectance per interface exceeding 36%. For this reason, the clinical use of germanium optics almost always requires advanced anti-reflective coatings, typically multilayer dielectric films or diamond-like carbon (DLC) coatings, which can reduce reflection losses to below 1% per surface and enhance overall transmittance (Savini et al., 2010).

Beyond its optical properties, germanium is valued for its chemical and environmental stability. Unlike hygroscopic materials such as calcium fluoride, germanium resists moisture-induced degradation and retains optical clarity under a range of clinical conditions. Its high density (5.33 g/cm^3), however, presents ergonomic challenges: lenses constructed from germanium are heavy, which can limit their use in portable, handheld biospectral cameras.

This constraint has been partially mitigated through ergonomic design innovations and hybrid systems combining germanium with lighter optical elements, but it remains a consideration when developing point-of-care diagnostic devices (Barker & Daniels, 2004).

Thermally, germanium maintains strong transmission properties up to approximately 100 °C but begins to suffer from bandgap-related opacity at higher temperatures due to free-carrier absorption. In clinical practice, this limitation is irrelevant, as imaging environments are typically stable and controlled. More relevant is the phenomenon of thermal lensing, where changes in temperature can slightly alter refractive index and lens performance.

For this reason, precision biospectral systems often incorporate environmental stabilization or real-time correction algorithms to account for temperature-related shifts in germanium optics (Hudson et al., 2008).

Germanium also demonstrates mechanical robustness, making it well suited for clinical devices subject to frequent handling, sterilization, and patient interaction. However, its expense remains one of its principal limitations. Germanium is a relatively scarce element, and its cost has increased in recent decades due to competing demands from fiber optics, semiconductor technology, and defense industries (Coleman et al., 2010).

This economic factor has stimulated the development of alternatives such as chalcogenide glasses, which aim to replicate germanium's infrared performance in a lighter and more cost-effective form.

In summary, germanium remains the optical gold standard for LWIR clinical imaging, combining spectral fidelity, chemical stability, and mechanical resilience. Its high refractive index, when paired with anti-reflective coatings, permits the precise focusing required for zone-based emissive mapping.

While heavy and costly, its unmatched performance in transmitting the most physiologically relevant portion of human infrared emission ensures that it continues to play a pivotal role in Biospectral Medicine.

Zinc Selenide (ZnSe)

Zinc Selenide (ZnSe) is one of the most versatile infrared optical materials and represents a widely adopted alternative to germanium in both industrial and biomedical imaging. Its most distinctive feature is its broad spectral transmission, which extends from the visible spectrum (~0.6 μm) through the entire long-wave infrared (LWIR) band up to approximately 20 μm.

This wide transparency window ensures that ZnSe optics can not only transmit the peak emissive wavelength of human skin (~9.4 μm) but also accommodate auxiliary imaging modalities or multispectral systems that combine near- and mid-infrared diagnostics with thermal mapping (Palik, 1998; Sanghera & Aggarwal, 1999).

Optically, ZnSe offers a moderate refractive index of approximately 2.4 at 10 μm, significantly lower than the ~4.0 index of germanium. This reduced refractive index translates into lower Fresnel reflection losses at each optical interface, simplifying lens assembly and allowing multi-element systems to be constructed with less dependence on complex anti-reflective coatings.

This characteristic is particularly advantageous for biospectral cameras employing compound optical trains, where multiple lenses and filters must be combined without degrading overall signal fidelity (Willemsen et al., 2011).

A further strength of ZnSe lies in its resistance to thermal shock and environmental fluctuations. Whereas certain infrared materials exhibit performance degradation in humid or variable conditions, ZnSe maintains transmission stability, making it well suited to clinical environments where equipment is frequently transported, sterilized, or exposed to variations in room temperature and humidity. Its chemical inertness also reduces the risk of corrosion or surface degradation, factors that are essential for long-term clinical deployment (Matsuura, 2004).

Clinically, ZnSe has proven to be particularly effective in diagnostic systems operating in dynamic environments, such as portable thermal cameras used in outpatient assessments or field-based medical applications. Because it is less dense than germanium (density 5.27 g/cm^3 vs. 5.33 g/cm^3) and is available in large, homogeneous crystals, ZnSe is also more amenable to the fabrication of lightweight, wide-aperture lenses.

This advantage supports the ongoing trend toward ergonomic, point-of-care biospectral devices, where portability and operator comfort are as critical as spectral fidelity (Zhou et al., 2019).

Another significant application of ZnSe lies in its dual compatibility with CO_2 laser systems (10.6 μm). This property allows ZnSe optics to be used in both diagnostic and therapeutic infrared instruments, creating continuity between imaging and treatment workflows.

For example, ZnSe windows are commonly integrated into medical laser devices, where their transparency in the LWIR spectrum enables simultaneous tissue visualization and photothermal application. Such cross-compatibility strengthens ZnSe's role in integrative biomedical platforms (Han et al., 2022).

Despite these advantages, ZnSe does carry certain limitations. It is mechanically softer than germanium, with a Knoop hardness of ~120 kg/mm^2 compared to germanium's ~780 kg/mm^2, making it more prone to scratching or abrasion during handling. This necessitates the application of protective hard coatings when ZnSe is used in clinical devices expected to undergo frequent cleaning or sterilization.

Furthermore, while its broad transparency window is beneficial for multispectral optics, its performance in the 8–14 µm diagnostic band is slightly lower than that of germanium, meaning a small compromise in transmission efficiency (Savini et al., 2006).

In summary, Zinc Selenide is a high-performance optical material whose broad transmission, reduced reflection losses, and environmental robustness make it a valuable component in biospectral systems.

While its mechanical softness and slightly lower LWIR efficiency must be managed through coatings and design considerations, ZnSe remains one of the most clinically adaptable materials, bridging diagnostic imaging with therapeutic infrared applications and supporting the portability and versatility required for modern Biospectral Medicine.

Chalcogenide Glasses

Chalcogenide glasses represent one of the most significant recent innovations in the field of infrared optics, marking a departure from reliance on crystalline materials such as germanium and zinc selenide. These glasses are composed primarily of the chalcogen elements sulfur, selenium, and tellurium, often combined with arsenic, germanium, or antimony to produce amorphous solids with tunable optical properties.

Their emergence has opened new possibilities for lightweight, low-cost, and moldable optical components that maintain functional transmission in the long-wave infrared (LWIR) spectrum critical to Biospectral Medicine (Sanghera & Aggarwal, 1999; Eggleton et al., 2011).

One of the principal advantages of chalcogenide glasses is their broad spectral transmission range, which typically extends from the mid-wave infrared (MWIR, ~2 µm) through the LWIR band up to ~14–16 µm, fully including the emissive peak of human skin.

While their absolute transmittance is slightly lower than germanium in the 8–14 µm window, this limitation can be offset by the application of optimized anti-reflective coatings. Importantly, their relatively low refractive index ($n \approx 2.3$–2.8 at 10 µm) reduces Fresnel reflection losses compared with germanium, facilitating their use in multi-element optical systems without excessive signal degradation (Wang et al., 2021).

From a manufacturing perspective, chalcogenide glasses offer transformative advantages. Unlike crystalline materials, which must be grown, cut, and polished under carefully controlled conditions, chalcogenide glasses are moldable and compatible with precision casting techniques.

This enables scalable, cost-effective production of complex lens geometries, diffractive surfaces, and miniaturized optical assemblies suitable for compact diagnostic devices.

In practical terms, this has accelerated the development of portable biospectral platforms and point-of-care diagnostic cameras, aligning with the broader trend in medicine toward decentralized and accessible technologies (Lucas et al., 2015).

Thermally, chalcogenide glasses exhibit stability across a wide range of operating conditions, although they are more susceptible to structural relaxation and crystallization than germanium or zinc selenide. Modern compositional engineering, however, has significantly improved their resistance to thermal shock and environmental degradation.

For clinical devices, protective coatings and hermetic packaging are frequently employed to safeguard optical integrity over repeated use and sterilization cycles (Zakery & Elliott, 2007).

Another important feature is the mechanical lightness of chalcogenide optics. With lower density than germanium, they substantially reduce the weight of imaging devices, improving ergonomics in handheld applications and enabling wearable or head-mounted infrared systems. This characteristic directly supports the miniaturization of Biospectral Medicine, making infrared imaging more adaptable for bedside monitoring, telemedicine, and home-based diagnostics (Calvez et al., 2012).

While still a relatively new entrant into clinical imaging, the trajectory of chalcogenide glass adoption suggests a growing role in the democratization of biospectral technologies. By combining adequate transmission in the LWIR spectrum with low cost, design flexibility, and reduced weight, chalcogenide glasses bridge the gap between high-performance crystalline optics and scalable clinical instrumentation.

Their rise reflects a broader trend in medical technology: shifting from heavy, laboratory-bound equipment toward lightweight, patient-centered systems that can extend advanced diagnostics beyond specialized centers into everyday healthcare environments.

Optical Design Considerations in Biospectral Systems

The reliability of Biospectral Medicine depends on the sensitivity of detectors, the transmission qualities of optical materials, and the design architecture of the optical system itself. Every lens, filter, and window represents a potential point of signal alteration.

Because quantitative emissive analysis relies on the faithful capture of subtle spectral differences across anatomical zones, even small imperfections in the optical train can introduce distortions that compromise diagnostic validity. For this reason, optical design in biospectral systems must be governed by principles that ensure maximum transmission efficiency, minimal reflection, and environmental protection throughout the acquisition process.

One of the central requirements is the application of anti-reflective (AR) coatings. Infrared optical materials such as germanium or zinc selenide have high intrinsic refractive indices, which, without coatings, can produce reflection losses exceeding 30% at each air–glass interface.

In a multi-element optical assembly, such losses accumulate and can reduce effective signal strength below clinically usable thresholds. Modern AR coatings, including multilayer dielectric films and diamond-like carbon (DLC) surfaces, have been shown to reduce Fresnel reflection to less than 1% per surface, dramatically improving signal-to-noise ratio and preserving the subtle biospectral contrasts required to detect vascular or autonomic asymmetries (Savini et al., 2010; López-Puente et al., 2020).

Equally important is the prevention of contamination and condensation on optical surfaces. Unlike visible light, where minor dust or smudges may only reduce image clarity, in the infrared spectrum such irregularities can attenuate or scatter radiation in ways that mimic pathological biosignals. A fingerprint oil residue on a lens can create a spurious cold spot, while a condensation layer can scatter emissive radiation and mask a genuine hyperemissive focus.

Clinical imaging protocols therefore mandate rigorous optical maintenance and environmental shielding, including humidity control and lens cleaning regimes, to ensure that captured signals reflect physiological reality rather than optical artifact (Hudson et al., 2008; Amiel et al., 2019).

The spectral matching of optics to detector sensitivity is another non-negotiable consideration. A detector array designed for long-wave infrared (8–14 μm) cannot operate at full capacity if coupled with optics that partially absorb or distort this spectral band. Material selection, coatings, and lens geometries must therefore be chosen to align perfectly with the detector's spectral response curve.

Failure to achieve this matching not only reduces transmission efficiency but also alters the effective emissive profile of the patient's skin, producing systematic errors that undermine both intra- and inter-patient comparability (Minkina & Dudzik, 2009).

Beyond transmission fidelity, optical design also determines the geometric parameters of imaging. Focal length, field of view (FOV), and magnification must be optimized for the anatomical regions under study. High-magnification germanium lenses may be required for facial imaging, where the detection of fine biospectral asymmetries in periorbital or perioral zones is essential.

Conversely, wide-angle chalcogenide optics are preferable for full-body scans, where the priority is to maintain global coverage of all 19 biospectral emission zones within a single frame. Clinical utility is therefore enhanced not by universal lens solutions, but by the availability of interchangeable optical modules adapted to specific diagnostic contexts (Calvez et al., 2012; Wilke et al., 2017).

Ultimately, optical design in Biospectral Medicine functions as both a technical foundation and a clinical safeguard. By ensuring that emissive signals are transmitted, focused, and recorded without distortion, optical engineering protects the diagnostic chain from artifacts that could be misinterpreted as vascular pathology, inflammatory activity, or autonomic inhibition.

The lens system is an active determinant of biospectral fidelity, directly shaping the capacity of clinicians to translate raw emission into meaningful diagnostic findings.

Sensor Resolution and Thermal Sensitivity

Quantitative Foundations for Diagnostic Precision in Biospectral Imaging

The diagnostic validity of Biospectral Medicine depends on a convergence of clinical reasoning and technological precision. On one side lies the interpretive framework: standardized zone mapping, comparative asymmetry analysis, and biosignal logic, which allow emissive patterns to be translated into physiological meaning.

On the other side lies the physical performance of the imaging hardware, which determines whether those signals are captured with sufficient clarity to permit reliable interpretation. If the instrumentation fails to resolve subtle emissive variations or cannot register faint contrasts above its internal noise threshold, the entire clinical model risks being undermined by technological limitation rather than by physiological ambiguity.

In this regard, the sensor array is the keystone of biospectral imaging. Its function is to produce a quantitatively stable and spatially accurate map of emissive behaviour, upon which diagnostic reasoning can be built.

Unlike classical thermography, which was often limited by low-resolution detectors and high system noise, Biospectral Medicine requires instrumentation capable of distinguishing millikelvin-level variations and resolving fine anatomical structures within the body's emissive terrain.

The standardization of imaging into nineteen emission zones amplifies this requirement: each zone must be captured with reproducibility, and subzone variations must remain visible rather than being blurred into undifferentiated averages (Ring et al., 2020).

Two hardware parameters define this capability most directly: spatial resolution and thermal sensitivity, the latter expressed as Noise-Equivalent Temperature Difference (NETD). Spatial resolution governs the ability of the system to accurately render the geometry of emissive regions.

Without sufficient pixel density, small but diagnostically critical features, such as lymphatic congestion in the axillary zones or subtle dermatomal asymmetries along the cervical spine, may be lost. Thermal sensitivity, by contrast, determines the system's capacity to detect minute emissive differences above background electronic noise.

This is critical in functional imaging, where subclinical dysfunction may present as emissive changes of less than 0.1 °C, invisible to lower-grade detectors but central to the biospectral diagnostic model (Nguyen et al., 2014; Fernández-Cuevas et al., 2015).

The interplay between these two parameters establishes the quantitative foundation of diagnostic precision in Biospectral Medicine. High spatial resolution ensures that emissive signals are correctly localized, preserving the anatomical integrity of the zone.

Low NETD ensures that even the faintest functional irregularities are captured, preventing early signs of vascular dysregulation or autonomic imbalance from being dismissed as noise. Together, they transform infrared imaging from a descriptive thermal map into a reproducible biosignal acquisition system, aligning the technology with the clinical requirements of functional medicine.

Spatial Resolution

Spatial resolution defines the ability of an infrared imaging system to represent emissive signals with sufficient anatomical fidelity to support the zone-based interpretive model of Biospectral Medicine. Resolution is determined by two interdependent factors: the number of pixels in the detector array (e.g., 320×240, 640×480, or higher) and the pixel pitch (the physical size of each sensing element).

Together, these parameters dictate whether the geometry of emissive patterns is faithfully reconstructed or blurred into approximations that obscure physiologically meaningful detail.

In the context of Biospectral Medicine, where interpretation often depends on identifying subtle asymmetries or subzone irregularities, insufficient resolution carries direct diagnostic risks. A low-density array may merge emissive patterns from adjacent anatomical structures, producing an averaged signal that conceals early signs of dysfunction.

This limitation is especially problematic in small but diagnostically rich territories such as the periorbital region, where microvascular changes can indicate systemic autonomic imbalance; the supraclavicular fossa, where lymphatic signals may emerge before palpable swelling; and the dermatomal distributions of the cervical spine, where subtle emissive asymmetries may correspond to neurogenic irritation (Nguyen et al., 2014).

Historically, clinical thermography operated with arrays offering resolutions as low as 160×120 pixels, which were adequate for gross screening but lacked the precision necessary for modern biospectral interpretation. Contemporary standards recognize 320×240 pixels (QVGA) as the minimal threshold for functional imaging, sufficient for global zone mapping and full-body scans but limited in capacity to resolve fine emissive gradients.

By contrast, systems with 640×480 pixels (VGA) or higher allow for subzone partitioning within the established 19 anatomical emission zones. This capability is particularly important in high-detail studies such as facial biosignal analysis, axillary lymphatic assessment, and microvascular terrain mapping, where emissive differences may cover only a few pixels in low-resolution arrays (Morales-Hernández et al., 2022).

Pixel pitch further refines spatial performance. Smaller pitch values (≤ 17 µm in modern uncooled microbolometers) increase the number of sensing elements per unit area, expanding field of view while maintaining high detail.

This enables clinicians to capture whole-body coverage without sacrificing the ability to detect local irregularities. Advances in fabrication have allowed even portable, uncooled systems to achieve this balance, thereby expanding high-resolution biospectral imaging into routine outpatient use (Han & Lee, 2018).

The clinical implications of resolution extend beyond static image quality. High-resolution detectors enable computational enhancements such as multi-frame averaging and emissive edge detection. Multi-frame averaging reduces random noise, sharpening emissive boundaries, while improved edge detection algorithms enhance the clinician's ability to delineate activose versus inhibose zones.

These refinements improve inter-observer reproducibility and diagnostic confidence, which are crucial in Biospectral Medicine, where subtle asymmetries may carry significant interpretive weight (Ring et al., 2020).

In sum, spatial resolution is a determinant of diagnostic granularity. High-density arrays and small pixel pitch ensure that emissive data retain their anatomical specificity, allowing the clinician to trace biosignals with precision across defined zones.

Without adequate resolution, the capacity of Biospectral Medicine to identify early, functional irregularities is compromised, reducing the method to coarse screening rather than a tool of refined diagnostic investigation.

Noise-Equivalent Temperature Difference (NETD)

If spatial resolution defines the structural fidelity of emissive imaging, thermal sensitivity determines its functional depth. Thermal sensitivity is quantified by the Noise-Equivalent Temperature Difference (NETD), a measure of the smallest temperature difference a sensor can detect above its intrinsic electronic noise floor.

Expressed in millikelvins (mK), this parameter represents the minimum emissive contrast required for a reliable signal. In Biospectral Medicine, where many clinically relevant anomalies manifest as variations of 0.1 °C or less, NETD is arguably the most decisive metric of sensor quality.

A detector with poor thermal sensitivity risks masking subtle vasoregulatory responses within background noise, thereby producing a false impression of symmetry or stability. By contrast, a low-NETD sensor can reveal faint differences in emissive intensity that correspond to early vascular compromise, subclinical lymphatic congestion, or sympathetic inhibition. For example, during a Spectrovascular Response Test (SVRT), transient emissive shifts of only a few hundredths of a degree may carry diagnostic weight.

If these microvariations cannot be resolved consistently, the functional profile of the zone is lost, and the biosignal reduced to artifact (Fernández-Cuevas et al., 2015).

Clinical thresholds have emerged from both technical and medical practice. An NETD of ≤100 mK is considered adequate for basic screening or non-specialized imaging. Such systems can reveal gross asymmetries but may miss microvascular patterns that define the biospectral method.

For functional diagnostics, the preferred standard is ≤50 mK (0.05 °C). At this level of sensitivity, imaging systems can capture subtle emissive irregularities, reproduce dynamic responses to cold provocation, and generate stable data across repeated acquisitions (Minkina & Dudzik, 2009; Ring et al., 2020).

Technological advances have pushed this boundary even further. Modern uncooled microbolometers now routinely achieve NETD values in the 30–40 mK range, even in compact, portable platforms (Han & Lee, 2018). This represents a transformative leap: where early medical thermography was limited to systems with NETD values above 100 mK, today's detectors can resolve fine emissive gradients invisible to the naked eye, thereby enabling reliable mapping of inhibitory and activose zones across the body.

Such precision is critical for the reproducibility of Biospectral Medicine, ensuring that identified asymmetries are genuine physiological signals rather than stochastic fluctuations.

The clinical significance of thermal sensitivity extends beyond early detection. By ensuring that minute emissive differences are consistently captured, low-NETD imaging strengthens longitudinal monitoring.

Patients undergoing therapeutic interventions can be re-imaged over time, and even slight improvements or deteriorations in vasomotor stability can be documented with confidence. This continuity is fundamental to the role of Biospectral Medicine as a functional imaging modality, enabling the tracking of regulatory balance before irreversible pathology emerges as well as the capture of disease once established. (Vardasca et al., 2018).

Thus, NETD serves as more than a hardware specification. It is a clinical enabler of functional imaging, anchoring the transition from descriptive temperature mapping to biosignal interpretation. Without high thermal sensitivity, the promise of Biospectral Medicine, to reveal invisible regulatory imbalances and guide early, functional intervention, would remain unrealized.

Integration in Diagnostic Protocols

In applied clinical settings, the diagnostic reliability of Biospectral Medicine arises from the integration of resolution and thermal sensitivity. Resolution defines the structural fidelity of emissive mapping, while thermal sensitivity dictates the system's ability to discern functional contrasts within that structure.

A high-resolution system with insufficient sensitivity may produce sharp anatomical outlines that nevertheless fail to capture the subtle gradients associated with early vasomotor dysregulation. Conversely, a detector with excellent NETD performance but limited pixel density may register emissive changes but misrepresent their spatial boundaries, leading to interpretive errors in zone-based mapping.

Only when these capabilities are balanced does the imaging platform produce a faithful visual substrate from which biospectral interpretation can proceed.

This balance is particularly evident in the placement of regions of interest (ROIs). Accurate subzone mapping depends on clear anatomical landmarks, whether in small facial regions, axillary zones, or lumbar dermatomes. Poor resolution risks diluting the emissive distinctions between adjacent territories, rendering ROI placement unreliable.

High pixel density, by contrast, permits precise segmentation, allowing clinicians to track subtle asymmetries with confidence. Yet without adequate NETD, even well-placed ROIs may yield inconclusive results if the underlying gradients fall below the sensor's detection threshold (Nguyen et al., 2014; Ring et al., 2020).

The integration of resolution and sensitivity also underpins the reliable detection of minimal ΔT (temperature differentials). In functional biosignal analysis, the most meaningful signatures are often those that deviate only slightly from baseline symmetry, fractions of a degree that mark the early stages of autonomic imbalance, microvascular stasis, or inflammatory activation.

Systems with insufficient NETD may average these contrasts into electronic noise, while systems with inadequate resolution may displace the anomaly into neighboring pixels, diluting its significance. Clinical-grade biospectral systems must therefore achieve a harmonic balance: spatial precision that anchors emissive gradients to the correct anatomical terrain, and sensitivity that ensures even the faintest biosignals are registered as diagnostically valid (Fernández-Cuevas et al., 2015; Vardasca et al., 2018).

Consistency represents the third axis of integration. Diagnostic imaging involves longitudinal monitoring and provocative testing, extending beyond a single snapshot. In follow-up protocols, resolution and sensitivity must remain stable across time, ensuring that observed changes reflect genuine physiological evolution rather than variation in sensor performance.

During stimulus-based protocols such as the Spectrovascular Response Test (SVRT), detectors must reproduce transient emissive changes consistently, even when differences are subtle and short-lived. Without this reproducibility, biospectral interpretation risks conflating physiological variability with instrumental noise, undermining its role as a functional diagnostic method (Machin & Cowie, 2013; Ring et al., 2020).

Ultimately, the integration of spatial resolution and NETD ensures the biosignal integrity of thermographic data. Resolution provides the structural grid, anchoring signals to defined anatomical territories; sensitivity reveals the functional contrasts that animate those structures.

Their interaction forms the technical foundation of Biospectral Medicine, transforming emissive radiation into a clinically interpretable map of physiological regulation. Without this equilibrium, imaging devolves into either aesthetically detailed but functionally blind representations, or sensitive but spatially ambiguous impressions. With it, biospectral imaging becomes a reliable clinical tool, capable of detecting dysfunction long before structural pathology emerges.

Calibration and Blackbody Reference Standards

Ensuring Signal Integrity in Biospectral Imaging

Calibration is a foundational requirement for any scientific imaging modality, and in Biospectral Medicine it acquires special significance. Unlike classical thermography, which often sought to equate emissive signals with absolute skin temperature, biospectral interpretation does not depend on assigning numerical values in degrees Celsius to each pixel.

Instead, its reliability derives from the reproducibility and integrity of biosignal patterns across zones, time, and stimulus conditions. Calibration ensures that these patterns are not distorted by instrumental drift, pixel-level variability, or environmental interference, thereby protecting the diagnostic validity of the imaging process.

All infrared imaging systems are subject to sources of error that accumulate over time. Focal plane arrays, particularly uncooled microbolometers, exhibit pixel non-uniformity, in which individual detector elements respond differently to identical radiation inputs. Electronic drift can alter sensitivity thresholds, while environmental conditions, such as ambient temperature changes or internal heating of the device. can shift the baseline signal.

Left uncorrected, these inconsistencies create the appearance of false asymmetries or conceal genuine functional differences, undermining the core comparative logic of zone-based analysis (Minkina & Dudzik, 2009).

Calibration addresses these challenges by providing a stable reference framework against which detector responses can be normalized. The process ensures that each pixel in the array corresponds consistently to the same level of radiant input, preserving the structural integrity of emissive patterns across the image.

In practical terms, this means that a hypoperfused supraclavicular zone or a localized activose signal in the axilla will be registered as such across repeated measurements, rather than fluctuating according to changes in sensor performance.

For longitudinal follow-up, where patients may be imaged weeks or months apart, calibration guarantees that apparent changes reflect true physiological evolution rather than instrumental variability (Machin & Cowie, 2013).

Furthermore, calibration is indispensable during provocative functional testing such as the Spectrovascular Response Test (SVRT). In these protocols, emissive changes often manifest as transient shifts of only a few hundredths of a degree. Without a calibrated system, these subtle variations could be absorbed into noise or misrepresented as uneven signal distribution.

Calibration thus underpins the ability of Biospectral Medicine to operate as a functional imaging discipline, capable of detecting regulatory responses that precede structural pathology (Fernández-Cuevas et al., 2015).

International standards in medical thermography increasingly emphasize calibration as a requirement for clinical validity. Traceability to recognized measurement protocols ensures that biospectral data can be compared across systems and institutions, supporting both clinical practice and scientific research.

By incorporating calibration into routine imaging workflows, Biospectral Medicine aligns itself with the broader principle of measurement science: that diagnostic reliability must rest on stable and verifiable technical foundations (Ring et al., 2020).

The instruments used to achieve this calibration are blackbody reference sources, engineered to provide emissive outputs of known stability and predictability across the infrared spectrum.

These devices serve as the physical anchor for calibration protocols, ensuring that biospectral imaging remains both internally consistent and externally traceable. Their specific role and design will be addressed in the following section.

Blackbody Sources: Definition and Function

At the core of calibration in infrared imaging lies the concept of the blackbody reference source, a device engineered to approximate the idealized emitter described by Planck's law of thermal radiation. A true blackbody absorbs all incident radiation and re-emits energy with unity emissivity across the electromagnetic spectrum.

While no material achieves this perfection, laboratory-engineered blackbodies can achieve emissivities greater than 0.995, producing outputs that are sufficiently close to the theoretical ideal for practical calibration purposes (Khlevnoy & Sapritsky, 2002).

In Biospectral Medicine, blackbody standards serve as the physical anchors of calibration, ensuring that emissive data acquired from the skin are stable, reproducible, and comparable over time. Their function is to provide a consistent emissive reference against which detector arrays can be corrected, rather than to validate absolute temperature readings.

When imaging systems are calibrated against such standards, pixel non-uniformities, sensor drift, and environmental fluctuations are normalized, allowing spectral patterns to be interpreted as true physiological signals rather than instrumental artifacts (Sapritsky & Khlevnoy, 1997; Machin et al., 2014).

The design of blackbody sources reflects this requirement for stability and traceability. Most clinical and research-grade systems employ cavity-type radiators, in which radiation undergoes multiple internal reflections within a conical or cylindrical cavity coated with high-emissivity material. This geometry minimizes reflection losses and produces a highly uniform output.

Precision heating and feedback control maintain the cavity at defined set-points, often with stability better than ±0.01 °C, ensuring that the emissive output remains predictable across long measurement intervals (Baldasano et al., 2016). Portable flat-plate blackbody sources are also employed in clinical environments, particularly for field calibration of compact biospectral systems, though their emissive uniformity is typically lower than cavity designs.

International metrology institutes such as NIST (USA), NPL (UK), and PTB (Germany) have established protocols for blackbody construction, characterization, and traceability. These standards specify emissivity performance and the uncertainty budgets associated with calibration, typically within 50 mK for high-grade sources.

For Biospectral Medicine, such traceability is crucial: it ensures that imaging performed in one clinical setting can be meaningfully compared with that performed elsewhere, thereby supporting reproducibility in research, multicenter trials, and long-term patient monitoring (Machin & Whittam, 2018; Machin & Cowie, 2013).

The clinical significance of blackbody standards lies in their ability to guarantee biosignal integrity. By anchoring detector calibration to a stable reference, they prevent spurious gradients from being misinterpreted as functional anomalies and ensure that subtle but genuine asymmetries remain visible.

In longitudinal protocols, blackbody-referenced calibration allows clinicians to track changes in vasomotor or lymphatic regulation with confidence, knowing that apparent shifts are physiological in origin rather than instrumental drift. In stimulus-based protocols such as the Spectrovascular Response Test (SVRT), blackbody calibration ensures that transient emissive changes, often measured in millikelvins, are faithfully captured against a stable baseline.

Thus, blackbody reference standards form the metrological backbone of Biospectral Medicine. They connect clinical practice to the universal framework of measurement science, embedding biosignal interpretation within a system of reproducible, traceable, and internationally recognized standards.

Without blackbody calibration, emissive imaging risks drifting into subjectivity; with it, Biospectral Medicine maintains the objectivity and reliability required of a functional diagnostic discipline.

Clinical Justification for Calibration in Biospectral Medicine

Although Biospectral Medicine does not depend on absolute temperature readings for diagnosis, instead favoring relative spectral patterns, zone-based asymmetries, and terrain-linked biosignals, calibration remains indispensable. The reasons include:

1. **Linearity Across the Dynamic Range**
   Calibration ensures that the camera's output signal is linearly proportional to radiative energy across the full thermal range relevant to human physiology (typically 28°C–40°C). This linearity is vital for detecting subtle intra-zone emission differentials, such as those observed during SVRT (Spectrovascular Response Testing).
2. **Spectral Palette Accuracy**
   Thermographic imaging in Biospectral Medicine relies on color palettes to visually represent emissive intensity. Calibrated systems maintain **consistent emission-to-color mapping**, so that changes observed across sessions or between patients reflect physiological differences rather than sensor drift or scale distortion (Ammer, 2018).
3. **Intra- and Inter-Patient Comparability**
   In longitudinal tracking or research-grade studies, data must be comparable across timepoints and between individuals. Without calibration, even small hardware inconsistencies or thermal sensor fatigue could introduce error into zone comparisons, potentially obscuring true clinical change (Ring & Ammer, 2020).
4. **Validation of Biospectral Maps**
   Because Biospectral Medicine applies comparative interpretation across 19 standardized anatomical zones, the validity of asymmetry detection depends on a stable reference signal. This is especially true in applications involving inhibose zones (spectrally suppressed areas) or activose zones (amplified regions) where signal deviation may be marginal.

Implementation Standards and Calibration Intervals

Infrared imaging systems designed for clinical use are generally delivered from the manufacturer with factory calibration, typically performed against dual-point or multi-point blackbody targets. This initial calibration establishes a baseline of uniformity and accuracy across the detector array, ensuring that pixel-to-pixel variability and electronic drift are corrected before the device reaches the clinic.

However, factory calibration alone is insufficient to guarantee long-term biospectral fidelity. Just as radiographic and ultrasound devices require regular quality assurance, infrared systems used in Biospectral Medicine must undergo periodic revalidation. This process maintains reproducibility and prevents subtle instrument drift from being mistaken for physiological change (Machin et al., 2014; Ring et al., 2020).

The frequency of revalidation depends on both usage intensity and system design. Devices used in daily clinical practice are exposed to greater thermal cycling, handling, and environmental variability, necessitating more frequent recalibration than systems employed only in controlled laboratory settings.

Some modern medical infrared cameras incorporate internal shutter-based calibration modules, which periodically block the optical path with a reference plate to correct for baseline drift. While this approach is effective for routine use, higher-end systems, particularly in research or multicenter clinical trials, rely on portable external blackbody sources.

These references allow operators to validate detector performance under the same conditions in which imaging occurs, reinforcing confidence in inter-session and inter-institutional comparability (Sapritsky & Khlevnoy, 1997; Machin & Whittam, 2018).

Operational standards further define how calibration should be executed to preserve the diagnostic value of emissive data. Revalidation is typically performed using incremental temperature steps of approximately 0.5–1.0 °C across the range relevant to human skin emission.

This practice ensures that the detector array remains stable across the spectrum of emissive variations likely to occur in zone-based imaging. In addition, blackbody surfaces used for calibration are required to exhibit emissivity values of at least 0.99, thereby minimizing reflection losses and ensuring that the calibration source closely approximates the ideal blackbody defined by Planck's radiation law.

By adhering to these standards, calibration procedures anchor biospectral imaging in reproducible physical principles rather than relative visual estimation (Khlevnoy & Sapritsky, 2002; Baldasano et al., 2016).

Another essential element of implementation is the stabilization period prior to each imaging session. Infrared detectors, particularly uncooled microbolometers, require time to thermally equilibrate with their environment. Without stabilization, residual electronic drift can produce image artifacts that confound baseline readings.

Allowing sufficient warm-up time before acquisition eliminates this variability and ensures that emission patterns reflect physiological rather than instrumental dynamics (Minkina & Dudzik, 2009).

Within the framework of the Computerized Biospectral Imaging (CBI) protocol, calibration conformity is treated as a clinical prerequisite. The interpretive logic of Biospectral Medicine rests on the assumption that spectral patterns are comparable across time, zones, and stimulus. Without calibration discipline, this assumption collapses, and the reliability of zone-based asymmetry analysis diminishes.

By enforcing rigorous calibration intervals and reference standards, the CBI protocol ensures that emissive data remain both internally consistent and externally traceable, thereby strengthening the clinical legitimacy of Biospectral Medicine as a diagnostic science (Reitz, 2025; Ring et al., 2020).

Palette Normalization and Zone-Based Contrast Integrity

Preserving Diagnostic Validity in Spectral Image Rendering

In Biospectral Medicine, imaging is interpreted as a spectral interface that renders emissive biosignals into a form perceivable by the human eye, rather than as an absolute record of temperature. The validity of diagnostic interpretation therefore depends critically on how infrared radiation, invisible to vision, is translated into visual maps through colour palettes and contrast algorithms.

Without rigorous control, these visual translations can distort or conceal clinical information. For example, automatic scaling that adjusts to the hottest and coldest points in a frame may suppress subtle emissive differences in diagnostically important zones, while over-enhancement of weak signals can generate spurious patterns that resemble pathology.

To safeguard reproducibility, the Computerized Biospectral Imaging (CBI) protocol requires that all systems support robust palette normalization and maintain zone-specific contrast integrity.

The challenge lies in the fundamental fact that false-color mapping is an abstraction: it substitutes human perception of hue and intensity for raw radiometric values.

While this translation is indispensable for clinical use, it introduces potential distortions unless the mapping process is rigorously standardized. Biospectral Medicine, which is founded on comparative logic across 19 emission zones, demands that emissive contrasts be preserved within and between zones without contamination from unrelated global extremes.

This requirement distinguishes it from industrial or security thermography, where global contrast is sufficient to identify overheating machinery or intruders but inadequate for detecting millikelvin-level asymmetries in human physiology (Lahiri et al., 2012).

To achieve this, manual range adjustment is a necessary capability. By allowing clinicians to set the upper and lower boundaries of the displayed range, manual scaling prevents single-pixel outliers from dictating the visualization of entire zones.

For instance, a bright reflection from jewelry or a cold artifact at the image periphery should not compress the contrast range to the point that subtle vascular asymmetries in the abdomen become invisible. Auto-range scaling with ROI locking represents a further refinement. This approach enables localized normalization of palettes within designated regions of interest, ensuring that comparisons remain clinically valid by restricting contrast scaling to anatomically relevant areas.

Such methods highlight emissive differences within and between zones while minimizing distortion from adjacent tissues or extraneous artifacts (Clark et al., 2021).

Finally, contrast rendering in Biospectral Medicine is based on relative emission, not absolute values. Since the discipline does not define pathology by fixed temperature thresholds, color mapping must prioritize the preservation of gradients and dynamics, rather than presenting absolute numerical temperatures.

A hotspot within the axillary zone, for example, is meaningful only in relation to the contralateral side or to its behavior under provocation. Palette normalization must therefore be designed to maintain the proportionality of these emissive gradients, ensuring that clinicians perceive the true biosignal pattern rather than a distorted visual exaggeration or suppression caused by software defaults (Ring et al., 2020).

Colour Palette Scaling and Emissive Fidelity

The rendering of emissive data into visible images requires the use of false-color palettes, which translate variations in infrared radiation into hues perceptible to the human eye. Although this process does not alter the raw sensor data, the choice of palette has profound implications for how emissive zones are perceived, compared, and ultimately interpreted in Biospectral Medicine.

What appears as a clinically significant activose hotspot under one palette may be visually minimized under another, while subtle inhibitory patterns may disappear entirely if contrast compression obscures gradients. Thus, palette selection is a determinant of diagnostic fidelity.

Historically, infrared thermography employed grayscale rendering, mapping colder regions to darker shades and warmer regions to lighter ones. Grayscale remains the most neutral and metrologically transparent palette, as it minimizes perceptual exaggeration and avoids introducing non-existent gradients through chromatic transitions.

However, grayscale has limitations when used in clinical contexts, particularly in differentiating subtle subzone asymmetries, since human visual perception is more sensitive to color variations than to gradations in luminance (Hoffman et al., 2010).

To address this limitation, a variety of chromatic palettes have been developed, ranging from the widely used ironbow scheme (where colder areas are mapped to purple/blue and hotter areas to yellow/white) to rainbow or high-contrast palettes that distribute emissive ranges across the visible spectrum.

In clinical use, ironbow-type palettes enhance the detection of localized activose regions, drawing attention to subtle hotspots by leveraging high perceptual sensitivity to red-yellow contrasts.

However, rainbow palettes have been criticized for introducing artificial boundaries: a gradual emissive gradient may appear as discrete zones of color change, misleading interpretation by exaggerating contrast that does not exist in the raw data (Borland & Taylor, 2007).

For this reason, the CBI (Computerized Biospectral Imaging) protocol emphasizes that palettes must be selected and standardized based on their ability to preserve proportional contrast within and between zones, rather than their visual appeal. Palette normalization ensures that small emissive differences are faithfully represented without artificial exaggeration or suppression.

Clinical studies have shown that when standardized palettes are used consistently, inter-observer agreement in zone asymmetry detection improves significantly, while inconsistent palette use introduces variability that reduces diagnostic reproducibility (Clark et al., 2021; Ring et al., 2020).

Furthermore, palette choice directly impacts longitudinal monitoring, an essential application of Biospectral Medicine. A patient imaged across multiple sessions must be rendered with the same palette normalization for valid comparison.

If the palette is altered between sessions, perceived changes in emissive intensity may reflect visualization differences rather than true physiological evolution. This risk underlines the need for strict protocol-driven palette selection, ideally supported by software that locks palette scaling to zone-based reference ranges (Vardasca et al., 2018).

In sum, colour palettes in biospectral imaging function as active determinants of clinical interpretation. Grayscale offers neutrality, iron bow enhances perceptual contrast for subtle hotspots, while rainbow and exaggerated palettes risk distortion.

By mandating palette normalization and consistent use across time and zones, the CBI framework ensures that emissive data are captured with fidelity and rendered in a manner that preserves their biosignal integrity.

Zone-Based Integrity and Internal Gain Control

Biospectral Medicine is structured around a standardized division of 19 anatomical emission zones, each selected for its physiological and diagnostic relevance. This segmentation underpins the comparative logic of the method: asymmetries between left and right zones may reveal vascular or autonomic imbalance, while emission suppression within a zone may suggest metabolic or circulatory dysfunction.

The integrity of this analytical framework depends on the raw sensitivity of the detector as well as on how emissive data are rendered and stabilized by the imaging system. Any processing step, whether palette scaling, contrast enhancement, or gain correction, must therefore preserve intra-zone fidelity and prevent cross-zone contamination, ensuring that visualized differences reflect true biosignals rather than software-induced distortions.

To maintain fidelity, modern systems must incorporate zone-lock contrast functions. This functionality enables clinicians to adjust and lock contrast normalization within a designated region of interest, rather than relying on the global image extremes.

Without this safeguard, a single hot pixel from jewellery reflection or a cold corner artefact could rescale the entire image, suppressing clinically significant microgradients within a zone. By localizing normalization, zone-lock functions protect the internal detail of emission fields, allowing precise visualization of subzone asymmetries such as periorbital activation, axillary lymphatic congestion, or dermatomal suppression along the spine (Clark et al., 2021).

Equally important is the presence of internal gain control algorithms. Infrared detectors are susceptible to ambient fluctuations, especially in clinical settings where sunlight, ventilation, or reflective surfaces may alter background load on the sensor.

Uncorrected, these shifts can bias pixel baselines, creating false gradients or erasing genuine ones. Internal gain control dynamically adjusts detector response to stabilize the baseline output, ensuring that emissive differences between zones are not contaminated by environmental variability. In essence, it acts as a buffer between the external environment and the internal biosignal, allowing reproducible imaging across different sessions and rooms (Ring & Ammer, 2020).

Another safeguard is the judicious application of frame averaging and noise filtering. Multiple frames can be combined to reduce random noise, improving signal-to-noise ratio without requiring excessive post-processing.

However, excessive filtering risks oversmoothing, blurring edge gradients and eliminating subtle emission anomalies that may carry diagnostic weight. In Biospectral Medicine, these fine emissive details often represent early functional irregularities, such as localized inhibition preceding vascular compromise.

The balance is therefore delicate: algorithms must suppress random noise while preserving micro-emissive structures, maintaining both global clarity and local detail (Watson et al., 2016).

Together, these measures, zone-locked contrast, gain control, and intelligent noise filtering, form the technical infrastructure for preserving zone-based integrity. They ensure that when clinicians interpret an asymmetric shoulder pattern or a focal inhibitory abdominal zone, they are responding to a true physiological biosignal rather than an artifact of contrast mis-scaling, ambient drift, or overprocessed imagery.

By embedding these controls into imaging systems, Biospectral Medicine establishes a diagnostic chain where each step, from acquisition to visualization, upholds the principle of signal fidelity within and between zones, the very foundation of comparative functional interpretation.

Avoiding Diagnostic Artifacts

In Biospectral Medicine, the greatest threat to diagnostic validity arises from systematic misrepresentation, including false amplification produced by aggressive auto-scaling and suppression caused when globally hot regions compress contrast across the rest of the frame. Either failure mode can tip a marginal activose or inhibose finding into a false positive or negative.

Because biospectral interpretation hinges on small, zone-bounded differences rather than large absolute swings, every link in the rendering chain, range selection, contrast mapping, denoising, and environmental compensation, must be engineered to preserve *proportional, zone-local* information rather than global extremes.

Reviews of infrared measurement science make this point repeatedly: visualization choices (e.g., histogram stretching, pseudo-colour mapping) can fabricate or hide gradients that are not present in the radiometric data, turning processing parameters into de facto clinical variables unless they are standardized and documented (Usamentiaga et al., 2014).

Longitudinal comparability is the first safeguard. Palette settings, range endpoints, and any normalization parameters must remain stable across serial exams so that observed changes reflect physiology rather than visualization drift.

Standards for clinical thermography and uncertainty management emphasize that traceable, repeatable configurations, and the explicit recording of those configurations, are prerequisites for between-session comparison and for inter-site reproducibility (IEC 80601-2-59, 2017; Machin & Cowie, 2013).

Practically, this means locking palettes and ranges at acquisition (or applying the same ROI-normalized presets during review), recording those values as part of the study record, and resisting global auto-scale when small hot or cold outliers would compress contrast in diagnostically relevant regions.

The imperative mirrors broader functional-imaging disciplines: fMRI and PET derive meaning from differential contrasts over time and condition; their reproducibility likewise depends on consistent preprocessing, scaling, and metadata capture (Gore, 2003; Cherry, 2006).

Second, biospectral systems should preserve *data primacy* by allowing export of raw radiometric frames (typically 14–16-bit) together with full calibration and acquisition metadata. Colorized screenshots are insufficient for audit or re-analysis because pseudo-colour and contrast decisions are already "baked in."

High-fidelity raw export enables independent verification of range, palette, emissivity assumptions, and noise filtering; it also supports later reprocessing with updated algorithms without re-imaging the patient.

Guidance drawn from infrared metrology and good-practice measurement texts treats raw radiometric access as essential for uncertainty analysis, emissivity compensation, and artifact investigation (ASTM E1933-14; Usamentiaga et al., 2014).

Third, the display layer should actively *prevent misinterpretation* by overlaying anatomy-aware information. Zone masks, ROI boundaries, palette/range readouts, and calibration tags (e.g., date/time of last reference, blackbody set-points, ambient/stabilization status) should be rendered alongside the thermogram so reviewers understand exactly how contrast was derived and to which anatomical container each emissive pattern belongs.

This mirrors safety-critical expectations in other medical image domains, where overlays and DICOM-level metadata reduce reader variance and support auditability (IEC 80601-2-59, 2017; Machin & Whittam, 2018).

Noise suppression requires equal nuance. Frame averaging and judicious denoising can elevate weak, but real, biosignals above the noise floor; yet over-smoothing erases micro-gradients at zone edges and can "round off" narrow activose streaks or focal inhibitory islands.

Classic image-processing work shows that aggressive global equalization or smoothing can exaggerate edges, promote banding, or amplify noise into false structure; in IR biomedical contexts, those artifacts become clinical errors (Pizer et al., 1987; Gonzalez & Woods, 2018). Filtering strategies in biospectral workflows should therefore be *edge-preserving* and validated against phantom or repeat-scan datasets to quantify whether fine gradients survive processing.

Finally, artifact prevention extends to the environment itself. Reflections from jewelry or glossy surfaces, solar loading through windows, HVAC drafts, and operator proximity can all inject structured error that global auto-scaling will dutifully "explain" as image contrast.

International guidance for human thermography stresses environmental stabilization, emissivity control, and background management precisely to stop these influences from cascading into the rendering pipeline, where they masquerade as physiology (IEC 80601-2-59, 2017; Machin & Cowie, 2013).

When such control is imperfect, as in mixed-light rooms or mobile settings, internal gain control and localized (zone-locked) normalization help decouple ambient drift from true biosignal by stabilizing pixel baselines and restricting contrast decisions to anatomically relevant ROIs.

In sum, artefact avoidance in Biospectral Medicine is a systems problem: palette consistency across sessions guards longitudinal validity; raw data export preserves auditability; anatomy-aware overlays contextualize contrast; edge-preserving denoising protects micro-structure; and environmental control plus gain stabilization prevent global conditions from overwhelming local truth.

Enforcing these practices ensures that the thermogram remains a faithful *biosignal interface* rather than an aesthetic rendering, aligning biospectral imaging with the rigor expected of functional modalities such as fMRI and PET, where visualization is carefully constrained to protect quantitative meaning (Gore, 2003; Cherry, 2006).

Technical Exclusions and Cautions

Defining the Operational Limits of Biospectral Imaging

Biospectral Medicine is a structured clinical modality that relies on the precise acquisition and interpretation of infrared spectral emission from human tissues. Its diagnostic validity rests on the ability of imaging systems to maintain optical fidelity, thermal sensitivity, and anatomical reproducibility across standardized protocols.

For this reason, not all infrared cameras, particularly those designed for industrial diagnostics, building inspection, or low-cost consumer wellness applications, are suitable for clinical use. Misapplication of such devices risks undermining both the scientific credibility and the clinical outcomes of biospectral analysis.

A principal exclusion involves the widespread class of industrial-grade infrared cameras. These instruments are typically optimized for detecting large temperature differentials in engineering contexts, such as identifying hotspots in electrical panels or structural heat leaks.

While they may offer broad temperature ranges (–20 °C to 650 °C or higher), their Noise-Equivalent Temperature Difference (NETD) often exceeds 100 mK, rendering them insensitive to the subtle emissive variations (<0.1 °C) that define early vascular or autonomic dysfunction in Biospectral Medicine.

Their calibration routines also prioritize absolute temperature accuracy across wide spans rather than fine-grained stability in the narrow thermal range relevant to human physiology (36–38 °C).

Consequently, while adequate for technical environments, they cannot reliably capture the millikelvin-level asymmetries necessary for zone-based biospectral analysis (Usamentiaga et al., 2014; Machin & Cowie, 2013).

A second category of exclusion is low-cost consumer infrared devices, such as smartphone add-ons and general wellness cameras. These products often employ very small focal plane arrays (e.g., 80×60 pixels) with poor spatial resolution, limited calibration features, and restricted spectral fidelity.

Their reliance on automatic scaling and fixed palettes makes them especially prone to diagnostic artifacts, such as false amplification or suppression of zones, leading to misinterpretation of activose or inhibose fields. Furthermore, their lack of access to raw radiometric data prevents clinical auditing and longitudinal reproducibility. In functional imaging disciplines, including PET and fMRI, such data transparency is non-negotiable; Biospectral Medicine requires the same level of traceability and auditability (Gore, 2003; Ring et al., 2020).

Another exclusion pertains to non-medical optical assemblies. Lenses made of materials unsuitable for long-wave infrared (LWIR), such as conventional silica glass, block the emissive wavelengths most relevant to human tissues (~8–14 μm). Devices employing such optics may still produce images through internal interpolation or alternative bands, but the captured data are spectrally mismatched and therefore physiologically misleading.

Only systems employing verified LWIR-compatible optics, such as germanium, zinc selenide, or advanced chalcogenide glasses, can ensure faithful transmission of the biosignal (Smith, 1993; Wilke et al., 2017).

Caution must also be exercised with environmentally unstable systems. Devices without internal gain control or blackbody-referenced calibration are highly susceptible to ambient drift, leading to fluctuating baselines that can obscure longitudinal patterns.

In Biospectral Medicine, where comparative follow-up across weeks or months is central to clinical logic, such instability invalidates the data. International standards for medical thermography emphasize that traceable calibration and environmental stability are prerequisites for clinical legitimacy, not optional enhancements (IEC 80601-2-59, 2017; Machin & Whittam, 2018).

In summary, the operational limits of Biospectral Medicine exclude any infrared system that lacks: (1) high thermal sensitivity (NETD ≤50 mK preferred), (2) adequate spatial resolution (≥320×240 pixels minimum), (3) access to raw radiometric data, (4) LWIR-compatible optics, and (5) robust calibration capability.

Industrial, consumer, and uncertified optical platforms fail to meet these requirements and must be excluded from clinical application. By clearly defining these exclusions, Biospectral Medicine safeguards its scientific integrity and prevents misapplication, ensuring that spectral imaging retains its role as a functional diagnostic modality aligned with the standards of advanced imaging sciences.

Exclusion of Industrial and Non-Medical Infrared Cameras

Infrared cameras originally developed for industrial or mechanical inspection are not suitable for clinical use in Biospectral Medicine. These devices, commonly employed in building thermography, electrical fault detection, or heating, ventilation, and air conditioning (HVAC) diagnostics, are engineered with fundamentally different design priorities.

Their purpose is to detect large-scale temperature gradients across machinery or infrastructure, not the millikelvin-level emissive variations that signify subtle vascular or autonomic dysfunction in human physiology. As a result, their specifications fall short of the technical and clinical requirements necessary for biospectral evaluation.

The most significant limitation lies in their calibration standards. Industrial cameras are typically calibrated for wide operational ranges, spanning from sub-zero to several hundred degrees Celsius, reflecting their role in detecting overheating components or thermal leaks.

Such calibration favors broad accuracy at extreme temperatures but neglects the fine stability required within the narrow physiological window of 30–40 °C. Without medical-grade calibration, these systems are incapable of producing consistent and reproducible emissive patterns across repeated patient assessments (Machin & Cowie, 2013).

A further deficiency is the lack of precise emissivity control. Human skin emissivity is approximately 0.98 in the long-wave infrared band, a value essential for accurate biosignal acquisition. Industrial devices often employ fixed emissivity presets, sometimes around 0.95, or provide only coarse adjustment.

This discrepancy, minor in engineering contexts, becomes critical in clinical imaging, where even small emissivity errors can distort subtle asymmetries or mask inhibitory fields (Minkina & Dudzik, 2009).

Optical incompatibility represents another exclusion criterion. Many industrial systems employ lenses not optimized for biological emissive ranges, relying instead on standard optical materials or coatings designed for durability and environmental resilience rather than spectral fidelity.

In some cases, these lenses do not transmit efficiently in the 8–14 μm long-wave infrared (LWIR) band, which corresponds to the emissive peak of human tissue (~9.4 μm at 33 °C). A device with undefined or broad spectral response may still produce images but fails to capture physiologically accurate emissive data, undermining the core logic of zone-based biospectral analysis (Lahiri et al., 2012; Ring & Ammer, 2020).

Finally, the imaging algorithms integrated into industrial systems are tuned for non-medical tasks, often prioritizing automatic scaling and contrast enhancement to highlight structural faults. These algorithms can artificially amplify or suppress emissive zones, creating patterns that resemble pathology but originate entirely from software processing. In Biospectral Medicine, where reproducibility and proportional contrast are paramount, such distortions are unacceptable.

For these reasons, the operational use of industrial and non-medical infrared cameras is excluded from Biospectral Medicine. Clinical biospectral systems must be specifically engineered with LWIR-compatible optics, fine emissivity adjustment, medical-grade calibration, and reproducible palette normalization. Only under these conditions can imaging serve as a functional biosignal interface rather than a coarse heat map designed for mechanical inspection.

Inadequacy of Low-Resolution Mobile Attachments

In recent years, the proliferation of smartphone-based infrared cameras and clip-on thermal imaging modules has made infrared visualization widely accessible to consumers. While these devices have value in educational demonstrations, wellness tracking, or basic environmental inspection, they are categorically excluded from clinical use in Biospectral Medicine. Their design priorities, low cost, portability, and ease of use, directly compromise the precision, stability, and reproducibility that biospectral diagnostics require.

The most fundamental limitation is spatial resolution. Many mobile thermal attachments operate at resolutions below 160×120 pixels, and some as low as 80×60. At such low densities, individual pixels may correspond to several square millimeters of skin surface, effectively averaging emissive detail across zones.

Subtle but diagnostically critical features, such as microvascular asymmetries in the periorbital region, inhibitory suppression along the cervical dermatomes, or fine gradients across the supraclavicular notch,

are lost in pixelation. These devices therefore cannot support the zone-to-zone comparative logic that underpins biospectral interpretation (Clark et al., 2021).

Noise performance further compounds the problem. Low-cost detectors integrated into mobile platforms often exhibit high Noise-Equivalent Temperature Difference (NETD), frequently >100 mK. In Biospectral Medicine, functional irregularities often manifest as emissive differences of 50 mK or less.

Such contrasts are imperceptible to sensors operating at higher noise floors, meaning early regulatory changes may remain invisible or be confounded with random fluctuations (Usamentiaga et al., 2014). The inability to discern these micrograd ients translates directly into false negatives, while coarse interpolation during image upscaling can generate false positives.

Equally problematic is the absence of calibration traceability. Clinical-grade systems employ blackbody-referenced calibration, emissivity adjustment, and quality assurance protocols traceable to metrological standards. Smartphone devices, by contrast, lack these capabilities and typically rely on factory presets designed for general-purpose thermal visualization.

Without calibration traceability, there is no assurance that zone-based differences represent physiological phenomena rather than sensor drift or algorithmic scaling. This absence of auditability places mobile attachments outside the standards required of functional imaging modalities such as fMRI, PET, or even high-resolution ultrasound (Machin & Cowie, 2013; IEC 80601-2-59, 2017).

It is acknowledged that such devices may hold value in educational or non-diagnostic contexts. For example, they can be employed for home self-monitoring to illustrate gross patterns of heat distribution, or in classroom demonstrations of emissive physics.

However, in a diagnostic context, their limitations pose an unacceptable risk of misclassification. False amplification of global gradients, loss of fine vascular or lymphatic detail, and lack of reproducibility make them incompatible with the standards of Biospectral Medicine.

In summary, smartphone-based infrared attachments cannot serve as clinical tools for biospectral imaging. Their low resolution, poor thermal sensitivity, and absence of calibration traceability preclude reliable visualization of the subtle biosignals that form the basis of diagnostic interpretation. While valuable as consumer technologies, their use in medical practice would undermine the scientific and clinical integrity of Biospectral Medicine.

Rejection of Non-LWIR Devices

The clinical foundations of Biospectral Medicine rest on the accurate capture of human tissue emission within the long-wave infrared (LWIR) spectrum, specifically the 8–14 μm window. This spectral band corresponds to the natural emissive peak of human skin, which radiates most strongly at approximately 9.5 μm under physiological conditions (33–35 °C), as predicted by Wien's displacement law.

Infrared sensors designed to operate outside this window, including mid-wave infrared (MWIR, 3–5 μm) systems or near-infrared (NIR, 0.7–1.4 μm) cameras, are fundamentally unsuited for biospectral imaging, as they fail to capture the biologically relevant emissions that form the basis of functional interpretation (Browne et al., 2015).

The inadequacy of non-LWIR devices can be traced to several interrelated factors. First, their signal-to-noise ratio for human tissues is inherently diminished. Because skin emits weakly in MWIR and negligibly in NIR, detectors tuned to these bands receive limited physiologically meaningful input, forcing reliance on electronic amplification.

The result is suboptimal contrast, elevated noise, and an inability to resolve subtle emissive gradients within the 19 standardized anatomical zones. In clinical terms, this leads to the suppression of biosignal fidelity and the masking of critical asymmetries that may represent vascular, autonomic, or metabolic irregularities (Holst & Lomheim, 2017).

Second, MWIR systems are typically engineered for non-medical applications, including aerospace imaging, missile guidance, and industrial inspection. To achieve their sensitivity, many employ cryogenic cooling mechanisms such as Stirling engines or liquid nitrogen reservoirs. These systems, while powerful in military or research settings, are impractical and unnecessary for routine clinical evaluation.

They introduce maintenance burdens, high costs, and safety risks incompatible with outpatient workflows. Moreover, their calibration protocols are optimized for wide dynamic ranges and rapid temporal resolution, not for the narrow, stable thermal window required in functional medical imaging (Holst & Lomheim, 2017; Hudson et al., 2008).

Third, NIR devices present an even greater mismatch. Since they primarily capture reflected rather than emitted radiation, NIR systems are more closely related to optical imaging than to emissive thermography. Reflections from ambient light, skin pigmentation, or topical substances dominate the signal, producing data that may be visually striking but biologically irrelevant in the context of emissive physiology.

Attempts to repurpose such devices for human thermal imaging risk conflating surface reflectivity with deep regulatory biosignals, undermining the interpretive logic of Biospectral Medicine (Holst & Lomheim, 2017).

For these reasons, the CBI (Computerized Biospectral Imaging) protocol explicitly excludes any infrared system that does not operate in the LWIR window. Only LWIR detectors, coupled with appropriate optics and calibration, can capture the physiologically meaningful radiation patterns of human tissues. This rejection ensures that biospectral interpretation remains anchored in spectral fidelity, preventing the introduction of data that may be technologically impressive but clinically misleading.

Lack of Emissivity and Palette Controls

A defining feature of Biospectral Medicine is its reliance on standardized, reproducible biosignal acquisition, anchored in precise emissivity calibration and zone-based visualization protocols. Any imaging device that lacks the ability to adjust emissivity, apply dynamic palette scaling, or manually control contrast parameters is therefore incompatible with the discipline. These features are structural requirements, essential to the comparative logic of Biospectral Medicine.

The first limitation involves fixed emissivity settings. Human skin emissivity in the long-wave infrared (LWIR) range is approximately 0.98, but this value can vary slightly with skin hydration, surface texture, or clinical context. Medical imaging systems must therefore allow emissivity adjustments to ensure signal fidelity.

Devices with factory-locked emissivity presets, often set to 0.95 for general industrial applications, introduce systematic underestimation of radiance, which can translate into false suppression of zones. In functional analysis, where inhibitory zones may only differ by fractions of a degree, such miscalibration renders biospectral interpretation unreliable (Minkina & Dudzik, 2009; Usamentiaga et al., 2014).

A second exclusion criterion is the absence of palette normalization controls. Infrared cameras designed for consumer or industrial use frequently default to global auto-scaling, where the hottest and coldest pixels define the entire color range. This mode may suffice for detecting overheating machinery or HVAC faults, but in clinical imaging it can obliterate subtle biosignals.

A single hot artifact, such as a reflection from jewelry, can shift the palette range, compressing contrast and masking vascular asymmetries within a zone. Conversely, cold outliers can exaggerate minor hotspots into apparent pathology. Without manual scaling or region-of-interest (ROI) locking, spectral patterns become software artifacts rather than physiological signals (Clark et al., 2021).

The third requirement is manual contrast control, which ensures that emissive gradients are preserved relative to their anatomical context. Automatic-only devices typically prioritize visual clarity over diagnostic precision, using proprietary algorithms that adjust brightness or contrast dynamically across frames. Such algorithms can blur intra-zone microgradients or exaggerate inter-zone differences, both of which compromise the R-CIIM interpretive model, where subtle contrasts and proportional asymmetries drive diagnostic reasoning.

In practice, this means that two scans of the same patient taken minutes apart could appear different simply because automatic scaling parameters shifted, not because the patient's physiology changed (Ring et al., 2020).

The consequences of these deficiencies extend to both intra-patient monitoring and inter-patient comparability. For follow-up evaluations, palette inconsistency prevents clinicians from tracking functional evolution reliably, eroding the longitudinal power of Biospectral Medicine. For comparative studies across patients or cohorts, fixed emissivity and auto-scaled palettes undermine reproducibility, making it impossible to establish standardized datasets for research or clinical validation.

By contrast, clinical-grade biospectral systems provide full access to emissivity settings, palette range controls, and raw radiometric export, thereby ensuring transparency and auditability (Watson et al., 2016; Vardasca et al., 2018).

In summary, devices without emissivity and palette controls transform infrared imaging into an aesthetic visualization tool rather than a scientific diagnostic interface. By distorting spectral information through fixed parameters and auto-only rendering, they compromise both the intra-zone fidelity and the inter-patient comparability upon which Biospectral Medicine depends. For this reason, such devices are categorically excluded from clinical application, preserving the discipline's commitment to reproducibility, traceability, and biosignal integrity.

Clinical and Legal Implications

The use of non-approved infrared imaging systems in a clinical setting carries consequences that extend beyond degraded interpretative accuracy. Substandard hardware undermines the biosignal fidelity on which Biospectral Medicine depends and introduces significant medicolegal risk. When interpretation is based on incomplete, distorted, or non-reproducible data, clinicians may inadvertently provide false reassurance or, conversely, provoke inappropriate concern.

In both cases, the impact on patient outcomes is tangible: early dysfunction may go undetected, or patients may be subjected to unnecessary anxiety, referrals, or interventions. Either outcome undermines confidence in the clinical process and places the practitioner in a position of potential liability.

Legal precedent across multiple imaging modalities reinforces that clinicians are accountable for both the act of interpretation and the technical adequacy of the equipment employed. Just as radiologists must confirm that CT or MRI scanners meet safety and performance standards, practitioners of Biospectral Medicine must verify that their infrared systems conform to established requirements.

Failure to do so exposes them to claims of negligence, as the chain of diagnostic reasoning can be challenged on the basis that the foundational data were flawed or invalid (Hudson et al., 2008; IEC 80601-2-59, 2017).

To mitigate these risks, the CBI (Computerized Biospectral Imaging) protocol defines a set of minimum technical specifications that are not optional enhancements but essential safeguards.

These include LWIR spectral alignment (8–14 μm), ensuring that detectors capture the emissive peak of human skin; thermal sensitivity with NETD ≤50 mK, allowing the detection of subclinical gradients; emissivity adjustability, with a default value of 0.98 to match human skin properties; spatial resolution of at least 320×240 pixels, preserving intra-zone detail; and full palette and contrast control, ensuring that visualization does not distort biosignal proportionality.

Together, these criteria establish the operational baseline for clinical legitimacy, aligning Biospectral Medicine with international measurement standards and functional imaging sciences (Ring et al., 2020; Vardasca et al., 2018).

From a legal standpoint, adherence to these standards provides practitioners with a defensible framework should diagnostic outcomes be questioned. Equipment that meets metrological and clinical benchmarks can be demonstrated to provide traceable, reproducible data, whereas the use of non-approved devices can be construed as a breach of duty of care.

In jurisdictions where imaging-based diagnostics are regulated, the absence of compliance may not only compromise patient safety but also constitute regulatory violation, further exposing clinicians or institutions to sanctions (Machin & Whittam, 2018).

In conclusion, the technical specifications mandated by the CBI protocol are simultaneously scientific imperatives and legal protections. By ensuring LWIR alignment, high sensitivity, emissivity control, adequate resolution, and palette flexibility, practitioners uphold the integrity of Biospectral Medicine as a functional imaging modality.

Compliance preserves both the clinical utility of the discipline and the professional security of those who practice it, underscoring that technology and liability are inseparably linked in modern diagnostic medicine.

Translational Bridge: From Infrared Physics to Clinical Biosignal Interpretation

The transition from physical theory to clinical application defines the core innovation of Biospectral Medicine. Unlike traditional thermography, which historically struggled with scientific rigor and clinical clarity, the biospectral model builds a translational continuum: beginning with the physics of infrared emission, refined through precision instrumentation, and culminating in zone-based functional interpretation.

This section synthesizes that continuum, demonstrating how blackbody radiation, emissivity, and detector technology are not abstract principles but direct enablers of diagnostic insight.

At the foundation lies the understanding that the human body emits infrared radiation as a predictable consequence of thermodynamic laws. Planck's Law and Wien's Displacement Law establish the spectral logic by which human skin, at approximately 33°C, emits most strongly in the long-wave infrared range, peaking near 9.5 μm.

This emission profile is not merely a passive release of heat, but a dynamic reflection of internal metabolic, vascular, autonomic, and inflammatory processes (Ma et al., 2019). Remarkably, human skin acts as a near-perfect blackbody in this range, with emissivity between 0.97 and 0.99, allowing infrared sensors to capture subtle differences with high fidelity (Vainer, 2020).

However, capturing these emissions in diagnostically meaningful ways depends on sensor technology that is both spectrally aligned and physiologically compatible. This requirement is met by uncooled microbolometer detectors, which operate in the 8–14 μm band, matching the natural emissive behaviour of skin tissue.

Their passive design, coupled with modern sensitivity thresholds of ≤50 mK NETD, allows the detection of fine emission gradients across anatomical regions, especially when structured into zone-based maps. While high-end photon detectors may surpass them in temporal resolution, their spectral mismatch and operational complexity render them inferior for biosignal analysis in clinical contexts (Gao et al., 2020; Alves et al., 2021).

These emissions are then filtered, focused, and interpreted through specialized optics, typically germanium or chalcogenide lenses, that allow transmission of long-wave infrared without distortion. Coupled with internal calibration against blackbody references, and supported by palette normalization protocols, the system transforms radiant flux into standardized, zone-specific visual outputs. This is the threshold at which physics ends and interpretation begins.

Biospectral Medicine then redefines the output: the captured emission is not merely "temperature data" but biosignal, a surface signature of deeper functional behaviour. This reclassification is critical.

For example, a symmetrical temperature elevation on both feet may be dismissed in a conventional model, but in the biospectral framework, one may exhibit activose behaviour (enhanced emissivity from vasomotor hyperactivity) while the other shows inhibose behaviour (flattened reactivity despite thermal elevation). Such distinctions emerge not from absolute temperatures, but from the context: spectral zone, lateral symmetry, regulation patterns, and response to challenge (e.g., via SVRT).

The physics of heat transfer, conduction, convection, radiation, is thus reinterpreted as physiology. A zone may radiate excess heat due to neurogenic overdrive, local hypoperfusion, or systemic hormonal effects. Another region may remain cool due to sympathetic overmodulation suppressing vascular dynamics. These are diagnostic messages encoded in biosignal form, not merely physical states.

Therefore, understanding emissive physics and instrumentation is not optional background knowledge; it is essential clinical literacy in Biospectral Medicine. As the field matures and begins to enter multidisciplinary care models, clinicians must be equipped to interpret thermal images, to understand how the image is formed, to recognize its physical constraints, and to identify how functional pathophysiology expresses itself through emission asymmetries.

This translational clarity prepares the reader for Part II, which introduces the Reitz Clinical Infrared Interpretation Model (R-CIIM), a 6-step system for decoding biospectral emissions into diagnostic meaning. It is here that physics becomes function, emission becomes narrative, and infrared medicine becomes a powerful tool for integrative clinical decision-making.

PART VI

TRANSLATIONAL BRIDGE

SCIENTIFIC REHABILITATION AND THE TRANSITION TO BIOSPECTRAL MEDICINE

Infrared thermography has undergone one of the most complex trajectories in the history of medical imaging, characterized by periods of rapid adoption, waves of skepticism, and eventual efforts toward rehabilitation. In its early clinical applications during the 1960s and 1970s, thermography was greeted with enthusiasm, particularly in oncology and vascular medicine, because it offered a non-invasive means of visualizing physiological change.

However, by the late 1970s and 1980s, the field began to drift into alternative medicine contexts where scientific standardization, anatomical consistency, and interpretive rigor were lacking. Thermograms were often interpreted subjectively, without reference to reproducible anatomical frameworks or validated diagnostic pathways (Ammer, 2008).

Exaggerated claims, especially regarding breast cancer screening, further damaged credibility. Some advocates proposed thermography as a stand-alone replacement for mammography, despite limited evidence and poor reproducibility in large-scale trials. These inflated expectations culminated in regulatory backlash.

By the early 1990s, critical reviews in the academic literature highlighted major limitations: over-reliance on arbitrary absolute temperature thresholds (such as the "1 °C rule"), high inter-operator variability, and low diagnostic specificity (Jones, 1998). These weaknesses fueled a narrative that thermography was a subjective and unreliable modality, incapable of meeting the evidentiary standards required of medical imaging.

Regulatory bodies reinforced this skepticism. The U.S. Food and Drug Administration (FDA) and the European Society of Breast Imaging (EUSOBI) issued strong statements restricting thermography's use, particularly in breast cancer screening, emphasizing that it should not replace evidence-based imaging such as mammography or MRI (FDA, 2019; EUSOBI, 2017).

These positions, though grounded in legitimate concerns, had the collateral effect of broadly discrediting thermography in academic and clinical communities, relegating it to niche use in alternative health practices.

In response, professional institutions such as the American Academy of Thermology (AAT) attempted to rehabilitate the field by publishing technical guidelines and recommending standardized acquisition environments, patient preparation protocols, and camera specifications (AAT, 2021).

These measures represented important progress, but they largely focused on technical conditions of image capture, stopping short of addressing the deeper issue of interpretation. Thermography continued to lack a coherent anatomical framework, diagnostic categories, and functional logic that could elevate it to the level of other functional imaging modalities such as fMRI or PET.

It was against this backdrop of both opportunity and failure that Biospectral Medicine emerged as a structured response. Developed by Felipe Reitz between 2005 and 2025, Biospectral Medicine originated in the practice of Computerized Thermographic Imaging (CTI) but evolved into a complete clinical discipline.

Unlike traditional thermography, which remained constrained by the pursuit of absolute temperatures, Biospectral Medicine redefined infrared emission as a biosignal, a zone-specific and physiologically contextual expression of vascular, autonomic, metabolic, or immune processes.

This transition was marked by the introduction of three foundational elements absent in earlier approaches. First, a standardized anatomical zoning system, dividing the body into 19 reproducible emission zones, provided the spatial logic for comparative interpretation. Second, a terrain-based model of analysis, mapping spectral behavior to systemic domains such as vascular, nervous, lymphatic, or endocrine, gave interpretive depth that aligned with functional physiology.

Third, the development of structured Interpretive categories and methodologies, embodied in the R-CIIM model, transformed thermographic imaging from an observational tool into a reproducible evaluative process.

By embedding emissive imaging within a framework of clinical systems logic, Biospectral Medicine represents the scientific rehabilitation of a field once dismissed as unreliable. It preserves the non-invasive strengths of infrared imaging while discarding its historical weaknesses of subjectivity and overreach.

In doing so, it establishes itself not as a rival to structural imaging modalities, but as a complementary functional system capable of detecting regulatory imbalances long before structural pathology is visible.

This reorientation fulfills the promise that thermography first hinted at but could not sustain: a reproducible, physiologically grounded imaging discipline that aligns with the rigor of contemporary medical science.

Functional Imaging and Biospectral Differentiation

In modern clinical diagnostics, imaging modalities can broadly be divided into two categories: anatomical imaging and functional imaging. Anatomical techniques such as ultrasonography, radiography, computed tomography (CT), and magnetic resonance imaging (MRI) provide high-resolution structural data and remain indispensable in lesion localization, surgical planning, and morphological assessment.

However, these modalities often fail to detect early-stage functional disturbances, such as inflammation, autonomic dysregulation, microvascular changes, or spectral emission abnormalities that may precede visible anatomical damage by years.

Functional imaging, by contrast, aims to detect physiological and biochemical changes within tissues, enabling earlier diagnosis, dynamic evaluation, and terrain-oriented interpretation. Technologies such as positron emission tomography (PET) and functional MRI (fMRI) illustrate the power of this approach.

PET can detect metabolic activity using radiolabeled tracers, while fMRI assesses neuronal activation through blood oxygenation level-dependent (BOLD) signals. However, both involve high operational costs, require exposure to radiation or contrast agents, and are largely inaccessible in integrative or preventive medicine settings.

A substantial body of research supports the conclusion that the majority of chronic pain conditions are rooted in functional or physiological dysregulation rather than discrete anatomical damage. Estimates suggest that up to 85% of patients presenting with low back pain, for example, show no clear structural abnormality on standard imaging modalities such as X-rays or MRI scans (Deyo & Weinstein, 2001).

This highlights a major limitation of anatomically focused diagnostic tools: they often fail to identify the physiological drivers of pain, such as autonomic imbalance, neurogenic inflammation, or myofascial dysfunction, that do not produce visible lesions. Consequently, anatomical imaging alone may overlook the true source of suffering in the vast majority of pain-related consultations.

It is in this context that Biospectral Medicine offers a clinically feasible, non-invasive, and radiation-free alternative. Unlike other functional modalities, Biospectral Medicine is based on the analysis of electromagnetic emissions naturally radiated by human tissues, captured through Computerized Biospectral Imaging (CBI). This technology does not rely on externally administered tracers, compression, or ionizing radiation, and can be applied repeatedly without harm.

Biospectral approach does not merely visualize superficial skin temperature, it interprets spectral activation patterns across defined anatomical zones, identifying areas of elevated, suppressed, or asymmetrical spectral emission.

The distinguishing feature of Biospectral Medicine lies in its **interpretive methodology**. Whereas thermographic imaging historically relied on **subjective visual assessment** or non-standardized thermal thresholds, the biospectral model introduces:

- A **19-zone anatomical framework**,
- A **multi-category interpretive structure** (vascular, neurological, musculoskeletal, etc.),
- The **R-CIIM interpretive model** (Reitz Clinical Infrared Interpretation Model), and
- Integration with **terrain analysis**, laboratory data, and clinical symptoms.

This structured approach enables the clinician to detect functional imbalances before anatomical lesions appear and to correlate findings with internal systemic dynamics such as autonomic stress, metabolic rigidity, or chronic regulatory disturbance. Recent studies have highlighted the value of functional imaging in pain, circulation, and oncology diagnostics.

For instance, Steketee (1973) and subsequent clinical works have demonstrated that inflammatory and neoplastic tissues emit more infrared radiation due to increased blood flow and metabolic activity. In oncology, angiogenesis, the formation of new blood vessels supporting tumour growth, can precede detectable tumours by 8–10 years, and may be visible as increased thermal emissions or vascular irregularities on biospectral imaging (Anbar, 1995; Head et al., 2000).

In contrast to mammography, which may cause discomfort, carry ionizing radiation risks, and exhibit false-positive or false-negative results in dense breast tissue, biospectral imaging offers a non-invasive, patient-friendly, and repeatable screening option. According to the FDA, while thermography is not approved as a replacement for mammography, it may serve as a complementary tool to monitor vascular activity and changes over time (FDA, 2019).

This is particularly important in young women or individuals with genetic risk factors, where cumulative radiation exposure is a concern.

The psychological dimension is also significant: biospectral imaging provides visual representation of physiological patterns, allowing patients to observe changes in real time. This visual feedback loop fosters engagement, compliance, and patient understanding, a key benefit in integrative and preventive care models.

Biospectral Medicine does not compete with traditional imaging but complements it by adding an entirely new interpretive dimension: the functional-emissive terrain of the body. It enables early detection, real-time monitoring, and individualized therapeutic strategies grounded in a clear interpretive structure.

Its clinical value lies in its precision, non-invasiveness, standardization, and its capacity to bridge subjective symptoms with objective spectral findings, a frontier that traditional imaging cannot yet fully address.

Biospectral Imaging: A Functional Interpretive System Bridging Infrared Emission and Integrative Medicine

The Biospectral interpretive system was developed by Felipe Reitz, who, between 2005 and 2025, advanced the clinical model of Computerized Thermographic Imaging (CTI), not as a technology, but as a protocol-based system of acquisition, anatomical division, and interpretive correlation. His early training with the Russian School of Medical Thermography, combined with concurrent specialization in ultrasonography, enabled real-time cross-validation of functional and structural findings.

Reitz observed that vascular, inflammatory, and neurological patterns could be seen spectrally before becoming detectable on ultrasound or conventional scans, especially in cases involving breast tissue, chronic pain, or vascular dysfunctions.

Biospectral Imaging uses high-sensitivity microbolometer sensors calibrated to detect emissivity changes across soft tissue surfaces. The analysis relies not on absolute temperatures but on pattern recognition, comparative zone behaviour, and systemic correlation. This places it in the broader field of functional imaging, similar in concept (though not in technology) to fMRI or PET, which detect tissue behaviour rather than structure (Phelps, 2000; Logothetis, 2008).

The non-contact, radiation-free nature of biospectral imaging allows for frequent repetition, longitudinal tracking, and preventive screening without harm, a distinct advantage over modalities such as mammography, which involve ionizing radiation and compression. Studies have shown that angiogenesis, often associated with malignant tumour formation, may be detected up to 8–10 years before tumour visibility on X-ray or ultrasound, owing to increased metabolic heat and vascularity (Anbar, 1995; Head et al., 2000).

Biospectral methods may identify such angiogenic patterns through subtle, zone-specific spectral activation, without exposure risks.

Visual biospectral reports allow patients to see their own physiological patterns, creating a psychophysiological feedback loop that improves therapeutic strategy adherence and emotional engagement. This patient-centered aspect aligns with the integrative philosophy of Biospectral Medicine, where the clinical picture includes both objective emission data and subjective experience.

While Biospectral Imaging draws on the well-established physics of infrared emission, it introduces a clinically transformative interpretive model. Through anatomically structured zones, terrain-based logic, and original interpretive terms, it shifts the paradigm from measuring surface heat to understanding how the body signals dysfunction through light.

This vision, pioneered by Reitz, positions Biospectral Medicine as a discipline in its own right, bridging functional physiology, advanced imaging, and integrative care.

Clinical Setup and Reproducibility Standards

Accurate biospectral evaluation depends on adherence to established environmental and procedural standards designed to ensure reproducibility and physiological reliability. Examinations are conducted under controlled conditions, including thermoregulatory stabilization and pre-imaging preparation.

While general principles are outlined, the complete set of clinical protocols, including room conditions, patient preparation, and acquisition procedures, is found on Biospectral Medicine Clinical Protocols to maximize quality and accuracy for the CBI

Imaging protocols follow structured anatomical sequencing, with standard angles and patient positioning. When appropriate, Spectrovascular Response Test (SVRT) may be applied to provoke vasoregulatory responses, enhancing contrast in emissive behaviour. Equipment is selected for sensitivity, emissivity calibration, and image fidelity, not for brand specificity. What defines Biospectral Medicine is not the hardware, but the clinical methodology applied to its data.

Strengths and Addressed Limitations

The strengths of Biospectral Medicine derive from its unique capacity to provide functional, non-invasive insight into human physiology. Unlike structural imaging modalities such as X-ray, CT, or MRI, which reveal anatomical alterations once pathology has manifested, biospectral imaging focuses on the dynamic regulatory processes that precede structural change.

Its safety profile further distinguishes it: infrared imaging involves no ionizing radiation and no physical contact, making it appropriate for repeated use across all populations, including children, pregnant individuals, and those requiring longitudinal monitoring (Lahiri et al., 2012).

This non-invasiveness allows clinicians to apply the modality interpretively and preventively, detecting subclinical imbalances before irreversible damage occurs.

A central strength is its ability to deliver functional insight, identifying disturbances in vascular tone, autonomic regulation, lymphatic activity, and inflammatory behavior well before conventional markers appear. This places Biospectral Medicine within the same paradigm as other functional imaging modalities such as fMRI or PET, but with distinct advantages: lower cost, wider accessibility, and greater safety (Ring & Ammer, 2020).

Its early warning potential has particular relevance in angiogenesis and inflammatory monitoring, where spectral anomalies may manifest years before conventional imaging demonstrates a detectable lesion or structural abnormality (Kennedy et al., 2009). By revealing microvascular and thermovascular patterns, Biospectral Medicine provides clinicians with actionable data at a stage when intervention can still prevent or mitigate long-term pathology.

Another major strength lies in its multisystem integration. Through its interpretive categories, vascular/circulatory, lymphatic/immune, metabolic/endocrine, neurological/spinal, musculoskeletal, and energetic/meridian systems, Biospectral Medicine transcends the single-organ focus of traditional imaging.

This systemic scope makes it particularly valuable for chronic, multisystem conditions, where dysfunction cannot be reduced to a single anatomical structure but reflects network-level imbalance. Such integrative capacity aligns Biospectral Medicine with modern systems biology and functional medicine, disciplines increasingly recognized as necessary complements to reductionist approaches (Vardasca et al., 2018).

Beyond technical and physiological strengths, Biospectral Medicine also promotes patient engagement. Because biospectral reports are visual and comparative, displaying activose and inhibose zones across defined anatomical territories, they provide patients with an intuitive representation of their condition.

This improves comprehension of complex findings, enhances adherence to therapeutic recommendations, and fosters trust in the evaluation process. Studies across imaging modalities have shown that visual evidence significantly improves patient adherence and engagement with treatment (Krol et al., 2015). In this sense, Biospectral Medicine functions as both an evaluation tool and a communicative bridge between clinician and patient.

The limitations that historically undermined medical thermography have also been systematically addressed within the framework of Biospectral Medicine. Environmental sensitivity, once a major criticism, has been neutralized through strict acquisition protocols, including controlled room temperature, patient acclimatization, shielding from drafts, and standardized calibration with blackbody references (Machin & Cowie, 2013).

Subjective interpretation, another longstanding critique, has been overcome through the structured methodology of the R-CIIM interpretive system, which provides a six-step, zone-based approach ensuring consistency and reproducibility across practitioners. Finally, while infrared emission is not a direct biochemical biomarker, its functional role as an early biosignal remains invaluable.

In many conditions, spectral behaviour, whether inhibitory suppression or activose amplification, emerges long before laboratory or structural findings, providing a temporal advantage in early diagnosis and preventive care (Clark et al., 2021).

In sum, Biospectral Medicine combines the safety and accessibility of non-contact imaging with the interpretive power of a structured, multisystem framework. Its capacity to reveal functional imbalances prior to structural systemic patter positions it as both an interpretive and preventive discipline, while its rigorous protocols and interpretive model have systematically addressed the limitations that once constrained thermography.

By transforming emissive imaging into a reproducible biosignal science, Biospectral Medicine re-establishes infrared imaging as a credible and clinically valuable modality within modern medicine.

The R-CIIM Interpretive Model

A Six-Step System for Functional Interpretation in Biospectral Medicine

A Structured Framework for Clinical Interpretation in Biospectral Medicine

In the evolving field of diagnostic imaging, the challenge has never been the acquisition of data alone, but the conversion of that data into clinically actionable knowledge. With infrared-based systems becoming increasingly accessible, the risk of superficial or inconsistent interpretation has also grown. In response to this, the Reitz Clinical Infrared Interpretation Model (R-CIIM) was developed to standardize the clinical application of biospectral imaging.

R-CIIM is not merely a reporting format, it is a structured interpretive methodology grounded in functional anatomy, physiology, and terrain-based medicine. It ensures that each image is interpreted through a reproducible, multi-layered lens, guided by logic and clinical correlation.

The R-CIIM model is the interpretive cornerstone of Biospectral Medicine, developed by Felipe Reitz after decades of integrative clinical work. It arose from the need to translate biospectral emission patterns, often complex, asymmetrical, and region-specific, into a coherent interpretive language.

At its core, R-CIIM provides a six-step analytical framework, allowing practitioners to move from image capture to differential diagnosis, and finally to clinical decision-making with consistency and depth.

Unlike traditional thermographic interpretations, which often rely on subjective colour pattern observation or simple temperature deltas, the R-CIIM model incorporates:

- Anatomical zoning,
- Functional system categorization,
- Terrain physiology,
- Confirmatory clinical correlations,
- And finally, integrative therapeutic guidance.

This model bridges the gap between physiological imaging and clinical logic, expanding the interpretive utility of infrared-based analysis while preserving clinical individuality and precision.

Step 1 – Refined Zone Description

Anatomical Precision as the Foundation of Functional Interpretation

The first step in the R-CIIM model establishes the indispensable basis for all subsequent interpretive reasoning: the precise anatomical definition of each emission zone. Unlike conventional thermography, which often renders the body as an undifferentiated surface field, Biospectral Medicine introduces a standardized zonal framework, dividing the body into 19 reproducible anatomical regions.

This segmentation is not arbitrary, but deliberately constructed so that each zone functions as a clinically coherent interpretive unit, including relationships that integrate vascular supply, neural pathways, musculoskeletal organization, lymphatic drainage, endocrine-metabolic influence, and even organ-reflective patterns.

By grounding interpretation within these clearly defined topographical containers, Biospectral Medicine transforms infrared imaging from a subjective visual exercise into a reproducible interpretive system capable of comparison over time, between bilateral sides, and across systemic categories (Ring & Ammer, 2020; Vardasca et al., 2018).

The development of these zones was the result of a long process of clinical refinement. Felipe Reitz, through the evaluation of thousands of patients between 2005 and 2025, identified consistent emission patterns that recurred within the same anatomical boundaries under a variety of clinical conditions.

These observations were not limited to static imaging, but included longitudinal follow-up, responses to therapeutic interventions, and controlled provocations such as the Spectrovascular Response Test (SVRT). Over time, the stability of these emission territories revealed them as physiologically meaningful units of regulation."

Their validity was further reinforced through correlation with comparative evaluations, such as Doppler ultrasound for vascular territories, laboratory markers for metabolic disturbances, and structural imaging modalities for musculoskeletal conditions. Inter-thermogram consistency across chronic cases, where the same emission anomalies recurred in the same defined zones, provided additional confirmation of reproducibility (Ammer, 2008; Lahiri et al., 2012).

The importance of this step lies in its ability to overcome the three major pitfalls that historically undermined thermographic interpretation. Without defined anatomical segmentation, imaging tends to become too general, producing descriptions such as "hot back" or "cold leg" that lack localization precision and cannot guide specific clinical action.

It also risks excessive subjectivity, with interpretation depending heavily on the experience or intuition of the practitioner, which produces significant inter-observer variability.

Finally, the absence of standardized segmentation makes longitudinal tracking unreliable, since comparisons across time are distorted if the zones of interest are not consistently delineated. By contrast, the zone-based interpretive language of Biospectral Medicine ensures cross-clinician reproducibility, educational standardization, reliable follow-up evaluation, and systemic correlation with organ and structural networks.

This provides not only a clinical advantage but also an academic framework that enables biospectral data to be studied, taught, and communicated with precision across institutions (Jones, 1998; Clark et al., 2021).

The integration of zone description with biospectral logic occurs on multiple levels. Each zone is first defined by topographical boundaries, often aligned with skeletal landmarks, muscle groups, or vertebral levels, which provide reproducibility in surface mapping.

Beyond this, each zone is also characterized by its underlying physiological relevance, reflecting the specific neural innervation, vascular supply, lymphatic drainage, or organ-reflective correspondence that gives clinical meaning to its spectral behaviour.

Over years of clinical observation, particular patterns of presentation have become associated with distinct zones, for example, tension and emissive amplification in the interscapular zone linked to postural strain and autonomic hyperactivity, or spectral suppression in the lateral abdominal zones reflecting digestive or reproductive organ dysfunction.

By anchoring these recurrent presentations within standardized zones, the interpretive model achieves both specificity and systemic integration (Fernández-Cuevas et al., 2015).

Equally critical is the recognition that each zone functions not in isolation but as part of a broader terrain interaction. A localized asymmetry may represent a vascular irregularity in one context, a neurological suppression in another, or a lymphatic stagnation in a third. The zone provides the structural base, but its meaning emerges from integration with the systemic terrain, whether neurovascular dynamics, endocrine regulation, or organ-reflective networks.

This step thus ensures that spectral interpretation remains anchored in physiology rather than drifting into surface description or purely visual impression (Ring et al., 2020; Vardasca et al., 2018).

By establishing this refined and standardized description of each of the 19 zones, Step 1 of the R-CIIM model lays the structural foundation upon which all subsequent steps rest. Without it, pattern recognition lacks the anatomical consistency required for evidence-based evaluations, correlation with systemic categories becomes speculative, and longitudinal evaluation loses reliability.

With it, Biospectral Medicine achieves what earlier generations of thermography could not: a coherent, reproducible, and clinically meaningful system of functional imaging, capable of bridging surface emissive patterns with internal physiological regulation.

Step 2 – Clinical Importance of the Zone

Understanding Each Zone's Interpretive and Systemic Significance

After the anatomical boundaries of a zone are established, the second step of the R-CIIM model requires the clinician to situate the zone within its clinical context. This step acknowledges that not all zones contribute equally to interpretive reasoning: some zones serve as primary expression sites where physiological dysfunction manifests directly, while others reveal secondary or compensatory patterns linked to systemic regulation.

The purpose of Step 2 is therefore to move beyond the geometry of segmentation and interpret each zone as a functional biosignal interface, integrating vascular, neurological, musculoskeletal, metabolic, and immune terrain relationships into a coherent diagnostic picture (Ammer, 2008; Ring & Ammer, 2020).

Each zone embodies a distinct set of physiological associations. Vascular pathways often define the first layer of relevance: emissive changes in the lower extremity zones, for example, can indicate venous stasis, microvascular obstruction, or impaired perfusion. Neurovegetative reflexes add a second layer, since dermatomal organization and sympathetic ganglia frequently produce segmental cutaneous manifestations of deeper dysfunctions.

This principle has long been recognized in the study of viscerocutaneous reflexes, where internal organ imbalances are reflected as localized cutaneous or subcutaneous changes (Kellgren, 1939; Wall & Woolf, 1999). Muscular and fascial pathways further reinforce the systemic integration of zones: patterns of emissive amplification along tension chains often reveal myofascial overload or postural compensations that cross multiple anatomical regions (Stecco et al., 2013).

Zones are also interpretively significant because of their segmental correspondence with visceral structures. For instance, changes in abdominal or paraspinal zones may represent the cutaneous expression of digestive, renal, or reproductive dysfunctions, depending on the sympathetic outflow and segmental overlap involved.

The supraclavicular and cervical zones are especially rich in organ-reflective relationships, often signaling thyroid, pulmonary, or lymphatic imbalance. Similarly, emissive changes in axillary or inguinal zones often reflect lymphatic drainage disturbances, immune activation, or compensatory load related to systemic inflammation (Fernández-Cuevas et al., 2015; Vardasca et al., 2018).

The interpretive task in Step 2 is to discern whether a biospectral alteration represents a local structural dysfunction, a referred systemic signal, a segmental reflex response, or a compensatory terrain adaptation.

For example, a finding in the dorsal lower leg zone may initially appear to represent venous insufficiency or fascial strain. Yet, when considered in the context of systemic physiology, it may instead reflect a segmental renal pattern, lumbar autonomic irritation, or compensatory redistribution of circulatory load. Similarly, spectral suppression in the lateral abdomen may not be a superficial hypoperfusion alone, but an externalized marker of deeper reproductive or gastrointestinal dysregulation.

By articulating each zone's interpretive relevance in this way, Step 2 transforms static surface mapping into a functional interpretive network. This process parallels the logic of functional imaging modalities such as fMRI or PET, where activity in a single anatomical region must be understood in relation to networks, systems, and temporal responses rather than isolated signals (Gore, 2003; Cherry, 2006).

In Biospectral Medicine, the zones serve as the structural vocabulary, while Step 2 provides the semantic meaning, allowing clinicians to move from mere pattern recognition to physiologically coherent interpretation.

Ultimately, the clinical importance of a zone cannot be reduced to its emissive appearance in isolation. It emerges from its anatomical boundaries, physiological associations, systemic correspondences, and terrain context, all of which must be considered in tandem. By situating each of the 19 zones within this integrative logic, Step 2 ensures that biospectral imaging achieves interpretive relevance, systemic coherence, and reproducibility across clinical settings.

Stratifying Interpretive Priority

Balancing Zone Reliability and Systemic Interpretation

Within the R-CIIM framework, interpretive reasoning is not a flat process where all zones are interpreted with equal weight. Instead, it recognizes the principle of interpretive priority, acknowledging that some anatomical zones consistently provide more stable, less environmentally reactive biosignals and are therefore more trustworthy for detecting early dysfunction.

Others, by contrast, are inherently more reactive or compensatory, often reflecting systemic adjustments rather than primary dysfunction. This stratification allows clinicians to assign proportional interpretive weight to each observation, thereby distinguishing primary from secondary findings and improving the overall coherence of biospectral interpretation.

Zones such as the anterior tibial surfaces or the supraclavicular fossae have been repeatedly shown to maintain emissive stability across varied acquisition conditions, making them highly reliable for detecting subclinical dysfunction. Their relative insulation from muscular activity, external thermal influences, and postural variability means that emission anomalies observed in these zones are less likely to represent transient noise and more likely to reflect persistent physiological imbalance.

By contrast, regions such as the axillae or abdominal surface may show greater reactivity to environmental or autonomic fluctuations, requiring contextualization within broader systemic patterns before being granted full diagnostic weight (Ammer, 2008; Fernández-Cuevas et al., 2015).

This hierarchy of reliability empowers the clinician to prioritize zones with higher interpretive yield, using them as anchors around which more variable findings can be interpreted. When consistent asymmetries are identified in stable zones, they lend authority to the overall interpretive picture, providing reference points against which more labile or compensatory patterns can be evaluated.

This principle is particularly valuable in multisystemic cases, where overlapping patterns may otherwise obscure the primary source of dysfunction. By applying interpretive priority, clinicians can correlate patterns logically across systems, ensuring that apparent anomalies in reactive zones are not misclassified as primary dysfunctions but are instead understood as secondary adjustments or systemic spillover phenomena (Jones, 1998; Ring & Ammer, 2020).

The concept of interpretive priority also enhances the efficiency of clinical workflow. By differentiating which zones offer the most reliable signals, practitioners can more effectively plan confirmatory assessments, directing laboratory, imaging, or functional tests toward the systems most likely implicated.

This not only increases the yield of follow-up testing but also reduces unnecessary investigations, aligning with modern principles of precision and personalized medicine (Vardasca et al., 2018).

Perhaps most importantly, this step shifts interpretation from a passive visual exercise to an active clinical dialogue with the biosignals. Rather than treating each thermogram as an aesthetic artifact, the physician engages with the image as a map of biological communication, in which each zone functions like a phrase in a systemic language. Stable zones provide grammatical anchors, while reactive zones offer contextual nuance.

The interpretive act lies not merely in seeing emissive patterns but in discerning their hierarchical meaning, assigning weight according to anatomical stability, systemic integration, and longitudinal reproducibility.

In this way, stratifying interpretive priority transforms Biospectral Medicine into a structured clinical reasoning process. It ensures that reproducible zones guide interpretation, reactive zones are integrated contextually, and systemic coherence is maintained throughout.

This approach not only safeguards against overinterpretation of reactive anomalies but also aligns biospectral imaging with the rigor of other functional modalities, where signals are evaluated according to their stability, reproducibility, and systemic significance (Gore, 2003; Cherry, 2006).

Step 3 – ROI Mapping and Pattern Recognition

From Emission Patterns to Functional Insight

The third step of the R-CIIM model moves beyond general zone description and clinical prioritization into the granular identification of Regions of Interest (ROIs) and the recognition of spectral patterns that reflect functional physiology. In traditional thermography, interpretation often depended on observing colour differences, typically framed as "hot" or "cold" spots, relative to adjacent tissues.

This simplistic reliance on colour gradients or temperature thresholds not only reduced interpretive reproducibility but also disconnected emissive findings from systemic physiology. Biospectral Medicine addresses this limitation by reframing ROIs as biospectral events, expressions of tissue function or dysfunction that are rooted in neurovascular regulation, inflammatory terrain, myofascial dynamics, and organ-specific physiology (Jones, 1998; Ring & Ammer, 2020).

ROI Mapping: Precision Beyond Surface Heat

An ROI in Biospectral Medicine is not simply any area of emissive variation. It is a defined micro-territory within a zone where spectral behaviour deviates meaningfully from expected patterns.

The process of identifying ROIs is guided by four interrelated criteria: (1) demonstrable asymmetry between bilateral zones, (2) focal emissions that diverge from established anatomical contours, (3) anomalies that persist across serial evaluations, and (4) mismatch between spectral findings and patient-reported symptoms, which may signal latent or subclinical dysfunction (Fernández-Cuevas et al., 2015).

Unlike in conventional thermography, ROI mapping in Biospectral Medicine is never arbitrary. The mapping follows anatomical and physiological logic, aligning with fascial planes, vascular pathways, nerve distributions, or viscerocutaneous reflex arcs.

For instance, a vertically oriented ROI extending medially from the scapula toward the lumbar spine might represent a myofascial tension chain, but it may also overlap with a renal segmental projection or reflect sympathetic irritation from the thoracolumbar outflow.

By anchoring ROI definition in anatomical reproducibility, the method ensures that imaging remains consistent, comparable, and clinically interpretable over time (Stecco et al., 2013; Kellgren, 1939).

Once defined, ROIs are further characterized by their biospectral consistency patterns, which classify whether the anomaly is acute, chronic-stable, or chronic-progressive. An acute ROI typically appears sharp and intense, often corresponding with recent inflammatory or vascular activation. Chronic-stable ROIs, by contrast, remain fixed but non-progressive, frequently reflecting long-standing compensatory states or scar-related emission suppression.

Chronic-progressive ROIs demonstrate expansion or intensification across serial studies and may indicate ongoing inflammatory activity, angiogenesis, or systemic organ-related dysfunction (Lahiri et al., 2012). This temporal characterization transforms ROI mapping into a functional timeline, linking surface emissive behaviour to the biological course of a condition.

Pattern Recognition: Reading Biological Communication

The recognition of patterns within and between ROIs elevates biospectral interpretation from static imaging to dynamic clinical reasoning. Pattern recognition in Biospectral Medicine does not equate to visual colour differentiation; instead, it deciphers systemic signals embedded in the emissive distribution.

Several archetypal patterns form the interpretive lexicon. Anisospectral distributions, bilateral asymmetries in emission, are the successor concept to "anisothermia," indicating lateralized dysfunction with neurovascular or autonomic origins (Ring & Ammer, 2012).

Segmental patterns follow dermatomes or viscerocutaneous projections, often revealing deep organ dysfunction expressed through sympathetic reflex arcs (Wall & Woolf, 1999). Radiated patterns, in which emissions spread centrifugally from a focal node, may indicate neurogenic irritation, lymphatic activation, or vascular spillage.

Finally, multifocal patterns, with scattered ROIs in non-contiguous zones, often signal metabolic, endocrine, or systemic inflammatory terrain imbalances (Vardasca et al., 2018).

Pattern interpretation requires integration not only with anatomical knowledge but also with clinical listening. A patient may present without overt symptoms in a region where a persistent ROI appears. such as the right iliac fossa, yet serial imaging could reveal that the anomaly is stable or progressive.

Correlation with subtle digestive irregularities or pelvic tension may then uncover subclinical appendiceal, ovarian, or lymphatic processes. In this way, ROIs act as early warnings of biological imbalance, highlighting dysfunction before structural changes or laboratory markers emerge.

Literature Support for Pattern-Based Interpretation

The literature strongly supports the emphasis on patterns over absolute values. Ring and Ammer (2012) demonstrated that thermal asymmetries, shape changes, and extension patterns often carry greater diagnostic significance than raw temperature differences, especially in chronic or inflammatory conditions.

Lahiri et al. (2012) similarly emphasized that consistent pattern recognition is more useful for detecting inflammation than reliance on simple temperature deltas. These findings directly align with the R-CIIM model, which treats ROIs as reproducible, anatomically grounded, and temporally trackable biosignals rather than as transient colour anomalies.

By integrating ROI mapping with structured pattern recognition, Step 3 transforms Biospectral Medicine into a language of biological communication. Emission anomalies are no longer "spots of heat or cold," but articulated signals that can be read, classified, and correlated with systemic physiology.

This process ensures that biospectral imaging not only visualizes dysfunction but contextualizes it as part of a dynamic interpretive narrative, enhancing both reproducibility and clinical meaning.

Step 4 – Key Interpretive Questions

Clinical Reasoning Guided by Biospectral Clues

The fourth step of the R-CIIM model represents the point at which biospectral data are transformed from visual anomalies into clinically actionable questions. Identifying a Region of Interest (ROI) and categorizing its spectral pattern provides the structural foundation, but the essence of Biospectral Medicine lies in interpreting what these signals mean for the patient's physiology.

Step 4 therefore bridges emissive findings with clinical reasoning, ensuring that each observed anomaly becomes the starting point for a line of inquiry that connects tissue-level biosignals to systemic processes and, ultimately, to the patient's lived experience.

This transition is critical because emissive patterns alone cannot determine etiology. A persistent activose ROI in the supraclavicular zone, for example, could represent lymphatic congestion, thyroid overactivation, or compensatory vascular load. Without context, the image risks remaining descriptive rather than interpretive.

The clinician must therefore ask: Which physiological processes could plausibly generate this emission? Is the anomaly consistent with the patient's reported symptoms? Does it align with known segmental, vascular, or organ-reflective relationships? Such questions operationalize the biospectral finding, linking it to hypotheses that can be confirmed or excluded through further testing (Fernández-Cuevas et al., 2015; Vardasca et al., 2018).

The process mirrors the logic applied in other functional imaging modalities. In fMRI, for instance, an area of cortical activation is never interpreted in isolation; it is evaluated in relation to task design, connectivity, and patient state.

Similarly, in PET, focal uptake must be contextualized against metabolic pathways and clinical history. In Biospectral Medicine, the ROI becomes a functional clue, which acquires meaning only when integrated with history, symptomatology, and physiological terrain (Gore, 2003; Cherry, 2006).

Key interpretive questions typically address four domains. First, they clarify whether the emission corresponds to a local dysfunction, such as vascular insufficiency, myofascial overload, or localized inflammation, or whether it reflects a referred systemic signal, such as viscerocutaneous reflex projection. Second, they probe the temporal dimension: is the anomaly acute, chronic-stable, or chronic-progressive, and how does this correlate with the patient's symptom timeline? Third, they assess systemic integration, asking whether the ROI is part of a broader pattern spanning multiple zones or terrains.

Finally, they seek to differentiate primary signals from compensatory adaptations, recognizing that spectral suppression or amplification in one zone may represent the body's effort to balance dysfunction elsewhere (Ammer, 2008; Ring & Ammer, 2020).

For example, an inhibose ROI in the lateral abdominal zone might prompt targeted questions regarding gastrointestinal function, reproductive health, or autonomic symptoms. A radiating activose pattern in the cervical spine region may lead to inquiries about headaches, dizziness, or neuromuscular tension. By framing such questions directly from the spectral findings, the clinician converts imaging into a dialogue with the patient's physiology, using visual data to guide deeper investigation and patient history.

Step 4 therefore represents the cognitive pivot of the R-CIIM process. The clinician does not merely observe emissive variation but interrogates it, translating image patterns into structured hypotheses that can be pursued through confirmatory testing. This ensures that Biospectral Medicine avoids the pitfalls of earlier thermographic practice, where images were often described but rarely integrated, and instead establishes itself as a reproducible, hypothesis-generating tool within evidence-based clinical reasoning.

From Image to Inquiry

In Biospectral Medicine, the interpretation of a Region of Interest (ROI) does not end with its identification or visual categorization. Instead, each ROI becomes the starting point for a sequence of targeted interpretive questions, grounded in anatomical, physiological, and systemic logic. These questions are never generic but are shaped by the ROI's zone location, emission pattern, and temporal behaviour.

For example, the presence of a linear ROI radiating inferiorly from the axillary zone immediately prompts inquiries into lymphatic stagnation, thoracic outlet vascular compromise, or autonomic dysregulation affecting the brachial plexus. In this way, the ROI serves as a visual hypothesis generator, channeling interpretive attention to structures and systems most likely implicated in the observed biospectral behaviour (Ring & Ammer, 2020; Fernández-Cuevas et al., 2015).

The first layer of inquiry concerns the anatomical substrate underlying the emission. Clinicians must consider which tissues lie within or beneath the ROI: is the pattern aligned with a vascular trajectory, a neural distribution, a fascial chain, or an organ-projection area? This anatomical anchoring reduces interpretive ambiguity, as the ROI cannot be considered in abstraction but only in relation to the body's structural organization.

A second layer addresses the physiological system most consistent with the emission: for example, does the pattern suggest a vascular irregularity such as venous stasis, or a neurogenic signal consistent with dermatomal radiation? The third dimension integrates clinical correlation, asking whether the patient reports symptoms corresponding to the emission site, pain, congestion, tension, or dysfunction that either confirms or challenges the spectral finding (Jones, 1998; Clark et al., 2021).

Temporal and lateral dimensions also shape inquiry. Determining whether an ROI is unilateral or bilateral, stable or evolving across serial imaging, is crucial for distinguishing between primary dysfunction and compensatory adjustment. A bilateral suppression in the lower extremities may point toward systemic vascular compromise, whereas a unilateral, progressive hotspot over the iliac fossa could suggest localized organ involvement.

Finally, the clinician must ask whether the emission represents a local disturbance or whether it is a referred expression of deeper dysfunction, such as a viscerocutaneous reflex arising from an organ in sympathetic distress (Kellgren, 1939; Wall & Woolf, 1999).

This line of structured questioning transforms what might otherwise remain a surface-level "hot" or "cold" observation into a multi-systemic hypothesis framework. By systematically exploring anatomical structures, physiological systems, symptom correlation, and systemic integration, the clinician is able to triage, prioritize, and focus interpretive attention, thereby preventing both under-interpretation and unnecessary over-testing.

Integration with the Nine Interpretive Categories

To avoid interpretive subjectivity, Biospectral Medicine anchors this questioning process within a standardized framework: the nine interpretive categories that structure biospectral reasoning. Each ROI is assessed through these categories to determine which functional system is most likely implicated and which pathways should be tested in the confirmatory phase of the R-CIIM model.

The vascular/circulatory category asks whether the emission reflects impaired venous return, microvascular overload, or arterial insufficiency, consistent with the known thermal correlates of altered perfusion (Lahiri et al., 2012). The muscular/myofascial category considers whether fascial adhesion, strain, or chronic tension explains the anomaly, linking ROI topography to myofascial chain anatomy (Stecco et al., 2013).

The skeletal/articular category raises questions about periosteal irritation, joint inflammation, or degenerative changes, where emissive suppression may correspond with reduced perfusion in arthritic processes (Ammer, 2008).

When the pattern follows dermatomal or neurogenic distribution, the nervous system/spine category is activated, highlighting possible radiculopathy, neuropathic irritation, or sympathetic segmental dysfunction (Ring & Ammer, 2020). In cases where emissions overlay lymphatic basins or drainage territories, the lymphatic/immune category guides inquiry toward stagnation, immune activation, or inflammatory reactivity (Vardasca et al., 2018).

The organs/GNM category prompts questions about visceral projections, viscerocutaneous reflexes, or the presence of active or healing phases described in German New Medicine, especially when emissions align with abdominal or thoracic zones (Fernández-Cuevas et al., 2015).

In zones where emission follows recognized energetic channels, the acupuncture/meridian category is engaged, correlating anomalies with classical Chinese medical pathways and their modern physiological interpretations (Yin et al., 2018). Where emissions are diffuse, radiating, or multifocal, clinicians may explore the energetic/frequency category, considering whether dysregulation in bioelectromagnetic coherence or systemic vibrational terrain is reflected in the pattern (Hammerschlag et al., 2012).

Finally, the metabolic/endocrine category evaluates whether ROI presentation reflects systemic dysregulation such as thyroid imbalance, adrenal strain, or altered mitochondrial metabolism, conditions known to affect emission dynamics even in the absence of overt structural change (Kennedy et al., 2009).

By applying the nine interpretive categories, Biospectral Medicine ensures that every ROI is contextualized not as a surface irregularity but as a multisystemic clue. Each category offers a structured pathway toward hypothesis formation, which can then be validated or excluded in Step 5 through targeted confirmatory testing.

This integration of structured questioning with systemic categorization exemplifies the distinctive strength of the biospectral approach: the capacity to transform surface emission data into a reproducible, physiologically grounded, and clinically actionable interpretive narrative.

Clinical Listening as a Compass

A central principle of Biospectral Medicine is that imaging findings cannot be disentangled from the lived experience of the patient. Felipe Reitz emphasizes that interpretive questioning must remain anchored in clinical listening, ensuring that biospectral anomalies are not interpreted as isolated data points but as part of a broader physiological and psychosocial context.

This approach recognizes that the meaning of a Region of Interest (ROI) is never fixed solely by its emissive pattern; it is dynamically shaped by the interplay between objective biosignals and subjective narrative.

For example, consider a persistent activose ROI over the left supraclavicular region. By itself, such an emission might suggest a vascular or lymphatic irregularity. However, the trajectory of questioning shifts considerably depending on the patient's reported experience. If the patient describes chronic neck tension, the clinician is guided toward the muscular or myofascial terrain, investigating fascial strain, postural overload, or neuromuscular compensation.

If the patient reports hormonal irregularities, such as thyroid dysfunction or metabolic fatigue, the same ROI may be interpreted primarily through the endocrine/metabolic category, prompting confirmatory testing of thyroid and adrenal function. Should the narrative reveal emotional repression, grief, or conflict in the domain of self-worth and heart coherence, the emission acquires further resonance within the GNM-organic framework, which links neurovegetative patterns to organ-reflective conflict phases (Hubbard & Kline, 1996; Schubring, 2014).

Finally, in cases where the ROI presents in the absence of any symptoms, the lack of narrative correlation does not negate its importance but rather invites exploratory reasoning, motivating longitudinal monitoring, terrain assessment, or targeted systemic testing to uncover latent dysfunction.

This integration of imaging with narrative establishes what can be described as a interpretive duet: a bidirectional relationship in which biospectral patterns provide objective anchors and the patient's story supplies interpretive context. Just as functional MRI or PET findings require correlation with behavioral or biochemical data to achieve interpretive significance, so too does biospectral imaging require the narrative compass of clinical listening to direct interpretation toward relevance rather than abstraction (Gore, 2003; Cherry, 2006).

Without this integration, imaging risks being overinterpreted as deterministic or dismissed as incidental, both of which undermine interpretative accuracy.

The importance of clinical listening is further reinforced by its capacity to individualize interpretive inquiry. Biospectral anomalies can manifest in diverse ways depending on the patient's terrain: the same supraclavicular emission may signal myofascial overload in one individual, endocrine strain in another, or unresolved psycho-organic conflict in a third. Only through attentive dialogue can the clinician discern which systemic terrain is most implicated.

This approach avoids the pitfalls of purely image-driven reasoning and aligns Biospectral Medicine with patient-centered evaluations, where technology serves to amplify rather than replace human interpretation (Epstein & Street, 2011).

Ultimately, Step 4 of the R-CIIM model reaches its full power only when biospectral questioning is fused with narrative exploration. The image provides the structural map, but the patient's account supplies the compass that directs inquiry toward meaningful terrain. Together, they ensure that Biospectral Medicine fulfills its role not merely as a functional imaging modality, but as a clinical method that unites the objectivity of emissive science with the subjectivity of human experience.

Scientific Context

The integration of imaging findings with clinical reasoning is not a speculative innovation of Biospectral Medicine, but a principle consistently emphasized in the broader thermographic and biomedical literature. Decades of research in medical infrared imaging have demonstrated that thermal anomalies, while visually compelling, are insufficient for interpretive certainty unless contextualized within anatomical, physiological, and patient-specific frameworks.

Lahiri et al. (2012), in their comprehensive review of medical thermography, conclude unequivocally that "clinical context is essential for the interpretation of thermal anomalies," warning that purely numerical or colourimetric evaluations risk false positives and diagnostic misdirection.

Similarly, Ring and Ammer (2012) reinforce that emissive data must always be "seen in anatomical and physiological coherence," arguing that reproducibility and clinical value arise only when imaging is embedded within a structured interpretive model rather than left to subjective visual judgment.

This evidence directly validates the methodology of the R-CIIM model, which operationalizes these principles into a stepwise system of reasoning. By anchoring ROI mapping and pattern recognition to anatomical boundaries, systemic terrains, and patient history, Biospectral Medicine avoids the reductionist pitfalls that contributed to the decline of classical thermography in the late 20th century.

Instead, it aligns with the standards expected of other functional imaging modalities such as fMRI or PET, where image-derived anomalies are always interpreted in the context of systemic physiology, experimental design, or metabolic pathways (Gore, 2003; Cherry, 2006). In this sense, Biospectral Medicine situates itself within a lineage of functional evaluations that prioritize integration of signal with context over raw measurement alone.

The significance of this integrative approach extends beyond interpretation. By transforming surface emissive behaviour into biospectral signals, the R-CIIM model provides clinicians with a reproducible framework for linking imaging data to therapeutic decisions. The literature underscores that the reliability of any imaging modality depends less on its technical sophistication than on the interpretive systems that guide its clinical application (Vardasca et al., 2018).

Biospectral Medicine contributes precisely this: a methodology that converts emissive anomalies into functional hypotheses, validates them through confirmatory tests, and integrates them into personalized therapeutic strategies.

Thus, the scientific context affirms that Biospectral Medicine is not only consistent with contemporary imaging science but also extends it. By uniting standardized imaging acquisition, zone-based segmentation, pattern recognition, and patient-centered inquiry, it ensures that thermographic data are not treated as isolated artifacts but as part of a clinically coherent interpretive narrative. This approach embodies the principle that imaging without context is descriptive, but imaging with structured reasoning is diagnostic and actionable.

Step 5 – Confirmatory Clinical Testing

From Hypothesis to Objective Correlation

The fifth step of the R-CIIM model marks the transition from pattern-based reasoning to evidence-based validation. Once a Region of Interest (ROI) has been mapped, categorized, and interrogated through structured interpretive questions, the clinician must seek objective confirmation to ensure that interpretation does not remain speculative.

This stage reflects the hybrid philosophy of Biospectral Medicine: it balances the interpretive power of Computerized Biospectral Imaging (CBI) with the rigor of established interpretive sciences, creating a dual-method system in which spectral signals guide inquiry and confirmatory tests substantiate conclusions.

This step is particularly important because functional anomalies often precede structural change. A spectral suppression in the lateral abdomen, for instance, may represent early autonomic inhibition long before endoscopic or imaging findings become visible. By subjecting such findings to confirmatory pathways, the clinician ensures that biospectral interpretation is anchored in measurable correlates while also maintaining its unique value as a precocious indicator of dysfunction (Lahiri et al., 2012; Ring & Ammer, 2020).

Matching Tests to Interpretive Categories

The confirmatory process is guided by the nine interpretive categories that structure Biospectral Medicine. Each category provides its own set of clinical tools to validate or exclude hypotheses generated from emissive findings.

In the vascular/circulatory domain, where ROIs often indicate venous stasis, arterial insufficiency, or microvascular overload, confirmatory testing may include Doppler ultrasound, ankle-brachial index (ABI), plethysmography, capillaroscopy, or vascular reactivity testing.

These tools quantify flow, perfusion, and vascular integrity, offering direct correlates to biospectral emission anomalies (Rossi et al., 2013).

For the muscular/myofascial system, where emissions often align with fascial chains or postural compensation, confirmatory assessment may involve palpation, range-of-motion evaluation, surface electromyography (EMG), or myofascial ultrasound. These methods provide biomechanical evidence of tension, adhesions, or altered activation patterns that correspond with spectral signals (Stecco et al., 2013).

In the skeletal/articular category, focal emissions over joints or periosteal regions may be confirmed with radiography, MRI, or ultrasound, as well as with functional tools such as joint stress testing or osteoarthritic scoring. Emissive suppression over joints has been correlated with degenerative or inflammatory changes in several thermographic studies (Jones, 1998).

When biospectral anomalies follow dermatomal or neurogenic patterns, the nervous system/spine category directs confirmatory testing toward nerve conduction studies, EMG, somatosensory evoked potentials, or spinal imaging. These tools can verify whether spectral asymmetries reflect radiculopathy, neuropathy, or sympathetic dysfunction (Fernández-Cuevas et al., 2015).

For the lymphatic/immune category, persistent hotspots in axillary, supraclavicular, or inguinal basins may require ultrasound of lymph nodes, lymphoscintigraphy, or laboratory immune markers such as C-reactive protein (CRP), white blood cell differentials, or cytokine panels (Vardasca et al., 2018).

In the organs/GNM category, confirmatory evaluation may include endoscopy, ultrasound, CT, or laboratory markers of organ function (e.g., liver enzymes, renal clearance tests). The integration of biospectral findings with viscerocutaneous reflex theory underscores the value of correlating emissions with deeper segmental processes (Kellgren, 1939).

For the metabolic/endocrine system, where spectral patterns often reflect systemic terrain, confirmatory tests may involve fasting insulin, HbA1c, thyroid function panels (TSH, free T3/T4), cortisol, vitamin D, homocysteine, or sex hormones, depending on the suspected imbalance (Kennedy et al., 2009).

In the acupuncture/meridian category, while conventional imaging may not always validate findings, correlations can be explored using heart rate variability (HRV), galvanic skin response, or electrophysiological meridian testing, which provide indirect confirmation of energy flow disruptions (Yin et al., 2018).

Finally, in the energetic/frequency category, where emissions may reflect biofield dysregulation or systemic vibrational imbalance, confirmatory pathways are more exploratory, often involving bioelectromagnetic assessments, frequency-based evaluations, or coherence analysis, fields still emerging within biomedical science but increasingly investigated for their role in systemic regulation (Hammerschlag et al., 2012).

Clinical Integration and Decision-Making

The value of Step 5 lies not in replacing biospectral interpretation with conventional diagnostics, but in creating a dialogue between modalities. A unilateral supraclavicular hotspot, for instance, interpreted within the lymphatic/immune terrain, may prompt ultrasound evaluation of axillary drainage.

If ultrasound confirms node reactivity, the ROI is validated as a true physiological signal; if it does not, longitudinal follow-up may still reveal early immune fluctuation not yet captured structurally. In this way, Step 5 balances precision with precaution, using confirmatory tools to validate without prematurely dismissing the early warnings inherent to biospectral signals.

This process also prevents over-testing, as ROI-derived hypotheses direct clinicians toward the most relevant confirmatory pathways. A bilateral leg suppression pattern, for example, suggests systemic vascular involvement, justifying systemic hemodynamic evaluation rather than localized joint imaging. By linking emission distribution with systemic logic, Step 5 optimizes evaluation efficiency and supports precision medicine principles.

Conclusion

Step 5 ensures that Biospectral Medicine remains both innovative and credible. By grounding spectral interpretation in confirmatory clinical tests, it strengthens interpretative accuracy, enhances reproducibility, and aligns the method with established biomedical standards. The integration of functional biosignals with objective validation situates Biospectral Medicine as a truly hybrid interpretive discipline, capable of detecting dysfunction earlier than conventional imaging while maintaining rigorous accountability through correlation with measurable findings.

Structuring the Confirmation

Step 5 of the R-CIIM model does not end with the suggestion of confirmatory testing. To preserve scientific rigor, each Region of Interest (ROI) must be integrated into a structured confirmation matrix that systematizes the pathway from spectral observation to clinical validation.

This matrix relies on four interrelated elements: what to test, why it matters, how to test, and what to expect. By formalizing these dimensions, Biospectral Medicine ensures that interpretation is never speculative but anchored in reproducible, evidence-based methodology.

The first dimension, *what to test*, identifies the suspected biomarker, physiological function, or anatomical system implicated by the ROI. For example, an emission over the left upper abdomen might implicate splenic involvement, whereas an inhibose ROI in the posterior neck suggests autonomic or spinal imbalance. This step aligns the ROI with a specific functional hypothesis, reducing the risk of diffuse or non-specific testing.

The second dimension, *why it matters*, highlights the clinical significance of the suspected disturbance. This ensures that testing is not pursued as an abstract exercise, but as a means of clarifying how the dysfunction may impact systemic health, patient well-being, or long-term prognosis.

In the case of splenic emission, relevance lies in its potential association with immune activity, hematological disorders, or systemic inflammation. For posterior neck suppression, the significance lies in its role as a marker of chronic sympathetic overdrive, a state linked with cardiovascular risk, endocrine dysregulation, and impaired resilience to stress (Thayer & Lane, 2000).

The third dimension, *how to test*, identifies the appropriate laboratory, imaging, or functional modality for confirmation. For splenic involvement, abdominal ultrasound, complete blood count (CBC) with differential, ferritin, and C-reactive protein (CRP) represent suitable confirmatory tools, each probing a different layer of systemic function.

For autonomic imbalance, methods such as heart rate variability (HRV) analysis, cold challenge provocation, or spinal thermocline mapping provide measurable correlates of sympathetic activity and recovery capacity (Shaffer & Ginsberg, 2017).

Finally, the fourth dimension, *expected findings*, defines what results would corroborate the biospectral expression. This step closes the loop, ensuring that spectral anomalies are not validated arbitrarily but only when measurable disturbances align with the hypothesis. In the splenic example, confirmation may include ultrasound evidence of splenomegaly, elevated inflammatory markers, or hematological changes suggestive of immune activation.

In the case of posterior neck inhibition, reduced HRV coherence, exaggerated sympathetic recovery after cold challenge, or persistent spinal emission suppression would support the interpretation of chronic autonomic strain.

This evidence-based triangulation is vital for both therapeutic safety and interpretative accuracy. By linking each ROI to a defined confirmatory pathway, clinicians reduce the risk of misinterpretation and prevent inappropriate or premature therapeutic interventions.

It also ensures that Biospectral Medicine aligns with the broader epistemology of biomedical imaging, where functional anomalies are always substantiated by objective correlates before informing treatment decisions (Gore, 2003; Vardasca et al., 2018).

Thus, structuring the confirmation transforms biospectral imaging into a closed-loop interpretive process, where spectral anomalies guide inquiry, confirmatory tests validate hypotheses, and clinical reasoning integrates both into therapeutic decision-making. This not only enhances reproducibility but also strengthens the medico-legal defensibility of Biospectral Medicine by demonstrating that interpretation is grounded in a systematic, verifiable methodology (Ring & Ammer, 2020).

Scientific Validation and Precedent

The integration of biospectral findings with confirmatory clinical testing is not only a methodological innovation of Biospectral Medicine but also a principle repeatedly emphasized in the broader thermographic literature. A persistent critique of classical thermography has been its tendency toward isolated interpretation, an approach in which emissive anomalies were presented as interpretive endpoints rather than as signals requiring corroboration.

This often led to overdiagnosis or false attribution of clinical meaning to what were, in some cases, environmentally influenced variations. By embedding confirmatory testing as a formalized step within the R-CIIM model, Biospectral Medicine directly addresses this historical shortcoming, ensuring that spectral anomalies are not treated as stand-alone evidence but as hypothesis-generating findings that demand validation.

Scientific precedent strongly supports this approach. Lahiri et al. (2012), in their comprehensive review of thermographic applications, emphasize that infrared imaging "should be integrated with standard diagnostics for maximum clinical reliability" (p. 240). They note that thermography achieves its highest clinical value not when used in isolation but when applied as a complementary tool that informs and refines subsequent testing.

Similarly, Ammer and Ring (2010) highlight that "infrared anomalies must be interpreted with correlation to clinical findings and laboratory results" to avoid misinterpretation and overextension of diagnostic claims. Their caution highlights that without structured integration, thermal imaging risks being misapplied as a definitive rather than contributory diagnostic modality.

Biospectral Medicine resolves this methodological gap by positioning Computerized Biospectral Imaging (CBI) as the first, risk-free layer of clinical triage. In this role, CBI provides non-invasive, radiation-free, and reproducible visualizations of functional disturbances, which can then be correlated with laboratory, imaging, or functional tests according to the nine interpretive categories.

This structured integration not only strengthens interpretive reliability but also aligns Biospectral Medicine with the evidentiary standards expected of functional imaging sciences such as fMRI, PET, or Doppler ultrasound, all of which rely on contextual correlation with systemic findings to achieve clinical validity (Gore, 2003; Cherry, 2006).

In doing so, Biospectral Medicine contributes a crucial methodological advance: it transforms emissive imaging from a descriptive tool with limited acceptance into a clinically anchored, evidence-based system that integrates seamlessly with biomedical diagnostics. By ensuring that every spectral anomaly is followed by targeted confirmatory testing, it upholds scientific rigor while preserving the modality's unique strength as an early, non-invasive detector of physiological imbalance.

The Role of Terrain

One of the most distinctive contributions of Biospectral Medicine is its terrain-based interpretive framework, which moves beyond organ-centered or reductionist models and considers health and dysfunction as the result of systemic networks.

While many medical imaging modalities rely on discrete structural abnormalities for confirmation, Biospectral Medicine emphasizes that functional anomalies often arise from terrain-level dysregulation, particularly in the metabolic, immunologic, and energetic domains. This emphasis ensures that interpretive confirmation is not restricted to isolated biomarkers, but instead incorporates multi-systemic contextualization.

For example, in cases where spectral anomalies implicate the digestive or immunological terrain, confirmatory evaluation may involve a comprehensive stool analysis to assess microbiome composition, digestive efficiency, inflammatory markers, and intestinal permeability. Such testing provides insight into the "gut terrain," which has been increasingly recognized as a central regulator of systemic physiology, influencing not only immune balance but also metabolic and neurological processes (Turnbaugh et al., 2007; Valdes et al., 2018).

Similarly, live blood analysis, though not universally standardized in conventional medicine, can provide functional insights into hematological terrain, revealing erythrocyte morphology, rouleaux formation, or oxidative stress markers that complement biospectral findings.

These assessments may be particularly relevant when spectral suppression or diffuse emissive anomalies suggest systemic stagnation, hypoperfusion, or terrain-level imbalance. The hemato-terrain thus becomes an important layer of confirmation, linking surface emission to blood microenvironment and rheological behavior (Ernst, 2006).

In metabolic and toxicological contexts, heavy metal panels serve as another dimension of terrain-oriented confirmation. Chronic low-level toxicant exposure can manifest in spectral anomalies such as diffuse suppression or multifocal hotspots, reflecting systemic oxidative stress or mitochondrial compromise. Confirming such patterns through toxicology not only strengthens the biospectral interpretation but also identifies modifiable environmental contributors to chronic disease processes (Patrick, 2003).

The biospectral model also accommodates frequency-based anomalies, where emission patterns appear less anatomically constrained and more diffuse, radiating, or multifocal. In such cases, confirmatory assessment may require vibrational or bioresonance testing, which, although still emerging in biomedical literature, aligns with growing evidence of bioelectromagnetic regulation in human physiology (Hammerschlag et al., 2012).

By considering the energetic/frequency terrain, Biospectral Medicine extends interpretive logic into domains that capture subtle regulatory dynamics often invisible to biochemical assays or structural imaging.

This terrain-based orientation underscores a central strength of the biospectral model: its ability to integrate diverse interpretive paradigms into a cohesive system. Confirmation does not rest solely on the presence or absence of discrete laboratory abnormalities, but instead on the coherence of findings across multiple terrains, vascular, neural, immune, metabolic, and energetic.

In this way, Biospectral Medicine mirrors the complexity of human physiology itself, offering a framework that is not only scientifically defensible but also clinically adaptable to the reality of chronic, multisystemic disorders (Vardasca et al., 2018).

Step 6 – Targeted Therapeutic Guidelines

Integrating Biospectral Insights into Strategic Clinical Interventions

The final stage of the R-CIIM model is the therapeutic response, where biospectral findings are no longer treated as abstract signals but as guides for precise clinical action. After an emission anomaly has been identified (Step 3), contextualized through interpretive questioning (Step 4), and validated with confirmatory testing (Step 5), the clinician enters Step 6: the translation of interpretive clarity into targeted, terrain-specific interventions.

This step represents the culmination of the biospectral process, transforming functional imaging from a evaluation modality into a platform for strategic therapeutic planning.

Unlike conventional medicine, which often emphasizes symptom suppression, Biospectral Medicine adopts a functional therapeutic strategy logic. This begins with the zone affected, proceeds through the physiological system implicated, and culminates in therapies directed at restoring systemic balance across the patient's unique terrain.

Therapeutic reasoning therefore flows from imaging to physiology, and from physiology to root-cause care plan, always prioritizing safety, coherence, and the layered resolution of dysfunction rather than short-term suppression (Ammer, 2008; Vardasca et al., 2018).

For example, when a focal ROI in the dorsal calf suggests venous congestion, therapeutic guidelines may emphasize vascular terrain strategies such as microcirculatory support, postural correction, and targeted movement therapies, confirmed by vascular diagnostics.

In contrast, a chronic inhibose ROI in the cervical spine zone, linked to autonomic suppression, might lead to interventions aimed at autonomic rebalancing, stress modulation, and neural integration, validated through heart rate variability (HRV) or cold challenge testing. In each case, the biospectral anomaly provides the starting point for a systemically coherent therapeutic plan rather than an isolated prescription.

Another distinctive strength of the biospectral approach lies in its terrain orientation, where interventions are selected not only for the system implicated but also for the patient's wider bio-individual context. A supraclavicular emission pattern interpreted as lymphatic stagnation, for instance, would direct therapy toward immune drainage support, inflammatory terrain modulation, and, where appropriate, detoxification strategies.

If confirmed metabolic imbalances are implicated in diffuse or multifocal ROIs, therapeutic strategy may incorporate endocrine regulation, nutritional optimization, and mitochondrial support. By linking imaging findings to the nine interpretive categories, Step 6 ensures that therapeutic strategy is always system-targeted and terrain-integrated (Fernández-Cuevas et al., 2015; Ring & Ammer, 2020).

The therapeutic logic of Biospectral Medicine also emphasizes layered intervention. Spectral anomalies often represent both primary dysfunctions and compensatory adaptations. An activose hotspot may indicate local inflammation, while an adjacent inhibose field reflects systemic protective suppression.

In such cases, care plans guidelines are carefully staged: first addressing the compensatory blockade to restore circulation and drainage, then gradually reducing inflammatory burden and stabilizing systemic terrain. This sequential and integrative approach avoids the risk of destabilizing the patient by prematurely removing compensatory adaptations, an error common in symptom-driven models of care (Thayer & Lane, 2000).

Finally, therapeutic guidance in the biospectral framework extends into longitudinal monitoring. Because spectral anomalies can precede structural systemic patters by months or years, therapeutic strategy efficacy can be tracked dynamically through follow-up imaging.

The resolution of a chronic ROI, stabilization of bilateral asymmetry, or normalization of terrain-linked emission patterns serves as an objective marker of therapeutic progress. This not only strengthens clinical accountability but also enhances patient engagement, as the visible evolution of biospectral images provides tangible evidence of functional improvement (Kennedy et al., 2009).

Thus, Step 6 is not an endpoint but a continuum of feedback and refinement. It integrates interpretive clarity with strategic, safe, and individualized interventions, always guided by the terrain context and reinforced through measurable clinical outcomes. In this way, Biospectral Medicine closes the loop of the R-CIIM model, uniting emission detection, systemic interpretation, confirmatory validation, and targeted therapeutic guidance into a comprehensive clinical methodology.

Principles of Therapeutic Targeting

Therapeutic reasoning within Biospectral Medicine rests on the principle that each emission anomaly is not only a marker of dysfunction but also a guidepost for clinical intervention. The R-CIIM model positions therapeutic strategies as the logical culmination of interpretive clarity, linking spectral behaviour to systemic physiology and patient-specific terrain.

To achieve this, therapeutic targeting is organized around the nine interpretive categories, each of which channels the biospectral finding into a distinct line of clinical reasoning. These categories do not function as rigid compartments but as interpretive lenses, through which interventions can be scaled from local correction to systemic regulation.

The first dimension of therapeutic targeting involves zone function and its physiological role. Every zone in the 19-part anatomical framework has reproducible links to vascular supply, neural innervation, fascial pathways, or viscerocutaneous reflexes. Thus, when an ROI presents in a given zone, therapeutic strategy must address not only the superficial emission but also the functional role of that zone in systemic physiology.

A hyperemissive anomaly in the calf, for example, cannot be managed as an isolated hotspot but must be interpreted in light of venous return, muscular load, and lymphatic drainage specific to that region (Ammer, 2008).

The second dimension emphasizes the biological terrain patterns that underlie the emission. Terrain-based reasoning recognizes that dysfunction may present as congestive, reactive, neurogenic, metabolic, or immune-mediated, and that therapeutic strategy must reflect this systemic ecology.

A congestive terrain may call for strategies that support drainage and circulation, while an inflammatory terrain may demand regulatory interventions to down-modulate immune activation. This terrain logic ensures that therapy does not simply suppress symptoms but addresses the systemic milieu that sustains dysfunction (Turnbaugh et al., 2007; Valdes et al., 2018).

The third dimension is derived directly from spectral emission characteristics. Whether a zone is activose (elevated emission) or inhibose (diminished emission) provides essential therapeutic direction. Activose zones often indicate acute inflammatory, vascular, or metabolic activation, calling for modulation and stabilization.

Inhibose zones, by contrast, may signify autonomic inhibition, hypoperfusion, or metabolic depletion, conditions in which reactivation and functional restoration become priorities. By interpreting emission not as static "hot" or "cold" but as functional expression of systemic tone, Biospectral Medicine creates a more precise therapeutic alignment (Ring & Ammer, 2020).

The final therapeutic dimension considers systemic involvement and comorbidity context. An ROI that presents in isolation may be addressed with localized interventions, but when emissive anomalies are multifocal or distributed across terrains, therapeutic strategy must prioritize systemic regulation.

For instance, a single axillary hotspot may be managed with lymphatic drainage support, but when paired with diffuse metabolic suppression and neurogenic asymmetry, therapy must expand to include endocrine stabilization, autonomic balance, and detoxification strategies. This layered reasoning ensures that care planning reflects both the local signal and the systemic network in which it resides (Kennedy et al., 2009).

By combining these dimensions, zone function, terrain ecology, spectral character, and systemic context, Biospectral Medicine constructs customized therapeutic strategies that are both individualized and physiologically grounded. In some cases, interventions may focus on local corrections, such as fascial release or vascular stimulation in a restricted region.

In others, particularly when multiple terrains are implicated, strategies extend toward systemic regulation, integrating metabolic rebalancing, immune modulation, or neurovegetative stabilization. The principle of therapeutic targeting is therefore not a prescriptive formula but a framework of reasoning, transforming spectral anomalies into clinical action plans that are safe, functional, and aligned with the patient's unique biosignal profile.

Clinical Strategies by Interpretive Category

Interpretive Category	Therapeutic Orientation
1. Vascular / Circulatory	Microcirculation enhancers (e.g., Ginkgo biloba, bioflavonoids), vasotonic phytotherapy, contrast therapy, movement-based vascular mobilization.
2. Muscular / Myofascial	Myofascial release, magnesium, proteolytic enzymes, trauma drainage (Arnica, Rhus tox.), structural osteopathy.
3. Skeletal / Articular	Anti-inflammatory phytocomplexes, collagen precursors, homeopathics for periosteal regeneration, vitamin D/K2.
4. Nervous System / Spine	Nervine adaptogens (e.g., Ashwagandha, Bacopa), neural therapy, vagal stimulation, HRV training, craniosacral therapy.

5. Lymphatic / Immune	Lymphagogues (e.g., Galium aparine, Phytolacca), immune modulators, drainage strategies (UNDA, Spagyric), fasting.
6. Organs / GNM	Organ-specific support (e.g., liver, pancreas, intestines), psychoemotional terrain mapping, GNM phase-based remedies.
7. Acupuncture / Meridians	Acupuncture, moxibustion, electrostimulation, auricular therapy, meridian-based phytotherapy.
8. Energetic / Frequency	Homeopathics, flower essences, frequency carriers (e.g., nosodes, isotherapics), bioresonance harmonization.
9. Metabolic / Endocrine	Terrain-corrective nutrition, trace minerals (zinc, selenium), hormonal modulators (e.g., Maca, Vitex), detox support.

Therapeutic decisions in Biospectral Medicine are not made solely from biochemical derangement but from functional pattern recognition aligned with physiology.

Strategic Layering and Clinical Judgment

Sequencing Therapeutic Phases in Complex Terrain

In clinical practice, biospectral anomalies rarely conform to a single interpretive category. Instead, zones often reveal multifactorial disturbances where vascular, lymphatic, neural, metabolic, and organ-reflective elements converge. This complexity demands a therapeutic approach that is neither linear nor reductionist, but layered and sequential, enabling the clinician to guide the body through phases of excretion, restoration, and regulation.

For example, emissive irregularities in the left hypochondrium may implicate vascular compromise related to splenic flow, lymphatic drainage limitations, and organ-level imbalances in the stomach–spleen terrain. Treating such a presentation as a single dysfunction would risk overlooking its systemic nature; instead, the therapeutic response must be strategically layered.

The first phase is drainage, focusing on clearing stagnation and reducing systemic burden. This may include strategies to support lymphatic drainage, hepatic clearance, and excretory function, ensuring that toxic load and immune congestion do not block subsequent restorative processes. The second phase is restoration, directed at strengthening the affected organ or system through trophorestoratives and terrain-specific interventions, such as splenic or gastrointestinal support when the hypochondrium is implicated. The third phase is regulation, addressing deeper terrain-level imbalances such as neurovegetative dysregulation, metabolic insufficiency, or emotional/psychosomatic patterns described in the GNM framework.

This triadic logic mirrors the therapeutic sequencing observed in anthroposophic and isopathic medicine, where treatment progresses from excretion to reconstitution and then to modulation, ensuring safety and systemic coherence (Schad, 2006; Kienle et al., 2013).

Role of the Terrain and Individualization

One of the most significant advances introduced by Biospectral Medicine is its ability to individualize therapy through visual terrain mapping. Unlike conventional diagnostics, which often present numerical values or structural images detached from systemic interpretation, biospectral imagery functions as a clinical compass. Each emission pattern not only guides the practitioner but also communicates meaning directly to the patient.

When patients see their emission zones mapped and contextualized within a terrain-based interpretive model, they gain an immediate and tangible understanding of their condition. This visibility fosters therapeutic compliance, engagement, and trust, since treatment is no longer abstract but visibly connected to the patient's unique physiology (Epstein & Street, 2011).

Another distinctive strength is the real-time follow-up capacity of Computerized Biospectral Imaging (CBI). Because many functional disturbances precede structural or biochemical changes, serial imaging provides a uniquely sensitive tool for monitoring the trajectory of therapeutic interventions.

Repeated scans can demonstrate whether drainage strategies are effectively reducing congestion, whether organ restoration is stabilizing emission zones, or whether regulatory therapies are achieving systemic balance. Just as importantly, CBI enables the clinician to detect compensatory strain in adjacent systems, highlighting the body's adaptive responses and preventing inadvertent destabilization (Vardasca et al., 2018).

As Lahiri et al. (2012) note, repeated thermographic evaluation "provides an objective measure of functional change over time" (p. 241). This principle, when extended into the structured interpretive logic of Biospectral Medicine, transforms CBI into a precision-care tool within functional medicine. It allows for ongoing calibration of strategy, ensuring that therapies remain both individualized and dynamically responsive to the patient's evolving terrain.

PART VII

OVERVIEW OF BIOSPECTRAL MEDICINE IN GLOBAL CONTEXT

The preceding parts have examined the history, physics, methodological standards, and translational bridge that shaped Biospectral Medicine. This concluding overview situates these elements within a global context, acknowledging the distinct contributions of different regions while clarifying how they converge in a unified, reproducible methodology.

By integrating Japanese, European, North American, and Latin American traditions, Biospectral Medicine emerges not as a local innovation but as a global discipline of functional imaging.

The evolution of Biospectral Medicine must be understood not as the isolated work of a single laboratory or region, but as the convergence of international traditions of thermology and functional evaluation.

Across continents, research groups and clinical societies pursued distinct but complementary priorities: some emphasized standardization of acquisition, others focused on governance and regulatory clarity, while still others advanced protocol-driven clinical expansion and longitudinal follow-up.

Taken together, these contributions reveal that emissive imaging achieved credibility only when it was embedded in reproducible conditions, when functional physiology rather than static surface maps was prioritized, and when results were correlated with confirmatory tests in an open interpretive ecosystem.

This international lineage underscores why a new synthesis was required. In Japan, thermology was advanced through strict control of environment and symmetry analysis, including the preservation of cold-challenge recovery protocols as probes of vasomotor function (Yamauchi, 1980; Shibata et al., 1989).

In Europe, radiological societies such as EUSOBI formalized the limits of emissive imaging in breast diagnostics, while academic scholars like Ring and Ammer reframed infrared emission as a physiological biosignal requiring standardization (Ring & Ammer, 2012; Sardanelli et al., 2017). In North America, practice guidelines were codified by the American Academy of Thermology, while federal agencies such as the U.S.

Food and Drug Administration communicated clearly to the public about both the potential and the limits of thermographic applications (FDA, 2019; AAT, 2024). In Latin America, clinical expansion flourished, particularly in Brazil, where thermography was applied in sports medicine, vascular assessment, and physiotherapy with strong attention to control variables and longitudinal monitoring (Moreira et al., 2017; Viegas et al., 2020; Passos et al., 2022).

The purpose of this Part is therefore twofold: first, to acknowledge and detail the unique contributions of each region to the modern rehabilitation of emissive imaging; and second, to demonstrate how Biospectral Medicine unifies these regional strands into a coherent methodology.

By situating the R-CIIM model within this international context, the Atlas emphasizes that what differentiates Biospectral Medicine is not only its structured interpretive logic, but its ability to act as a clinical bridge, linking radiative physics, global methodological heritage, and integrative patient care into one reproducible interpretive system.

JAPAN: Standardization, Symmetry, and Dynamic Provocation

Japan's thermology community advanced medical infrared imaging by insisting on strict acquisition control, contralateral (left–right) symmetry analysis, and dynamic provocation paradigms that transform static surface maps into physiological biosignals.

Three pillars recur across the Japanese lineage: (1) reproducible environments (room conditioning, acclimatization, draught control), (2) intra-individual comparison through symmetry norms, and (3) reactivity testing (cooling/rewarm curves) that probe vasomotor regulation and autonomic tone.

Collectively, these elements anticipate the operational logic of Biospectral Medicine, where emissive patterns are interpreted as regulated functions rather than mere temperatures. (Ring & Ammer, 2012).

Acquisition standardization. Early and sustained Japanese work linked credibility in infrared imaging to environmental stability and patient preparation.

Contemporary standardization chapters that synthesize international practice trace multiple fundamentals, ambient temperature control (≈18–25 °C), avoidance of draughts, camera warm-up, fixed working distances/fields-of-view, and a minimum acclimatization period (~10–15 min), to the same methodological emphasis on physiological steadiness before capture (Ammer, "Standard Procedures for Infrared Imaging in Medicine").

The same sources note that acclimatization shorter than ~10 min or poorly controlled rooms increases variance and degrades repeatability, while longer times may be required for specific cameras or populations; these requirements align with human thermoregulatory dynamics and reduce artifactual asymmetries. (Ammer, ch. "Standard Procedures"; see sections on ambient control, pre-imaging equilibration).

Symmetry as a clinical comparator. A crucial Japanese contribution was the elevation of contralateral symmetry to a first-line interpretive comparator. Uematsu's seminal report, "Symmetry of skin temperatures comparing one side of the body to the other" (Thermology, 1985), quantified side-to-side differences by body region, establishing that healthy individuals exhibit tight bilateral similarity, with deviations suggesting neural, vascular, or inflammatory perturbations; Goodman and colleagues extended these findings for back and extremities (1986).

Subsequent European confirmations (e.g., Ring's work on the lower leg) reinforced symmetry as a robust anchor for intra-individual interpretation and follow-up. In modern reviews, bilateral symmetry appears as a general population characteristic and a practical biomarker of dysregulation when disrupted, precisely the logic exploited in zone-based Biospectral analysis. (Uematsu, 1985; Goodman et al., 1986; Ring, 1986; Symons et al., 2015).

Dynamic provocation and recovery (cold challenge). Japanese investigators preserved and developed cold-provocation/recovery paradigms in clinical and occupational contexts (e.g., hand–arm vibration syndrome), where finger/hand rewarm kinetics serve as a window into microvascular function and autonomic control.

Dynamic thermography after standardized cold stress distinguishes fast vs. slow rewarmers and reveals patterns consistent with vasospasm or endothelial dysfunction, principles later formalized in Biospectral Medicine's Spectrovascular Response Test (SVRT).

Even outside Japan, the strongest methodological threads (standardized water-immersion or air-cooling, fixed exposure times, recovery modeling) echo this tradition and appear in Japanese journals (e.g., *Journal of Occupational Health*). (Jankovic, 2008; Norheim et al., 2018).

Japanese biomedical engineering and emissivity insights. A second line of Japanese work, exemplified by Togawa and Saito, moved beyond static temperature to thermal property imaging (non-contact estimation of skin thermal parameters under controlled radiative shifts).

This research highlighted that emissive behavior is heterogeneous across the skin and can be interrogated with controlled radiative environments, reinforcing why controlled acquisition is not optional and why palette normalization and emissivity assumptions must be explicit in clinical protocols.

These engineering studies underpin Biospectral Medicine's insistence on LWIR windows (8–14 µm), palette integrity, and zone-specific contrast fidelity when interpreting functional terrain. (Togawa & Saito, 1994; Ammer, "Standard Procedures").

Institutional continuity and acceptance. Historically, Japanese sources document formal acceptance of medical thermography as a diagnostic procedure early in the modern era, alongside workshops that proposed procedures for physiological function analysis and neuromuscular thermogram interpretation under the Japanese Society of Biomedical Thermology.

This institutional framing, discipline-specific journal (*Biomedical Thermology*), workshop-derived criteria, and neuromuscular evaluation proposals, shows that Japan not only refined technique but also embedded thermology within a society-governed clinical discourse, a template echoed in today's Biospectral framework. (Atsumi, 1985; Fujimasa et al., 1986; Fujimasa, 1991; summarized in Ammer's standardization chapter).

Why this matters for Biospectral Medicine. Japan's methodological DNA, stable environments, symmetry-first comparison, and dynamic provocation, maps directly onto the Biospectral workflow: standardized acquisition ensures emissive fidelity; contralateral/zone-based comparison yields functionally meaningful differentials; and SVRT-style probing converts an image into a biosignal over time.

These features are precisely those identified in international reviews as prerequisites for credibility: proper equipment use, rigorous recording methods, and interpretation grounded in thermal physiology. (Ring & Ammer, 2012).

EUROPE: Governance Boundaries and Methodological Rehabilitation

In Europe, thermology matured under the dual influence of radiological governance and methodological refinement. On one hand, pan-European societies clarified the boundaries of emissive imaging in sensitive domains such as breast cancer screening; on the other, academic groups reframed infrared imaging as a credible physiological tool by enforcing reproducibility and functional interpretation.

Together, these contributions prevented misuse, preserved credibility, and laid much of the methodological groundwork for what Biospectral Medicine formalizes today.

Governance in Breast Diagnostics

The most visible European intervention was the issuance of formal position papers on breast imaging. The European Society of Breast Imaging (EUSOBI), supported by related radiological associations, reaffirmed mammography as the gold standard for population screening, with MRI indicated for women at high genetic or familial risk (Sardanelli et al., 2017).

Thermography was explicitly excluded as a stand-alone or substitute screening tool, reflecting decades of unstandardized claims and patient risk when used outside validated protocols.

This governance boundary was crucial: it discouraged thermography's promotion as a competitive replacement for structural imaging and instead situated emissive methods as potential adjuncts, functional assessments capable of detecting asymmetry, regulatory instability, or vascular activity, but always to be correlated with confirmatory structural tests.

By drawing these boundaries, European societies established a safety-first regulatory context in which emissive imaging could be rehabilitated rather than dismissed outright.

Methodological Rehabilitation

Parallel to governance, European academic scholarship worked to rescue medical infrared from marginalization. The most influential contributions came from Ernst Ring and Kurt Ammer, whose reviews and monographs provided structured evidence for the medical use of infrared thermal imaging (Ring & Ammer, 2012; Ring, 2014). Their work highlighted three methodological imperatives:

1. Standardized acquisition - stable ambient temperature, subject acclimatization, and reproducible protocols as non-negotiable conditions.
2. Functional interpretation - moving beyond "hot/cold spots" to analyze patterns, asymmetries, and dynamics reflective of underlying physiology.

3. Clinical integration - thermography as an adjunct within a broader diagnostic and therapeutic framework, not as a stand-alone exam.

Ring and Ammer's reviews synthesized hundreds of studies and systematically addressed critiques from radiology and oncology. They demonstrated that many failures attributed to thermography were failures of protocol, interpretation, and instrumentation, not of emissive physics itself.

Their rehabilitation strategy aligned thermology with biomedical optics, physiology, and clinical imaging sciences, a transition Biospectral Medicine now completes by formalizing emissive signals as structured biospectral data.

European Research Tradition

Beyond breast imaging and methodological reviews, European research also contributed in applied clinical areas. Studies in rheumatology, musculoskeletal disorders, and peripheral vascular assessment emphasized zone-specific repeatability and intra-individual baselines, reinforcing the importance of longitudinal monitoring.

Academic centers in Germany, the UK, and Austria integrated emissive imaging into occupational health and rehabilitation, often in collaboration with biomedical engineering departments, thereby consolidating the physiological rather than purely thermal framing of the discipline.

Relevance for Biospectral Medicine

The European legacy is twofold: it protected patients and public health through governance (preventing misuse in breast cancer screening) and restored credibility through rigorous methodological rehabilitation.

These contributions map directly onto the principles of Biospectral Medicine, where emissive imaging functions as a clinical adjunct requiring strict reproducibility, zone-based logic, and integration into practice.

In this sense, Biospectral Medicine represents the logical extension of European thermology, a discipline that retains standardization and safety while advancing the interpretive model into the structured six-step R-CIIM sequence.

NORTH AMERICA: Guidelines, Regulation, and Clinical Niches

In North America, the trajectory of medical infrared imaging was shaped by a dual structure: professional societies established practice guidelines for legitimate applications, while federal agencies, most notably the U.S. Food and Drug Administration (FDA), issued regulatory communications to protect patients from unsubstantiated claims.

This combination of codified standards and public-facing warnings defined the credibility space in which emissive imaging could survive, evolve, and eventually converge with the broader integrative diagnostics reflected in Biospectral Medicine.

Professional Guidelines and Clinical Codification

The American Academy of Thermology (AAT) played the central role in North America by publishing formal practice guidelines that defined how and when medical infrared imaging could be legitimately employed. These documents outlined acquisition controls, reporting structures, and diagnostic contexts where infrared contributed useful information, particularly in neuro-musculoskeletal medicine, pain management, reflex sympathetic dystrophy, and sympathetic skin response studies (AAT, 2024).

The AAT guidelines stressed that infrared imaging must be:

1. **Protocol-driven**, with standardized environment and acclimatization.
2. **Integrated with clinical context**, never used in isolation.
3. **Focused on functional interpretation**, particularly in vascular and neural territories.

This codification of practice paralleled European methodological rehabilitation but was more practitioner-facing, offering clinicians a structured way to incorporate infrared imaging into diagnostic decision-making.

Regulatory Oversight and FDA Communications

At the same time, the FDA acted as a public guardian against misuse. The agency released repeated advisories reminding patients and clinicians that thermography is not a substitute for mammography or other structural breast imaging modalities (FDA, 2019).

These communications were direct, sometimes even appearing in consumer-oriented outlets, reflecting concern about clinics marketing thermography as a stand-alone breast cancer screening test.

FDA warnings had a dual impact: they limited inappropriate breast cancer claims but also discouraged broader adoption in contexts where thermography could have provided functional adjunctive value.

From a historical standpoint, these regulatory interventions explain why emissive imaging in the U.S. became marginalized in oncology but retained legitimacy in niche clinical settings (neurology, sports medicine, rehabilitation).

Applied Clinical Niches in North America

Despite regulatory caution, North American research and practice sustained emissive imaging in several applied domains:

- **Neurology and pain medicine -** infrared was used to evaluate sympathetic dysfunction, complex regional pain syndrome (CRPS), and peripheral neuropathies, where emissive asymmetries correlated with autonomic dysregulation.
- **Sports and rehabilitation -** centers employed infrared to monitor injury recovery, muscular strain, and peripheral vascular performance.
- **Occupational health -** dynamic thermography was used in the evaluation of hand–arm vibration syndrome and repetitive strain injuries, often in collaboration with physiology departments.

These niches reflected the U.S. emphasis on functional assessment of specific syndromes rather than broad population screening.

Relevance for Biospectral Medicine

The North American legacy lies in the contrast between caution and codification. On one side, the FDA narrowed thermography's permissible scope, effectively preventing its misuse in oncology. On the other, the AAT guidelines preserved legitimate niches and codified standards for musculoskeletal and neural applications.

This dual legacy maps onto the principles of Biospectral Medicine, where emissive imaging complements structural imaging and, when standardized and clinically contextualized, provides unique biosignals of vascular, neural, and autonomic regulation.

In this way, Biospectral Medicine can be seen as the continuation of the American guideline tradition, extending beyond neuro-musculoskeletal care to a structured, zone-based, and reproducible system applicable across nine diagnostic categories.

LATIN AMERICA: Protocol Expansion and Longitudinal Clinical Care

In Latin America, most prominently in Brazil, thermography developed along a trajectory distinct from the governance-heavy approaches of Europe or the niche-focused frameworks of North America. Here, clinical uptake flourished across multiple disciplines, supported by a strong emphasis on control variables, protocol-driven methodology, and longitudinal patient monitoring.

These contributions have been particularly visible in sports medicine, vascular diagnostics, and rehabilitation, where infrared imaging was positioned as a functional adjunct embedded in follow-up protocols.

Emphasis on Control Variables

Brazilian groups recognized early that the reliability of thermography depended on consistent management of environmental and patient-related variables. Systematic reviews have identified standardized control factors, including room acclimatization, activity restriction before imaging, avoidance of stimulants, and control of circadian influences, as prerequisites for valid data capture (Viegas et al., 2020).

By consolidating these methodological safeguards, Latin American research provided reproducibility frameworks comparable in rigor to those developed in Japan and Europe, but anchored in applied clinical practice.

Expansion into Sports and Exercise Medicine

Thermography gained substantial visibility in sports and exercise medicine, where Brazilian and Latin American researchers used emissive imaging to monitor muscular strain, overload, and recovery.

Delphi consensus processes and applied trials confirmed that thermal asymmetry and dynamic changes correlate with fatigue, microtrauma, and risk of injury (Moreira et al., 2017). This positioned thermography as a non-invasive monitoring tool in elite athletic settings, where repeated measures across training cycles demanded both sensitivity and reproducibility.

Applications in Vascular and Rehabilitation Medicine

Beyond sports, Latin American teams extended thermography into vascular diagnostics, demonstrating its utility in peripheral arterial disease (PAD). Pilot studies using portable thermography showed that emissive asymmetry could track microcirculatory compromise and monitor therapeutic response (Passos et al., 2022).

In rehabilitation and physiotherapy, infrared imaging became a tool to document progress, stratify interventions, and provide visual biofeedback for patients. These applications reinforced the method's role in longitudinal care, where intra-individual follow-up is more informative than single time-point comparisons.

Latin American Methodological Culture

What distinguished Latin American contributions was the marriage of methodological rigor with clinical pragmatism. Unlike in North America, where regulatory caution narrowed thermography's niche, Latin America embraced protocol-driven expansion, ensuring reproducibility while embedding emissive imaging into broader therapeutic strategies ecosystems.

This generated a body of literature describing thermography as a functional monitoring tool, aligned with integrative and rehabilitative care models.

Relevance for Biospectral Medicine

The Latin American legacy highlights the value of reproducible follow-up and terrain-oriented monitoring. Biospectral Medicine inherits this ethos by formalizing zone-based longitudinal comparisons: each patient becomes their own control, and emissive changes are interpreted against individualized baselines rather than population norms.

In this sense, Latin America's emphasis on applied, repeated-measure thermography provides a practical bridge for the Atlas, demonstrating that emissive imaging thrives when integrated into therapeutic trajectories rather than isolated diagnostic events.

The Clinical Bridge: From Emissive Signal to Decision

The international lineage of thermology demonstrates that emissive imaging only achieves clinical relevance when signals are standardized, contextualized, and translated into decision pathways.

Japan emphasized reproducible acquisition and dynamic provocation; Europe reinforced governance boundaries and methodological rehabilitation; North America codified legitimate niches through professional guidelines while preventing misuse via regulatory oversight; and Latin America operationalized protocol-driven monitoring in sports, vascular, and rehabilitative care.

Biospectral Medicine integrates these strands into a clinical bridge: a reproducible sequence by which infrared emission is transformed from raw surface gradients into actionable interpretive and therapeutic guidance.

Step 1 – Standardized Acquisition

Every credible thermology tradition insisted on controlled environments, patient preparation, and calibration. Biospectral Medicine formalizes this into acquisition standards: acclimatization (10–15 min minimum), ambient temperature control, palette normalization, and zone-based integrity checks. Without this foundation, emissive asymmetries cannot be distinguished from artifact (Ammer, 2008; Ring & Ammer, 2012).

Step 2 – Functional Provocation

Where Japan contributed cold challenge recovery and Latin America operationalized follow-up protocols, Biospectral Medicine introduces the Spectrovascular Response Test (SVRT). This structured provocation transforms static emissive mapping into a dynamic curve of vascular regulation, analogous to stress tests in cardiology or autonomic reflex testing in neurology. Functional provocation makes regulation visible, not just morphology.

Step 3 – Structured Interpretation

Building on European methodological rehabilitation, Biospectral Medicine abandons simplistic "hot/cold" descriptors. Instead, it uses a zone-based lexicon (activose, inhibose, anisospectral, equibose) to define emission patterns across 19 anatomical zones. This structured interpretation ensures consistency, reproducibility, and scalability for training and credentialing.

Step 4 – Hypothesis Formation by Interpretive Category

In North America, emissive imaging persisted as a functional adjunct in neurology and musculoskeletal care. Biospectral Medicine extends this logic across nine interpretive categories: vascular, neural, metabolic, immune, endocrine, skeletal, muscular, organ/GNM, and meridian/energetic. Each emission pattern is interpreted as a hypothesis generator that guides the next step in clinical reasoning.

Step 5 – Confirmatory Testing

Global consensus emphasizes that emissive imaging cannot substitute structural definition when required. The clinical bridge therefore mandates targeted confirmation:

- Vascular asymmetry → **Doppler ultrasound or ABI**
- Neural emission shifts → **sensory mapping, reflex testing, HRV**
- Endocrine or metabolic terrain → **laboratory assays**
- Skeletal/joint hypotheses → **X-ray or MRI correlation**

This ensures that emissive signals are never misused in isolation, but instead serve as functional guides to appropriate testing.

Step 6 – Therapeutic Strategy and Longitudinal Monitoring

Latin America's contributions demonstrated the power of longitudinal thermography: repeated measures tracking rehabilitation, athletic load, or vascular therapy. Biospectral Medicine incorporates this into the R-CIIM sequence, where emissive follow-up is used to evaluate therapeutic impact over time. Care plan becomes iterative: interventions are guided by baseline asymmetry, adjusted by confirmatory tests, and reassessed through emissive recovery patterns.

Why This Bridge Matters

The clinical bridge protects against the two historical extremes of thermology: uncritical promotion as a stand-alone diagnostic, and wholesale dismissal as unscientific. By embedding emissive imaging inside a reproducible, hypothesis-driven, confirmatory framework, Biospectral Medicine preserves the non-invasive, functional strengths of long-wave infrared while ensuring alignment with modern evidence-based practice.

It answers the central question posed by regulators and academics alike: *how can emissive signals be made clinically reliable?* The answer is through bridging, from emission to biosignal, from biosignal to hypothesis, and from hypothesis to tested, individualized therapy.

Research and Education Agenda

The international rehabilitation of medical infrared imaging requires a coordinated research and education agenda. The lessons from Japan, Europe, North America, and Latin America converge on a single imperative: emissive imaging acquires lasting credibility only when protocols are harmonized, validation studies are terrain-specific, and training is standardized across disciplines. Biospectral Medicine crystallizes this trajectory but also opens a future roadmap for scientific consolidation and academic dissemination.

1. Harmonization of Acquisition and Provocation Protocols

Across all regions, the most consistent barrier to reproducibility has been heterogeneity in acquisition conditions. Ambient temperature control, subject acclimatization, camera calibration, and color palette integrity are widely mentioned in protocols, but international variation remains significant (Ammer, 2008; Ring & Ammer, 2012).

Likewise, provocation tests such as cold challenge or SVRT differ in timing, exposure, and recovery modeling across research groups. A coordinated effort to publish multicenter consensus protocols, specifying environmental conditioning, minimum acclimatization time, and standardized SVRT parameters, will be essential for inter-laboratory comparability and eventual guideline-level acceptance.

2. Validation Studies by Interpretive Category

Global scholarship confirms that emissive imaging should never be marketed as a "screening tool" in isolation, but it also demonstrates that terrain-linked validation is feasible. Future research must pre-register and stratify hypotheses by the nine interpretive categories of Biospectral Medicine. For example:

- **Vascular / circulatory terrain:** Correlating calf-zone asymmetry with Doppler ultrasound or ankle–brachial index (ABI).
- **Neural / spinal terrain:** Relating cervical emissive differentials to segmental sensory thresholds, mechanosensory testing, or HRV metrics.
- **Endocrine / metabolic terrain:** Linking supraclavicular emission changes to thyroid hormone panels or metabolic assays.
- **Musculoskeletal terrain:** Tracking joint emission zones against MRI or radiographic inflammation markers.

These studies will provide the scientific validation regulators demand and demonstrate the translational power of the R-CIIM model.

3. Training and Credentialing Frameworks

Another global challenge is the absence of formal training pathways for emissive imaging. The Japanese Society of Biomedical Thermology, the American Academy of Thermology, and European consensus groups each proposed standards, but there is no unified curriculum (Uematsu, 1985; AAT, 2024). Biospectral Medicine proposes a tiered training approach:

- **Level 1 – Technician competence:** mastery of acquisition, acclimatization, and artifact control.
- **Level 2 – Clinical interpreter:** zone-based interpretation, symmetry assessment, integration with the nine interpretive categories.
- **Level 3 – Biospectral clinician:** application of the full R-CIIM model, integration with laboratory/structural testing, and individualized therapeutic planning.

Such a credentialing framework will allow institutions to ensure consistency, protect patients, and professionalize the field.

4. Integration into Multimodal Evaluations

The Atlas makes clear that the future of emissive imaging lies in integration with CT, MRI, and ultrasound.The role of emissive imaging is to detect regulation, asymmetry, instability, dynamic reactivity, while structural imaging defines morphology.

Future research must demonstrate the additive value of combining emissive biosignals with conventional modalities in vascular disease, pain syndromes, endocrine dysfunction, and immune/lymphatic dysregulation (Sardanelli et al., 2017; Spalding et al., 2008).

5. Longitudinal and Digital Health Applications

Latin America's applied research highlights the potential of emissive imaging as a longitudinal monitoring tool. The next step is integration into digital health platforms, where emissive data is combined with wearables, HRV sensors, and laboratory panels to track patient terrain dynamically over time. This will enable personalized medicine workflows, where therapies are titrated against continuous biospectral feedback.

Closing Perspective

The rehabilitation of thermography into Biospectral Medicine represents both a recovery of neglected scientific value and a forward-looking transformation. The international agenda is clear: protocols must be harmonized, validation pursued by interpretive category, training standards established, and integration with multimodal evaluations achieved.

Through these steps, emissive imaging will claim its rightful place as a reproducible, scientifically anchored discipline for mapping human regulation.

The strongest traditions developed in Japan, Europe, North America, and Latin America, yet contributions from other regions are emerging. Research initiatives in China, India, and Africa, particularly within engineering, infectious disease, and public health fields, reflect a growing international convergence toward the principles that strengthen Biospectral Medicine, positioning it to evolve into a truly global practice."

These efforts will mature by adopting the standardized methodologies and international frameworks consolidated in this Atlas.

Biospectral Medicine complements established imaging modalities by visualizing regulation, asymmetry, and dynamic recovery.

By integrating the methodological legacies of the past with a forward-looking research and education agenda, this Atlas defines Biospectral Medicine as the first global discipline of emissive functional evaluations.

CHAPTER 2

THE R-CIIM INTERPRETATIVE MODEL

A Six-Step System for Functional Interpretation in Biospectral Medicine

A Structured Framework for Clinical Interpretation in Biospectral Medicine

In the evolving field of diagnostic imaging, the difficulty has never been limited to the acquisition of data, but to its transformation into knowledge that can be used in clinical practice. As infrared-based systems become increasingly available, the ability to obtain biospectral images has multiplied, yet so has the danger of misinterpretation.

Without a coherent interpretive system, images risk being reduced to superficial impressions, where striking colour contrasts are mistaken for diagnostic certainty. The challenge lies in moving from raw imagery to structured reasoning, where functional disturbances are identified with clarity and therapeutic relevance.

It was to address this need that the Reitz Clinical Infrared Interpretation Model (R-CIIM) was conceived. Developed by Felipe Reitz after decades of integrative clinical work, the model emerged from the necessity of translating biospectral emission patterns, often irregular, asymmetrical, and region-specific, into a clinical language that is both logical and reproducible.

R-CIIM is not a template for reporting but an interpretative methodology, grounded in functional anatomy, physiology, and terrain-based medicine. Its purpose is to ensure that every image is approached through a structured, multi-layered lens, guiding the clinician step by step from observation to therapeutic decision-making with consistency and depth.

The interpretive depth of R-CIIM comes from the way it integrates five essential dimensions into one coherent process. The first of these is anatomical zoning, where every emissive finding is located within a precise structural map of the body. By doing so, interpretation avoids the ambiguity of vague visual impressions, since each irregularity is examined within the topography of its region, creating an immediate link between image and structure.

From this anatomical base, the reasoning advances to functional system categorization. Each zone is related to one or more physiological systems, so that what appears on the surface is not seen as an isolated anomaly but as an expression of circulatory, muscular, skeletal, or neural dynamics. This systemic view expands interpretation from local irregularity to integrated function, connecting surface findings with deeper regulatory processes.

The model further refines interpretation through terrain physiology, which acknowledges that every patient presents a unique biological landscape. Emissive signals are therefore read not as universal patterns but as reflections of terrain qualities such as congestion, metabolic imbalance, or neurogenic strain. This perspective individualizes the analysis, ensuring that the same biospectral sign may carry different meaning depending on the terrain in which it arises.

R-CIIM strengthens its rigor through confirmatory clinical correlations, requiring that findings be interpreted alongside patient history, symptomatology, and when available, complementary tests. By anchoring interpretation to clinical reality, this step prevents the isolation of imaging from lived experience and secures the reliability of biospectral reasoning.

The model leads naturally into integrative therapeutic guidance. Interpretation does not remain descriptive; it extends into action, translating the evaluative narrative into strategies of care. By doing so, R-CIIM ensures that emissive images reveal dysfunction and orient resolution, linking the act of interpretation directly to the therapeutic path.

By weaving these five dimensions into a continuous interpretive sequence, R-CIIM bridges the longstanding divide between physiological imaging and clinical logic. It expands the utility of infrared-based analysis from visual description to evaluation precision, while safeguarding the individuality of each patient. In this balance of standardization and personalization, R-CIIM secures its place as the interpretive foundation of Biospectral Medicine.

STEP 1

REFINED ZONE DESCRIPTION

Anatomical Precision as the Foundation of Functional Interpretation

The first step in the R-CIIM model is the establishment of anatomical precision. Interpretation begins not with color scales or surface impressions, but with the exact definition of the zone under examination.

While most infrared imaging systems generate free-form visualizations that offer a wide view of surface emissions, Biospectral Medicine introduces a structured zonal framework that divides the body into reproducible, anatomically grounded regions. This approach allows the clinician to conduct systematic comparisons across time, between contralateral sides, and within interconnected physiological systems.

The design of these zones was not arbitrary. Each of the nineteen regions employed in Biospectral Imaging has been delineated as a functionally coherent unit, in which vascular, neural, musculoskeletal, metabolic, and organ-reflective elements converge. Their definition arose from thousands of clinical evaluations conducted by Felipe Reitz, where recurrent emissive patterns revealed consistent anatomical boundaries.

These observations were subsequently validated by longitudinal follow-up, by comparative diagnostics such as Doppler ultrasound and laboratory testing, and by the repeated consistency of inter-image findings in chronic conditions. In this way, the zonal model provides a structural foundation that transforms biospectral imagery from a descriptive surface phenomenon into a disciplined instrument of clinical reasoning.

Without defined anatomical segmentation, interpretation risks losing its clinical sharpness. When emissive patterns are read without zonal boundaries, they become excessively general, reducing the capacity to localize dysfunction with precision. Such generalization undermines the interpretative value of the image, leaving the practitioner with a broad impression but without the detail required to connect findings to specific structures or systems.

Equally problematic is the danger of subjectivity. In the absence of clear anatomical segmentation, interpretation relies heavily on the practitioner's personal familiarity or experience, which inevitably varies.

What one observer perceives as significant, another may dismiss, and this variability weakens the reliability of biospectral analysis. By anchoring interpretation in a zonal framework, subjectivity is replaced with structured consistency, making the reading less dependent on individual perception and more aligned with reproducible clinical logic.

A further limitation arises when images cannot be reliably compared over time. Without stable zones, longitudinal follow-up becomes uncertain, as the regions under analysis may shift or overlap from one session to the next. This compromises the ability to measure progress, track therapeutic outcomes, or identify subtle changes in chronic conditions. Reproducibility is therefore essential for evaluation clarity and for monitoring the trajectory of care.

By addressing these three risks, generalization, subjectivity, and lack of reproducibility, the refined zonal description of Step 1 provides the essential foundation for all subsequent stages of the R-CIIM model. It ensures that interpretation begins with anatomical discipline, allowing every emissive signal to be situated with clarity, consistency, and long-term clinical value.

The Value of a Zone-Based Interpretative Language

Establishing a Common Interpretive Structure

One of the most significant contributions of the R-CIIM framework is the creation of a zone-based interpretative language. This innovation transforms biospectral imaging from a descriptive visual tool into a structured interpretive system. By defining and naming reproducible anatomical regions, R-CIIM provides clinicians with a common reference point, ensuring that findings are communicated with precision and consistency.

The language of zones does not attempt to label disease, but rather establishes a shared framework in which biospectral signals can be described, compared, and taught with clarity. In this way, what might otherwise remain a subjective impression becomes part of an organized vocabulary that can be applied across disciplines and clinical settings.

Advancing Reproducibility, Education, and Clinical Application

This zone-based language strengthens the field in several interconnected ways. First, it encourages cross-clinician reproducibility by ensuring that different practitioners, working in different contexts, can interpret the same emissive patterns with comparable logic. When zones are standardized, interpretation becomes less dependent on individual style and more aligned with structured reasoning, which enhances both reliability and credibility.

It also supports educational standardization, offering students and new practitioners a clear system through which to learn and apply biospectral interpretation. Instead of depending on years of subjective experience, the language of zones provides a scaffold for teaching, allowing clinical training to progress systematically from basic recognition of emissive fields to more advanced integrative reasoning.

The framework further allows correlation with organ systems and structural networks, creating a natural bridge between the surface image and deeper functional processes. Each zone carries relationships to vascular, musculoskeletal, neural, or visceral domains, and by anchoring emissive findings within this map, the interpretation gains functional depth without making diagnostic claims.

A zone-based language facilitates consistent follow-up and care plan evaluation. Because the same zones can be compared over time, clinicians can monitor changes in emissive activity with greater confidence, evaluating whether therapeutic strategies are producing functional shifts.

This consistency is vital for long-term care, as it allows patients and clinicians alike to see tangible evidence of change, reinforcing both confidence in the process and adherence to therapeutic strategies recommendations.

Through these interrelated functions, the R-CIIM language transforms biospectral imagery into a reproducible, teachable, and clinically adaptable system. It ensures that the interpretation of images is methodologically sound and transferable across practitioners, educational settings, and therapeutic contexts, establishing a standard that supports both scientific integrity and individualized care.

Integration with Biospectral Logic

Establishing the Basis for Interpretation

For the R-CIIM model to function as a structured interpretative system, each zone must be described in anatomical terms and integrated with the broader logic of biospectral interpretation. This integration ensures that surface findings are never read as isolated irregularities but as signals embedded within a network of structure, physiology, and terrain.

The mapping of zones therefore creates more than a visual grid; it forms the foundation upon which all subsequent interpretive steps rest. Without such refinement and standardization, pattern recognition would risk becoming inconsistent, correlation would weaken, and interpretation would lack the coherence expected in evidence-based clinical reasoning.

From Boundaries to Systemic Relevance

In practice, each zone is defined first by its topographical boundaries, which may follow muscular compartments, vertebral levels, or other reproducible anatomical landmarks. These boundaries establish the structural clarity needed for consistent comparison, whether across sides of the body, between patients, or over time within the same case.

Beyond surface boundaries, zones are characterized by their underlying physiological relevance. This includes patterns of innervation, vascular pathways, and drainage routes that give functional depth to what might otherwise be a superficial field. By anchoring emissive findings to these physiological substrates, interpretation gains both logic and plausibility.

Each zone is also enriched by knowledge of its common clinical presentations. Over thousands of observations, recurrent phenomena such as muscular tension, asymmetry, or reactive patterns have been consistently associated with specific regions.

These recurring presentations provide an experiential layer of interpretation, reminding the clinician that biospectral signals are not abstract but correlate with functional disturbances often encountered in practice.

Zones are understood in terms of their interaction with systemic terrain. No region exists in isolation; each reflects and participates in broader dynamics such as neurovascular regulation, lymphatic flow, or segmental organ relationships. Recognizing these interactions prevents the error of localism and ensures that interpretation accounts for the systemic context in which the emissive signal appears.

Through the integration of boundaries, physiological depth, clinical observation, and systemic interaction, each zone acquires a coherent identity within biospectral logic. This identity transforms the surface image into a structured foundation, allowing subsequent R-CIIM steps, classification, correlation, and therapeutic reasoning, to unfold with clarity and reproducibility.

STEP 2

CLINICAL IMPORTANCE OF THE ZONE

Understanding Each Zone's Interpretative and Systemic Significance

Once the anatomical boundaries of a zone have been defined, the next step in the R-CIIM model is to clarify its clinical importance. This transition from structure to function is essential, because not all zones contribute equally to evaluation reasoning.

Some regions serve as primary expression areas where physiological dysfunction becomes directly visible, while others reveal more indirect, compensatory patterns that emerge as the body adapts to systemic stress. The ability to distinguish between primary and secondary signals protects the clinician from misinterpretation and ensures that the most relevant findings guide the evaluation process.

In Biospectral Medicine, the clinical importance of a zone is never reduced to superficial deviations of surface temperature. Instead, each region is evaluated through the lens of functional and integrative physiology, where emission signals are understood as markers of deeper regulatory dynamics.

This step positions the zone as more than a surface field, it becomes a interpretative interface that connects emissive patterns with the physiology of circulation, innervation, tissue tone, organ correspondence, and drainage.

Zone-Specific Physiological Relationships

Every zone possesses its own network of physiological relationships, which explain why emissive changes in that region carry specific interpretative weight. A central consideration is the presence of vascular pathways, since both arterial supply and venous return determine how well tissues are nourished and how effectively metabolic byproducts are cleared. Alterations in vascular flow often leave a distinct emissive signature, and zones with dense vascular connections provide particularly meaningful insights.

Equally significant are neurovegetative reflexes, which include the influence of sympathetic ganglia and dermatomal patterns. These reflexive circuits link the skin and deeper organs through autonomic pathways, allowing emissive changes to reveal regulatory imbalances that extend beyond the immediate surface.

Zones are also tied to muscular tension chains and fascial pathways, which create structural lines of stress and compensation throughout the body. Because these connective networks transmit both mechanical and regulatory forces, emissive irregularities often reflect chronic postural loading or myofascial restriction that extends across distant regions.

Another dimension is the organ segmental correspondence, where zones reflect viscerocutaneous relationships. In these cases, the skin acts as a projection field for deeper organ states, a phenomenon well documented in the study of reflex pathways. Recognition of these correspondences allows the clinician to connect localized surface findings with systemic organ regulation, while maintaining interpretive caution and functional neutrality.

Zones may hold particular relevance for lymphatic drainage, as in axillary or inguinal fields. When lymphatic flow is compromised, emissive mapping often reveals signs of stagnation that affect the region itself and influence the dynamics of adjacent systems.

Together, these relationships demonstrate why each zone must be evaluated not simply as an isolated surface area, but as an integrative field where vascular, neural, musculoskeletal, organ-related, and lymphatic factors converge.

By situating emissive findings within this physiological web, the clinician can recognize both the interpretative and systemic significance of each zone, ensuring that interpretation remains both functionally grounded and clinically meaningful.

Interpreting Biospectral Associations

From Observation to Functional Meaning

Once the physiological relationships of a zone have been established, the next interpretive step is to determine what type of disturbance the emissive alteration may represent. Not every biospectral signal carries the same meaning. Some reflect immediate local dysfunction, while others reveal systemic adaptation or deeper organ correspondence.

The role of the clinician is to position each finding within its functional context, so that the image is not over-read as physiological response nor under-read as trivial variation. By framing emissive changes within categories of association, the R-CIIM model provides a disciplined way to move from raw signal to functional meaning.

Categories of Interpretation

In certain situations, an emissive alteration reflects a local structural dysfunction, where the irregularity corresponds directly to changes in the tissues beneath the zone, muscular overload, fascial restriction, or localized circulatory strain. In other cases, the signal points toward a referred systemic pattern, in which the surface field acts as a projection site for stresses distributed along vascular or fascial pathways.

There are also circumstances where the finding represents a segmental response to deep organ imbalance. Through viscerocutaneous reflexes, disturbances within internal organs may manifest as specific emissive changes in related cutaneous zones, highlighting the interconnectedness of somatic and visceral physiology.

Beyond these relationships, emissive findings can also embody a compensatory metabolic terrain signal, expressing the body's adaptive efforts in the face of systemic strain such as congestion, endocrine load, or lymphatic stagnation.

By distinguishing among these interpretive possibilities, local, referred, segmental, or compensatory, the clinician ensures that each emissive finding is situated within a structured logic. This approach prevents reductionism, maintains clinical neutrality, and secures the value of biospectral imaging as a functional, evidence-based guide to individualized care.

For example, changes in the dorsal lower leg zone may indicate impaired venous return or fascial strain, but could also reflect segmental renal or lumbar dysfunction, depending on lateralization and zone overlap.

Stratifying Interpretive Priority

The Principle of Interpretive Weight

An essential refinement introduced by the R-CIIM model is the concept of interpretive weight. Not all zones contribute equally to clinical interpretation, and some carry greater stability and reliability than others. Regions such as the anterior tibial surfaces or the supraclavicular areas are less influenced by external variables, making them particularly valuable for detecting subtle or early dysfunctions.

By contrast, other regions may demonstrate higher reactivity, reflecting compensatory changes or short-term adaptations rather than primary alterations. Understanding this hierarchy of reliability allows the clinician to give greater emphasis to zones that consistently mirror functional imbalance while approaching reactive areas with interpretive caution.

In this way, the model balances sensitivity with specificity, ensuring that the richness of biospectral imagery translates into structured interpretive reasoning.

Applying Functional Importance to Clinical Reasoning

When interpretive weight is considered from the outset, the clinician gains a clearer path for decision-making. Stable zones with high interpretive yield can be prioritized, forming the backbone of interpretation and serving as anchors against which more variable findings are compared.

This anchoring effect allows emissive anomalies to be correlated across multiple systems in a logical way, revealing patterns that extend beyond isolated zones and pointing toward systemic coherence or systemic imbalance.

With this layered perspective, it becomes possible to distinguish primary findings from those that are secondary or compensatory. Primary findings, often revealed in zones of greater stability, indicate areas where dysfunction originates or consolidates. Secondary findings, more common in reactive fields, may reflect the body's attempts to adapt or redistribute strain.

Differentiating between the two prevents misinterpretation and directs therapeutic strategies toward root causes rather than surface effects.

The weighting of zones also improves the efficiency of confirmatory assessments. When priority zones highlight probable dysfunctions, complementary tests such as laboratory analysis or imaging can be planned more strategically, reducing unnecessary procedures and focusing resources where they are most likely to yield meaningful confirmation.

Through the integration of interpretive weight into the interpretive process, the R-CIIM model provides clinicians with a hierarchy of reliability. This structured stratification refines both the accuracy of biospectral interpretation and the efficiency of subsequent clinical actions, reinforcing the model's role as a rigorous and practical framework for functional evaluations.

Integrating Clinical Judgment

Within the R-CIIM model, biospectral imaging is not regarded as a static visual artifact but as a medium of biological communication.

Each image becomes a map in which emissive signals are arranged like phrases in a systemic language, conveying information about how the organism regulates, compensates, and adapts. The interpretive act is therefore not limited to observing shapes or color contrasts; it requires discerning meaning from the placement of signals within defined zones.

Clinical judgment arises when the physician connects these zone-specific findings to their functional relevance, appreciating that the same emissive variation may hold different significance depending on whether it occurs in a stable anchor region, a reactive surface, or a compensatory field.

By reading the image in this way, the clinician translates biospectral data into a coherent narrative of functional regulation, transforming what appears as surface emission into clinically meaningful communication.

STEP 3

ROI MAPPING AND PATTERN RECOGNITION

From Emission Patterns to Functional Insight

The third step in the R-CIIM model advances from defining zones of interest to a more refined process of mapping and recognizing emissive patterns within those zones. These Regions of Interest (ROIs) are the specific sites where biospectral deviations emerge with greater intensity or persistence, offering clues about the organism's regulatory state.

In conventional thermography, practitioners have often relied on colour variations alone to suggest hyper- or hypothermic states, managing the image primarily as a temperature gradient.

Biospectral Medicine, however, views these same signals as spectral expressions of tissue function and dysfunction, grounded in the interplay of neurovascular regulation, metabolic load, reactive terrain, and organ-related physiology. This broader interpretive frame elevates ROIs from simple hot or cold spots into meaningful markers of functional dynamics.

Precision Beyond Surface Heat

The identification of ROIs requires careful discrimination, since not every visual irregularity carries equal clinical value. One of the most reliable markers is asymmetry between bilateral zones, where one side demonstrates a consistent emissive divergence from its contralateral counterpart. Such asymmetries, when reproducible, often reflect localized dysfunction or unbalanced systemic regulation.

Another key feature is the presence of focal emissions that do not conform to expected anatomical contours. These stand out because they resist explanation by underlying muscular, vascular, or skeletal boundaries, suggesting instead a regulatory or functional imbalance that requires further exploration.

ROIs also gain significance when they appear as persistent anomalies across serial evaluations. Transient emissive variations may reflect environmental influence or momentary regulation, but persistence over repeated sessions indicates a stable functional disturbance. This temporal consistency gives weight to the finding and reinforces its interpretive importance.

The clinician must attend to discrepancies between an ROI and patient-reported symptoms. When the emissive finding diverges from subjective complaints, it may reveal subclinical dysfunction or compensatory processes that the patient has not yet perceived. Conversely, alignment between ROI and symptom location strengthens clinical correlation, confirming that the image is reflecting lived experience.

By integrating these criteria, ROI mapping becomes far more than an exercise in visual inspection. It evolves into a structured method of identifying focal points of functional imbalance, ensuring that emissive anomalies are interpreted with rigor and tied meaningfully to the patient's physiological narrative. This transformation, of surface deviation into functional insight, marks the distinctive contribution of Step 3 within the R-CIIM model.

Biospectral ROI mapping is always guided by anatomical logic. Regions of Interest are not chosen arbitrarily but are identified in accordance with the body's structural and physiological organization. They frequently align with fascial planes, vascular trajectories, or nerve distributions, which anchor the emissive signal in recognizable pathways.

For example, a vertically oriented ROI that extends medially from the scapula toward the lower back may represent tension along a myofascial chain or, in certain contexts, reflect a segmental renal reflex projection. Such anatomical consistency greatly enhances the reproducibility of findings.

It also provides a foundation for longitudinal follow-up, allowing clinicians to evaluate whether a signal maintains the same location and form over time, shifts into new regions, or resolves under therapeutic influence.

Biospectral Consistency Patterns

Within this framework, the concept of biospectral consistency patterns becomes central. Each ROI is evaluated for its presence and its temporal behavior, whether it remains stable, fluctuates, or progressively expands. This classification provides insight into the functional timeline of the disturbance.

An ROI that is sharp, intense, and of recent onset often reflects an acute presentation, suggesting a dynamic regulatory response in its early stages. When an ROI persists over multiple evaluations without change, it is more consistent with a chronic-stable state, indicating a long-standing functional adaptation that, while not worsening, has not resolved.

In contrast, an ROI that gradually enlarges or intensifies signals a chronic-progressive course, where the underlying imbalance is advancing despite compensatory efforts.

These dynamic profiles are not interpreted in isolation but correlated with functional physiology. Acute ROIs frequently align with heightened reactive or neurovascular responses, whereas chronic-stable signals often point toward structural adaptation or fixed terrain imbalance.

Chronic-progressive findings may be associated with vascular insufficiency, persistent metabolic burden, or organ system dysregulation that fails to stabilize. By discerning these temporal dynamics, the clinician gains a practical timeline of dysfunction, moving beyond static observation to an appreciation of how the body is actively responding, adapting, or deteriorating.

Through this approach, Step 3 transforms ROI mapping into a process of both spatial and temporal pattern recognition. The emphasis on anatomical coherence ensures reproducibility, while the classification of consistency patterns adds depth by revealing the trajectory of functional disturbance. Together, these elements secure ROI analysis as one of the most clinically powerful aspects of the R-CIIM framework.

Pattern Recognition: Reading Biological Communication

In Biospectral Medicine, the art of pattern recognition extends far beyond the surface impression of colour visualization. What the practitioner learns to detect is not simply contrast but structured forms of biological communication, each carrying a distinct functional meaning. One important dimension is the presence of anisospectral distributions, where asymmetric emissions emerge between paired regions of the body.

These asymmetries often suggest unilateral dysfunction and represent an evolution of the older concept of "anisothermia," reframed here as spectral imbalance rather than mere temperature difference.

Equally significant are segmental patterns, in which emissions align with dermatomes or with organ-related viscerocutaneous projections. These bands follow known neurological or reflexive pathways, linking surface signals with deeper systemic processes and revealing how organ states can project outward into the cutaneous landscape.

The clinician must also be attuned to radiated patterns, where emissive signals spread outward from a central node. These configurations frequently indicate a neurogenic or vascular source, suggesting that the disturbance originates at a focal point and then distributes along neural or circulatory channels. Such radiations highlight dynamic processes rather than fixed abnormalities, showing how regulation itself creates identifiable biospectral forms.

A further dimension involves multifocal patterns, characterized by scattered ROIs in non-contiguous zones. Unlike localized disturbances, these dispersed signals often point toward metabolic or terrain-driven imbalances, in which the body expresses systemic strain through multiple, seemingly unrelated emission sites. Recognizing this type of distribution allows the clinician to move from local interpretation to a broader appreciation of terrain physiology.

The interpretive act does not end with visual classification; it requires integration with anatomical knowledge and clinical listening. A patient may present with no overt complaints yet reveal a persistent ROI over the right iliac fossa. If this finding is observed consistently across serial imaging and accompanied by subtle digestive irregularities or pelvic tension, it may prompt further investigation.

Such exploration could uncover functional issues involving the appendix, ovaries, or regional lymphatics, imbalances that may remain clinically silent in early stages but are nonetheless visible in biospectral mapping.

In this way, pattern recognition becomes one of the most powerful aspects of R-CIIM, transforming emissions from surface anomalies into early signals of biological imbalance. What begins as a visual irregularity is revealed as a form of communication, an intelligible sign that the body is signalling adaptation, compensation, or dysfunction before these processes consolidate into obvious functional change.

Supporting Literature

The principles of ROI mapping and pattern recognition within the R-CIIM model are supported by a growing body of literature that underscores the interpretive value of stability and asymmetry over isolated numerical data.

In their comprehensive review, Ring and Ammer (2012) concluded that *"the pattern is more important than the temperature value,"* pointing to the fact that consistent asymmetries, or variations in shape and extension, often carry greater interpretive weight than simple point measurements of temperature difference. Their work reinforces the view that imaging should be understood less as a tool of quantification and more as a tool of functional pattern recognition.

This perspective is echoed by Lahiri et al. (2012), who emphasized that thermal imaging proves particularly useful in detecting reactive or regulatory activity when interpretation is grounded in consistent pattern recognition rather than numerical deltas alone.

By shifting the emphasis from absolute values to relative distributions and repeated findings, these authors highlight the importance of reproducibility and anatomical logic in elevating thermography from visual screening to a reliable interpretive adjunct.

Such observations resonate directly with the philosophy of Biospectral Medicine and the R-CIIM framework. By prioritizing pattern stability, respecting anatomical boundaries, and incorporating terrain-based reasoning, the model ensures that Regions of Interest are evaluated in a way that is both systematic and clinically relevant.

This alignment between published literature and the structured methodology of R-CIIM reinforces its validity as an interpretive system capable of transforming biospectral images into reproducible and actionable clinical insights.

STEP 4

KEY INTERPRETIVE QUESTIONS

Clinical Reasoning Guided by Biospectral Clues

Once a Region of Interest (ROI) has been identified and its emissive pattern categorized, the fourth step of the R-CIIM model is to translate this visual signal into targeted clinical inquiry. At this stage, the image no longer functions as a static record but as a catalyst for dialogue between physiology and patient history.

The strength of Biospectral Medicine does not lie in the mere recognition of anomalies, but in the disciplined process of asking what these anomalies suggest about underlying function.

Through this process, passive observation is transformed into active reasoning. The clinician interprets each ROI not as an isolated irregularity but as a biospectral clue pointing toward vascular dynamics, neuromuscular adaptation, metabolic strain, or organ-related regulation.

This interpretive shift requires the practitioner to formulate precise questions: Why does this zone demonstrate persistent asymmetry? Could the emission reflect compensatory load rather than primary dysfunction? Does the patient's history confirm, contradict, or add nuance to the emissive finding? In this way, the image itself becomes a guide that directs the line of questioning.

Equally important is the connection to the patient's lived experience. An ROI gains its true significance only when interpreted alongside the narrative of symptoms, functional limitations, or subtle complaints described during consultation.

A localized emissive anomaly that at first appears incidental may acquire interpretive importance when the patient recalls intermittent discomfort, digestive irregularities, or fatigue linked to the corresponding physiological system. On the other hand, an ROI unaccompanied by evident symptoms may point toward subclinical processes, inviting closer observation and longitudinal follow-up.

Step 4 thus represents a pivotal transition in the R-CIIM framework. It bridges the technical act of image analysis with the human dimension of clinical care, ensuring that biospectral findings are never read in isolation but always contextualized through dialogue, reasoning, and corroboration.

By embedding targeted interpretive questions into the interpretive process, the model preserves both scientific discipline and patient individuality, positioning the image as an active partner in the search for functional clarity.

From Image to Inquiry

Every Region of Interest (ROI) becomes the starting point for a series of targeted clinical questions. These inquiries are not generic checklists, but precise prompts shaped by the location of the ROI, the type of pattern it displays, and the way the emission behaves over time.

For example, a linear ROI radiating from the axillary region naturally directs attention to possible lymphatic congestion, vascular compromise, or autonomic involvement in the thoracic outlet, guiding the clinician to consider these systems in relation to the image.

To achieve this depth of reasoning, the clinician first considers what anatomical structures lie beneath the ROI, evaluating whether veins, nerves, fasciae, or organ reflections may account for the observed emission. The next step is to determine whether the pattern is characteristic of a specific physiological system, such as vascular, neural, immune, or musculoskeletal regulation. This systemic perspective prevents superficial interpretation and anchors the signal in a functional framework.

The clinician then evaluates whether the patient's symptoms correlate with the emissive finding, since alignment between lived experience and biospectral signals adds interpretive weight. At the same time, the pattern itself is analysed for its distribution, whether it appears unilaterally or bilaterally, and whether it is stable, fluctuating, or progressively evolving. These temporal and spatial features contribute critical information about the trajectory of the underlying imbalance.

The practitioner reflects on whether the emission represents a local disturbance or whether it could be referred from deeper dysfunction. By maintaining this dual perspective, the image is not reduced to surface appearance but connected to potential systemic processes.

Through such structured inquiry, each ROI becomes a functional hypothesis generator. This process allows the clinician to triage and prioritize which systems may be involved, focusing subsequent assessments where they are most likely to be informative. In doing so, R-CIIM strengthens clinical precision, minimizes unnecessary testing, and transforms biospectral imaging into an active partner in interpretive reasoning.

Integration with the 9 Interpretive Categories

Each Region of Interest (ROI) identified through the R-CIIM model becomes meaningful only when transformed into targeted questions. To systematize this process, Biospectral Medicine employs nine interpretive categories, each of which directs inquiry toward a distinct functional system.

When a finding is considered within the vascular and circulatory category, the clinician may ask whether the ROI reflects impaired venous return, early capillary overload, or signs of arterial insufficiency. If the pattern suggests structural or mechanical strain, the focus shifts to the muscular and myofascial category, where the central questions involve tension chains, postural compensation, or the presence of chronic fascial adhesion.

In zones that project closer to the skeleton, the clinician asks whether the ROI points to the skeletal and articular category, exploring the possibility of joint irritation, degenerative changes, or periosteal involvement.

Patterns that align with dermatomes or radiating neural trajectories guide questioning into the nervous system and spine category, where the key inquiry is whether the emission reflects a segmental neural pathway or a neurogenic projection. When the ROI occurs in recognized drainage fields, the lymphatic and immune category raises questions of stagnation, immune reactivity, or impaired clearance.

In certain contexts, the finding may direct attention to the organs and GNM category, prompting questions about viscerocutaneous reflexes, neurovegetative segmental zones, or expressions consistent with an active-phase organ response.

Other emissions track along energetic lines, leading to the acupuncture and meridians category, where the inquiry centers on whether the ROI follows the path of a known meridian or reveals a blocked energetic pathway. Broader and less localized disturbances may point toward the energetic and frequency category, prompting the clinician to ask whether the emission could signal terrain-level dysregulation in the body's electromagnetic or biofield domains.

Systemic or diffuse signals often direct inquiry into the metabolic and endocrine category, where the central questions involve whether the ROI arises from hormonal imbalance, terrain instability, or altered cellular metabolism.

By aligning each ROI with the nine interpretive categories in the form of questions, the clinician is guided toward precise lines of reasoning rather than vague speculation. These inquiries do not determine a diagnosis on their own but establish a structured foundation for Step 5, where confirmatory clinical testing validates or rules out the hypotheses generated.

In this way, the nine categories function as a questioning framework that translates biospectral signals into targeted, system-specific exploration.

Clinical Listening as a Compass

Felipe Reitz emphasizes that interpretive questioning within the R-CIIM model must remain inseparably linked to the patient's subjective narrative. An image may present a striking ROI, yet its meaning crystallizes only when read in dialogue with the patient's lived experience.

A clear example is an emissive finding over the left supraclavicular zone. The direction of inquiry changes profoundly depending on what the patient describes. If long-standing neck tension is reported, the ROI may be approached through a musculoskeletal lens, raising questions of muscular strain or fascial overload.

If the patient instead speaks of endocrine irregularities, the same ROI invites consideration of hormonal influences, placing the finding within a metabolic and regulatory framework. When the narrative centres on emotional repression or a sense of unresolved conflict in the chest, the interpretation extends toward organ-related or GNM-linked reflections, suggesting that the ROI may express deeper psycho-physiological dynamics.

And if the patient is entirely asymptomatic, the ROI becomes a prompt for exploratory reasoning, encouraging the clinician to investigate subclinical processes or to follow the finding longitudinally for signs of progression.

In this way, the image and the narrative form a true interpretive duet. The biospectral signal provides objective structure, while the patient's voice adds subjective depth, and only through their integration does interpretation achieve accuracy.

This combination prevents the detachment of imaging from lived reality and ensures that each ROI is mapped and meaningfully contextualized within the full spectrum of clinical reasoning.

Scientific Context

The integrative character of the R-CIIM model is firmly supported in the scientific literature. Lahiri et al. (2012) have emphasized that *"clinical context is essential for the interpretation of thermal anomalies,"* underscoring that emissive findings acquire meaning only when correlated with the broader physiological and patient narrative.

Ring and Ammer (2012) further note that *"a pattern must be seen in anatomical and physiological coherence,"* reminding practitioners that isolated surface changes cannot be read in abstraction from the structures and systems they represent.

Together, these observations validate the interpretive discipline embedded in R-CIIM. By insisting on anatomical grounding, physiological plausibility, and contextual reasoning, the model ensures that biospectral images are not reduced to descriptive visuals but are transformed into clinically relevant insights.

This structured approach positions R-CIIM as a bridge between imaging and therapeutic logic, showing how scientific principles and clinical reasoning converge to guide decision-making in a reproducible and evidence-oriented manner.

STEP 5

CONFIRMATORY CLINICAL TESTING

From Hypothesis to Objective Correlation

After the formulation of key interpretive questions in Step 4, the interpretive process of R-CIIM progresses toward validation. The fifth step shifts the focus from hypothesis generation to clinical confirmation, requiring the practitioner to move beyond image-based reasoning and establish correlation with objective findings.

This transition ensures that biospectral interpretation does not remain in the realm of speculation but is anchored in data that can be measured, reproduced, and integrated into broader clinical decision-making.

Confirmatory testing may involve a range of complementary methods, including laboratory analysis, imaging modalities such as Doppler ultrasound or MRI, functional assessments of circulation or neuromuscular performance, and targeted physical examination. The selection of tests is never random; it is guided by the zone involved, the category of interpretation, and the interpretive questions generated in the earlier step.

For instance, a biospectral ROI linked to possible vascular overload may prompt Doppler investigation of venous return, while an emission associated with suspected myofascial tension might lead to palpatory assessment or structural imaging. In each case, the confirmatory tool serves to test the plausibility of the biospectral hypothesis.

This step creates balance within the model. On one side lies the interpretive power of Computerized Biospectral Imaging (CBI), which reveals patterns of regulation and adaptation invisible to conventional tools.

On the other side stand established diagnostic sciences, which provide quantifiable data and recognized standards of evidence. Step 5 integrates these two perspectives, forming a hybrid model of investigative diagnosis. The image generates the question, the clinical reasoning directs the inquiry, and the confirmatory test provides the measurable answer.

By embedding confirmatory testing into the interpretive sequence, R-CIIM secures both scientific rigor and clinical safety. The model emphasizes that biospectral findings are not replacements for conventional diagnostics but catalysts for their targeted use.

This approach reduces unnecessary testing by directing investigations toward the most relevant systems, while simultaneously protecting patients from over-reliance on imaging alone. In doing so, Step 5 transforms the process of interpretation into a cycle of hypothesis, correlation, and verification, aligning Biospectral Medicine with the highest standards of functional and integrative evaluations.

Matching Tests to Interpretive Categories

The nine interpretive categories of Biospectral Medicine orient interpretation and provide a framework for selecting appropriate confirmatory tests. By aligning emissive findings with system-specific assessments, the clinician ensures that each hypothesis generated by R-CIIM is evaluated with rigor and objectivity.

When an ROI is interpreted through the vascular and circulatory category, confirmatory tools may include Doppler ultrasound to assess venous return, Ankle-Brachial Index (ABI) for arterial sufficiency, capillaroscopy for microvascular status, or reactivity testing to evaluate dynamic vascular responses. These examinations help determine whether the biospectral signal corresponds to measurable circulatory strain or impaired perfusion.

In cases where emissive findings point toward the metabolic and endocrine category, laboratory analysis provides the most relevant confirmation. Markers such as fasting insulin, HbA1c, thyroid hormones (TSH, free T3, free T4), cortisol, vitamin D, or homocysteine allow the clinician to assess metabolic balance, endocrine regulation, and systemic terrain quality. Such testing clarifies whether diffuse or multifocal emissive patterns have a biochemical correlate.

For ROIs associated with the muscular and myofascial category, confirmation often relies on functional and structural assessment. Palpation and range-of-motion testing remain valuable clinical tools, while electromyography (EMG) or targeted ultrasound can provide objective evidence of muscular overload, fascial adhesion, or myofascial trigger activity. These methods allow surface emissions to be correlated with verifiable biomechanical dysfunction.

The decision of which test to employ is not determined by category alone but also by the characteristics of the emissive pattern itself. Symmetry, distribution, and patient-reported experience all guide the process.

A bilateral finding often points toward systemic involvement, suggesting the need for metabolic, endocrine, or vascular investigation. A sharply localized unilateral hotspot, by contrast, may suggest focal vascular entrapment, neuromuscular strain, or reactive activity, directing testing toward the specific structures beneath the ROI.

By matching confirmatory tools to both interpretive categories and pattern features, the clinician avoids indiscriminate testing and focuses investigative effort where it will be most meaningful. This method preserves efficiency, protects patients from unnecessary procedures, and reinforces the R-CIIM model's commitment to reproducibility, logic, and integrative precision.

Structuring the Confirmation

In practical application, every Region of Interest initiates a structured pathway of verification. The first dimension of this process is to determine what to test, identifying the biomarker, physiological parameter, or structural feature most likely implicated by the ROI. This step ensures that confirmatory investigations are not arbitrary but directed toward specific hypotheses generated by the biospectral finding.

The next dimension clarifies why the test matters, situating the suspected disturbance within a framework of clinical relevance. A proposed biomarker or functional parameter gains significance only when its alteration would meaningfully explain the patient's symptoms, regulatory imbalance, or terrain expression. In this way, testing is tied to clinical logic rather than to rote data collection.

Once the rationale is established, the clinician selects how to test, choosing the laboratory method, imaging modality, or functional assessment that offers the most reliable confirmation. This decision balances precision with accessibility, ensuring that the investigative tool is both technically valid and feasible within the clinical context.

The process considers what findings would be expected if the ROI reflects the hypothesized dysfunction. Establishing anticipated outcomes before testing prevents misinterpretation of results, as it forces the clinician to articulate how a given laboratory value, imaging feature, or functional parameter would corroborate or contradict the biospectral observation.

Through this structured sequence, the act of confirmation becomes a disciplined extension of the interpretive model. Each ROI is mapped, questioned, and followed into a chain of logical verification, where the selection, rationale, methodology, and anticipated outcome are all aligned. This approach reinforces reproducibility, strengthens clinical reasoning, and ensures that biospectral imaging functions as a catalyst for evidence-based investigation rather than as an isolated technique.

Practical Examples of Confirmation

To illustrate how confirmatory testing aligns with biospectral interpretation, consider a focal high-emission finding in the upper left abdominal zone. Within the framework of the organs and GNM category, such a signal may direct inquiry toward splenic physiology.

Confirmation in this case might involve abdominal ultrasound to evaluate structural changes, together with laboratory measures such as a complete blood count with differential, ferritin, and C-reactive protein. Should these tests reveal splenomegaly or elevated reactive markers, the biospectral clue gains objective support, reinforcing its relevance in the clinical picture.

A different scenario involves a cold or inhibose ROI appearing over the posterior cervical region. This pattern can be functionally associated with chronic sympathetic overdrive within the nervous system and spine category.

Objective correlation may then be sought through measures of autonomic regulation, such as heart rate variability analysis, evaluation of vascular response under a cold challenge, or assessment of spinal thermocline dynamics. Consistency between these findings and the biospectral anomaly strengthens the interpretive conclusion and guides therapeutic orientation.

These examples demonstrate how triangulation between biospectral signals, clinical reasoning, and confirmatory testing secures both safety and accuracy in therapeutic decision-making. The process ensures that surface emissions are not accepted in isolation but are translated into actionable insights through a rigorous sequence of observation, inquiry, and verification.

Scientific Validation and Precedent

The integrative emphasis of the R-CIIM model is strongly supported by existing scientific literature. In their comprehensive review, Lahiri et al. (2012) stressed that thermal imaging *"should be integrated with standard diagnostics for maximum clinical reliability"* (p. 240).

This position highlights the fact that emissive findings, while valuable, gain true clinical weight only when correlated with objective diagnostic methods. Ammer and Ring (2010) similarly observed that *"infrared anomalies must be interpreted with correlation to clinical findings and laboratory results"* in order to avoid both overdiagnosis and the misinterpretation of surface variations. Together, these perspectives underscore the necessity of positioning thermal analysis within a larger investigative framework.

The Biospectral model directly addresses this longstanding limitation of conventional thermography. By embedding confirmatory testing into its methodology, it resolves the problem of isolated interpretation and situates Computerized Biospectral Imaging (CBI) as the opening stage of a broader interpretive sequence.

Within this structure, CBI serves as a non-invasive, risk-free triage tool that identifies functional irregularities, which are then examined further through laboratory, imaging, or functional assessment. This layered process ensures that biospectral insights are consistently validated and transformed into clinically reliable knowledge.

In doing so, the R-CIIM model strengthens both the scientific credibility and the practical safety of biospectral interpretation, integrating innovative imaging with established interpretive standards.

Terrain Dynamics

A defining strength of Biospectral Medicine lies in its emphasis on terrain-based interpretation, which becomes particularly relevant when emissive findings point toward metabolic, immunologic, or energetic domains.

Unlike conventional diagnostic models that rely exclusively on biochemical confirmation, the terrain perspective acknowledges that systemic imbalances often manifest across multiple physiological layers. This approach naturally broadens the scope of confirmatory assessment and encourages the clinician to look beyond isolated laboratory values.

In practical application, certain findings may direct inquiry toward the gastrointestinal terrain, where comprehensive stool analysis offers insights into microbial ecology, digestive efficiency, and mucosal health. Other cases call for live blood analysis, which provides a hemato-terrain perspective by revealing rheological patterns, cellular stress markers, and circulatory dynamics not visible in routine blood counts.

When biospectral signals raise suspicion of toxic load or metabolic congestion, targeted evaluation may include heavy metal panels, clarifying whether environmental burden contributes to the observed terrain imbalance. In situations where emissive anomalies appear to resonate with frequency-based patterns, bioresonance or vibrational response testing may provide complementary information, situating the ROI within the body's broader energetic field.

In these contexts, confirmation is not derived from a single biomarker but from a constellation of findings that require cross-system interpretation. The strength of the biospectral model lies precisely in this ability to contextualize signals across biochemical, structural, and energetic domains.

By integrating diverse forms of evidence into a coherent interpretive framework, Biospectral Medicine provides a level of interpretive depth that captures the complexity of terrain physiology while maintaining clinical safety and reproducibility.

STEP 6

TARGETED THERAPEUTIC GUIDELINES

Integrating Biospectral Insights into Strategic Clinical Interventions

Once spectral anomalies have been identified in Step 3, questioned interpretively in Step 4, and corroborated through confirmatory testing in Step 5, at this stage, the clinician enters a decisive phase, the therapeutic response. Step 6 of the R-CIIM model translates interpretive clarity into targeted, terrain-specific interventions, strategically aligned with the functional category of disturbance and with the unique bio-individual profile of the patient.

This moment of translation is fundamental, for it bridges the purely investigative dimension of Biospectral Medicine with the pragmatic dimension of care, ensuring that discovery evolves into precise, clinically effective action.

Unlike conventional symptom-based prescribing, which often seeks only to suppress discomfort or normalize isolated markers, Biospectral Medicine proposes a functional Therapeutic strategy logic.

This logic begins with the anatomical zone where the emissive signal was first detected, extends into the physiological system most directly implicated, and culminates in a therapeutic plan that engages the biological terrain in its full complexity.

Such an approach ensures that intervention is layered, safety-conscious, and root-cause oriented. Resolution is sought not through suppression, but through regulatory harmonization that allows the organism to re-establish its natural balance.

Principles of Therapeutic Targeting

The formulation of therapy in Biospectral Medicine is guided by a set of interpretive principles that integrate structural anatomy, systemic physiology, and bio-emissive patterns. The first principle is that each of the nine interpretive categories invites a corresponding therapeutic logic.

A vascular or circulatory alteration, for example, directs attention to strategies of improving flow dynamics, endothelial resilience, and microcirculatory efficiency.

A muscular or myofascial finding, by contrast, will orient interventions toward releasing contractile tension, restoring fascial elasticity, and recalibrating neuro-muscular coordination.

The second principle is that the zone itself must be respected in terms of its functional role. The frontal abdomen cannot be addressed in the same way as the dorsal cervical region, for their structural contributions to visceral stability and neurovascular relay are profoundly different.

Therapeutic reasoning, therefore, is anchored in both the local function of the emission zone and the systemic consequences that radiate from its dysregulation.

A third principle concerns the patterns of the biological terrain. The biospectral reading does not stop at recognizing an emission increase or decrease; it reveals whether the terrain is congestive, neurogenic, metabolic, or lymphatic in character. A congestive terrain requires a strategy that promotes drainage and circulation, whereas a neurogenic terrain calls for modulation of excitability and synaptic regulation.

The specific spectral signature, whether elevated, diminished, or fluctuating, guides the polarity of therapeutic action, indicating whether stimulation, dispersion, or stabilization is required.

Therapeutic targeting must consider systemic involvement and comorbidity context. Rarely is a spectral disturbance isolated; more often it coexists with metabolic strain, emotional tension, or postural dysfunctions.

For this reason, interventions must be custom-formulated, ranging from precise local applications designed to resolve focal overload, to systemic measures aimed at long-term regulation and resilience.

Through this multilayered reasoning, Step 6 provides the structural bridge between interpretive intelligence and applied care. It secures the uniqueness of Biospectral Medicine as a methodology capable of guiding clinicians beyond description, into the domain of targeted, rational, and terrain-oriented therapeutic action.

Clinical Strategies by Interpretive Category

Interpretive Category	Therapeutic Orientation
1. Vascular / Circulatory	Microcirculation enhancers (e.g., Ginkgo biloba, bioflavonoids), vasotonic phytotherapy, contrast therapy, movement-based vascular mobilization.
2. Muscular / Myofascial	Myofascial release, magnesium, proteolytic enzymes, trauma drainage (Arnica, Rhus tox.), structural osteopathy.
3. Skeletal / Articular	Anti-reactive phytocomplexes, collagen precursors, homeopathics for periosteal regeneration, vitamin D/K2.
4. Nervous System / Spine	Nervine adaptogens (e.g., Ashwagandha, Bacopa), neural therapy, vagal stimulation, HRV training, craniosacral therapy.
5. Lymphatic / Immune	Lymphagogues (e.g., Galium aparine, Phytolacca), immune modulators, drainage strategies (UNDA, Spagyric), fasting.

6. Organs / GNM	Organ-specific support (e.g., liver, pancreas, intestines), psychoemotional terrain mapping, GNM phase-based remedies.
7. Acupuncture / Meridians	Acupuncture, moxibustion, electrostimulation, auricular therapy, meridian-based phytotherapy.
8. Energetic / Frequency	Homeopathics, flower essences, frequency carriers (e.g., nosodes, isotherapics), bioresonance harmonization.
9. Metabolic / Endocrine	Terrain-corrective nutrition, trace minerals (zinc, selenium), hormonal modulators (e.g., Maca, Vitex), detox support.

Therapeutic decisions in Biospectral Medicine are not made solely from biochemical derangement but from functional pattern recognition aligned with physiology.

Strategic Layering and Clinical Judgment

In complex clinical scenarios, it is common for biospectral zones to reveal anomalies that traverse more than one interpretive category simultaneously. A single emission zone may represent the intersection of circulatory compromise, lymphatic congestion, and organ terrain dysfunction, creating a multifactorial pattern that demands nuanced therapeutic reasoning.

The left hypochondrium, for instance, frequently illustrates this principle. Irregular emission in this zone may correspond to vascular phenomena involving splenic perfusion, lymphatic stasis linked to impaired drainage pathways, and organ-specific changes affecting the stomach–spleen terrain. In such a constellation, the therapeutic response cannot be singular or linear; rather, it requires a deliberate sequence of layered interventions that progressively address the biological hierarchy of disturbance.

The first stage in this hierarchy is the phase of drainage. Before the organism can be strengthened or regulated, it must be unburdened of accumulated stasis and metabolic residues. Drainage in this context includes the facilitation of lymphatic flow, hepatic clearance, and in some cases renal or intestinal excretion.

By prioritizing excretory function, the biospectral logic acknowledges that an overloaded terrain cannot respond effectively to restorative inputs. The objective is not aggressive detoxification, which risks destabilization, but rather the opening of physiological channels of elimination so that subsequent measures may find receptivity within the organism.

Once drainage has been established, the second stage of intervention is directed toward restoration. Here the focus shifts from removing burden to rebuilding integrity. Organ-specific trophorestorative strategies are introduced to enhance the resilience of the tissues most implicated in the emissive pattern.

In the example of the left hypochondrium, this may include supportive measures for splenic vitality, gastric mucosal equilibrium, or pancreatic metabolic balance, depending on the spectrum of findings.

Restoration is not conceived merely as replacement but as nourishment and reconstitution, allowing the organ system to recover structural and functional coherence. This phase ensures that the biological substrate regains enough vitality to sustain long-term regulation.

The third stage is that of regulation. After clearance and strengthening, the deeper terrains that shape systemic balance can be addressed. At this level, the therapeutic focus extends toward neuroendocrine coordination, metabolic rhythm, and even the psycho-emotional dynamics emphasized within German New Medicine and related fields.

Regulation includes modulation of excitatory patterns in the nervous system, stabilization of metabolic oscillations, and alignment of the individual's emotional and existential posture with their physiological functioning. It is in this stage that the long-term resilience of the patient is secured, as the organism's capacity for self-regulation is progressively restored.

This sequential layering, drainage, restoration, and regulation, follows a therapeutic logic long employed in traditions such as anthroposophic and isopathic medicine, yet is here refined through the precision of biospectral mapping. The order is not arbitrary; it reflects the biological necessity of moving from excretion to reconstitution and finally to modulation.

To reverse this order would risk reinforcing imbalance, much as attempting to regulate an organ still burdened by toxic load would fail to achieve stability. Strategic layering thus represents both a philosophical stance and a clinical safeguard, ensuring that interventions are delivered in the order most aligned with the organism's intrinsic healing intelligence.

Terrain as the Basis for Individualization

One of the most significant advances introduced by Biospectral Medicine is its capacity to individualize therapy through visual terrain mapping. Rather than offering a static or generic diagnosis, the imagery reveals the patient's unique physiological and regulatory patterns, transforming the act of observation into a direct dialogue with the terrain itself.

The image serves as interpretive confirmation and as a dynamic clinical compass, guiding both the practitioner and the patient toward a truly personalized strategy. When the patient is invited to see the image and to understand its interpretive model, the therapeutic relationship is transformed. Compliance improves markedly, not through persuasion, but because the patient now perceives the logic of intervention as an extension of their own body's signal.

The real power of terrain mapping lies in its longitudinal capacity. Computerized Biospectral Imaging (CBI) does not simply record a snapshot of dysfunction; it allows the clinician to track adaptive or maladaptive processes as they evolve over time. This enables the monitoring of therapeutic strategies responses in real time, ensuring that interventions are not applied rigidly but are continually adjusted in accordance with physiological shifts.

When a congestive terrain begins to open under drainage strategies, or when muscular emissive overload diminishes after regulatory work, the imagery confirms the effectiveness of the chosen path and offers the practitioner the confidence to refine or intensify the plan.

At the same time, repeated biospectral imaging plays a preventive role by identifying compensatory strain in adjacent systems before it consolidates into symptomatic systemic patter. A patient presenting with localized emission irregularities may, for example, show secondary adaptations in vascular or musculoskeletal zones that, if left unchecked, could evolve into new sources of imbalance.

The early detection of these compensations provides the clinician with the opportunity to intervene at a formative stage, preserving systemic integrity and avoiding future chronicity.

As Lahiri et al. (2012) emphasize, repeated imaging "provides an objective measure of functional change over time," a feature that distinguishes functional and integrative models of care from static diagnostic frameworks (p. 241).

In Biospectral Medicine, this objectivity translates into precision care, a care plan process that is not linear but adaptive, not imposed but co-created with the patient's terrain. By aligning therapeutic pathways with real-time visual evidence, the methodology secures its place as a modern reference for individualized, functionally intelligent medicine.

CHAPTER 3

THE 19 EMISSION ZONES
ANATOMICAL MAP AND SPECTRAL LOGIC FOR CLINICAL ANALYSIS

Infrared thermography has long been recognized as a powerful, non-invasive imaging modality capable of visualizing subtle physiological phenomena through surface emission. Its application, however, has often lacked a standardized interpretive framework. In this Atlas, the physical principles of infrared emission are advanced into the methodology of Biospectral Medicine. Here, raw emissive data is no longer viewed as temperature alone, but as a structured biosignal, mapped, categorized, and interpreted through defined anatomical zones and systemic logic.

The *Atlas of Infrared Thermography* addressed this need historically by segmenting the body into 19 discrete thermographic zones, each representing anatomically and functionally distinct regions with specific clinical significance (Ring & Ammer, 2012; Lahiri et al., 2012). As Ring & Ammer note, "infrared imaging can detect changes in cutaneous blood flow and metabolism, providing useful clinical information on underlying pathology" (p. R33).

Building on this foundation, Biospectral Medicine defines these same regions as emission zones, advancing them from descriptive thermographic segments into the structured framework of a biosignal language. To enhance usability and interpretive precision, the 19 zones are organized into four major anatomical and functional groups. This grouping serves multiple purposes: it enables professionals to contextualize emissive findings within relevant anatomical systems, facilitates recognition of complex regulatory imbalances, and streamlines the interpretive workflow by clustering related structures.

Furthermore, these groups align with the principles of the Reitz Clinical Infrared Interpretation Model (R-CIIM), a comprehensive seven-step methodology designed to guide practitioners systematically from image acquisition through to care planning and intervention strategies (Reitz, 2024).

This chapter introduces these four major groups in detail, emphasizing their anatomical boundaries, physiological relevance, and interpretive implications. It also explicates how these groups integrate with the R-CIIM model to provide a structured, reproducible approach to biospectral interpretation and care strategies across diverse clinical contexts.

1. The Four Major Anatomical and Functional Groups of Biospectral Zones

1.1 Lower Extremities Group

The first major group includes Zones 1 to 8, incorporating the frontal and dorsal aspects of the lower and upper legs, including both medial and lateral compartments. The lower extremities represent a complex and highly vascularized region fundamental to locomotion, weight-bearing, and venous return.

Peripheral vascular conditions are prevalent in this region and have been correlated with emissive asymmetries in conventional imaging literature (Norgren et al., 2007). Rockson (2001) further describes how lymphatic dysfunction frequently affects the lower limbs, producing emission patterns consistent with lymphedema and tissue-level inflammatory responses.

From a biospectral standpoint, this group serves as a primary field for evaluating vascular, lymphatic, musculoskeletal, and neurological regulation. The R-CIIM model directs practitioners to assess biospectral asymmetries, hyperemission indicating congestion or ractive behavior, and hypoemission reflecting hypoperfusion states, in order to generate interpretive hypotheses grounded in biosignal interpretation.

Subsequent methodological steps involve applying category-specific clinical inquiries, conducting confirmatory procedures such as Doppler ultrasound or angiographic imaging, and developing care strategies targeted to vascular, neuromuscular, lymphatic, or neuroregulatory dysfunctions.

Clinically, this grouping enables the early detection of circulatory dysregulation, reactive activity, and neuropathic shifts, supporting timely and strategic intervention. It also enhances differentiation between localized and systemic processes by providing a coherent biospectral overview of the limb's vascular and neurofunctional condition.

1.2 Abdominal and Lumbar Group

Zones 9 through 12 cover the frontal abdomen, lateral flanks, and lumbar regions. This group represents a structural and regulatory convergence of visceral organs, musculoskeletal stabilization, and autonomic innervation. Biospectral patterns observed in these zones frequently reflect multifactorial dynamics such as visceral activation, neurofluidic retention, myofascial overload, and autonomic imbalance. Vinik et al. (2013) emphasize the physiological integration between neural and visceral systems in these regions, highlighting their influence on regional regulatory behavior and systemic communication.

The R-CIIM methodology utilizes this grouping to guide interpretive differentiation across nine diagnostic categories: vascular, muscular, skeletal, nervous, lymphatic, organ-related (GNM), acupuncture/meridian, energetic, and metabolic/endocrine. For example, hyperemissive biosignals in the abdominal zones may correlate with heightened visceral reactivity, while hypoemissive fields may denote diminished vascular perfusion or autonomic suppression.

Confirmatory evaluation is an essential component of this stage and may include laboratory analysis of regulatory markers, organ-focused imaging, and functional assessments. Care strategies often integrate naturopathic, rehabilitative, and conventional elements, tailored to address the specific regulatory domains involved.

Given the anatomical density and regulatory complexity of this group, its precise identification supports accurate biospectral interpretation and enhances clinical decision-making in both localized and systemic conditions.

1.3 Thorax and Axillary Group

Zones 13 through 16 incorporate the anterior chest, sternum, bilateral axillary regions, and upper back. This group is essential for comprehensive evaluation of cardiorespiratory regulation, upper musculoskeletal coordination, lymphatic flow dynamics, and breast tissue biosignal behavior.

Historical literature on infrared thermographic imaging in this region emphasized its role in differentiating angiogenesis, vasodilation, calcifications, and nodular formations within breast tissue (Gautherie & Gros, 1980). As they noted, *"The thermal anomalies detected by infrared imaging are primarily due to increased vascularization (angiogenesis) associated with malignant tumors, allowing differentiation from non-malignant lesions"* (p. 22). Subsequent reports observed that thermographic methods could reveal vascular changes associated with tumor development earlier than mammography or ultrasound, without radiation or compression (Head & Wang, 2011). *"Infrared imaging of the breast provides functional information that precedes anatomical changes detected by mammography or ultrasound, offering a valuable adjunct in early cancer detection without radiation exposure"* (p. 106).

Building upon this historical context, Biospectral Medicine redefines these thoracic and axillary regions as structured emission zones, shifting the focus from isolated pathological screening to a comprehensive mapping of vascular, lymphatic, musculoskeletal, and neuroregulatory signaling. The R-CIIM model enhances interpretive precision by guiding ROI classification, zone-specific inquiry, and pattern differentiation across upper-torso biosignal categories, including cardiopulmonary, lymphatic, and musculoskeletal systems, as well as breast-related biospectral behaviors.

Confirmatory evaluations may include cardiac imaging, pulmonary function studies, lymphoscintigraphy, mammography, or structural assessments, depending on the clinical context. Care strategies emphasize integrative regulatory support for circulatory and respiratory coherence, myofascial balance, lymphatic release, and breast tissue equilibrium.

1.4 Neck and Face Group

The final group comprises Zones 17 through 19, including the frontal neck and supraclavicular area, cervical spine and nuchal zone, and the facial region. These zones overlay a highly complex anatomical network involving vascular, neuroregulatory, endocrine, lymphatic, and psychophysiological systems. Rubik (2002) describes this region as a biofield zone where *"vascular, nervous, endocrine, and psychosomatic interactions create dynamic thermal patterns"* (p. 705).

Historical studies employing infrared thermography in this group identified associations with neurovascular compromise, lymphatic congestion, endocrine gland activity (notably thyroid and parathyroid), and psychosomatic or energetic variables, highlighting its sensitivity to multi-systemic dynamics.

In Biospectral Medicine, these regions are reinterpreted as structured emission zones that reflect the intersection of regulatory hierarchies. The R-CIIM methodology emphasizes an integrated interpretive model, incorporating energetic and psychological categories alongside vascular, nervous, endocrine, lymphatic, and structural domains.

Given the systems involved, this group benefits from a multimodal clinical strategy that combines detailed biospectral analysis, zone-specific inquiry, confirmatory laboratory and imaging assessments, and individualized therapeutic planning. Care strategies may include natural, functional, psychoregulatory, or bioenergetic interventions, tailored to the patient's integrative diagnostic profile.

2. The Nine Interpretive Categories in The R-CIIM Model

Their Rationale and Clinical Significance in Biospectral Medicine

Historical literature describes infrared thermography as a tool that captures thermal variations reflecting underlying tissue physiology (Ring & Ammer, 2012). Ring and Ammer note that infrared imaging can register changes in skin temperature associated with alterations in blood flow and metabolism, making it a non-invasive adjunct for exploring functional states.

Biospectral Medicine, as formalized in the Reitz Clinical Infrared Interpretation Model (R-CIIM), builds upon and redefines this background by establishing a structured set of nine interpretive categories. Each category represents a major regulatory domain that influences emissive patterning and surface biosignal expression. These categories; vascular/circulatory, muscular, skeletal, nervous, lymphatic, organ-related (GNM), acupuncture/meridian, energetic, and metabolic/endocrine, form the core diagnostic framework of emissive zone-based analysis.

Each category corresponds to a distinct but interrelated system contributing to the complexity of biospectral signatures. Reitz (2024) outlines these categories as integral to the R-CIIM methodology, emphasizing their convergence as essential to advanced biospectral interpretation and clinical decision-making.

1. **Vascular / Circulatory**
   Vascular and circulatory regulation exerts one of the most fundamental influences on biospectral imaging. Since blood flow is the primary vehicle for surface emission, any alteration, arterial insufficiency, venous congestion, or microcirculatory dysregulation, produces characteristic biospectral asymmetries. Hyperemission reflects congestive or reactive activity, whereas hypoemission denotes ischemic or hypoperfusion behavior.

   Historical literature emphasized that thermography could detect such patterns early in conditions such as peripheral arterial disease, venous thrombosis, or Raynaud-type

presentations (Norgren et al., 2007; Rockson, 2001). Norgren et al. (2007) highlighted the vascular implications observable in limb thermography, while Rockson (2001) described lymphatic alterations producing thermal asymmetries.
Within the R-CIIM framework, this category establishes a systematic evaluation of circulatory regulation as a cornerstone of biospectral interpretation.

2. **Muscular / Myofascial**
The muscular system contributes significantly to local biospectral activity due to its metabolic demands. Myofascial activation, spasmodic contractions, or trigger-zone reactivity manifest as focal hyperemission, while chronic hypoperfusion or fibrotic adaptation is expressed through hypoemission. Recognizing these biospectral signatures enables early identification of musculoskeletal overload or dysregulation, guiding interpretive reasoning within rehabilitation and regulatory care contexts.

Vinik et al. (2013) describe how muscular alterations affect tissue metabolism and blood flow, changes which thermography has historically documented. In Biospectral Medicine, this category organizes muscular contributions to emissive signals within a systemic terrain analysis, ensuring their integration into the broader interpretive framework of the R-CIIM model.

3. **Skeletal / Articular**
Although skeletal tissue itself is relatively low in emissive output, degenerative activity and articular processes involving bones and joints exert secondary effects on surrounding soft tissues. These influences emerge as biospectral asymmetries, which may reveal fractures, arthro-articular degeneration, or intervertebral disc involvement through their regulatory impact on adjacent myofascial and vascular systems.

Lahiri et al. (2012) note that skeletal disorders influence thermographic signatures primarily through changes in neighboring tissues. Within the R-CIIM model, this category emphasizes practitioner vigilance for subtle yet clinically meaningful skeletal contributions to the overall biospectral field, ensuring they are not overlooked in systemic interpretation.

By integrating skeletal patterns into zone-based analysis, Biospectral Medicine extends beyond structural pathology to reveal how osseous and articular changes can modulate emissive behavior, providing understanding into the dynamic interaction of skeletal stability, soft tissue adaptation, and systemic regulation.

4. **Nervous System / Spine**
The nervous system exerts a primary influence over circulation, metabolism, and overall regulation. Through its autonomic, sensory, and motor divisions, it directs vascular tone, glandular activity, and tissue function. Neuropathic irritation, compressive changes, or degenerative processes disturb these mechanisms, producing biospectral asymmetries that indicate altered neuroregulation. Hyperemission reflects neurogenic activation, while hypoemission reflects reduced autonomic drive or conduction weakness.

Vinik et al. (2013) highlighted the importance of the autonomic nervous system in shaping vascular tone and metabolic balance, providing a foundation for interpreting emissive asymmetries. Nervous system disturbances may also influence other categories, including circulatory, muscular, and metabolic domains, extending their clinical relevance.

In Biospectral Medicine, the nervous system category brings attention to how neurovascular and neuroendocrine connections shape biosignal patterns across multiple regions. Within the R-CIIM framework, practitioners can recognize both localized neuropathic findings and broader regulatory changes, ensuring these signals are integrated into clinical interpretation.

5. **Lymphatic / Immune**

The lymphatic system sustains immune regulation and fluid homeostasis, acting as a bridge between local tissue environments and systemic defense. When lymphatic flow is obstructed or slowed, congestion, stasis, and tissue stress develop, creating biospectral asymmetries that signal underlying dysregulation. These signals may appear as hyperemission in zones of fluid accumulation or hypoemission when lymphatic flow is chronically reduced.

Historically, thermography demonstrated sensitivity to lymphatic alterations, supporting clinical monitoring of lymphatic burden (Rockson, 2001). *Rockson described how lymphatic changes produce detectable shifts in surface temperature patterns,* confirming the relationship between lymphatic dysfunction and surface emissive signatures.

Within the R-CIIM framework, this category organizes lymphatic findings as a distinct domain of biospectral interpretation. Practitioners are guided to assess how immune activation, impaired drainage, or fluid retention influence systemic balance. Because the lymphatic network closely interacts with vascular, immune, and inflammatory mechanisms, its emissive patterns often provide an early signal of immune challenge or tissue overloading before structural changes are clinically evident.

By incorporating lymphatic signatures into zone-based analysis, Biospectral Medicine expands the ability to interpret immune competence and fluid dynamics as part of whole-system regulation. This ensures that subtle biospectral findings, whether local or diffuse, are recognized as contributors to systemic adaptation and patient resilience.

6. **Organs / GNM**

The organ-related category, informed by German New Medicine (GNM), introduces a psychosomatic and biological-conflict dimension into biospectral interpretation. It recognizes that unresolved emotional or psychological stressors can lead to biological adaptations, expressed as distinct emissive patterns within organ-related zones. These signatures highlight the intimate relationship between emotional regulation and physical expression, extending the interpretive scope beyond structural or vascular processes alone.

Reitz (2024) emphasizes that psychosomatic influences leave recognizable traces in biospectral signatures, particularly when viewed through the zone-based mapping of Biospectral Medicine. By incorporating GNM principles, the R-CIIM framework integrates mind-body regulation into systemic analysis, allowing practitioners to identify when organ-related emissions reflect deeper psychological or conflict-driven processes.

Within this category, biospectral findings are not interpreted as isolated events but as part of the body's broader adaptive strategy. This perspective supports a clinical approach where organ-related signals are assessed both in their local context and in connection to the patient's emotional and psychological terrain, creating a more complete understanding of systemic regulation.

7. **Acupuncture / Meridian**

Traditional concepts of energy flow are represented in the acupuncture/meridian category, reflecting how imbalances in meridian dynamics influence physiological regulation and appear as biospectral irregularities. Historically, thermographic imaging was applied to explore these pathways non-invasively, offering early visual correlations with acupuncture-based strategies.

In Biospectral Medicine, this category connects classical meridian frameworks with contemporary integrative models, expanding interpretive scope within the R-CIIM methodology (Reitz, 2024). Reitz (2024) describes how biospectral patterns align with meridian pathways, enabling correlation with acupuncture practice and supporting investigation of how regulatory signals extend beyond structural anatomy.

By integrating this category, the R-CIIM framework acknowledges the role of subtle regulatory systems in shaping emissive behavior. This validates classical observations of meridian influence and provides a structured means to analyze them within a modern biosignal model, reinforcing Biospectral Medicine's capacity to integrate diverse physiological traditions into a unified interpretive logic.

8. **Energetic / Frequency**

The energetic category examines bioelectromagnetic fields and systemic frequency dynamics as contributors to regulation and adaptation. Variations in these fields influence tissue responsiveness, repair capacity, and systemic coherence, often emerging as biospectral signatures before structural changes appear on conventional imaging. This perspective highlights how frequency-based processes can shape both localized emissive patterns and broader systemic regulation.

Rubik (2002) presented evidence of biofield effects and their correlation with emissive imaging, supporting the relevance of this category within a broader scientific context.

Rubik described how subtle field interactions create measurable shifts in thermal patterns, suggesting that energy dynamics form part of the body's regulatory language.

Within Biospectral Medicine, this category integrates frequency-related findings into the R-CIIM framework, allowing practitioners to assess how subtle energetic influences interact with vascular, nervous, endocrine, and psychological systems. By including energetic analysis, Biospectral Medicine extends beyond visible structures to account for the invisible but measurable forces that shape regulatory behavior, resilience, and systemic adaptation.

9. **Metabolic / Endocrine**
The metabolic and endocrine category addresses how hormonal and metabolic regulation shape tissue function, circulation, and systemic adaptation. Variations in endocrine output influence perfusion, reparative capacity, and immune balance, producing characteristic biospectral patterns that reveal systemic regulatory status. Diabetes, thyroid imbalance, and other metabolic conditions often generate recognizable emissive signatures through their impact on vascular, muscular, and connective tissue domains.

Historical thermographic studies emphasized early recognition of metabolic and endocrine influences, noting their measurable effect on emissive presentation. *Vinik et al. (2013) described how endocrine and metabolic alterations affect vascularization and metabolic activity, changes reflected in surface imaging.*

Within Biospectral Medicine, this category organizes metabolic and endocrine regulation as a core interpretive domain of the R-CIIM framework. By integrating these influences, practitioners can identify how systemic hormonal and metabolic states interact with other categories, such as vascular, nervous, and immune, shaping both localized emissions and overall biosignal coherence. This category therefore supports both early recognition of systemic imbalance and targeted clinical correlation, reinforcing the integrative scope of biospectral interpretation.

Unified Framework for Biospectral Interpretation

Together, these nine categories establish a structured and integrated interpretive framework that captures the complexity of human regulatory dynamics as expressed in biospectral imaging. They guide practitioners beyond superficial review toward a system-based understanding of biospectral findings.

Through this comprehensive perspective, the R-CIIM model enables precise differentiation, structured confirmatory evaluation, and individualized care planning, positioning emissive imaging as an essential method for functional biosignal assessment (Reitz, 2024).

By uniting vascular, muscular, skeletal, nervous, lymphatic, organ-related, meridian, energetic, and endocrine dimensions within a single model, Biospectral Medicine provides a complete interpretive map for human regulation. This unified approach ensures that no biosignal is viewed in isolation, but always in relation to the wider physiological and psychosomatic terrain. In doing so, it transforms emissive imaging from a descriptive technique into a language of regulation, capable of guiding both investigative reasoning and therapeutic strategy.

3. Clinical Workflow Based on the CTI and Zone-Category Model

Effective interpretation of emissive imaging depends on a structured and repeatable workflow. The combined framework of Computerized Thermographic Imaging (CTI) and the Zone–Category Model ensures that findings are not viewed in isolation but assessed within a systematic map of regulatory domains.

The Reitz Clinical Infrared Interpretation Model (R-CIIM) organizes this process into a six-step sequence, guiding practitioners from image acquisition through to interpretive synthesis and the development of care strategies. Each step links emissive observations to the broader clinical context, enabling a consistent approach that combines biospectral signals with patient history, confirmatory evaluation, and therapeutic planning.

By following this workflow, practitioners can maintain interpretive precision, reduce variability, and ensure that care decisions are anchored in both objective biospectral findings and the individual's systemic presentation.

Step 1: Biospectral Zones and Functional Anatomy

The first step emphasizes acquiring high-quality emissive images across all 19 predefined Biospectral Zones of the body. Clear and precise visualization of each zone's functional anatomy is essential, since this mapping forms the foundation for reliable biospectral interpretation. Only with accurate delineation of anatomical regions can emissive signals be correctly classified, compared, and integrated into systemic analysis.

Historical literature reinforced the same requirement. *Ring and Ammer (2012) noted that precise anatomical localization was necessary in thermography to interpret thermal changes reliably and to differentiate normal from pathological patterns.* Similarly, *Lahiri et al. (2012) emphasized that image quality and anatomical clarity were critical for meaningful analysis.*

Within Biospectral Medicine, this principle is expanded into a zone-based framework where anatomical precision is inseparable from functional interpretation. By anchoring emissive findings to well-defined Biospectral Zones, practitioners ensure that subsequent steps in the workflow rest on a clear and reproducible foundation.

Step 2: ROI Classification (Hyperemission / Hypoemission)

Following image acquisition, practitioners identify Regions of Interest (ROIs) that demonstrate biospectral asymmetries. These ROIs are classified as hyperemissive (increased emissive activity) or hypoemissive (reduced emissive activity). This binary classification provides the first layer of structured interpretation, separating zones of heightened regulation from those of diminished output.

Ammer (2008) noted that emissive asymmetry, measured as differences between corresponding anatomical sites, offers early clues of underlying regulatory alterations. *He described hyperemission as frequently linked to congestion or inflammatory activity, and hypoemission as suggestive of ischemic or perfusion-related limitations.*

Within Biospectral Medicine, ROI classification is not an end in itself but a transitional step. By mapping asymmetries onto the predefined Biospectral Zones, practitioners anchor observed signals to anatomical and functional context, ensuring that subsequent steps, category determination, patient history correlation, and confirmatory evaluation, are grounded in precise, reproducible findings.

Step 3: Category Determination

Each ROI and its corresponding zone are assessed through the nine interpretive categories: vascular/circulatory, muscular, skeletal, nervous, lymphatic, organ-related (GNM), acupuncture/meridian, energetic, and metabolic/endocrine. This stage ensures that emissive findings are not viewed in isolation but are systematically linked to the body's major regulatory domains.

Reitz (2024) explains that integrating these categories aligns emissive data with complex regulatory mechanisms, enabling a comprehensive systems-based perspective. *Robinson et al. (2020) likewise emphasize that a multi-category framework is essential for moving beyond superficial review toward deeper clinical utility.*

Within Biospectral Medicine, category determination transforms emissive asymmetries into structured biosignal classifications, setting the foundation for subsequent steps of patient history correlation and confirmatory evaluation. By applying this step, practitioners move from descriptive observation to a functional map of systemic regulation, giving clinical meaning to emissive signals within the R-CIIM process.

Step 4: Interpretive Questions

To refine the interpretive impression, practitioners apply targeted differential questions to each ROI. This step synthesizes patient history, reported experience, and physical findings to differentiate among regulatory patterns identified in the previous step.

Robinson et al. (2020) describe how structured questioning, when combined with emissive findings, improves interpretive specificity and directs further evaluation while reducing unnecessary investigations. Within Biospectral Medicine, this process anchors emissive signals to the patient's subjective and objective context, ensuring that biospectral classifications are clinically relevant rather than abstract.

By aligning biospectral findings with patient responses, this step transforms initial categorizations into individualized interpretive profiles, creating a bridge between imaging data and confirmatory evaluation.

Step 5: Confirmatory Evaluation

Based on the biospectral hypothesis, appropriate confirmatory evaluations are selected, which may include laboratory assays, imaging studies, or functional assessments. These evaluations provide objective data that either reinforce or refine the interpretive impression derived from emissive findings.

Lahiri et al. (2012) emphasized that *thermographic methods should complement, not replace, other diagnostic approaches,* providing physiological context that guides test selection and interpretation. In line with this perspective, Biospectral Medicine incorporates confirmatory evaluation as a safeguard against over-reliance on imaging alone, ensuring that findings are anchored in a broader clinical framework.

This step contextualizes biospectral signals within the larger clinical picture, supporting both accuracy of interpretation and the development of individualized care strategies. By linking emissive analysis with confirmatory evaluation, practitioners establish a more reliable foundation for therapeutic planning.

Step 6: Care Strategies and Intervention Pathways

With confirmatory alignment, care is tailored according to the zone and its category-based findings. Intervention pathways may draw on naturopathic, biomedical, rehabilitative, or bioenergetic approaches, selected according to the regulatory systems most involved. This ensures that care addresses both local signals and their connection to the patient's systemic profile.

Reitz (2024) highlights the value of adaptive strategies that respond to evolving regulatory patterns, rather than fixed protocols. Within Biospectral Medicine, therapeutic planning is viewed as a dynamic process, in which interventions are continually informed by follow-up imaging, patient response, and the broader clinical context.

This approach strengthens the relevance of each intervention and supports more effective outcomes. By closing the interpretive workflow with individualized care application, Step 6 completes the R-CIIM process, ensuring that emissive analysis directly informs actionable strategies for patient regulation and recovery.

Important Step: Iteration and Reassessment

Although positioned outside the formal six-step workflow, iterative reassessment is critical for continuity of care. Emissive signals are not static but evolve in response to interventions, lifestyle adjustments, and the body's own adaptive processes. Periodic reassessment allows practitioners to track these changes and refine interpretive conclusions accordingly.

Ring and Ammer (2012) recommended periodic reevaluation to monitor regulatory progression and adaptive responses. *Ammer (2008) further emphasized that documenting changes over time supports interpretive decision-making and maintains clinical continuity.* Reitz (2024) adds that adaptive management depends on longitudinal integration of emissive and clinical data, ensuring that therapeutic strategies remain relevant as the patient's regulatory profile evolves.

By embedding reassessment into practice, Biospectral Medicine ensures that findings are not viewed as isolated events but as part of an ongoing process of systemic regulation and adaptation. This approach strengthens interpretive precision and helps align care with the patient's real-time biological responses.

GROUP 1

LOWER EXTREMITIES

The lower extremities provide a revealing field for observing peripheral vascular regulation and gravitational drainage dynamics. As biospectral regions, these zones frequently demonstrate anispectral expression, vascular stasis, and myofascial asymmetry, making them valuable for identifying tendencies toward venous insufficiency, postural strain, or peripheral manifestations of metabolic overload.

A defining feature of this group is its predictable bilateral symmetry in healthy individuals. This makes even subtle deviations clinically meaningful, such as unilateral hyperemissive strips along the course of the great saphenous vein or medial hypoemissive fields reflecting reduced perfusion. ROI evaluation in these zones often benefits from gravity-sensitive analysis, including emissive changes that fluctuate with time of day or orthostatic positioning.

Practitioners may also observe that lymphatic stasis and neurovascular syndromes, such as meralgia paresthetica, appear biospectrally in these regions earlier than they are detected by structural imaging. In addition, the lower extremities often respond to systemic factors such as hydration, electrolyte balance, and microcirculatory regulation during prolonged standing, establishing them as a key terrain for functional interpretation within clinical practice.

Zones 1 to 8: Frontal and Dorsal Legs – Internal, External, and Proximal Regions

Emissive imaging of the lower extremities offers foundational insights into multiple physiological domains. These regions are functionally demanding, contributing to postural stability, locomotion, peripheral circulation, and compensatory adaptation in response to systemic influences.

Because of their biomechanical exposure, gravitational demand, and vascular distance from central regulation, the lower limbs frequently manifest early indicators of regulatory imbalance across several systems. *Ring and Ammer (2012) emphasized that these regions often display distinctive thermal patterns due to vascular and neurological influences related to their peripheral location and functional load.*

Within Biospectral Medicine, the lower extremities are viewed as a sensitive biosignal field, where emissive findings reveal both local strain and systemic adaptation. This dual perspective makes them an essential starting point for functional interpretation and zone-based analysis.

This group includes eight zones:

1. Frontal Lower Legs
2. Dorsal Lower Legs
3. Internal Left Leg
4. Internal Right Leg
5. External Left Leg
6. External Right Leg
7. Frontal Upper Legs
8. Dorsal Upper Legs

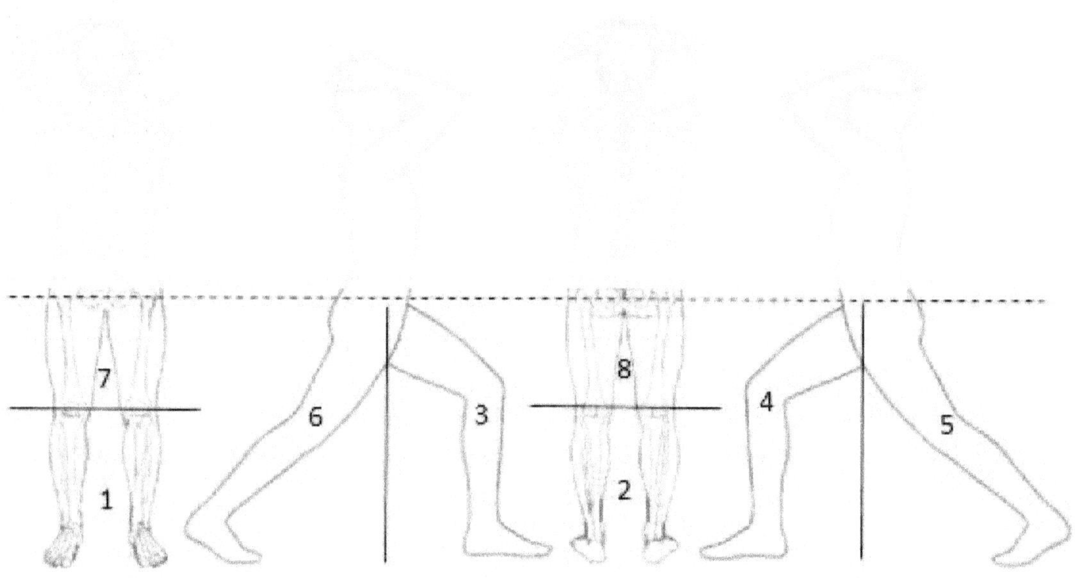

Each of these zones represents a distinct anatomical and functional compartment of the lower extremity. The division into anterior (frontal), posterior (dorsal), medial (internal), and lateral (external) planes allows for precise mapping of localized biospectral patterns, enabling recognition of asymmetric regulation, compensatory strain, circulatory congestion, and myofascial restriction.

Lahiri et al. (2012) highlighted that such detailed anatomical segmentation improves the sensitivity and specificity of thermographic assessment by allowing focused analysis of regional variations. The lower extremities demonstrate rich emissive variation due to their role in venous return and microvascular perfusion, the complexity of overlapping muscular chains, and their sensitivity to autonomic (particularly sympathetic) regulation.

Ammer (2008) noted that peripheral vasculature and muscle metabolism contribute significantly to emissive signals in these regions, while Myers (2014) described how fascial continuity and muscular chains create biomechanical influences on emissive distribution. Reitz (2024) further explains that metabolic, lymphatic, and energetic factors also modulate emissive responses, reinforcing the interpretive importance of the lower extremities within Biospectral Medicine.

Hyperemissive and hypoemissive patterns in the lower extremity zones often correspond to specific regulatory disturbances. Vascular stasis or ischemic tendencies may be expressed as localized hypoemission, while peripheral neuropathies can generate focal asymmetries linked to impaired neuroregulation. Myofascial overload or deactivation frequently manifests in compartmental patterns, reflecting strain or weakness within muscular chains.

Articular processes may be visualized through emissive irregularities in joint regions, while sympathetic dominance or regulatory failure produces broader shifts across entire limb segments. In addition, these zones may reveal viscerosomatic reflex fields, particularly those associated with pelvic or renal organ influence, highlighting the interconnected nature of lower limb biospectral expression.

When interpreted through the R-CIIM model, biospectral signals gain specificity and clinical orientation. Each zone is examined through anatomical framing, emissive polarity analysis, and systemic attribution across the nine interpretive categories. This multidimensional approach supports both localized evaluation and systemic reasoning, enabling practitioners to differentiate structural overload, circulatory insufficiency, neurogenic contribution, and terrain-related influences.

Robinson et al. (2020) emphasized that integrating thermographic data with clinical history and functional anatomy improves interpretive accuracy and guides confirmatory evaluation.

In this Atlas, the zones are organized into four major anatomical groups, each containing specific emission fields. For every zone, the six-step interpretive process is applied, showing how relevant categories from the nine total interpretive domains shape emissive expression.

In the sections that follow, each zone is examined in detail, presenting interpretive pathways that integrate functional anatomy, emissive physiology, and biospectral insights to support clinical reasoning and care planning. *Ring and Ammer (2012) and Lahiri et al. (2012) described structured grouping as essential for systematic clinical application of infrared thermography.*

For clarity, the organ-related category (Category 6) is generally excluded from this section, as visceral organs exert minimal direct influence on the emissive profile of the anterior lower leg.

GROUP 1

ZONE 1 – FRONTAL LOWER LEG

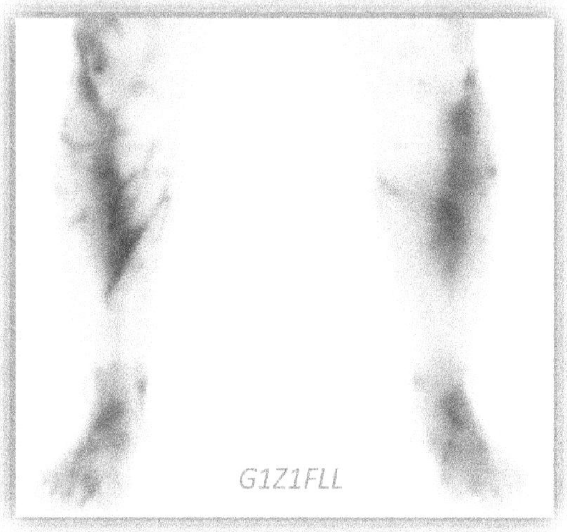

The frontal lower legs are among the most emission-stable regions of the body due to their minimal subcutaneous fat and high vascular exposure. This stability makes even slight biospectral asymmetries or ROI deviations clinically significant, since what manifests here is rarely incidental. Most patterns in this zone relate to circulatory regulation, fascial strain, or tibial periosteal activation, yet the diagnostic potential extends far beyond local physiology.

The anterior tibial artery runs superficially across this region, providing one of the most accessible vascular corridors of the lower extremities (Standring, 2016). Because of this anatomical characteristic, emissive irregularities in the frontal shin often precede clinical recognition of circulatory disturbances elsewhere in the limb. Studies of exertional compartment syndrome have shown that nearly 40% of cases present initial alterations in the anterior tibial compartment, where the fascial sheath is among the least compliant in the body, amplifying minor circulatory changes into significant functional stress (Styf & Körnerberg, 1986).

In athletes, tibial stress reactions can account for 10–15% of lower limb overuse injuries, with subtle changes in the anterior shin sometimes visible weeks before bone scans confirm pathology (Fredericson & Jennings, 2007). Even in non-athletes, the anterior shin has been noted as a region where vascular adaptations to postural load are disproportionately expressed, reflecting microvascular sensitivity long before overt pathology emerges (Mickle et al., 2009).

From a biospectral perspective, this zone can reveal early terrain-level regulatory imbalances ranging from peripheral vascular strain to myofascial overload. Particularly in runners, dancers, and individuals with unexplained shin tightness or paresthesia, the anterior compartment's emissive profile functions as a silent sentinel of circulatory and fascial coherence.

What appears to be a plain and stable surface in everyday observation is, in fact, an early-warning field for systemic regulation and one of the most reliable entry points for functional interpretive analysis.

Zone 1 – Frontal Lower Legs: Biospectral Relevant Structures

Category	Relevant Structures	Emission Relevance
1. Vascular / Circulatory	Great saphenous vein (medial) - Anterior tibial vein - Capillary plexuses along tibial crest	Hyperemission reflects congestion in superficial veins. Hypoemission reflects ischemia, arterial spasm, or reduced capillary perfusion from sympathetic dominance.
2. Muscular / Myofascial	Tibialis anterior - Extensor digitorum longus - Extensor hallucis longus - Peroneus tertius - Fascia cruris (anterior deep fascia of the leg)	Hyperemission reflects postural overload, repetitive strain, or acute exertion. Hypoemission reflects immobilization, hypotonia, or fascial compartment tension.
3. Skeletal / Articular	Tibia (anterior crest) - Fibula (lateral border) - Patella (superior reference) - Medial/lateral malleoli (inferior boundary markers)	Localized hyperemission reflects periosteal stress or structural activation. Hypoemission reflects chronic degeneration, disuse, or systemic hyporegulation.
4. Nervous System / Spine	Deep peroneal nerve (motor/sensory anterior leg) - Saphenous nerve (medial cutaneous) - L4–L5 dermatomes	Hyperemission reflects nerve irritation or neuropathic activation. Hypoemission reflects chronic suppression or reduced conduction.
5. Lymphatic / Immune	Pre-tibial lymphatic microcirculation - Drainage via medial route toward inguinal chain	Hyperemission reflects lymphatic stagnation or lymphatic burden. Hypoemission reflects immune hyporegulation, drainage failure, or scarring.
6. Organs / GNM	*(Not applicable for this zone)*	-
7. Acupuncture / Meridians	Stomach Meridian (ST) – runs centrally over anterior leg - Spleen Meridian (SP) – medial influence on anterior-medial boundary - Gallbladder Meridian (GB) – lateral influence	Hyperemission reflects Qi stagnation or Yang excess in the Stomach or Gallbladder meridians. Hypoemission reflects Spleen Qi deficiency, Damp-Cold retention, or Yang depletion.deficiency, Damp-Cold accumulation, or Yang collapse.
8. Energetic / Frequency	Reflex zones for personal direction, forward motion, and stability (bioenergetic interpretation) - Lower limb frequency disruptions linked to fatigue, overwhelm, or disconnection	Hyperemission reflects overexertion, emotional tension, or Yang discharge. Hypoemission reflects adrenal hyporegulation, stagnation, or energetic disconnection.
9. Metabolic / Endocrine	Peripheral mitochondrial activity zones in lower limb muscle - Sites of glucose uptake and lactic acid metabolism - Reflex terrain of adrenal function	Hypoemission reflects thyroid hyporegulation, adrenal hyporegulation, or metabolic suppression. Hyperemission reflects lactic retention, hypermetabolic drive, or detox-related activity.

GROUP 1 - ZONE 1 – FRONTAL LOWER LEG

Category 1: *Vascular / Circulatory*

Step 1: **Functional Anatomy and Interpretive Importance**

The anterior tibial artery arises from the popliteal artery at the lower border of the popliteus and passes through the interosseous membrane to descend on its anterior surface, supplying the tibialis anterior, extensor hallucis longus, extensor digitorum longus, fibularis tertius, the anterior interosseous structures, and overlying skin. Venous return is carried by paired anterior tibial veins that ascend to the popliteal vein, with additional drainage through superficial tributaries connecting to the great saphenous vein (Standring, 2016).

Vascular studies emphasize the anterior tibial system as a critical pathway in revascularization and circulatory assessment, underscoring its role in maintaining anterior compartment perfusion (Hiatt et al., 2015). This vascular arrangement generates emissive fields along the anterior shin that are highly sensitive to circulatory variation.

On spectral surface reading, asymmetries in this region often reflect reduced inflow, venous stasis, or subtle regulatory changes in the microcirculation. Given the constant mechanical demand of propulsion and balance, the zone frequently provides early evidence of peripheral circulatory stress.

Step 2,3,4: **ROI Classification and Interpretive Questions**

Hyperemission reflects venous congestion or microvascular activation, indicated by increased local blood volume and metabolic activity (Chrubasik et al., 2011).

- Any heaviness, swelling, warmth, or pain after long standing/walking?
- Are varicosities or skin changes visible?

Hypoemission signals arterial insufficiency or vasospasm, reflecting reduced perfusion and diminished emissive output consistent with vascular compromise *(Norgren et al., 2007).*

- Is there coldness, numbness, pallor, or intermittent claudication?
- Is wound healing delayed?

Step 5: **Confirmatory Evaluations**

Test	Purpose & Justification	Relevance to Emissive Pattern
Doppler ultrasound	Evaluates arterial and venous blood flow; confirms venous insufficiency or PAD (Brant et al., 2016).	Confirms hyperemissive venous congestion and hypoemissive arterial insufficiency.
Ankle-Brachial Index (ABI)	Quantifies arterial perfusion; ABI <0.9 confirms PAD severity (Norgren et al., 2007).	Validates hypoemissive arterial insufficiency.

Capillary refill time	Assesses microcirculation; delayed refill indicates microvascular dysfunction.	Supports hypoemissive microcirculatory stagnation.
Blood tests (CBC, CRP, coagulation profile)	Detect systemic inflammation and coagulopathy contributing to vascular disease (Brennan et al., 2014).	Supports hyperemissive microvascular activation or thrombotic processes.

Step 6: Care Strategies and Intervention Pathways

Naturopathic Approach

Botanical venotonics such as *Aesculus hippocastanum* and *Centella asiatica* strengthen venous tone and capillary integrity, reducing venous congestion (Chrubasik et al., 2011). Hydrotherapy, including contrast foot baths, improves circulation and reduces edema (Sutkowy et al., 2019). An anti-inflammatory diet rich in bioflavonoids, vitamin C, and omega-3 fatty acids supports vascular health and reduces systemic inflammation (Calder, 2017). Nitric oxide boosters (e.g., beetroot, arginine) and omega-3 fatty acids enhance arterial perfusion and endothelial function (Moncada & Higgs, 1993; Calder, 2017). Limb elevation and walking promote venous return. For arterial insufficiency, circulatory stimulants such as *Ginkgo biloba* and warming compresses improve perfusion. Supplementation with iron, B12, and folate supports oxygen delivery as needed.

Standard Medical Approaches

Doppler ultrasound and ABI guide treatment with graduated compression stockings, venoactive drugs, and NSAIDs for venous disease. Sclerotherapy or ablation may be necessary in advanced cases (Brant et al., 2016). Arterial disease treatment includes antiplatelet therapy, statins, supervised exercise, and revascularization (Norgren et al., 2007). Wound care is crucial in ischemic ulcers.

Specialty / Practitioner Care Strategies Table

Specialty Group	Practitioners Included	Hyperemissive Strategies	Hypoemissive Strategies
Biochemistry	Nutritionists, Orthomolecular, Herbalists, Naturopaths	Botanical venotonics, anti-inflammatory diet, antioxidants, vitamins C, E, selenium, CoQ10, bioflavonoids, omega-3s	Circulatory stimulants (*Ginkgo*, cayenne), blood-building nutrients (iron, B12, folate), magnesium, arginine, nitrate-rich diet
Rehabilitation	Physiotherapists, Massage Therapists, Osteopaths / Chiropractors	Lymphatic drainage, calf pump exercises, postural retraining, gentle Swedish massage, myofascial release	Graded aerobic exercise, gait training, emissive protection, foot care, warming massage, reflexology, ergonomic guidance
Energetics	Acupuncturists (TCM), Bioenergetic Therapists	Acupuncture (SP6, ST36), moxibustion, herbal formulas, Qi and Blood tonics, bioresonance, PEMF	Warming acupuncture, Qi and Blood tonics, PEMF, energy healing
Psychological	GNM practitioners, Psychotherapists, Vibrational therapists, Family constellation facilitators	GNM conflict protocols, psychotherapy, bioresonance, mindfulness, energy clearing	Psychosomatic conflict resolution, vibrational medicine, stress reduction, emotional balancing

Educational Pearls & Considerations.

- Exclude deep vein thrombosis or critical ischemia before heat, massage, or exercise.
- Botanical venotonics combined with hydrotherapy synergistically reduce venous congestion.
- Nitric oxide boosters and omega-3 fatty acids enhance arterial perfusion and endothelial function.
- Compression therapy is contraindicated in severe arterial disease.
- Early mobilization and limb elevation prevent chronic vascular complications.

GROUP 1 - ZONE 1 – FRONTAL LOWER LEG

Category 2: *Muscular*

Step 1: Functional Anatomy and Interpretive Importance

The anterior compartment of the lower leg contains the tibialis anterior, extensor hallucis longus, and extensor digitorum longus, innervated by the deep fibular nerve and stabilized by the extensor retinacula. These muscles drive dorsiflexion and toe extension for foot clearance and stance stability, while the tibialis anterior also contributes to inversion and fine balance adjustments (Standring, 2016).

Overuse syndromes such as tibialis anterior tendinopathy and chronic exertional compartment syndrome are common in runners, leading to pain, stiffness, and reduced endurance (Styf & Körner, 1986). The same strain that predisposes to dysfunction also alters emissive patterns along the anterior shin, where fascial tension and repetitive contraction reshape the biospectral signature. These changes are often evident before clinical symptoms, making this compartment a sensitive zone for detecting early imbalance in locomotor dynamics.

Step 2,3,4: ROI Classification and Interpretive Questions

Hyperemission indicates acute muscle strain, tissue activation, or reactive myopathy characterized by increased blood flow and metabolic activity.

- Has the patient experienced recent trauma, overuse, or exercise-induced pain?
- Is there localized tenderness, swelling, or muscle spasms?

Hypoemission suggests chronic perfusion reduction, compartment adaptation, or neurogenic suppression causing reduced perfusion and lower metabolic activity.

- Are there symptoms of numbness, weakness, or cramping at rest or with exertion?
- Is muscle bulk decreased or is gait altered?

Step 5: Confirmatory Evaluations

Test	Purpose & Justification	Relevance to Emissive Pattern
Creatine kinase (CK), LDH	Detect muscle fiber damage or inflammation (Maffulli et al., 2014).	Elevated in hyperemissive muscular activation.
MRI	Visualizes muscle edema, inflammation, ischemia, or atrophy.	Supports hyperemissive vascular or tissue activation, or hypoemissive ischemia/atrophy
Compartment pressure measurement	Diagnoses compartment syndrome by assessing increased intracompartmental pressure.	Relevant to hypoemissive ischemic presentations.
Nerve conduction studies (NCS), Electromyography (EMG)	Evaluate neurogenic causes of muscle weakness or atrophy.	Hypoemission related to neurogenic dysfunction.
Blood tests (CBC, inflammatory markers)	Detect systemic inflammation or infection contributing to myositis.	Supports hyperemissive regulatory or vascular activation.

Step 6: Care Strategies and Intervention Pathways

Naturopathic Approach

Management aims to reduce inflammation, support tissue repair, and improve circulation. Anti-inflammatory botanicals such as *Curcuma longa* (turmeric) and *Boswellia serrata* reduce muscle inflammation (Hewlings & Kalman, 2017). Magnesium supplementation supports muscle relaxation and function. Hydrotherapy with alternating warm and cold compresses enhances circulation and reduces edema (Sutkowy et al., 2019). Gentle stretching and graded strengthening exercises restore muscle function. Nutritional support includes antioxidant-rich foods and adequate protein for repair.

Standard Medical Approaches

Rest, NSAIDs, and physical therapy form the cornerstone of acute muscle injury management (Maffulli et al., 2014). In compartment syndrome, urgent surgical fasciotomy is required. Neurogenic causes demand targeted neurological evaluation and rehabilitation.

Specialty / Practitioner Care Strategies Table

Specialty Group	Practitioners Included	Hyperemissive Strategies	Hypoemissive Strategies
Biochemistry	Nutritionists, Orthomolecular, Herbalists, Naturopaths	Anti-inflammatory botanicals, magnesium supplementation, antioxidant-rich diet, protein support	Circulatory stimulants, neurotrophic nutrients, protein supplementation
Rehabilitation	Physiotherapists, Massage Therapists, Osteopaths / Chiropractors	Myofascial release, trigger point therapy, gentle massage, postural retraining	Graded aerobic exercise, gait training, neurorehabilitation, ergonomic guidance
Energetics	Acupuncturists (TCM), Bioenergetic Therapists	Acupuncture (ST36, LI10), moxibustion, PEMF, energy balancing	Warming acupuncture, frequency therapy, energy healing
Psychological	GNM practitioners, Psychotherapists, Vibrational therapists, Family constellation facilitators	Psychotherapy, bioresonance, mindfulness, energy clearing	Psychosomatic conflict resolution, vibrational medicine, emotional balancing

Educational Pearls & Considerations.

- Early recognition of compartment syndrome is critical; delayed treatment risks permanent damage.
- Magnesium supports muscle relaxation and prevents cramps.
- Hydrotherapy protocols must be adapted to avoid worsening acute inflammation.
- Neurogenic muscle weakness requires comprehensive neurological assessment.
- Graded rehabilitation prevents chronic dysfunction.

GROUP 1 - ZONE 1 – FRONTAL LOWER LEG

Category 3: *Skeletal*

Step 1: Functional Anatomy and Interpretive Importance

The anterior compartment of the lower leg is dominated by the tibial shaft, accompanied laterally by the fibula and extending distally into the ankle mortise (Standring, 2016). These osseous elements stabilize posture and serve as rigid levers for muscular insertion, transmitting forces essential for dorsiflexion and forward propulsion.

The tibial surface, with minimal soft tissue covering, is particularly exposed to repetitive loading, explaining its frequent involvement in stress-related syndromes. Bennell et al. (1999) highlight the high prevalence of tibial stress reactions in athletes, where remodeling responses occur before fracture lines are evident radiographically.

Such skeletal loading patterns influence peripheral regulation, and their imprint emerges on spectral surface readings as focused biospectral asymmetries aligned with the tibial crest. Rather than diffuse muscular expressions, these signals delineate the precise interaction of bone, periosteum, and adjacent soft tissue, providing an externalized image of early structural adaptation.

Step 2,3,4: ROI Classification and Interpretive Questions

Hyperemission indicates acute bone injury, periosteal activation, or reactive remodeling with increased local blood flow.

- Has the patient experienced trauma or repetitive stress?
- Is there localized tenderness, swelling, or joint stiffness?

Hypoemission may reflect chronic structural change, articular adaptation, or vascular underperfusion with reduced perfusion and metabolic activity.

- Are there symptoms of chronic pain, stiffness, or reduced joint mobility?
- Is there a history of joint deformity or instability?

Step 5: Confirmatory Evaluations

Test	Purpose & Justification	Relevance to Emissive Pattern
X-ray imaging	Detects fractures, stress reactions, and joint space alterations.	Confirms hyperemissive acute injuries or hypoemissive chronic degenerative changes.
MRI	Visualizes bone marrow edema, occult fractures, and soft tissue involvement.	Supports hyperemissive tissue activation or hypoemissive chronic pathology.
Bone scan	Assesses bone metabolism and detects stress fractures or infection.	Correlates with areas of hyperemission reflecting active bone involvement.
Blood tests (inflammatory markers)	Detect systemic inflammation related to bone injury or infection.	Supports hyperemissive regulatory or vascular activation.

Step 6: Care Strategies and Intervention Pathways

Naturopathic Approach

Management includes supporting bone healing and reducing inflammation. Nutrients such as calcium, vitamin D, magnesium, and vitamin K are essential for bone metabolism (Heaney, 2006). Anti-inflammatory botanicals like *Boswellia serrata* may reduce periosteal inflammation. Rest and immobilization prevent further injury. Therapeutic ultrasound and pulsed electromagnetic fields (PEMF) may stimulate bone repair (Gordon et al., 2016).

Standard Medical Approaches

Imaging guides immobilization, casting, or surgical intervention for fractures (Khan et al., 2012). NSAIDs and physical therapy manage pain and restore function. Osteoarthritis requires analgesics, anti-inflammatory drugs, and joint support strategies.

Specialty / Practitioner Care Strategies Table

Specialty Group	Practitioners Included	Hyperemissive Strategies	Hypoemissive Strategies
Biochemistry	Nutritionists, Orthomolecular, Herbalists, Naturopaths	Bone-supportive nutrients, anti-inflammatory botanicals	Nutritional support for bone remodeling and joint health
Rehabilitation	Physiotherapists, Massage Therapists, Osteopaths / Chiropractors	Joint mobilization, therapeutic ultrasound, myofascial release	Joint stabilization, graded strengthening, ergonomic guidance
Energetics	Acupuncturists (TCM), Bioenergetic Therapists	Acupuncture, PEMF, herbal formulas for inflammation	Warming acupuncture, energy balancing
Psychological	GNM practitioners, Psychotherapists, Vibrational therapists, Family constellation facilitators	Mind-body therapies supporting pain management and healing	Psychosomatic support, emotional balancing

Educational Pearls & Considerations.

- Early immobilization is critical in fractures to prevent displacement.
- Nutritional support accelerates bone healing.
- PEMF shows promise but requires proper clinical application.
- Chronic joint Hypoemission may reflect degenerative changes requiring multidisciplinary management.
- Psychological support improves pain perception and recovery outcomes.

GROUP 1 - ZONE 1 – FRONTAL LOWER LEG

Category 4: *Nervous*

Step 1: Functional Anatomy and Interpretive Importance

The anterior lower leg is supplied by the deep peroneal nerve and superficial peroneal branches, coordinating dorsiflexion, toe extension, and sensory input from the dorsum of the foot (Standring, 2016). These neural circuits are fundamental for balance and stride clearance, as conduction delay or compression readily alters motor timing and proprioceptive acuity.

Clinical reports on anterior tarsal tunnel syndrome demonstrate how deep peroneal entrapment produces pain, paresthesia, and weakness that emerge gradually with mechanical loading (Singh et al., 2012).

Such disturbances extend beyond isolated neural transmission, influencing vascular tone and muscular recruitment in the anterior compartment. The resulting regulatory shifts are externally expressed as narrow emissive fields tracking the tibial crest toward the dorsum, distinct from the diffuse patterns of muscular activation.

In this way, the neurophysiological burden of peroneal dysfunction translates directly into surface biosignals, allowing clinicians to visualize early neural compromise through emissive expression rather than waiting for advanced motor deficit.

Step 2,3,4: ROI Classification and Interpretive Questions

Hyperemission may indicate nerve irritation or neurogenic activation with increased regional blood flow due to signal-driven vascular response.

- Does the patient report burning, tingling, or shooting pain?
- Are there signs of local swelling or hypersensitivity?

Hypoemission suggests nerve compression, perfusion reduction, or denervation causing reduced autonomic regulation and lower biosignal output.

- Is there numbness, weakness, muscle atrophy, or coldness?
- Are there symptoms exacerbated by position or activity?

Step 5: Confirmatory Evaluations

Test	Purpose & Justification	Relevance to Emissive Pattern
Nerve conduction studies (NCS), Electromyography (EMG)	Evaluate nerve function and muscle innervation status (Campbell & Meyer, 2006).	Correlates with hypoemissive neurogenic dysfunction.

Quantitative sensory testing (QST)	Measures sensory nerve function and thresholds.	Supports both hyper- and hypoemissive neuropathic activity.
MRI / Ultrasound	Detect nerve compression or structural lesions.	Identifies neurogenic involvement linked to emission changes.
Blood tests (glucose, HbA1c, vitamin B12)	Rule out metabolic causes of neuropathy such as diabetes or deficiency.	Supports neuropathic involvement affecting biospectral regulation.

Step 6: Care Strategies and Intervention Pathways

Naturopathic Approach

Treatment aims to reduce neuroinflammation, support nerve repair, and restore autonomic balance. Nutrients such as B-complex vitamins, alpha-lipoic acid, and Acetyl-L-carnitine aid nerve regeneration (Papanas & Ziegler, 2014). Herbal anti-inflammatories like *Hypericum perforatum* (St. John's Wort) may alleviate neuropathic pain (Kasper et al., 2010). Physical therapies including neural mobilization and gentle stretching support functional recovery. Mind-body techniques, bioresonance, and acupuncture modulate pain and neurovascular regulation.

Standard Medical Approaches

Pharmacological treatments include anticonvulsants, antidepressants, and analgesics for neuropathic pain. Physical therapy and surgical decompression are considered where appropriate. Metabolic control is essential in diabetic neuropathy.

Specialty / Practitioner Care Strategies Table

Specialty Group	Practitioners Included	Hyperemissive Strategies	Hypoemissive Strategies
Biochemistry	Nutritionists, Orthomolecular, Herbalists, Naturopaths	Neurotrophic vitamins, alpha-lipoic acid, anti-inflammatory botanicals	Circulatory stimulants, metabolic support, neuroprotective nutrients
Rehabilitation	Physiotherapists, Massage Therapists, Osteopaths / Chiropractors	Neural mobilization, myofascial release, gentle massage	Neural gliding exercises, ergonomic guidance, neurorehabilitation
Energetics	Acupuncturists (TCM), Bioenergetic Therapists	Acupuncture, moxibustion, PEMF, energy balancing	Warming acupuncture, frequency therapy, energy healing
Psychological	GNM practitioners, Psychotherapists, Vibrational therapists, Family constellation facilitators	Psychotherapy, bioresonance, mindfulness, energy clearing	Psychosomatic conflict resolution, vibrational medicine, emotional balancing

Educational Pearls & Considerations.

- Early identification of nerve compression prevents permanent damage.
- Nutritional support is essential for nerve regeneration.
- Mind-body therapies may significantly reduce neuropathic pain perception.
- Careful assessment of metabolic contributors improves outcomes.
- Avoid aggressive physical therapies in acute nerve inflammation.

GROUP 1 - ZONE 1 – FRONTAL LOWER LEG

Category 5: *Lymphatic*

Step 1: Functional Anatomy and Interpretive Importance

The anterior lower leg contains superficial and deep lymphatic vessels that converge toward the inguinal lymph nodes, draining interstitial fluid, immune cells, and metabolic byproducts (Standring, 2016). This network operates in concert with venous channels, ensuring fluid homeostasis and rapid immune surveillance.

Rockson (2001) emphasized that impairment of lymphatic transport leads to tissue congestion and altered local defense, a process that often begins subtly in distal extremities. In the anterior tibial region, even minor stasis disrupts neurovascular balance and modifies fascial tension, producing externally perceptible changes.

On surface imaging, these alterations frequently appear as localized emissive variations running longitudinally along the tibial crest, where containment and geometric clarity distinguish them from diffuse muscular or vascular fields. Such biospectral asymmetries reveal the silent burden of impaired lymphatic clearance, allowing clinicians to detect early immune activation or stagnation before overt edema becomes clinically apparent.

Step 2,3,4: ROI Classification and Interpretive Questions

Hyperemission indicates immune node activation, acute tissue reactivity, or lymphatic congestion associated with increased local emissive output.

- Are there signs of redness, warmth, and tenderness?
- Is there sudden swelling or a history of infection?

Hypoemission suggests chronic lymphatic stagnation with tissue rigidity or reduced drainage leading to decreased perfusion.

- Is the swelling persistent, firm, or associated with skin thickening?
- Are there recurrent infections or slow wound healing?

Step 5: Confirmatory Evaluations

Test	Purpose & Justification	Relevance to Emissive Pattern
Lymphoscintigraphy	Assesses lymphatic flow and identifies obstruction or insufficiency.	Validates lymphatic burden or hypoperfusion.
Doppler ultrasound	Excludes venous insufficiency contributing to lymphatic dysfunction.	Differentiates vascular from lymphatic causes.

Blood tests (CBC, inflammatory markers)	Detect infection or systemic inflammation impacting lymphatics.	Supports hyperemissive regulatory activation.
Physical examination (Stemmer's sign, limb circumference)	Evaluates clinical signs of lymphedema.	Confirms lymphatic dysfunction associated with emission changes.

Step 6: Care Strategies and Intervention Pathways

Naturopathic Approach

Treatment focuses on reducing inflammation, supporting lymphatic drainage, and preventing infection. Herbal lymphagogues such as *Hedera helix* (ivy leaf) and *Vitis vinifera* (grape seed extract) improve lymph flow and vessel tone (Godoy et al., 2012). Manual lymphatic drainage by trained therapists promotes fluid movement. Compression therapy is recommended but must be individualized. Nutritional support includes antioxidants and anti-inflammatory nutrients. Hydrotherapy with alternating warm and cool water improves lymphatic circulation.

Standard Medical Approaches

Lymphedema management includes manual lymph drainage, compression garments, and physical therapy. Infection requires prompt antibiotic therapy. Severe cases may benefit from surgical intervention.

Specialty / Practitioner Care Strategies Table

Specialty Group	Practitioners Included	Hyperemissive Strategies	Hypoemissive Strategies
Biochemistry	Nutritionists, Orthomolecular, Herbalists, Naturopaths	Herbal lymphagogues, antioxidants, anti-inflammatory nutrients	Circulatory support, nutritional support for tissue repair
Rehabilitation	Physiotherapists, Massage Therapists, Osteopaths / Chiropractors	Manual lymphatic drainage, gentle massage, postural retraining	Compression therapy, graded exercise, ergonomic guidance
Energetics	Acupuncturists (TCM), Bioenergetic Therapists	Acupuncture, herbal formulas, PEMF	Warming acupuncture, energy balancing
Psychological	GNM practitioners, Psychotherapists, Vibrational therapists, Family constellation facilitators	Mind-body therapies supporting immune function and healing	Psychosomatic conflict resolution, emotional balancing

Educational Pearls & Considerations.

- Early intervention prevents progression to chronic lymphedema.
- Manual lymphatic drainage must be performed by trained professionals to avoid complications.
- Compression therapy should be customized and monitored carefully.
- Nutritional support enhances tissue repair and reduces inflammation.
- Monitor for recurrent infections, which worsen lymphatic dysfunction.

GROUP 1 - ZONE 1 – FRONTAL LOWER LEG

Category 7: *Acupuncture / Meridian*

Step 1: Functional Anatomy and Interpretive Importance

The anterior lower leg contains the tibialis anterior, extensor digitorum longus, and extensor hallucis longus, stabilized by the tibia and fibula with vascular and neural input (Standring, 2016). In acupuncture mapping, this zone aligns with the Stomach (ST) meridian coursing along the tibial crest and the Gallbladder (GB) meridian running more laterally.

Flaws (2000) emphasized their influence on digestive regulation, muscular tone, and pain mediation in the leg. Deadman et al. (2007) described how needling points along ST36 to ST40 relieve local symptoms and affect systemic energy distribution, highlighting their broad physiological role.

Clinically, disturbances of these meridians are reported as cramping, anterior leg pain, or weakness. In biosignal imaging, such dysfunctions appear as linear emissive fields of hypo- or hyperactivation tracking the path of these channels, providing external evidence of energetic imbalance superimposed upon anatomical structures.

Step 2,3,4: ROI Classification and Interpretive Questions

Hyperemission suggests active Qi stagnation or meridian reactivity along the pathway.

- Is there localized tenderness, swelling, or acute pain following the meridian?
- Are symptoms aggravated by movement or pressure on specific acupuncture points?

Hypoemission indicates Qi deficiency or chronic stagnation contributing to reduced energy flow and localized perfusion decline.

- Does the patient experience weakness, coldness, numbness, or chronic dull pain?
- Are there signs of chronic fatigue or poor circulation?

Step 5: Confirmatory Evaluations

Test	Purpose & Justification	Relevance to Emissive Pattern
Pulse diagnosis and tongue examination	Traditional diagnostic tools assessing Qi and blood status (Flaws, 2000).	Correlate with biospectral findings to refine meridian interpretation.
Biospectral imaging	Detects emissive asymmetries corresponding to meridian imbalances.	Direct visualization of hyper- or hypoemissive meridian zones.
Patient symptom questionnaire	Evaluates patterns of pain, fatigue, and other subjective signs.	Supports differentiation between Qi stagnation and deficiency.

Step 6: Care Strategies and Intervention Pathways

Naturopathic Approach

Acupuncture targeting points along the Stomach and Gallbladder meridians (e.g., ST36, GB34) improves Qi flow, reduces inflammation, and enhances circulation (Lao et al., 2004). Moxibustion provides warming and tonifying effects for hypoemissive patterns. Herbal formulas such as *Dang Gui* and *Chuan Xiong* nourish blood and regulate Qi (Bensky et al., 2004). Nutritional support with Qi-building foods and antioxidants supports therapeutic outcomes.

Standard Medical Approaches

While acupuncture is primarily naturopathic, integration with physical therapy and pain management optimizes outcomes in musculoskeletal conditions related to meridian dysfunction.

Specialty / Practitioner Care Strategies Table

Specialty Group	Practitioners Included	Hyperemissive Strategies	Hypoemissive Strategies
Biochemistry	Nutritionists, Orthomolecular, Herbalists, Naturopaths	Herbal formulas to regulate Qi and blood, antioxidants	Qi tonics, blood nourishing supplements
Rehabilitation	Physiotherapists, Massage Therapists, Osteopaths / Chiropractors	Trigger point therapy complementary to acupuncture	Gentle mobilization, warming massage
Energetics	Acupuncturists (TCM), Bioenergetic Therapists	Acupuncture, moxibustion, PEMF	Warming acupuncture, Qi tonics, energy healing
Psychological	GNM practitioners, Psychotherapists, Vibrational therapists, Family constellation facilitators	Mind-body therapies, bioresonance, energy clearing	Psychosomatic conflict resolution, emotional balancing

Educational Pearls & Considerations.

- Proper point selection is essential to balance hyper- and hypoemissive meridian imbalances.
- Moxibustion should be used cautiously in patients with heat sensitivity or inflammation.
- Herbal formulas require careful diagnosis to avoid overstimulation or contraindications.
- Combining acupuncture with physical therapy enhances functional recovery.

GROUP 1 - ZONE 1 – FRONTAL LOWER LEG

Category 8: *Energetic*

Step 1: Functional Anatomy and Interpretive Importance

The anterior lower leg includes the tibialis anterior and extensor muscles, positioned between tibial and fibular shafts and supplied by the anterior tibial neurovascular bundle (Standring, 2016).

From an energetic perspective, this region reflects longitudinal conduction pathways essential for coordinated locomotion and systemic balance. Oschman (2016) emphasized that connective tissue behaves as a semi-conductive matrix, propagating subtle signals that influence vascular and muscular regulation.

Clinically, disturbances may appear as tension or fatigue not fully explained by structural assessment. Spectral surface imaging often reveals narrow hyperemissive streaks suggesting overactive regulation or hypoemissive depressions indicating conduction block along fascial trajectories.

These emissive features provide clinicians with an externalized map of subtle energetic dynamics, clarifying how anterior leg fields serve as an index of systemic coherence or depletion.

Step 2,3,4: ROI Classification and Interpretive Questions

Hyperemission indicates localized energetic congestion, reactivity, or overactivity.

- Are there sensations of heat, tingling, or localized discomfort without clear physical cause?
- Is there an emotional or stress-related component exacerbating symptoms?

Hypoemission suggests energy underexpression, reduced flow, or stagnation.

- Does the patient report coldness, numbness, fatigue, or low vitality?
- Are symptoms chronic, with poor response to conventional treatments?

Step 5: Confirmatory Evaluations

Test	Purpose & Justification	Relevance to Emissive Pattern
Bioresonance testing	Assesses energetic imbalances and frequencies in tissues.	Correlates with hyper- or hypoemissive emission zones.
Electrodermal screening (EDS)	Measures skin conductance related to energetic pathways.	Supports interpretation of energetic imbalances.
Patient symptom and emotional history	Provides context for energy-related dysfunction.	Aids differentiation of energetic dynamics.

Step 6: Care Strategies and Intervention Pathways

Naturopathic Approach

Energetic therapies include bioresonance, pulsed electromagnetic fields (PEMF), and herbal formulas aimed at restoring energetic balance and supporting physiological healing (Matsumoto et al., 2010). Nutritional support includes adaptogens and antioxidants to enhance systemic resilience. Mindfulness and stress reduction techniques complement energetic rebalancing.

Standard Medical Approaches

These therapies are adjunctive and integrated with conventional treatments addressing structural or biochemical dysfunctions for comprehensive care.

Specialty / Practitioner Care Strategies Table

Specialty Group	Practitioners Included	Hyperemissive Strategies	Hypoemissive Strategies
Biochemistry	Nutritionists, Orthomolecular, Herbalists, Naturopaths	Adaptogens, antioxidants, herbal energetics	Nutritional support for energy deficiency
Rehabilitation	Physiotherapists, Massage Therapists, Osteopaths / Chiropractors	Energy-based manual therapies, PEMF, therapeutic touch	Gentle stimulation, mobilization
Energetics	Acupuncturists (TCM), Bioenergetic Therapists	Bioresonance, PEMF, acupuncture	Warming acupuncture, energy balancing
Psychological	GNM practitioners, Psychotherapists, Vibrational therapists, Family constellation facilitators	Psychotherapy, bioresonance, mindfulness	Emotional balancing, vibrational medicine

Educational Pearls & Considerations.

- Energetic therapies are complementary and should be used alongside conventional diagnostics.
- Practitioner skill and patient receptivity affect outcomes significantly.
- Monitor for symptomatic changes that may indicate shifts in energy balance requiring treatment adaptation.
- Always consider psychological and physical factors when addressing energetic disturbances.

GROUP 1 - ZONE 1 – FRONTAL LOWER LEG

Category 9: *Metabolic / Endocrine*

Step 1: Functional Anatomy and Interpretive Importance

The frontal lower leg is defined by the tibial surface, anterior musculature, and fascial planes linking knee and ankle stability (Standring, 2016). Endocrine and metabolic regulation strongly influence this region, as systemic glycoregulatory and thyroid activity modulate circulation, nerve conduction, and reparative capacity.

Vinik et al. (2003) demonstrated that diabetic neuropathy and microvascular complications frequently manifest as altered lower limb physiology, often preceding overt ulceration or skin change. Patients may report numbness, burning pain, or poor wound healing in this field, reflecting metabolic stress.

Spectral surface readings reveal hypoemissive depressions linked with reduced perfusion or neural suppression, contrasted with patchy hyperemissive foci indicating reparative activation.

These signals often follow fascial and vascular trajectories, mapping systemic metabolic strain into visible surface signatures. Clinically, the anterior lower leg serves as an external indicator of glycoregulatory balance and peripheral endocrine resilience.

Step 2,3,4: ROI Classification and Interpretive Questions

Hyperemission may indicate localized tissue activation, immune response, or metabolic overactivity.

- Are there signs of redness, warmth, or edema?
- Is the patient's metabolic condition poorly controlled?

Hypoemission reflects impaired perfusion, neural suppression, or perfusion reduction secondary to metabolic/endocrine regulatory shifts.

- Does the patient experience coldness, numbness, or non-healing wounds?
- Are there systemic signs such as fatigue, weight changes, or temperature intolerance?

Step 5: Confirmatory Evaluations

Test	Purpose & Justification	Relevance to Emissive Pattern
HbA1c, fasting glucose	Monitor glycemic control in diabetes mellitus.	Links to hypoemissive neuropathic or ischemic areas.
Thyroid function tests (TSH, Free T4)	Detect thyroid dysfunction affecting metabolism and circulation.	Associated with altered emission regulation.

Lipid profile	Assess risk for vascular disease influencing tissue perfusion.	Supports understanding of metabolic vascular impact.
Inflammatory markers (CRP, ESR)	Identify systemic inflammation influencing tissue health.	Correlates with hyperemissive regulatory activation

Step 6: Care Strategies and Intervention Pathways

Naturopathic Approach

Optimize metabolic control through diet emphasizing low glycemic index foods, antioxidants, and micronutrients supporting insulin sensitivity (Alberti et al., 2006). Herbal adaptogens like *Panax ginseng* and *Gymnema sylvestre* may support endocrine balance. Supplementation with chromium, magnesium, and alpha-lipoic acid assists glucose metabolism and nerve protection. Regular moderate exercise improves circulation and metabolic parameters.

Standard Medical Approaches

Strict glycemic control using pharmacotherapy and lifestyle modification is critical in diabetes management. Thyroid hormone replacement or modulation addresses endocrine causes. Management of dyslipidemia and hypertension reduces vascular complications.

Specialty / Practitioner Care Strategies Table

Specialty Group	Practitioners Included	Hyperemissive Strategies	Hypoemissive Strategies
Biochemistry	Nutritionists, Orthomolecular, Herbalists, Naturopaths	Antioxidants, adaptogens, insulin sensitizers, micronutrients	Metabolic support, neuroprotective nutrients, dietary management
Rehabilitation	Physiotherapists, Massage Therapists, Osteopaths / Chiropractors	Exercise therapy, circulation enhancement	Neuromuscular re-education, aerobic conditioning
Energetics	Acupuncturists (TCM), Bioenergetic Therapists	Acupuncture supporting metabolic function	Energy balancing, PEMF
Psychological	GNM practitioners, Psychotherapists, Vibrational therapists, Family constellation facilitators	Mind-body therapies supporting metabolic regulation	Stress reduction, emotional balancing

Educational Pearls & Considerations.

- Monitor metabolic parameters regularly to prevent progression of vascular and neuropathic complications.
- Integrate lifestyle interventions with clinical management for best outcomes.
- Adaptogens can support but not replace conventional endocrine therapies.
- Patient education on wound care and foot protection is critical.

GROUP 1

ZONE 2 – DORSAL LOWER LEG

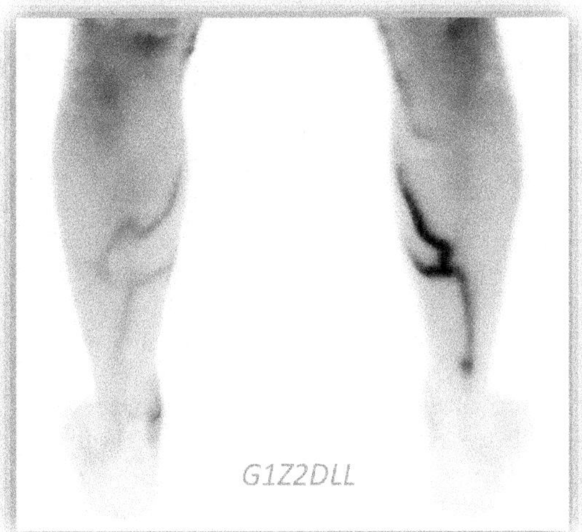

The posterior lower legs frequently express emissive changes related to venous stasis and lymphatic backflow, particularly in the gastrocnemius–soleus complex and along the Achilles tendon. Unlike the anterior shin, where hypoemissive tendencies often correspond to circulatory restriction, dorsal patterns typically reflect overload conditions such as venous pooling, fascial strain, or impaired lymphatic return.

Anatomically, the calf serves as the "peripheral heart" of the lower limb, with the gastrocnemius–soleus muscle pump responsible for propelling venous blood back toward the heart (Standring, 2016). When this pump is compromised, whether by inactivity, prolonged standing, or fascial constriction, emissive disturbances often appear before symptomatic varicosities are established.

Epidemiological data show that up to 25–30% of adults develop chronic venous disease, and early alterations often manifest first in the posterior calf region (Beebe-Dimmer, 2005). Persistent hyperemission medial to the Achilles tendon has been clinically correlated with pre-varicose states, a finding supported by imaging studies linking calf venous pressure and local soft-tissue adaptations (Raju & Neglén, 2009).

This region is also highly responsive to lymphodynamic shifts, with emissive asymmetries frequently associated with impaired calf lymphatic drainage or compensatory postural strain. From a functional interpretive perspective, the dorsal calf may reveal signs of overload, circulatory stagnation, or fascial rigidity even in patients who are asymptomatic, providing a window into preclinical vascular stress.

For athletes, this zone can also demonstrate lactic acid accumulation after intense exertion, with hyperemissive activity reflecting local metabolic strain, while in sedentary individuals, hypoactive drainage fields may reveal early lymphatic stasis.

Taken together, the posterior lower leg offers unique insight into peripheral vascular and lymphatic coherence, serving both as a marker of venous resilience and as a practical terrain indicator of systemic circulatory health.

Zone 2 – Dorsal Lower Legs: Emission-Relevant Structures

Category	Relevant Structures	Emission Relevance
1. Vascular / Circulatory	- Small saphenous vein (posterior midline) - Posterior tibial vein - Peroneal vein - Perforators connecting superficial to deep systems	Hyperemission often signals venous reflux or overload, especially in varicosity-prone individuals. Hypoemission may reflect vascular collapse, peripheral insufficiency, or stasis.
2. Muscular / Myofascial	- Gastrocnemius (medial and lateral heads) - Soleus - Plantaris - Flexor digitorum longus - Flexor hallucis longus - Crural and Achilles fascia	Overuse and postural strain in calf muscles frequently result in dorsal hyperemission. Hypoemission may follow disuse, fascial tightness, or chronic myofascial inhibition.
3. Skeletal / Articular	- Calcaneus (heel) - Tibia (posterior surface) - Fibula (posterolateral shaft) - Popliteal fossa landmarks	Hyperemission may signal bony activation, enthesopathy, or microtrauma. Hypoemissive fields suggest joint hypoactivity, systemic underuse, or vascular–bone disconnection.
4. Nervous System / Spine	- Tibial nerve (deep posterior compartment) - Sural nerve (cutaneous lateral calf) - S1–S2 dermatomes	Neural irritation may drive hyperemission in dermatomal or nerve-trace distribution. Hypoemission indicates sensory hypoactivity, neuropathy, or spinal compression syndromes.
5. Lymphatic / Immune	- Posterior tibial lymphatic pathways - Popliteal lymph nodes (drain calf and foot posterior compartments)	Lymphatic stagnation, especially post-infectious or due to chronic lymphatic burden, may present with persistent dorsal leg hyperemission. Hypoemissive zones indicate immune hyporegulation or drainage block.
6. Organs / GNM	*(Not applicable in this zone)*	
7. Acupuncture / Meridians	- Bladder Meridian (BL) – primary posterior leg meridian - Kidney Meridian (KD) – deeper medial-posterior line (less visually evident niospectrally)	Hyperemissive fields along the Bladder channel often reflect stress-axis activation or Yang excess. Hypoemission suggests Kidney Yang deficiency or Qi depletion.
8. Energetic / Frequency	- Reflex zones for backflow, exhaustion, and postural stability (bioenergetic readings) - Chronic dorsal cold in burnout syndromes	Dorsal Hyperemission may reflect sympathetic stress, fear tension, or unresolved somatic memory. Hypoemission indicates adrenal depletion, postural collapse, or chronic fatigue.
9. Metabolic / Endocrine	- Mitochondrial zones in calf musculature - Glucose and ATP turnover pathways - Peripheral thyroid/adrenal terrain zones	Hypometabolic states reduce posterior leg emissive activity, especially in thyroid or insulin-resistant presentations. Local hyperemission can follow intense exertion or lactic overload.

GROUP 1 - ZONE 2 – DORSAL LOWER LEG

Category 1: *Vascular / Circulatory*

Step 1: Functional Anatomy and Interpretive Importance

The posterior tibial artery, together with the fibular (peroneal) artery, provides inflow to the posterior calf, perfusing the gastrocnemius, soleus, and deep flexor compartment. Venous return occurs through paired posterior tibial veins draining into the popliteal system and through the small saphenous vein for the superficial posterior tissues (Standring, 2016).

Epidemiological analyses identify the posterior tibial segment as one of the most reliable sites for detecting peripheral arterial disease progression, underscoring its value in vascular assessment (Criqui & Aboyans, 2015).

Spectral surface readings of the posterior calf often reveal emissive asymmetries along these vascular tracks. Such patterns may represent venous pooling, impaired calf pump efficiency, or restricted posterior tibial inflow. Because this zone sustains both propulsion and venous return, emissive irregularities here are particularly informative for early vascular evaluation.

Step 2,3,4: ROI Classification and Interpretive Questions

Hyperemission indicates venous congestion or microvascular activation, accompanied by increased local blood flow and metabolic activity.

- Are symptoms of swelling, warmth, heaviness, or pain present?
- Is there visible venous dilation or skin changes?

Hypoemission suggests arterial underperfusion, vasospasm, or microvascular flow restriction causing decreased perfusion.

- Is there coldness, numbness, intermittent claudication, or delayed wound healing?
- Are pulses diminished?

Step 5: Confirmatory Evaluations

Test	Purpose & Justification	Relevance to Emissive Pattern
Doppler ultrasound	Assesses arterial and venous flow; confirms vascular pathology (Brant et al., 2016).	Correlates with hyperemissive venous and hypoemissive arterial patterns.
Ankle-Brachial Index (ABI)	Quantifies arterial perfusion; ABI <0.9 indicates peripheral arterial disease (Norgren et al., 2007).	Validates hypoemissive arterial insufficiency.
Capillary refill time	Evaluates microcirculation and perfusion status.	Supports microvascular dysfunction in Hypoemission.
Blood tests (CBC, CRP, coagulation)	Detect systemic inflammation and thrombotic risk factors.	Supports venous activation patterns.

Step 5: **Care Strategies and Intervention Pathways**

Naturopathic Approach

Botanical venotonics such as *Aesculus hippocastanum* and *Centella asiatica* improve venous tone (Chrubasik et al., 2011). Hydrotherapy stimulates circulation and reduces edema (Sutkowy et al., 2019). Anti-inflammatory diet rich in antioxidants and omega-3 fatty acids supports vascular integrity (Calder, 2017). Nitric oxide boosters enhance arterial perfusion (Moncada & Higgs, 1993). Limb elevation and movement promote venous return. Circulatory stimulants such as *Ginkgo biloba* support arterial flow. Nutritional supplementation with iron, B12, and folate optimizes oxygen transport.

Standard Medical Approaches

Doppler and ABI guide use of compression stockings, venoactive drugs, NSAIDs, sclerotherapy, or revascularization as indicated (Brant et al., 2016; Norgren et al., 2007). Wound care is essential in ischemic ulcers.

Specialty / Practitioner Care Strategies Table

Specialty Group	Practitioners Included	Hyperemissive Strategies	Hypoemissive Strategies
Biochemistry	Nutritionists, Orthomolecular, Herbalists, Naturopaths	Botanical venotonics, anti-inflammatory diet, antioxidants, vitamins C, E, selenium, CoQ10, bioflavonoids, omega-3s	Circulatory stimulants (*Ginkgo*, cayenne), blood-building nutrients (iron, B12, folate), magnesium, arginine, nitrate-rich diet
Rehabilitation	Physiotherapists, Massage Therapists, Osteopaths / Chiropractors	Lymphatic drainage, calf pump exercises, postural retraining, gentle Swedish massage, myofascial release	Graded aerobic exercise, gait training, emission protection, foot care, warming massage, reflexology, ergonomic guidance
Energetics	Acupuncturists (TCM), Bioenergetic Therapists	Acupuncture (SP6, ST36), moxibustion, herbal formulas, Qi and Blood tonics, bioresonance, PEMF	Warming acupuncture, Qi and Blood tonics, PEMF, energy healing
Psychological	GNM practitioners, Psychotherapists, Vibrational therapists, Family constellation facilitators	GNM conflict protocols, psychotherapy, bioresonance, mindfulness, energy clearing	Psychosomatic conflict resolution, vibrational medicine, stress reduction, emotional balancing

Educational Pearls & Considerations.

- Exclude deep vein thrombosis or critical ischemia before heat, massage, or exercise.
- Botanical venotonics combined with hydrotherapy synergistically reduce venous congestion.
- Nitric oxide boosters and omega-3 fatty acids enhance arterial perfusion and endothelial function.
- Compression therapy contraindicated in severe arterial disease.
- Early mobilization and limb elevation prevent chronic complications.

GROUP 1 - ZONE 2 – DORSAL LOWER LEG

Category 2: *Muscular*

Step 1: Functional Anatomy and Interpretive Importance

The posterior compartment of the leg includes a superficial group, gastrocnemius, soleus, and plantaris, and a deep group with tibialis posterior, flexor hallucis longus, and flexor digitorum longus, all innervated by the tibial nerve. These muscles generate plantar flexion, drive gait propulsion, and contribute to postural stability, with the Achilles tendon forming the most powerful tendinous structure of the limb (Standring, 2016).

Clinical literature identifies the calf as one of the most frequent sites of muscle injury, with gastrocnemius strains common in running and jumping activities, particularly among middle-aged athletes (Del Buono et al., 2012).

Because these muscles also support venous return, their overload disrupts propulsion and modifies circulatory efficiency, producing emissive asymmetries across the calf These signals, often paramedian or band-like, reveal early stages of muscular fatigue and fascial rigidity, offering a biospectral window into both mechanical and vascular stress during locomotion.

Step 2,3,4: ROI Classification and Interpretive Questions

Hyperemission suggests acute muscle strain, myofascial activation, or reactive overload with increased blood flow and metabolic activity.

- Has the patient experienced recent trauma or repetitive strain?
- Is there localized tenderness, swelling, or spasms?

Hypoemission indicates chronic perfusion decline, compartment adaptation, or neurogenic signal reduction causing decreased perfusion and metabolism.

- Are there symptoms of numbness, weakness, cramping, or muscle wasting?
- Is gait altered or muscle bulk reduced?

Step 5: Confirmatory Evaluations

Test	Purpose & Justification	Relevance to Emissive Pattern
Creatine kinase (CK), LDH	Detect muscle damage or inflammation (Maffulli et al., 2014).	Elevated in hyperemissive muscle activation.
MRI	Visualizes edema, inflammation, ischemia, or atrophy.	Supports hyperemissive tissue activation or hypoemissive ischemia.
Compartment pressure measurement	Diagnoses compartment syndrome by measuring intracompartmental pressure.	Relevant for hypoemissive ischemic presentations.

Nerve conduction studies (NCS), Electromyography (EMG)	Evaluates neurogenic muscle dysfunction.	Hypoemission related to neurogenic causes.
Blood tests (CBC, inflammatory markers)	Detect systemic inflammation or infection.	Supports hyperemissive regulatory activation.

Step 6: Care Strategies and Intervention Pathways

Naturopathic Approach

Management focuses on reducing inflammation and supporting muscle repair. Anti-inflammatory botanicals such as *Curcuma longa* (turmeric) and *Boswellia serrata* reduce inflammation (Hewlings & Kalman, 2017). Magnesium supplementation supports muscle function. Hydrotherapy with alternating warm and cold compresses improves circulation (Sutkowy et al., 2019). Gentle stretching and graded strengthening aid functional recovery. Adequate protein and antioxidant-rich nutrition support repair.

Standard Medical Approaches

Rest, NSAIDs, and physical therapy remain standard treatments for acute injuries (Maffulli et al., 2014). Compartment syndrome requires urgent surgical intervention. Neurogenic dysfunction requires neurological evaluation and rehabilitation.

Specialty / Practitioner Care Strategies Table

Specialty Group	Practitioners Included	Hyperemissive Strategies	Hypoemissive Strategies
Biochemistry	Nutritionists, Orthomolecular, Herbalists, Naturopaths	Anti-inflammatory botanicals, magnesium, antioxidants, protein	Circulatory support, neurotrophic nutrients, protein support
Rehabilitation	Physiotherapists, Massage Therapists, Osteopaths / Chiropractors	Myofascial release, trigger point therapy, gentle massage	Graded aerobic exercise, neurorehabilitation, ergonomic advice
Energetics	Acupuncturists (TCM), Bioenergetic Therapists	Acupuncture, moxibustion, PEMF	Warming acupuncture, frequency therapy
Psychological	GNM practitioners, Psychotherapists, Vibrational therapists, Family constellation facilitators	Psychotherapy, bioresonance, mindfulness	Psychosomatic conflict resolution, emotional balancing

Educational Pearls & Considerations.

- Early diagnosis of compartment syndrome is vital to prevent permanent damage.
- Magnesium aids muscle relaxation and prevents cramps.
- Hydrotherapy protocols must be tailored to inflammation status.
- Neurogenic muscle weakness requires thorough evaluation.
- Graded rehabilitation prevents chronic dysfunction.

GROUP 1 - ZONE 2 – DORSAL LOWER LEG

Category 3: *Skeletal*

Step 1: Functional Anatomy and Interpretive Importance

The dorsal lower leg comprehendes the posterior tibia and fibula, which articulate with the talus and calcaneus to maintain ankle stability (Standring, 2016). These bones are subject to axial and torsional forces during walking and running, often acting as conduits for load transmission through the ankle and foot arch.

When repetitive stress exceeds adaptive capacity, periosteal responses and joint microinstability may develop, particularly along the posterior tibial margin where soft tissue protection is limited. Matheson et al. (1987) described how posterior tibial stress fractures often emerge in high-demand activities, preceding overt radiological changes.

Such skeletal adaptations influence emissive regulation, and spectral surface readings frequently reveal elongated biospectral asymmetries tracing the dorsal tibial contour. These emissive signatures, sharper and more localized than muscular fields, externalize the osseous response to repetitive loading, offering a noninvasive window into early structural adaptation before it manifests clinically.

Step 2,3,4: ROI Classification and Interpretive Questions

Hyperemission suggests acute bone injury, periosteal activation, or structural reactivity with increased blood flow.

- Has the patient suffered trauma or repetitive stress?
- Is there localized tenderness, swelling, or joint stiffness?

Hypoemission may indicate chronic articular adaptation, reduced perfusion, or structural decline affecting metabolic activity.

- Is there chronic pain, stiffness, or reduced joint mobility?
- Is there a history of joint deformity or instability?

Step 5: Confirmatory Evaluations

Test	Purpose & Justification	Relevance to Emissive Pattern
X-ray imaging	Detects fractures, stress reactions, and joint space changes.	Confirms hyperemissive acute injuries or hypoemissive degenerative changes.
MRI	Visualizes bone marrow edema, occult fractures, and soft tissue.	Supports hyperemissive tissue activation or hypoemissive chronic pathology.
Bone scan	Assesses bone metabolism and detects stress fractures or infection.	Correlates with hyperemissive bone involvement.
Blood tests (inflammatory markers)	Detects systemic inflammation related to bone injury or infection.	Supports hyperemissive regulatory activation

Step 6: Care Strategies and Intervention Pathways

Naturopathic Approach

Supports bone healing and reduces inflammation. Nutrients including calcium, vitamin D, magnesium, and vitamin K are vital for bone metabolism (Heaney, 2006). Anti-inflammatory botanicals such as *Boswellia serrata* reduce periosteal inflammation. Therapeutic ultrasound and pulsed electromagnetic fields (PEMF) stimulate bone repair (Gordon et al., 2016). Rest and immobilization prevent further injury.

Standard Medical Approaches

Imaging guides immobilization, casting, or surgical repair of fractures (Khan et al., 2012). NSAIDs and physical therapy manage pain and restore function. Osteoarthritis treatment includes analgesics, anti-inflammatory drugs, and joint support.

Specialty / Practitioner Care Strategies Table

Specialty Group	Practitioners Included	Hyperemissive Strategies	Hypoemissive Strategies
Biochemistry	Nutritionists, Orthomolecular, Herbalists, Naturopaths	Bone-supportive nutrients, anti-inflammatory botanicals	Nutritional support for bone remodeling and joint health
Rehabilitation	Physiotherapists, Massage Therapists, Osteopaths / Chiropractors	Joint mobilization, therapeutic ultrasound, myofascial release	Joint stabilization, graded strengthening, ergonomic guidance
Energetics	Acupuncturists (TCM), Bioenergetic Therapists	Acupuncture, PEMF, herbal formulas for inflammation	Warming acupuncture, energy balancing
Psychological	GNM practitioners, Psychotherapists, Vibrational therapists, Family constellation facilitators	Mind-body therapies supporting pain management and healing	Psychosomatic support, emotional balancing

Educational Pearls & Considerations.

- Immobilization is essential in fractures to prevent displacement.
- Nutritional support accelerates bone healing.
- PEMF therapy should be applied carefully under professional supervision.
- Chronic hypoemissive joint patterns may indicate degenerative disease requiring multidisciplinary management.
- Psychological support can improve pain and recovery outcomes.

GROUP 1 - ZONE 2 – DORSAL LOWER LEG

Category 4: *Nervous*

Step 1: Functional Anatomy and Interpretive Importance

Innervation of the dorsal lower leg arises from the superficial and deep branches of the peroneal nerve, which provide motor control for dorsiflexion and sensory distribution across the dorsum of the foot (Standring, 2016).

The nerve's trajectory around the fibular neck creates a natural site of vulnerability, where compression or repetitive strain frequently provokes neuropathic changes. Styf (1989) noted that athletes exposed to repetitive ankle motion often develop peroneal entrapment presenting as pain, paresthesia, or progressive weakness.

When conduction falters, autonomic regulation of perfusion and muscular tone is also altered, producing secondary patterns of imbalance. These regulatory consequences become perceptible at the surface as elongated emissive fields following the tibial contour, their sharply defined geometry reflecting the linear course of the nerve.

Unlike diffuse myofascial signals, these patterns map directly onto the neural distribution, providing a visual correlate of peroneal stress that refines diagnostic interpretation in this zone.

Step 2,3,4: ROI Classification and Interpretive Questions

Hyperemission may indicate nerve irritation or neurogenic activation associated with increased local blood flow.

- Are there burning, tingling, or shooting pains?
- Is there localized hypersensitivity or swelling?

Hypoemission suggests nerve compression, perfusion decline, or denervation leading to decreased autonomic regulation and reduced emissive output.

- Is numbness, weakness, muscle wasting, or coldness present?
- Do symptoms worsen with activity or certain positions?

Step 5: Confirmatory Evaluations

Test	Purpose & Justification	Relevance to Emissive Pattern
Nerve conduction studies (NCS), Electromyography (EMG)	Assess nerve and muscle function (Campbell & Meyer, 2006).	Correlate with hypoemissive neurogenic dysfunction.
Quantitative sensory testing (QST)	Measures sensory nerve thresholds and function.	Supports neuropathic activation.

MRI / Ultrasound	Visualizes nerve compression or lesions.	Identifies neurogenic involvement
Blood tests (glucose, vitamin B12)	Rules out metabolic neuropathies.	Supports interpretive correlation with neuropathic patterns.

Step 6: Care Strategies and Intervention Pathways

Naturopathic Approach

Nutritional support with B-complex vitamins, alpha-lipoic acid, and Acetyl-L-carnitine aids nerve repair (Papanas & Ziegler, 2014). Anti-inflammatory herbs like *Hypericum perforatum* may alleviate neuropathic pain (Kasper et al., 2010). Physical therapies including neural mobilization and gentle stretching promote functional recovery. Mind-body techniques, bioresonance, and acupuncture modulate pain and improve neurovascular regulation.

Standard Medical Approaches

Pharmacologic management includes anticonvulsants, antidepressants, and analgesics. Physical therapy and surgical decompression may be required. Metabolic control is crucial in diabetic neuropathy.

Specialty / Practitioner Care Strategies Table

Specialty Group	Practitioners Included	Hyperemissive Strategies	Hypoemissive Strategies
Biochemistry	Nutritionists, Orthomolecular, Herbalists, Naturopaths	Neurotrophic vitamins, alpha-lipoic acid, anti-inflammatory botanicals	Circulatory stimulants, metabolic support, neuroprotective nutrients
Rehabilitation	Physiotherapists, Massage Therapists, Osteopaths / Chiropractors	Neural mobilization, myofascial release, gentle massage	Neural gliding exercises, ergonomic guidance, neurorehabilitation
Energetics	Acupuncturists (TCM), Bioenergetic Therapists	Acupuncture, moxibustion, PEMF	Warming acupuncture, frequency therapy, energy healing
Psychological	GNM practitioners, Psychotherapists, Vibrational therapists, Family constellation facilitators	Psychotherapy, bioresonance, mindfulness	Psychosomatic conflict resolution, vibrational medicine

Educational Pearls & Considerations.

- Early diagnosis and intervention prevent permanent nerve damage.
- Nutritional therapies support regeneration but do not replace medical treatment.
- Mind-body and energetic therapies can modulate pain perception.
- Monitor metabolic factors such as diabetes.
- Avoid aggressive therapies during acute inflammation.

GROUP 1 - ZONE 2 – DORSAL LOWER LEG

Category 5: *Lymphatic*

Step 1: Functional Anatomy and Interpretive Importance

The dorsal compartment of the lower leg is traversed by superficial lymphatic vessels that course with the saphenous system and deep collectors accompanying posterior tibial veins, directing flow toward popliteal and inguinal nodes (Standring, 2016). These pathways are central for maintaining posterior compartment fluid balance and immune traffic.

Mortimer and Levick (2004) noted that lymphatic dysfunction in the lower limbs frequently coexists with venous insufficiency, compounding tissue congestion and reducing immune efficiency. When such alterations occur dorsally, they influence surrounding vascular tone and muscular compliance, creating emissive irregularities that extend vertically toward the popliteal fossa.

The biospectral patterns generated in this region often demonstrate elongated fields aligned with the posterior tibia, reflecting the directional compromise of lymphatic transport. These visible signals provide clinicians with an externalized marker of posterior lymphatic strain, supporting differentiation between venous overload and primary lymphatic insufficiency in the dorsal lower leg.

Step 2,3,4: ROI Classification and Interpretive Questions

Hyperemission reflects acute immune activation, infectious response, or lymphatic congestion with localized warmth and swelling.

- Is there redness, tenderness, or acute swelling?
- Has there been recent injury or infection?

Hypoemission indicates chronic lymphatic stagnation with tissue rigidity, poor drainage, or reduced oxygenation.

- Is swelling persistent and firm?
- Are there recurrent infections or slow healing wounds?

Step 5: Confirmatory Evaluations

Test	Purpose & Justification	Relevance to Emissive Pattern
Lymphoscintigraphy	Assesses lymphatic drainage and identifies obstruction.	Validates lymphatic burden or hypoperfusion.
Doppler ultrasound	Excludes venous insufficiency contributing to lymphatic issues.	Differentiates vascular from lymphatic causes.

Blood tests (CBC, inflammatory markers)	Detect infection or systemic inflammation.	Supports hyperemissive regulatory activation.
Physical examination (Stemmer's sign, limb circumference)	Identifies clinical lymphedema signs.	Confirms lymphatic dysfunction correlated with emissive analysis.

Step 6: Care Strategies and Intervention Pathways

Naturopathic Approach

Treatment emphasizes enhancing lymphatic flow and reducing inflammation. Herbal lymphagogues such as *Hedera helix* (ivy leaf) and *Vitis vinifera* (grape seed extract) improve lymphatic vessel tone (Godoy et al., 2012). Manual lymphatic drainage performed by trained therapists facilitates fluid movement. Compression therapy, when indicated, supports lymphatic return. Nutritional antioxidants and anti-inflammatory nutrients support tissue health. Hydrotherapy with alternating warm and cold water stimulates lymphatic circulation.

Standard Medical Approaches

Standard care includes manual lymph drainage, compression garments, physical therapy, and prompt treatment of infections. Severe or refractory cases may require surgical intervention.

Specialty / Practitioner Care Strategies Table

Specialty Group	Practitioners Included	Hyperemissive Strategies	Hypoemissive Strategies
Biochemistry	Nutritionists, Orthomolecular, Herbalists, Naturopaths	Herbal lymphagogues, antioxidants, anti-inflammatory nutrients	Circulatory support, nutritional tissue repair support
Rehabilitation	Physiotherapists, Massage Therapists, Osteopaths / Chiropractors	Manual lymphatic drainage, gentle massage, postural retraining	Compression therapy, graded exercise, ergonomic guidance
Energetics	Acupuncturists (TCM), Bioenergetic Therapists	Acupuncture, herbal formulas, PEMF	Warming acupuncture, energy balancing
Psychological	GNM practitioners, Psychotherapists, Vibrational therapists, Family constellation facilitators	Mind-body therapies supporting immune function and healing	Psychosomatic conflict resolution, emotional balancing

Educational Pearls & Considerations.

- Early intervention prevents progression to chronic lymphedema.
- Manual lymph drainage should only be performed by qualified practitioners.
- Compression therapy requires individualized fitting and monitoring.
- Nutritional support enhances lymphatic function and tissue repair.
- Monitor for recurrent infections, which exacerbate lymphatic dysfunction.

GROUP 1 - ZONE 2 – DORSAL LOWER LEG

Category 7: *Acupuncture / Meridian*

Step 1: Functional Anatomy and Interpretive Importance

The posterior lower leg includes the gastrocnemius, soleus, and plantaris, all converging into the Achilles tendon, supported by venous plexuses and fascial planes (Standring, 2016). This zone corresponds primarily to the Bladder (BL) meridian, descending through the posterior leg, and to secondary pathways of the Gallbladder (GB) meridian.

Maciocia (2015) highlighted that the Bladder meridian governs water metabolism and defensive Qi, while also modulating spinal and muscular stability. Langevin and Yandow (2002) proposed a structural model in which meridians parallel connective tissue planes, offering a biophysical explanation for observed effects.

Patients with disruptions along these channels often present with calf pain, tension, or postural fatigue. On emissive assessment, the posterior leg reveals vertical fields of altered intensity following BL trajectories, their pattern distinct from diffuse muscular activation, thus reflecting both energetic and structural influences.

Step 2,3,4: ROI Classification and Interpretive Questions

Hyperemission suggests active Qi stagnation or meridian reactivity along the pathway.

- Is there localized tenderness, swelling, or sharp pain along specific acupuncture points?
- Are symptoms aggravated by movement or pressure?

Hypoemission indicates Qi deficiency or chronic stagnation contributing to reduced energy flow and localized oxygenation decline.

- Does the patient experience weakness, coldness, or numbness?
- Are there signs of chronic fatigue or poor circulation?

Step 5: Confirmatory Evaluations

Test	Purpose & Justification	Relevance to Emissive Pattern
Pulse diagnosis and tongue examination	Traditional TCM tools assessing Qi and blood status (Flaws, 2000).	Correlate with emissive findings to refine interpretation.
Biospectral imaging	Detects emissive asymmetries corresponding to meridian imbalances.	Direct visualization of hyper- or hypoemissive meridian zones.
Patient symptom questionnaire	Assesses pain patterns and functional status.	Supports differentiation between Qi stagnation and Qi deficiency.

Step 6: Care Strategies and Intervention Pathways

Naturopathic Approach

Acupuncture targeting key points such as ST36 and GB34 improves Qi flow, reduces inflammation, and enhances circulation (Lao et al., 2004). Moxibustion provides warming and tonifying effects for hypoemissive patterns. Herbal formulas like *Dang Gui* and *Chuan Xiong* nourish blood and regulate Qi (Bensky et al., 2004). Nutritional support with Qi-building foods complements therapy.

Standard Medical Approaches

Acupuncture is used adjunctively with physical therapy and pain management to optimize outcomes in musculoskeletal disorders related to meridian dysfunction.

Specialty / Practitioner Care Strategies Table

Specialty Group	Practitioners Included	Hyperemissive Strategies	Hypoemissive Strategies
Biochemistry	Nutritionists, Orthomolecular, Herbalists, Naturopaths	Herbal formulas to regulate Qi and blood, antioxidants	Qi tonics, blood nourishing supplements
Rehabilitation	Physiotherapists, Massage Therapists, Osteopaths / Chiropractors	Trigger point therapy complementary to acupuncture	Gentle mobilization, warming massage
Energetics	Acupuncturists (TCM), Bioenergetic Therapists	Acupuncture, moxibustion, PEMF	Warming acupuncture, Qi tonics, energy healing
Psychological	GNM practitioners, Psychotherapists, Vibrational therapists, Family constellation facilitators	Mind-body therapies, bioresonance, energy clearing	Psychosomatic conflict resolution, emotional balancing

Educational Pearls & Considerations.

- Accurate point selection is crucial to balance hyper- and hypoemissive patterns.
- Use moxibustion cautiously in patients' sensitive to heat or inflammation.
- Herbal formulas require appropriate diagnosis and supervision.
- Combining acupuncture with rehabilitation optimizes recovery.

GROUP 1 - ZONE 2 – DORSAL LOWER LEG

Category 8: *Energetic*

Step 1: Functional Anatomy and Interpretive Importance

The posterior lower leg is dominated by the gastrocnemius–soleus complex, plantaris, and the Achilles tendon, forming a powerful lever system stabilized by venous plexuses and fascial compartments (Standring, 2016).

Energetically, this region relates to propulsion and grounding forces, where coherent energy circulation ensures functional strength and recovery. Hunt (1996) documented measurable field fluctuations around the calves correlating with pain, fatigue, and circulatory stress.

On emissive evaluation, posterior fields frequently display diffuse hypoemission reflecting stagnation, punctuated by focal hyperemissive nodes that indicate compensatory activation.

These patterns follow fascial and vascular lines rather than muscular boundaries, underscoring their energetic rather than purely structural origin. Integrating these observations allows clinicians to interpret calf disturbances within a broader energetic regulatory framework.

Step 2,3,4: ROI Classification and Interpretive Questions

Hyperemission reflects localized energetic congestion or reactivity.

- Are there sensations of heat, tingling, or discomfort without clear physical cause?
- Does stress or emotional distress exacerbate symptoms?

Hypoemission indicates energy underexpression or stagnation.

- Does the patient report coldness, numbness, fatigue, or low vitality?
- Are symptoms chronic and refractory to conventional treatments?

Step 5: Confirmatory Evaluations

Test	Purpose & Justification	Relevance to Emissive Pattern
Bioresonance testing	Evaluates energetic imbalances and tissue frequencies.	Correlates with hyper- or hypoemissive zones.
Electrodermal screening (EDS)	Measures skin conductance related to energy pathways.	Supports interpretation of energetic dynamics.
Patient emotional and symptom history	Provides context for energy-related dysfunction.	Assists in differential assessment.

Step 6: Care Strategies and Intervention Pathways

Naturopathic Approach

Energetic therapies include bioresonance, pulsed electromagnetic fields (PEMF), and herbal support aimed at restoring energetic balance and supporting physiological healing (Matsumoto et al., 2010). Nutritional adaptogens and antioxidants enhance systemic resilience. Mindfulness and stress reduction complement these therapies.

Standard Medical Approaches

Energetic therapies serve as adjuncts alongside conventional structural and biochemical treatments to optimize patient outcomes.

Specialty / Practitioner Care Strategies Table

Specialty Group	Practitioners Included	Hyperemissive Strategies	Hypoemissive Strategies
Biochemistry	Nutritionists, Orthomolecular, Herbalists, Naturopaths	Adaptogens, antioxidants, herbal energetics	Nutritional support for energy deficiency
Rehabilitation	Physiotherapists, Massage Therapists, Osteopaths / Chiropractors	Energy-based manual therapies, PEMF, therapeutic touch	Gentle stimulation, mobilization
Energetics	Acupuncturists (TCM), Bioenergetic Therapists	Bioresonance, PEMF, acupuncture	Warming acupuncture, energy balancing
Psychological	GNM practitioners, Psychotherapists, Vibrational therapists, Family constellation facilitators	Psychotherapy, bioresonance, mindfulness	Emotional balancing, vibrational medicine

Educational Pearls & Considerations.

- Use energetic therapies as complementary treatments integrated with conventional care.
- Patient receptivity and practitioner expertise affect efficacy.
- Monitor for clinical changes and adjust therapies accordingly.
- Consider psychological and physical factors when treating energetic imbalances.

GROUP 1 - ZONE 2 – DORSAL LOWER LEG

Category 9: *Metabolic / Endocrine*

Step 1: Functional Anatomy and Interpretive Importance

The dorsal lower leg incorporates the gastrocnemius–soleus complex, posterior tibial vessels, and fascial compartments central to propulsion and venous return (Standring, 2016). Metabolic and endocrine disturbances, particularly diabetes and thyroid dysregulation, frequently alter circulatory dynamics and reparative physiology here.

DeFronzo & Ferrannini (1991) described insulin resistance as a driver of microvascular and muscular impairment, offering a mechanistic link to changes observed in this region. Clinically, patients may present with cramping, fatigue, or delayed healing, especially under systemic metabolic strain.

Spectral surface readings highlight hypoemissive fields aligned with perfusion decline and, at times, hyperemissive arcs suggesting adaptive vascular reactivity. These emissive expressions extend across myofascial planes rather than isolated muscles, underscoring the systemic origin of local signals. The dorsal lower leg is thus a key field for visualizing early metabolic imbalance before structural pathology emerges.

Step 2,3,4: ROI Classification and Interpretive Questions

Hyperemission may indicate tissue activation, immune response, or metabolic overactivity.

- Is there localized redness, warmth, or edema?
- Is the patient's metabolic condition uncontrolled?

Hypoemission reflects impaired circulation, neural suppression, or perfusion reduction due to metabolic/endocrine regulatory shifts.

- Does the patient experience numbness, coldness, or chronic wounds?
- Are systemic symptoms such as fatigue or temperature intolerance present?

Step 5: Confirmatory Evaluations

Test	Purpose & Justification	Relevance to Emissive Pattern
HbA1c, fasting glucose	Monitors diabetic control.	Links hypoemissive neuropathic or ischemic areas.
Thyroid function tests (TSH, Free T4)	Detect thyroid dysfunction affecting metabolism and circulation.	Associated with altered emission regulation.
Lipid profile	Assesses vascular risk influencing tissue perfusion.	Supports metabolic vascular impact.
Inflammatory markers (CRP, ESR)	Identifies systemic inflammation.	Correlates with hyperemissive regulatory activation.

Step 6: Care Strategies and Intervention Pathways

Naturopathic Approach

Focuses on optimizing metabolic control with a low glycemic diet, antioxidants, and micronutrients that improve insulin sensitivity (Alberti et al., 2006). Adaptogenic herbs like *Panax ginseng* and *Gymnema sylvestre* support endocrine function. Supplements such as chromium, magnesium, and alpha-lipoic acid aid glucose metabolism and nerve protection. Regular exercise improves circulation and metabolism.

Standard Medical Approaches

Strict glycemic and metabolic control through medication and lifestyle modification is essential. Thyroid hormone therapy and management of dyslipidemia reduce complications.

Specialty / Practitioner Care Strategies Table

Specialty Group	Practitioners Included	Hyperemissive Strategies	Hypoemissive Strategies
Biochemistry	Nutritionists, Orthomolecular, Herbalists, Naturopaths	Antioxidants, adaptogens, insulin sensitizers, micronutrients	Metabolic support, neuroprotective nutrients, dietary management
Rehabilitation	Physiotherapists, Massage Therapists, Osteopaths / Chiropractors	Exercise therapy, circulation enhancement	Neuromuscular re-education, aerobic conditioning
Energetics	Acupuncturists (TCM), Bioenergetic Therapists	Acupuncture supporting metabolic function	Energy balancing, PEMF
Psychological	GNM practitioners, Psychotherapists, Vibrational therapists, Family constellation facilitators	Mind-body therapies supporting metabolic regulation	Stress reduction, emotional balancing

Educational Pearls & Considerations.

- Regular metabolic monitoring is vital to prevent tissue complications.
- Integrate lifestyle and dietary changes with clinical management.
- Adaptogens support but do not replace conventional treatments.
- Patient education on foot care and wound prevention is advisable.

GROUP 1

ZONE 3 – INTERNAL LEFT LEG

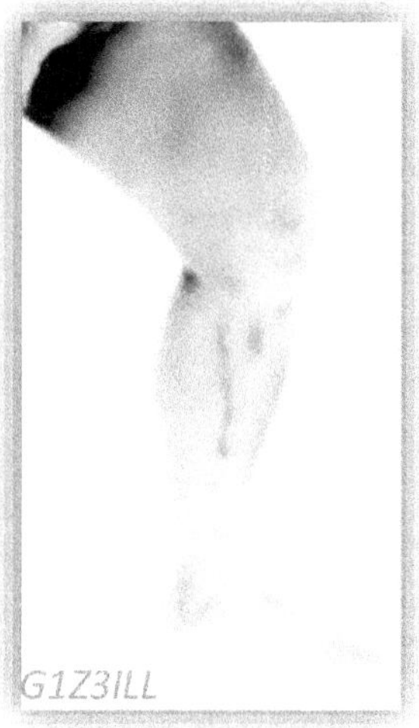

The internal left leg is among the most clinically sensitive terrains of the lower limb due to its lymphatic and hormonal–metabolic responsiveness. Unlike the lateral and frontal surfaces, this medial compartment often reflects systemic influences before overt pathology appears.

The region includes the great saphenous vein, deep lymphatic channels, and the adductor compartment musculature, all contributing to its biospectral reactivity (Standring, 2016). Asymmetrical hyperemissive activity here frequently correlates with pelvic and gynecologic influences, particularly in women, where patterns may indicate ovarian or uterine field activity despite the absence of direct anatomical continuity.

Studies show that 20–30% of women in postpartum or sedentary states present impaired pelvic drainage that secondarily influences emissive expression along the medial thigh (Cignini et al., 2012). Medial thigh lymph nodes form a critical drainage route for both limb and pelvis, and chronic overload predisposes to edema, venous hypertension, or delayed recovery (Mortimer & Rockson, 2014). The medial left leg often retains hyperemissive activity in these contexts, serving as an early cue of systemic burden long before swelling develops.

In endocrine contexts, subtle biospectral asymmetries here have been linked to metabolic stress, particularly in perimenopausal women where estrogen fluctuations alter vascular tone and lymphatic flow (Stachenfeld, 2008). These findings reinforce the value of this zone for musculoskeletal interpretation and as a reflex terrain marker of systemic influences.

Functionally, what appears as a narrow anatomical strip becomes a sensitive diagnostic landscape that reveals hormonal, metabolic, and lymphatic coherence, with relevance for early recognition of pelvic and endocrine strain and indispensable for integrative biospectral interpretation.

Zone 3 – Internal Left Leg: Emission-Relevant Structures.

Category	Relevant Structures	Emission Relevance
1. Vascular / Circulatory	- Great saphenous vein (runs along entire medial leg and thigh) - Perforating branches to femoral vein	Hyperemission may reflect venous overload, early varicosities, or valve incompetence. Hypoemission may indicate impaired flow, postural collapse, or lymphovenous stagnation.
2. Muscular / Myofascial	- Sartorius - Gracilis - Semitendinosus (upper medial thigh) - Tibialis posterior (lower medial leg) - Medial intermuscular septum fascia	Local hyperemissive activity may suggest muscular compensation, overuse due to pelvic imbalance, or fascial adhesion. Hypoemission is linked to disuse, pelvic instability, or hypotonic fascial pull.
3. Skeletal / Articular	- Medial tibial surface - Medial femoral condyle - Pubic ramus (proximally)	Bone-related hyperemission may signal periostitis, enthesopathy, or mechanical overload. Hypoemissive zones are commonly linked with chronic pelvic misalignment or degenerative hip mechanics.
4. Nervous System / Spine	- Saphenous nerve (cutaneous sensory, medial leg) - Obturator nerve (adductors/thigh) - L3–L4 dermatomes	Hyperemission of neuropathic type may result from femoral or obturator nerve irritation. Hypoemission may occur from prolonged tension, root compression, or low spinal drive to this quadrant.
5. Lymphatic / Immune	- Superficial lymphatic channels draining to inguinal nodes - Medial calf and thigh zones for fluid retention and toxin burden	Hyperemission suggests lymphatic congestion, detox stress, or hormonal overflow (e.g., estrogen). Hypoemissive fields may point to lymphatic collapse or immune suppression in lower extremity.
6. Organs / GNM	*(Typically excluded for direct organ mapping in this zone)*	
7. Acupuncture / Meridians	- Spleen Meridian (SP) – travels up medial leg and thigh - Liver Meridian (LR) – medial leg to groin - Kidney Meridian (KD) – medial-posterior blend	Hyperemission suggests Spleen or Liver meridian overload, especially tied to emotional stagnation, blood/Qi stasis, or metabolic taxation. Hypoemission indicates chronic depletion or Yin deficiency.
8. Energetic / Frequency	- Reflex area for internal security, stability, and nourishment (bioenergetic interpretation) - Links to reproductive terrain (feminine polarity zones)	Hyperemissive patterns may relate to pelvic emotional tension or maternal/relational stress fields. Hypoemission may reflect adrenal hyporegulation, hormonal burnout, or suppressed root-level energetic activity.
9. Metabolic / Endocrine	- Reflex zones for spleen-pancreas metabolism, estrogen/androgen terrain, and peripheral thyroid influence	Hypoemission may reflect endocrine slowing, insulin resistance, or liver load. Hyperemission may suggest metabolic compensation, dysregulation, or detox drainage in the thigh-pelvis path.

GROUP 1 - ZONE 3 – INTERNAL LEFT LEG

Category 1: *Vascular / Circulatory*

Step 1: Functional Anatomy and Interpretive Importance

The medial lower leg is supplied by the posterior tibial artery, which descends into the tarsal tunnel before continuing into plantar branches. It nourishes the tibialis posterior, flexor hallucis longus, flexor digitorum longus, and adjacent cutaneous areas. Venous return follows paired posterior tibial veins with support from the great saphenous vein along the medial border (Standring, 2016). International consensus identifies the posterior tibial system as a key axis for revascularization and limb salvage in advanced ischemia, confirming its central role in clinical management (Conte et al., 2019).

Medial emissive patterns in this zone often reflect venous retention or reduced inflow. Because deep and superficial systems converge here, even minor circulatory adjustments can amplify into visible emissive asymmetries, making this region highly responsive in functional evaluation.

Step 2,3,4: ROI Classification and Interpretive Questions

Hyperemission often indicates venous congestion or microvascular activation, presenting with increased local emissive output and visible redness.

- Are there complaints of leg heaviness, swelling, warmth, or pain?
- Is varicosity or skin discoloration observed?

Hypoemission reflects arterial underperfusion, vasospasm, or flow restriction causing reduced perfusion and diminished biosignal expression.

- Are there coldness, numbness, or intermittent claudication?
- Is there a history of delayed wound healing or ulcers?

Step 5: Confirmatory Evaluations

Test	Purpose & Justification	Relevance to Emissive Pattern
Doppler ultrasound	Assesses arterial and venous blood flow to confirm insufficiency or obstruction (Brant et al., 2016).	Correlates with hyperemissive venous congestion and hypoemissive arterial disease.
Ankle-Brachial Index (ABI)	Quantifies arterial perfusion; values below 0.9 suggest peripheral arterial disease (Norgren et al., 2007).	Validates hypoemissive arterial insufficiency.
Capillary refill time	Evaluates microvascular perfusion.	Supports hypoemissive microcirculatory compromise.
Blood tests (CBC, CRP, coagulation)	Detect systemic inflammation or thrombophilia contributing to vascular pathology.	Supports hyperemissive vascular or thrombotic activity.

Step 6: **Care Strategies and Intervention Pathways**

Naturopathic Approach

Use botanical venotonics such as *Aesculus hippocastanum* and *Centella asiatica* to strengthen venous tone (Chrubasik et al., 2011). Hydrotherapy with contrast baths enhances circulation and reduces edema (Sutkowy et al., 2019). An anti-inflammatory diet rich in bioflavonoids, vitamin C, and omega-3 fatty acids supports vascular health (Calder, 2017). Nitric oxide donors like beetroot and arginine improve arterial perfusion (Moncada & Higgs, 1993). Limb elevation and exercise promote venous return. Supplement iron, B12, and folate as needed.

Standard Medical Approaches

Doppler and ABI guide treatment with compression stockings, venoactive agents, NSAIDs, sclerotherapy, or revascularization (Brant et al., 2016; Norgren et al., 2007). Wound care is vital in ischemic ulcers.

Specialty / Practitioner Care Strategies Table

Specialty Group	Practitioners Included	Hyperemissive Strategies	Hypoemissive Strategies
Biochemistry	Nutritionists, Orthomolecular, Herbalists, Naturopaths	Botanical venotonics, anti-inflammatory diet, antioxidants, vitamins C, E, selenium, CoQ10, bioflavonoids, omega-3s	Circulatory stimulants (*Ginkgo*, cayenne), blood-building nutrients (iron, B12, folate), magnesium, arginine, nitrate-rich diet
Rehabilitation	Physiotherapists, Massage Therapists, Osteopaths / Chiropractors	Lymphatic drainage, calf pump exercises, postural retraining, gentle Swedish massage, myofascial release	Graded aerobic exercise, gait training, emission protection, foot care, warming massage, reflexology, ergonomic guidance
Energetics	Acupuncturists (TCM), Bioenergetic Therapists	Acupuncture (SP6, ST36), moxibustion, herbal formulas, Qi and Blood tonics, bioresonance, PEMF	Warming acupuncture, Qi and Blood tonics, PEMF, energy healing
Psychological	GNM practitioners, Psychotherapists, Vibrational therapists, Family constellation facilitators	GNM conflict protocols, psychotherapy, bioresonance, mindfulness, energy clearing	Psychosomatic conflict resolution, vibrational medicine, stress reduction, emotional balancing

Educational Pearls & Considerations.

- Exclude deep vein thrombosis or critical ischemia before heat, massage, or exercise.
- Botanical venotonics combined with hydrotherapy synergistically reduce venous congestion.
- Nitric oxide boosters and omega-3 fatty acids enhance arterial perfusion and endothelial function.
- Compression therapy is contraindicated in severe arterial disease.
- Early mobilization and limb elevation prevent chronic complications.

GROUP 1 - ZONE 3 – INTERNAL LEFT LEG

Category 2: *Muscular*

Step 1: Functional Anatomy and Interpretive Importance

The medial thigh, represented here in the internal left leg, contains the adductor longus, brevis, magnus, gracilis, and contributions from the sartorius. Supplied primarily by the obturator nerve, these muscles act in hip adduction, pelvic stabilization, and medial knee control, transmitting load across the pelvis and lower limb (Standring, 2016). Adductor injuries are a leading cause of chronic groin pain in athletes, particularly in sports such as soccer and ice hockey that demand repetitive changes of direction, where overload fosters weakness, fibrosis, and pain (Petersen & Holmich, 2005).

This same mechanical environment often produces medial emissive asymmetries aligned with fascial compartments or tendon insertions. On spectral evaluation, such irregularities signal regions of heightened load transfer and function as indicators of kinetic chain imbalance involving pelvis, hip, and lumbar stabilizers.

Step 2,3,4: ROI Classification and Interpretive Questions

Hyperemission indicates acute muscle strain, myofascial activation, or reactive overload with increased perfusion and metabolic activity.

- Has the patient experienced trauma, overuse, or exercise-related pain?
- Is localized tenderness, swelling, or spasm present?

Hypoemission suggests chronic perfusion decline, compartment adaptation, or neurogenic signal reduction causing reduced perfusion and metabolism.

- Are there numbness, weakness, or muscle wasting symptoms?
- Is gait or limb function impaired?

Step 5: Confirmatory Evaluations

Test	Purpose & Justification	Relevance to Emissive Pattern
Creatine kinase (CK), LDH	Detect muscle fiber damage or inflammation (Maffulli et al., 2014).	Elevated in hyperemissive tissue activation.
MRI	Visualizes edema, inflammation, ischemia, or atrophy.	Supports hyperemissive or hypoemissive states.
Compartment pressure measurement	Diagnoses compartment syndrome by intracompartmental pressure.	Relevant in hypoemissive ischemic presentations.
Nerve conduction studies (NCS), Electromyography (EMG)	Evaluates neurogenic muscle dysfunction.	Hypoemission linked to neurogenic causes.
Blood tests (CBC, inflammatory markers)	Detect systemic inflammation or infection.	Supports hyperemissive regulatory activation.

Step 6: Care Strategies and Intervention Pathways

Naturopathic Approach

Management focuses on reducing inflammation and enhancing repair. Anti-inflammatory botanicals such as *Curcuma longa* and *Boswellia serrata* have demonstrated efficacy (Hewlings & Kalman, 2017). Magnesium supplementation supports muscle relaxation. Hydrotherapy with alternating warm and cold compresses improves circulation (Sutkowy et al., 2019). Gentle stretching and progressive strengthening exercises restore function. Adequate protein and antioxidants support healing.

Standard Medical Approaches

Rest, NSAIDs, and physical therapy are standard for acute injuries (Maffulli et al., 2014). Compartment syndrome requires urgent surgical management. Neurogenic dysfunction warrants neurological evaluation and rehabilitation.

Specialty / Practitioner Care Strategies Table

Specialty Group	Practitioners Included	Hyperemissive Strategies	Hypoemissive Strategies
Biochemistry	Nutritionists, Orthomolecular, Herbalists, Naturopaths	Anti-inflammatory botanicals, magnesium, antioxidants, protein	Circulatory support, neurotrophic nutrients, protein support
Rehabilitation	Physiotherapists, Massage Therapists, Osteopaths / Chiropractors	Myofascial release, trigger point therapy, gentle massage	Graded aerobic exercise, neurorehabilitation, ergonomic guidance
Energetics	Acupuncturists (TCM), Bioenergetic Therapists	Acupuncture, moxibustion, PEMF	Warming acupuncture, frequency therapy
Psychological	GNM practitioners, Psychotherapists, Vibrational therapists, Family constellation facilitators	Psychotherapy, bioresonance, mindfulness	Psychosomatic conflict resolution, emotional balancing

Educational Pearls & Considerations.

- Early identification and treatment of compartment syndrome is critical.
- Magnesium aids in preventing muscle cramps and spasms.
- Hydrotherapy protocols must be tailored to inflammation stage.
- Neurogenic muscle weakness requires comprehensive assessment.
- Graded rehabilitation prevents chronic dysfunction.

GROUP 1 - ZONE 3 – INTERNAL LEFT LEG

Category 3: *Skeletal*

Step 1: Functional Anatomy and Interpretive Importance

The medial compartment of the distal femur, including the medial condyle and tibial plateau, forms the principal weight-bearing surface of the knee (Standring, 2016). These skeletal elements are responsible for transmitting compressive forces that are concentrated medially during ambulation.

Clinical studies have shown that this compartment is disproportionately affected by degenerative and overload syndromes, where subchondral stress and osteochondral remodeling are common precursors to more advanced pathology (Sharma et al., 2001).

As these skeletal reactions unfold, periarticular tissues undergo secondary regulatory adjustments, and their imprint can be visualized through spectral surface readings. Biospectral asymmetries at the medial knee often appear as focused intensifications that parallel the underlying joint line, reflecting articular stress and the compensatory modulation of adjacent tissues.

In this way, emissive expression translates the invisible burden of skeletal load distribution into a surface-accessible signal, highlighting early articular compromise before irreversible remodeling occurs.

Step 2,3,4: ROI Classification and Interpretive Questions

Hyperemission suggests acute fracture, periosteal activation, or joint fluid accumulation with increased local perfusion.

- Has the patient experienced recent trauma or overuse?
- Is there localized pain, swelling, or joint stiffness?

Hypoemission indicates chronic articular remodeling, structural degeneration, or vascular underperfusion resulting in reduced perfusion.

- Are there chronic joint pains, stiffness, or mobility restrictions?
- Is there a history of joint deformity or instability?

Step 5: Confirmatory Evaluations

Test	Purpose & Justification	Relevance to Emissive Pattern
X-ray imaging	Detects fractures, stress injuries, and joint space narrowing.	Confirms hyperemissive acute injuries or hypoemissive degenerative changes.
MRI	Visualizes bone marrow edema, occult fractures, cartilage, and soft tissue.	Supports hyperemissive tissue activation or hypoemissive chronic pathology.

Bone scan	Assesses bone metabolism and detects stress fractures or infection.	Correlates with hyperemissive bone involvement.
Blood tests (inflammatory markers)	Detects systemic inflammation related to bone injury or infection.	Supports hyperemissive regulatory activation.

Step 6: Care Strategies and Intervention Pathways

Naturopathic Approach

Supporting bone repair includes adequate calcium, vitamin D, magnesium, and vitamin K intake (Heaney, 2006). Anti-inflammatory botanicals such as *Boswellia serrata* reduce periosteal inflammation. Therapeutic ultrasound and PEMF stimulate bone healing (Gordon et al., 2016). Rest and immobilization prevent further injury.

Standard Medical Approaches

Imaging guides immobilization or surgery for fractures (Khan et al., 2012). NSAIDs and physical therapy manage symptoms. Osteoarthritis requires analgesics and supportive therapies.

Specialty / Practitioner Care Strategies Table

Specialty Group	Practitioners Included	Hyperemissive Strategies	Hypoemissive Strategies
Biochemistry	Nutritionists, Orthomolecular, Herbalists, Naturopaths	Bone-supportive nutrients, anti-inflammatory botanicals	Nutritional support for bone remodeling and joint health
Rehabilitation	Physiotherapists, Massage Therapists, Osteopaths / Chiropractors	Joint mobilization, therapeutic ultrasound, myofascial release	Joint stabilization, graded strengthening, ergonomic guidance
Energetics	Acupuncturists (TCM), Bioenergetic Therapists	Acupuncture, PEMF, herbal formulas for inflammation	Warming acupuncture, energy balancing
Psychological	GNM practitioners, Psychotherapists, Vibrational therapists, Family constellation facilitators	Mind-body therapies supporting pain management and healing	Psychosomatic support, emotional balancing

Educational Pearls & Considerations.

- Immobilize fractures promptly to prevent displacement.
- Adequate nutrition accelerates bone healing.
- PEMF therapy requires professional guidance.
- Chronic hypoemissive joint changes may require multidisciplinary care.
- Psychological support aids recovery.

GROUP 1 - ZONE 3 – INTERNAL LEFT LEG

Category 4: *Nervous*

Step 1: Functional Anatomy and Interpretive Importance

The medial thigh and knee region is supplied by the obturator nerve, responsible for adductor strength and sensory relay from the medial thigh (Standring, 2016). The nerve's narrow passage through the obturator canal predisposes it to entrapment, particularly in activities involving repetitive hip loading.

Bradshaw and McCrory (2007) described obturator neuropathy as a source of groin and medial thigh pain in athletes, often accompanied by weakness and gait disturbance. Neural irritation compromises motor drive, alters vascular dynamics, and modifies fascial recruitment, creating changes in the surface biosignal profile.

These influences often appear externally as contained emissive asymmetries localized to the medial femoral line, bounded more sharply than vascular or muscular emissions. Such patterns provide a tangible correlate of neural dysfunction, revealing the obturator nerve's burden on regional biomechanics and allowing clinicians to detect early neuropathic compromise through surface emissive mapping.

Step 2,3,4: ROI Classification and Interpretive Questions

Hyperemission may indicate nerve irritation or neurogenic activation with increased local blood flow.

- Are there burning, tingling, or shooting pains along the medial thigh?
- Is there localized hypersensitivity or swelling?

Hypoemission suggests nerve compression, perfusion decline, or denervation causing decreased autonomic regulation and reduced biosignal output.

- Are numbness, weakness, or muscle atrophy present?
- Do symptoms worsen with movement or pressure?

Step 5: Confirmatory Evaluations

Test	Purpose & Justification	Relevance to Emissive Pattern
Nerve conduction studies (NCS), Electromyography (EMG)	Assess nerve and muscle function (Campbell & Meyer, 2006).	Correlate with hypoemissive neurogenic dysfunction.
Quantitative sensory testing (QST)	Measures sensory thresholds and nerve function.	Supports neuropathic activation.
MRI / Ultrasound	Detects nerve compression or structural abnormalities.	Identifies neurogenic involvement
Blood tests (glucose, vitamin B12)	Evaluates metabolic causes of neuropathy.	Supports interpretation of neuropathic patterns.

Step 6: **Care Strategies and Intervention Pathways**

Naturopathic Approach

Nutrients such as B-complex vitamins, alpha-lipoic acid, and Acetyl-L-carnitine support nerve repair (Papanas & Ziegler, 2014). Herbal anti-inflammatories like *Hypericum perforatum* may alleviate neuropathic pain (Kasper et al., 2010). Physical therapies including neural mobilization and gentle stretching promote functional recovery. Mind-body therapies and bioresonance modulate pain and neurovascular regulation.

Standard Medical Approaches

Pharmacological treatments include anticonvulsants, antidepressants, and analgesics. Surgical decompression may be necessary. Metabolic control is vital in systemic neuropathies.

Specialty / Practitioner Care Strategies Table

Specialty Group	Practitioners Included	Hyperemissive Strategies	Hypoemissive Strategies
Biochemistry	Nutritionists, Orthomolecular, Herbalists, Naturopaths	Neurotrophic vitamins, alpha-lipoic acid, anti-inflammatory botanicals	Circulatory stimulants, metabolic support, neuroprotective nutrients
Rehabilitation	Physiotherapists, Massage Therapists, Osteopaths / Chiropractors	Neural mobilization, myofascial release, gentle massage	Neural gliding exercises, ergonomic guidance, neurorehabilitation
Energetics	Acupuncturists (TCM), Bioenergetic Therapists	Acupuncture, moxibustion, PEMF	Warming acupuncture, frequency therapy, energy healing
Psychological	GNM practitioners, Psychotherapists, Vibrational therapists, Family constellation facilitators	Psychotherapy, bioresonance, mindfulness	Psychosomatic conflict resolution, vibrational medicine

Educational Pearls & Considerations.

- Early diagnosis prevents irreversible nerve damage.
- Nutritional support aids regeneration but does not replace medical treatment.
- Mind-body and energetic therapies reduce pain perception.
- Monitor metabolic contributors.
- Avoid aggressive therapies during acute inflammation.

GROUP 1 - ZONE 3 – INTERNAL LEFT LEG

Category 5: *Lymphatic*

Step 1: Functional Anatomy and Interpretive Importance

The internal left leg is supplied by a rich plexus of lymphatic vessels that accompany the great saphenous vein and drain medially into inguinal lymph nodes (Standring, 2016). This pathway plays a key role in returning interstitial fluid and facilitating immune surveillance of the lower limb.

Keeley (2008) highlighted that medial limb lymphedema is among the earliest and most persistent presentations in chronic lymphatic dysfunction, often preceding visible swelling. Subtle disruption in this drainage modifies local mechanical properties and autonomic regulation, projecting its effects outward.

On surface assessment, biospectral asymmetries tend to concentrate as focal emissive zones along the medial femoral line, sharply bounded in contrast to broader vascular patterns. These externally visible signatures embody the functional state of medial lymphatic transport, offering clinicians a tool for identifying early immune congestion in the inguinal-directed channels of the internal leg.

Step 2,3,4: ROI Classification and Interpretive Questions

Hyperemission indicates acute immune activation, infectious response, or lymphatic congestion with warmth and swelling.

- Is there redness, tenderness, or sudden swelling?
- Has the patient experienced recent injury or infection?

Hypoemission suggests chronic lymphatic stagnation with tissue rigidity or poor drainage causing decreased perfusion.

- Is swelling persistent, firm, or accompanied by skin changes?
- Are infections recurrent or wounds slow to heal?

Step 5: Confirmatory Evaluations

Test	Purpose & Justification	Relevance to Emissive Pattern
Lymphoscintigraphy	Evaluates lymphatic drainage and detects obstruction.	Confirms lymphatic burden or hypoperfusion.
Doppler ultrasound	Excludes venous insufficiency as a cause of swelling.	Differentiates vascular and lymphatic causes.

Blood tests (CBC, inflammatory markers)	Detect infection or systemic inflammation.	Supports hyperemissive regulatory activation
Physical exam (Stemmer's sign, limb measurements)	Assesses clinical signs of lymphedema.	Correlates with emissive findings.

Step 6: Care Strategies and Intervention Pathways

Naturopathic Approach

Treatment focuses on improving lymphatic flow and reducing inflammation. Herbal lymphagogues such as *Hedera helix* (ivy leaf) and *Vitis vinifera* (grape seed extract) support lymph vessel tone (Godoy et al., 2012). Manual lymphatic drainage by trained therapists promotes fluid movement. Compression therapy aids lymph return but must be customized. Nutritional antioxidants and anti-inflammatory nutrients support tissue health. Hydrotherapy with alternating warm and cold water stimulates lymphatic circulation.

Standard Medical Approaches

Standard care includes manual lymph drainage, compression garments, physical therapy, and antibiotics for infections. Severe cases may require surgical intervention.

Specialty / Practitioner Care Strategies Table

Specialty Group	Practitioners Included	Hyperemissive Strategies	Hypoemissive Strategies
Biochemistry	Nutritionists, Orthomolecular, Herbalists, Naturopaths	Herbal lymphagogues, antioxidants, anti-inflammatory nutrients	Circulatory support, nutritional tissue repair support
Rehabilitation	Physiotherapists, Massage Therapists, Osteopaths / Chiropractors	Manual lymphatic drainage, gentle massage, postural retraining	Compression therapy, graded exercise, ergonomic guidance
Energetics	Acupuncturists (TCM), Bioenergetic Therapists	Acupuncture, herbal formulas, PEMF	Warming acupuncture, energy balancing
Psychological	GNM practitioners, Psychotherapists, Vibrational therapists, Family constellation facilitators	Mind-body therapies supporting immune function and healing	Psychosomatic conflict resolution, emotional balancing

Educational Pearls & Considerations.

- Early treatment prevents progression to chronic lymphedema.
- Manual lymph drainage must be performed by skilled therapists.
- Compression therapy requires careful fitting and monitoring.
- Nutritional support enhances lymphatic and tissue health.
- Monitor and promptly treat infections.

GROUP 1 - ZONE 3 – INTERNAL LEFT LEG

Category 7: *Acupuncture / Meridian*

Step 1: Functional Anatomy and Interpretive Importance

The medial aspect of the leg integrates the femur's condyles, adductor attachments, and deep fascial septa with vascular channels coursing toward the pelvis (Standring, 2016). This region corresponds to the Spleen (SP) and Liver (LV) meridians, which ascend along the inner leg to the trunk.

Kaptchuk (2000) emphasized their systemic role in harmonizing digestion, blood storage, and emotional regulation, linking peripheral stagnation with central imbalance. Cheng (1987) further described classical associations between medial leg pain and disruptions in SP–LV flow.

Clinically, dysfunction manifests as heaviness, edema, or medial knee discomfort. On biosignal imaging, emissive changes emerge as sharply aligned vertical patterns along the inner thigh and knee, distinguishing them from vascular or myofascial overload. These findings support the view that emissive fields can externalize the functional state of SP and LV channels, bridging meridian theory with observable biospectral expression.

Step 2,3,4: ROI Classification and Interpretive Questions

Hyperemission suggests Qi stagnation or meridian reactivity along the pathway.

- Is there localized tenderness, swelling, or acute pain along the meridian?
- Are symptoms aggravated by movement or pressure?

Hypoemission indicates Qi deficiency or chronic stagnation, resulting in decreased energy flow and localized oxygenation decline.

- Does the patient report weakness, coldness, numbness, or chronic dull pain?
- Are there signs of poor circulation or fatigue?

Step 5: Confirmatory Evaluations

Test	Purpose & Justification	Relevance to Emissive Pattern
Pulse diagnosis and tongue examination	Traditional TCM methods assessing Qi and blood status (Flaws, 2000).	Correlates with emissive findings to refine interpretation
Biospectral imaging	Detects emissive asymmetries along meridian pathways.	Directly visualizes hyper- or hypoemissive meridian zones.
Patient symptom questionnaire	Evaluates pain patterns, energy levels, and functional status.	Supports differentiation between Qi stagnation and Qi deficiency.

Step 6: Care Strategies and Intervention Pathways

Naturopathic Approach

Acupuncture targeting key points like SP6 and LV3 improves Qi and blood flow, reducing inflammation and restoring function (Lao et al., 2004). Moxibustion warms and tonifies hypoemissive meridians. Herbal formulas such as *Dang Gui* and *Chuan Xiong* nourish blood and regulate Qi (Bensky et al., 2004). Nutritional support with Qi-building foods complements treatment.

Standard Medical Approaches

Acupuncture is used adjunctively with physical therapy and pain management for musculoskeletal disorders related to meridian imbalance.

Specialty / Practitioner Care Strategies Table

Specialty Group	Practitioners Included	Hyperemissive Strategies	Hypoemissive Strategies
Biochemistry	Nutritionists, Orthomolecular, Herbalists, Naturopaths	Herbal formulas regulating Qi and blood, antioxidants	Qi tonics, blood nourishing supplements
Rehabilitation	Physiotherapists, Massage Therapists, Osteopaths / Chiropractors	Trigger point therapy complementary to acupuncture	Gentle mobilization, warming massage
Energetics	Acupuncturists (TCM), Bioenergetic Therapists	Acupuncture, moxibustion, PEMF	Warming acupuncture, Qi tonics, energy healing
Psychological	GNM practitioners, Psychotherapists, Vibrational therapists, Family constellation facilitators	Mind-body therapies, bioresonance, energy clearing	Psychosomatic conflict resolution, emotional balancing

Educational Pearls & Considerations.

- Accurate point selection is crucial for balancing meridian imbalances.
- Moxibustion should be applied cautiously in patients with heat sensitivity.
- Herbal treatments require diagnosis and professional supervision.

GROUP 1 - ZONE 3 – INTERNAL LEFT LEG

Category 8: *Energetic*

Step 1: Functional Anatomy and Interpretive Importance

The medial leg containes the femoral condyle, adductor insertions, and fascial planes guiding neurovascular channels toward the pelvis (Standring, 2016). Subtle energetic frameworks associate this area with circulatory coherence, immune defense, and systemic equilibrium. Becker and Selden (1985) described how low-level electrical potentials regulate tissue healing, suggesting that medial compartments act as conduits for broader systemic signals.

Clinically, patients may present with swelling, heaviness, or unexplained weakness of the medial knee. Biospectral imaging reveals elongated hypoemissive tracts corresponding to stagnation, or localized hyperemissive foci indicative of reparative activity.

These signals provide an externalized representation of medial energy dynamics, positioning this region as both a structural and energetic interface between limb and systemic physiology.

Step 2,3,4: ROI Classification and Interpretive Questions

Hyperemission reflects localized energy congestion or reactivity.

- Are there sensations of heat, tingling, or unexplained discomfort?
- Does stress or emotional distress influence symptoms?

Hypoemission indicates energy underexpression or stagnation.

- Does the patient report coldness, fatigue, numbness, or low vitality?
- Are symptoms chronic and resistant to conventional therapies?

Step 5: Confirmatory Evaluations

Test	Purpose & Justification	Relevance to Emissive Pattern
Bioresonance testing	Assesses tissue energy frequencies and imbalances.	Correlates with emission patterns.
Electrodermal screening (EDS)	Measures skin conductance linked to energy pathways.	Supports interpretation of energetic dynamics.
Patient emotional and symptom history	Provides context for energy-related dysfunction.	Assists differential assessment.

Step 6: Care Strategies and Intervention Pathways

Naturopathic Approach

Includes bioresonance, PEMF, and herbal adaptogens to restore energetic balance and support physiological healing (Matsumoto et al., 2010). Nutritional antioxidants and adaptogens improve systemic resilience. Mindfulness and stress reduction complement treatment.

Standard Medical Approaches

Energetic therapies are adjunctive, integrated with conventional medical and rehabilitative care.

Specialty / Practitioner Care Strategies Table

Specialty Group	Practitioners Included	Hyperemissive Strategies	Hypoemissive Strategies
Biochemistry	Nutritionists, Orthomolecular, Herbalists, Naturopaths	Adaptogens, antioxidants, herbal energetics	Nutritional support for energy deficiency
Rehabilitation	Physiotherapists, Massage Therapists, Osteopaths / Chiropractors	Energy-based manual therapies, PEMF, therapeutic touch	Gentle stimulation, mobilization
Energetics	Acupuncturists (TCM), Bioenergetic Therapists	Bioresonance, PEMF, acupuncture	Warming acupuncture, energy balancing
Psychological	GNM practitioners, Psychotherapists, Vibrational therapists, Family constellation facilitators	Psychotherapy, bioresonance, mindfulness	Emotional balancing, vibrational medicine

Educational Pearls & Considerations.

- Energetic therapies complement conventional treatments.
- Practitioner skill and patient receptivity affect results.
- Monitor clinical changes to adapt therapy.
- Address psychological and physical factors for holistic care.
- Combined acupuncture and rehabilitation improve outcomes.

GROUP 1 - ZONE 3 – INTERNAL LEFT LEG

Category 9: *Metabolic / Endocrine*

Step 1: Functional Anatomy and Interpretive Importance

The medial aspect of the left leg includes the distal femur, knee articulation, and fascial continuity extending into the adductor compartment (Standring, 2016). This region is highly sensitive to endocrine regulation of vascular tone and connective tissue metabolism.

Reaven (1988) identified metabolic syndrome as a systemic pattern influencing vascular compliance and tissue repair, directly relevant to medial leg physiology. Clinically, patients may describe heaviness, instability, or delayed healing in the medial field. Spectral surface readings often reveal hypoemissive depressions tracing venous or lymphatic trajectories, indicative of suppressed circulatory drive, while focal hyperemissive zones appear with reparative or inflammatory activity.

These biospectral dynamics reinforce the medial leg as a sensitive indicator of systemic metabolic load, where energy-intensive tissues provide early external signals of endocrine imbalance.

Step 2,3,4: ROI Classification and Interpretive Questions

Hyperemission may indicate tissue activation, immune response, or metabolic overactivity.

- Is there redness, warmth, or edema?
- Is the patient's metabolic/endocrine condition poorly controlled?

Hypoemission reflects impaired perfusion, neural suppression, or perfusion reduction due to metabolic/endocrine regulatory shifts.

- Does the patient report coldness, numbness, or chronic wounds?
- Are there systemic symptoms like fatigue or temperature intolerance?

Step 5: Confirmatory Evaluations

Test	Purpose & Justification	Relevance to Emissive Pattern
HbA1c, fasting glucose	Monitors glycemic control in diabetes.	Links hypoemissive neuropathic or ischemic areas.
Thyroid function tests (TSH, Free T4)	Detect thyroid disorders affecting metabolism and circulation.	Associated with altered emission regulation.
Lipid profile	Assesses vascular risk factors impacting tissue perfusion.	Supports metabolic vascular impact.
Inflammatory markers (CRP, ESR)	Identifies systemic inflammation influencing tissue health.	Correlates with hyperemissive regulatory activation.

Step 6: Care Strategies and Intervention Pathways

Naturopathic Approach

Optimizes metabolic function through low glycemic diet, antioxidants, and micronutrients supporting insulin sensitivity (Alberti et al., 2006). Adaptogenic herbs such as *Panax ginseng* and *Gymnema sylvestre* support endocrine balance. Supplementation with chromium, magnesium, and alpha-lipoic acid aids glucose metabolism and nerve protection. Regular moderate exercise enhances circulation and metabolism.

Standard Medical Approaches

Strict metabolic control using pharmacotherapy and lifestyle modification is essential. Thyroid hormone replacement and lipid management reduce complications.

Specialty / Practitioner Care Strategies Table

Specialty Group	Practitioners Included	Hyperemissive Strategies	Hypoemissive Strategies
Biochemistry	Nutritionists, Orthomolecular, Herbalists, Naturopaths	Antioxidants, adaptogens, insulin sensitizers, micronutrients	Metabolic support, neuroprotective nutrients, dietary management
Rehabilitation	Physiotherapists, Massage Therapists, Osteopaths / Chiropractors	Exercise therapy, circulation enhancement	Neuromuscular re-education, aerobic conditioning
Energetics	Acupuncturists (TCM), Bioenergetic Therapists	Acupuncture supporting metabolic function	Energy balancing, PEMF
Psychological	GNM practitioners, Psychotherapists, Vibrational therapists, Family constellation facilitators	Mind-body therapies supporting metabolic regulation	Stress reduction, emotional balancing

Educational Pearls & Considerations.

- Regular metabolic monitoring prevents progression of complications.
- Lifestyle and dietary changes complement clinical care.
- Adaptogens support but do not replace conventional therapies.
- Patient education on wound care is critical.

GROUP 1

ZONE 4 – INTERNAL RIGHT LEG

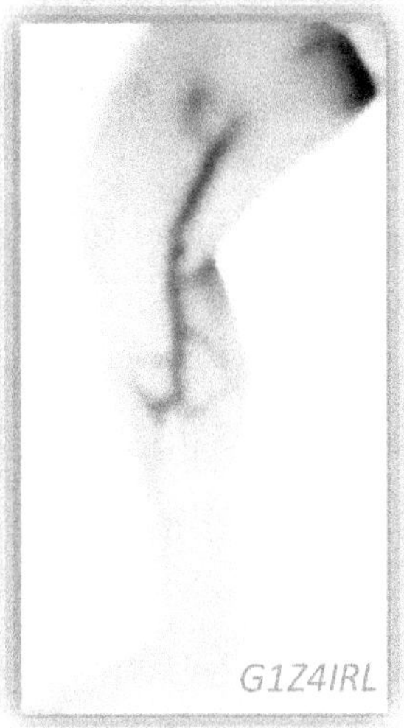

The internal right leg carries interpretive weight that extends beyond local musculoskeletal function, serving as a peripheral window into visceral regulation. This region contains the same venous and lymphatic pathways as its contralateral counterpart, yet clinically it demonstrates a greater association with hepatic, biliary, and right-sided colonic fields (Standring, 2016).

Anatomical studies have shown that right-sided lymphatic drainage often interacts more directly with hepatic and portal circulation, which may explain why emissive alterations here are frequently linked with hepatic regulatory burden (Gashev, 2008). A distinct clinical observation is that hypoemissive streaks on the right inner thigh, when unilateral, can correspond with early hepatic overload or bowel terrain imbalance, sometimes appearing before laboratory markers detect liver enzyme fluctuation.

In metabolic research, hepatic stress has been associated with altered microvascular reactivity, with peripheral markers sometimes detectable weeks before biochemical confirmation (Blendis & Wong, 2001). Biospectrally, this translates into interpretive findings where the right medial thigh expresses functional changes reflective of systemic terrain rather than localized dysfunction.

In gastrointestinal contexts, correlations have also been drawn between emissive asymmetries on the right medial leg and altered colonic motility, particularly in patients presenting with chronic constipation or right-sided abdominal tension (Camilleri, 2001). The lymphatic proximity of this zone further reinforces its systemic importance, as right-sided overload patterns often reveal congestion that extends beyond the limb into visceral drainage.

Functionally, persistent hyperemission in this region may also align with gallbladder sensitivity or biliary strain, offering subtle but valuable cues of visceral compensation. For integrative analysis, the strength of this zone lies in its ability to reveal systemic regulatory states, hepatic, biliary, or bowel-related, through a peripheral and non-invasive observation point.

By connecting limb emissive patterns with visceral physiology, the internal right leg serves as a functional barometer of metabolic and digestive coherence, providing interpretive insight well before structural or biochemical diagnosis.

Zone 4 – Internal Right Leg: Emission-Relevant Structures.

Category	Relevant Structures	Emission Relevance
1. Vascular / Circulatory	- Great saphenous vein (runs along medial leg and thigh) - Communicating perforators to femoral system	Hyperemission here often suggests venous reflux, overload, or liver-related drainage pressure. Hypoemission may indicate postural constriction, chronic hypoflow, or venous valve failure.
2. Muscular / Myofascial	- Sartorius - Gracilis - Semitendinosus - Tibialis posterior - Medial fascial interconnections and pelvic tension lines	Hyperemissive activity often follows pelvic rotation, muscular overload (e.g., in leg dominance), or fascial anchoring. Hypoemission may signal underuse, core disconnection, or chronic restriction.
3. Skeletal / Articular	- Medial tibia - Femoral medial condyle - Pubic ramus	Hyperemission may relate to joint overload, enthesopathy, or misalignment. Hypoemission can occur with degeneration, regulatory strain, or iliopubic imbalance.
4. Nervous System / Spine	- Saphenous nerve - Obturator nerve - L3–L4 dermatomes (innervating medial thigh and leg)	Hyperemission may reflect active neural strain due to tension or compression. Hypoemission may indicate femoral nerve hypoactivation, L4 impingement, or sympathetic hypoactivity.
5. Lymphatic / Immune	- Inguinal lymph nodes - Superficial and deep medial channels	Hyperemission is often linked to lymphatic congestion due to liver burden, hormonal shifts, or toxic load. Hypoemission reflects lymphatic insufficiency or immune hyporegulation.
6. Organs / GNM	*(Typically excluded from direct interpretation here)*	
7. Acupuncture / Meridians	- Liver Meridian (LR) – medial lower limb and thigh - Spleen Meridian (SP) - Kidney Meridian (KD)	Hyperemission commonly indicates Liver Qi stagnation, frustration, or anger held in the pelvic root. Hypoemission may reflect adrenal or kidney depletion, or weakened Spleen–Liver axis.
8. Energetic / Frequency	- Bioenergetic field for direction, confidence, reproductive identity, and masculine polarity zones	Hyperemission suggests emotional overload, performance anxiety, or goal frustration. Hypoemission may reflect burnout, adrenal hyporegulation, or constitutional Yang deficiency.
9. Metabolic / Endocrine	- Zones reflexively linked to liver metabolism, insulin regulation, and androgen pathways	Hypoemission may indicate hypometabolic patterns, liver stagnation, or testosterone decline. Hyperemission may be linked to detox efforts, hormonal fluctuations, or metabolic strain.

GROUP 1 - ZONE 4 – INTERNAL RIGHT LEG

Category 1: *Vascular / Circulatory*

Step 1: Functional Anatomy and Interpretive Importance

The medial right leg follows the same anatomical plan: the posterior tibial artery and its venae comitantes descend to join the popliteal vein, while the great saphenous vein provides superficial drainage.

This circulation sustains the posterior compartment musculature and cutaneous territories (Standring, 2016). Classic vascular classifications identify the posterior tibial artery as a major reference point for staging disease severity and guiding intervention in peripheral arterial disorders (Dormandy & Rutherford, 2000).

Altered emissive signatures in this zone often correspond to venous pooling, slowed clearance, or constricted arterial supply. Because of the constant biomechanical stress of gait, the medial calf frequently demonstrates early emissive evidence of circulatory adjustment.

Step 2,3,4: ROI Classification and Interpretive Questions

Hyperemission suggests venous congestion, microvascular activation, or vascular reactivity with increased perfusion.

- Is swelling, warmth, or discomfort present?
- Are varicose veins or skin changes visible?

Hypoemission indicates arterial underperfusion, vasospasm, or flow restriction associated with decreased biosignal output.

- Is there coldness, numbness, or intermittent claudication?
- Are peripheral pulses diminished?

Step 5: Confirmatory Evaluations

Test	Purpose & Justification	Relevance to Emissive Pattern
Doppler ultrasound	Assesses arterial and venous flow, detecting insufficiency (Brant et al., 2016).	Correlates with hyperemissive venous congestion and hypoemissive arterial disease.
Ankle-Brachial Index (ABI)	Quantifies arterial perfusion; ABI <0.9 indicates peripheral arterial disease (Norgren et al., 2007).	Validates hypoemissive arterial insufficiency.
Capillary refill time	Evaluates microcirculation.	Supports hypoemissive microvascular compromise.
Blood tests (CBC, CRP, coagulation)	Detects systemic inflammation or thrombotic risk factors.	Supports vascular activation patterns.

Step 6: Care Strategies and Intervention Pathways

Naturopathic Approach

Botanical venotonics such as *Aesculus hippocastanum* and *Centella asiatica* improve venous tone (Chrubasik et al., 2011). Hydrotherapy stimulates circulation and reduces edema (Sutkowy et al., 2019). Anti-inflammatory diets rich in antioxidants and omega-3 fatty acids support vascular health (Calder, 2017). Nitric oxide boosters enhance arterial perfusion (Moncada & Higgs, 1993). Limb elevation and exercise promote venous return. Nutritional support with iron, B12, and folate optimizes oxygen transport.

Standard Medical Approaches

Doppler and ABI guide use of compression stockings, venoactive drugs, NSAIDs, sclerotherapy, or revascularization (Brant et al., 2016; Norgren et al., 2007). Wound care is vital for ischemic ulcers.

Specialty / Practitioner Care Strategies Table

Specialty Group	Practitioners Included	Hyperemissive Strategies	Hypoemissive Strategies
Biochemistry	Nutritionists, Orthomolecular, Herbalists, Naturopaths	Botanical venotonics, anti-inflammatory diet, antioxidants, vitamins C, E, selenium, CoQ10, bioflavonoids, omega-3s	Circulatory stimulants (*Ginkgo*, cayenne), blood-building nutrients (iron, B12, folate), magnesium, arginine, nitrate-rich diet
Rehabilitation	Physiotherapists, Massage Therapists, Osteopaths / Chiropractors	Lymphatic drainage, calf pump exercises, postural retraining, gentle Swedish massage, myofascial release	Graded aerobic exercise, gait training, emission protection, foot care, warming massage, reflexology, ergonomic guidance
Energetics	Acupuncturists (TCM), Bioenergetic Therapists	Acupuncture (SP6, ST36), moxibustion, herbal formulas, Qi and Blood tonics, bioresonance, PEMF	Warming acupuncture, Qi and Blood tonics, PEMF, energy healing
Psychological	GNM practitioners, Psychotherapists, Vibrational therapists, Family constellation facilitators	GNM conflict protocols, psychotherapy, bioresonance, mindfulness, energy clearing	Psychosomatic conflict resolution, vibrational medicine, stress reduction, emotional balancing

Educational Pearls & Considerations.

- Exclude deep vein thrombosis or critical ischemia before heat, massage, or exercise.
- Botanical venotonics combined with hydrotherapy synergistically reduce venous congestion.
- Nitric oxide boosters and omega-3 fatty acids enhance arterial perfusion and endothelial function.
- Compression therapy is contraindicated in severe arterial disease.
- Early mobilization and limb elevation prevent chronic complications.

GROUP 1 - ZONE 4 – INTERNAL RIGHT LEG

Category 2: *Muscular*

Step 1: Functional Anatomy and Interpretive Importance

The internal right thigh mirrors the left, with adductor longus, brevis, magnus, gracilis, and sartorius providing hip adduction, pelvic alignment, and medial knee stabilization. These muscles, innervated primarily by the obturator nerve, are mechanically integrated with both femoral and sciatic contributions, ensuring controlled gait and stance stability (Standring, 2016).

Prospective cohort studies demonstrate that reduced adductor strength or flexibility is one of the strongest predictors of groin injury, confirming their importance in athletic performance and prevention strategies (Emery et al., 2001).

In functional imaging, the same predisposition manifests as emissive asymmetries along the medial thigh, with signal variation more pronounced in the dominant leg. These findings, when interpreted in context, often reveal compensatory asymmetry of pelvic stabilizers, making the medial thigh an early biospectral marker of systemic postural imbalance.

Step 2,3,4: ROI Classification and Interpretive Questions

Hyperemission indicates acute muscle strain, myofascial activation, or reactive overload with increased blood flow.

- Has the patient suffered trauma or overuse?
- Is there localized tenderness, swelling, or muscle spasm?

Hypoemission suggests chronic perfusion reduction, compartment adaptation, or neurogenic signal suppression causing decreased perfusion.

- Are there numbness, weakness, or muscle wasting?
- Is gait or limb function impaired?

Step 5: Confirmatory Evaluations

Test	Purpose & Justification	Relevance to Emissive Pattern
Creatine kinase (CK), LDH	Detects muscle damage or inflammation (Maffulli et al., 2014).	Elevated in hyperemissive tissue activation.
MRI	Visualizes edema, inflammation, ischemia, or atrophy.	Supports hyperemissive or hypoemissive findings.
Compartment pressure measurement	Diagnoses compartment syndrome by measuring intracompartmental pressure.	Relevant in hypoemissive ischemic presentations.

Nerve conduction studies (NCS), Electromyography (EMG)	Evaluates neurogenic muscle dysfunction.	Correlates with hypoemissive neurogenic causes.
Blood tests (CBC, inflammatory markers)	Detects systemic inflammation or infection.	Supports hyperemissive inflammatory states.

Step 6: Care Strategies and Intervention Pathways

Naturopathic Approach

Use anti-inflammatory botanicals like *Curcuma longa* and *Boswellia serrata* to reduce inflammation (Hewlings & Kalman, 2017). Magnesium supports muscle relaxation. Hydrotherapy with alternating warm and cold compresses improves circulation (Sutkowy et al., 2019). Gentle stretching and graded strengthening restore function. Protein and antioxidants aid repair.

Standard Medical Approaches

Rest, NSAIDs, and physical therapy are standard for acute muscle injuries (Maffulli et al., 2014). Compartment syndrome requires urgent surgical intervention. Neurogenic dysfunction necessitates neurological assessment and rehabilitation.

Specialty / Practitioner Care Strategies Table

Specialty Group	Practitioners Included	Hyperemissive Strategies	Hypoemissive Strategies
Biochemistry	Nutritionists, Orthomolecular, Herbalists, Naturopaths	Anti-inflammatory botanicals, magnesium, antioxidants, protein	Circulatory support, neurotrophic nutrients, protein support
Rehabilitation	Physiotherapists, Massage Therapists, Osteopaths / Chiropractors	Myofascial release, trigger point therapy, gentle massage	Graded aerobic exercise, neurorehabilitation, ergonomic guidance
Energetics	Acupuncturists (TCM), Bioenergetic Therapists	Acupuncture, moxibustion, PEMF	Warming acupuncture, frequency therapy
Psychological	GNM practitioners, Psychotherapists, Vibrational therapists, Family constellation facilitators	Psychotherapy, bioresonance, mindfulness	Psychosomatic conflict resolution, emotional balancing

Educational Pearls & Considerations.

- Early diagnosis of compartment syndrome is critical.
- Magnesium supports muscle relaxation and reduces cramps.
- Hydrotherapy should be tailored to the inflammation phase.
- Neurogenic muscle weakness requires comprehensive evaluation.
- Graded rehabilitation prevents chronic dysfunction.

GROUP 1 - ZONE 4 – INTERNAL RIGHT LEG

Category 3: *Skeletal*

Step 1: Functional Anatomy and Interpretive Importance

The internal right leg mirrors the skeletal framework of the contralateral medial femoral condyle and tibial plateau, forming the load-bearing axis of the knee (Standring, 2016). This region plays a decisive role in stabilizing gait and absorbing repetitive ground reaction forces.

Medial joint overload has been linked to progressive cartilage thinning and osseous remodeling, processes that often begin subclinically with subtle stiffness or discomfort (Felson et al., 2000). These changes alter local vascular and periosteal signaling, producing emissive variations that extend beyond the confines of the bone itself.

On spectral surface readings, biospectral asymmetries typically present as contained focal fields overlying the medial joint, sometimes projecting distally toward the tibial metaphysis. The clarity of these patterns contrasts with diffuse muscular emissions, underscoring their skeletal origin and enabling the clinician to distinguish articular load adaptation from soft-tissue sources. Such integration positions surface emissive analysis as a sensitive marker of early osseous maladaptation.

Step 2,3,4: ROI Classification and Interpretive Questions

Hyperemission indicates acute fractures, periosteal activation, or joint fluid accumulation with increased local blood flow.

- Has the patient experienced recent trauma or overuse?
- Are there signs of swelling, tenderness, or joint stiffness?

Hypoemission suggests chronic structural adaptation, articular decline, or vascular underperfusion causing reduced perfusion.

- Is there chronic joint pain, stiffness, or limited mobility?
- Is there a history of joint deformity or instability?

Step 5: Confirmatory Evaluations

Test	Purpose & Justification	Relevance to Emissive Pattern
X-ray imaging	Detects fractures, stress injuries, and joint space narrowing.	Confirms hyperemissive acute injuries or hypoemissive degenerative changes.
MRI	Visualizes bone marrow edema, occult fractures, cartilage, and soft tissue pathology.	Supports hyperemissive tissue activation or hypoemissive chronic changes.

Bone scan	Assesses bone metabolism and detects stress fractures or infection.	Correlates with hyperemissive bone involvement.
Blood tests (inflammatory markers)	Detect systemic inflammation related to bone injury or infection.	Supports hyperemissive regulatory activation.

Step 6: Care Strategies and Intervention Pathways

Naturopathic Approach

Bone healing is supported by adequate intake of calcium, vitamin D, magnesium, and vitamin K (Heaney, 2006). Anti-inflammatory botanicals like *Boswellia serrata* reduce periosteal inflammation. Therapeutic ultrasound and PEMF stimulate bone repair (Gordon et al., 2016). Immobilization protects injured structures.

Standard Medical Approaches

Imaging guides immobilization or surgical intervention for fractures (Khan et al., 2012). NSAIDs and physical therapy manage symptoms. Osteoarthritis requires analgesics and supportive care.

Specialty / Practitioner Care Strategies Table

Specialty Group	Practitioners Included	Hyperemissive Strategies	Hypoemissive Strategies
Biochemistry	Nutritionists, Orthomolecular, Herbalists, Naturopaths	Bone-supportive nutrients, anti-inflammatory botanicals	Nutritional support for bone remodeling and joint health
Rehabilitation	Physiotherapists, Massage Therapists, Osteopaths / Chiropractors	Joint mobilization, therapeutic ultrasound, myofascial release	Joint stabilization, graded strengthening, ergonomic guidance
Energetics	Acupuncturists (TCM), Bioenergetic Therapists	Acupuncture, PEMF, herbal formulas for inflammation	Warming acupuncture, energy balancing
Psychological	GNM practitioners, Psychotherapists, Vibrational therapists, Family constellation facilitators	Mind-body therapies supporting pain management and healing	Psychosomatic support, emotional balancing

Educational Pearls & Considerations.

- Prompt immobilization prevents further injury.
- Nutrition accelerates bone healing.
- PEMF therapy requires skilled application.
- Chronic hypoemissive patterns suggest degenerative disease needing multidisciplinary care.
- Psychological support enhances recovery.

GROUP 1 - ZONE 4 – INTERNAL RIGHT LEG

Category 4: *Nervous*

Step 1: Functional Anatomy and Interpretive Importance

The internal right thigh mirrors the contralateral distribution of the obturator nerve, stabilizing gait and coordinating medial thigh motion (Standring, 2016). Entrapment or irritation of this pathway, frequently reported in cases of pelvic instability or fascial narrowing, can result in adductor weakness, sensory disturbance, and restricted hip control.

Neary et al. (2003) emphasized that obturator entrapment is an underdiagnosed cause of chronic medial thigh pain, with many cases misattributed to muscular strain. Neural stress of this nature influences vascular tone and periarticular recruitment, projecting an external emissive signature that follows the medial femoral shaft or knee line.

These sharply bounded signals differ from broader capsular or tendinous fields, underscoring their neurogenic character. In clinical interpretation, such emissive expressions provide a noninvasive means of distinguishing nervous system involvement from purely musculoskeletal sources, clarifying the neural contribution to medial thigh dysfunction.

Step 2,3,4: ROI Classification and Interpretive Questions

Hyperemission may indicate nerve irritation or neurogenic activation with increased blood flow.

- Does the patient report burning, tingling, or sharp pains?
- Is there localized hypersensitivity or swelling?

Hypoemission suggests nerve compression, perfusion decline, or denervation causing reduced autonomic regulation and diminished biosignal expression.

- Are numbness, weakness, or muscle wasting present?
- Do symptoms worsen with certain movements or positions?

Step 5: Confirmatory Evaluations

Test	Purpose & Justification	Relevance to Emissive Pattern
Nerve conduction studies (NCS), Electromyography (EMG)	Assess nerve and muscle function (Campbell & Meyer, 2006).	Correlate with hypoemissive neurogenic dysfunction.
Quantitative sensory testing (QST)	Measures sensory thresholds and nerve function.	Supports neuropathic activity.
MRI / Ultrasound	Visualizes nerve compression or lesions.	Identifies neurogenic involvement
Blood tests (glucose, vitamin B12)	Evaluates metabolic causes of neuropathy.	Supports interpretation of metabolic neuropathic patterns

Step 6: Care Strategies and Intervention Pathways

Naturopathic Approach

Neurotrophic vitamins (B-complex), alpha-lipoic acid, and Acetyl-L-carnitine support nerve repair (Papanas & Ziegler, 2014). Herbal anti-inflammatories like *Hypericum perforatum* may alleviate neuropathic pain (Kasper et al., 2010). Neural mobilization and gentle stretching aid recovery. Mind-body therapies and bioresonance modulate pain and neurovascular function.

Standard Medical Approaches

Pharmacologic treatments include anticonvulsants, antidepressants, and analgesics. Surgical decompression may be necessary. Metabolic control is essential in systemic neuropathies.

Specialty / Practitioner Care Strategies Table

Specialty Group	Practitioners Included	Hyperemissive Strategies	Hypoemissive Strategies
Biochemistry	Nutritionists, Orthomolecular, Herbalists, Naturopaths	Neurotrophic vitamins, alpha-lipoic acid, anti-inflammatory botanicals	Circulatory stimulants, metabolic support, neuroprotective nutrients
Rehabilitation	Physiotherapists, Massage Therapists, Osteopaths / Chiropractors	Neural mobilization, myofascial release, gentle massage	Neural gliding exercises, ergonomic guidance, neurorehabilitation
Energetics	Acupuncturists (TCM), Bioenergetic Therapists	Acupuncture, moxibustion, PEMF	Warming acupuncture, frequency therapy, energy healing
Psychological	GNM practitioners, Psychotherapists, Vibrational therapists, Family constellation facilitators	Psychotherapy, bioresonance, mindfulness	Psychosomatic conflict resolution, vibrational medicine

Educational Pearls & Considerations.

- Early diagnosis prevents irreversible nerve damage.
- Nutritional support aids nerve regeneration but complements medical treatment.
- Mind-body and energetic therapies reduce pain perception.
- Monitor metabolic factors such as diabetes.
- Avoid aggressive therapies during acute inflammation.

GROUP 1 - ZONE 4 – INTERNAL RIGHT LEG

Category 5: *Lymphatic*

Step 1: Functional Anatomy and Interpretive Importance

The internal right leg mirrors its contralateral counterpart, with lymphatic vessels accompanying the great saphenous system en route to the inguinal nodes (Standring, 2016). Efficient clearance here is critical, as disruption promotes localized stasis and compromises immune surveillance.

International consensus statements on lymphedema management highlight the frequency of medial limb involvement, particularly following trauma or infection that challenges lymphatic integrity (International Society of Lymphology, 2013). Such disturbances reshape local tissue compliance and vascular signaling, creating emissive patterns that extend along the medial knee and femoral shaft.

These biospectral asymmetries, defined by their compact geometry and correspondence to lymphatic drainage lines, provide external evidence of impaired clearance. Their presence refines interpretation by linking medial emissive fields to vascular load and immune transport dynamics, positioning spectral surface imaging as an adjunctive method for identifying early lymphatic stress.

Step 2,3,4: ROI Classification and Interpretive Questions

Hyperemission reflects acute immune activation, infectious response, or lymphatic congestion with warmth and swelling.

- Is there redness, tenderness, or sudden swelling?
- Has there been recent trauma or infection?

Hypoemission indicates chronic lymphatic stagnation with tissue rigidity and poor drainage causing reduced perfusion.

- Is swelling persistent, firm, or accompanied by skin changes?
- Are infections recurrent or wounds slow to heal?

Step 5: Confirmatory Evaluations

Test	Purpose & Justification	Relevance to Emissive Pattern
Lymphoscintigraphy	Evaluates lymphatic drainage and identifies obstruction.	Confirms lymphatic burden or hypoperfusion.
Doppler ultrasound	Excludes venous insufficiency contributing to swelling.	Differentiates vascular from lymphatic causes.

Blood tests (CBC, inflammatory markers)	Detect infection or systemic inflammation.	Supports hyperemissive regulatory activation
Physical exam (Stemmer's sign, limb circumference)	Identifies clinical signs of lymphedema.	Correlates with emissive findings.

Step 6: Care Strategies and Intervention Pathways

Naturopathic Approach

Enhance lymphatic flow and reduce inflammation with herbal lymphagogues like *Hedera helix* and *Vitis vinifera* (Godoy et al., 2012). Manual lymphatic drainage by trained therapists facilitates fluid movement. Compression therapy supports lymphatic return. Nutritional antioxidants and anti-inflammatory nutrients promote tissue health. Hydrotherapy with alternating warm and cold water stimulates lymph circulation.

Standard Medical Approaches

Standard care includes manual lymph drainage, compression garments, physical therapy, and prompt infection treatment. Surgery may be necessary in severe cases.

Specialty / Practitioner Care Strategies Table

Specialty Group	Practitioners Included	Hyperemissive Strategies	Hypoemissive Strategies
Biochemistry	Nutritionists, Orthomolecular, Herbalists, Naturopaths	Herbal lymphagogues, antioxidants, anti-inflammatory nutrients	Circulatory support, nutritional tissue repair support
Rehabilitation	Physiotherapists, Massage Therapists, Osteopaths / Chiropractors	Manual lymphatic drainage, gentle massage, postural retraining	Compression therapy, graded exercise, ergonomic guidance
Energetics	Acupuncturists (TCM), Bioenergetic Therapists	Acupuncture, herbal formulas, PEMF	Warming acupuncture, energy balancing
Psychological	GNM practitioners, Psychotherapists, Vibrational therapists, Family constellation facilitators	Mind-body therapies supporting immune function and healing	Psychosomatic conflict resolution, emotional balancing

Educational Pearls & Considerations.

- Early intervention prevents chronic lymphedema progression.
- Manual lymph drainage should be performed by qualified therapists.
- Compression therapy requires individualized fitting and monitoring.
- Nutritional support enhances lymphatic and tissue health.
- Promptly treat infections to avoid worsening lymphatic dysfunction.

GROUP 1 - ZONE 4 – INTERNAL RIGHT LEG

Category 7: *Acupuncture / Meridian*

Step 1: Functional Anatomy and Interpretive Importance

The internal right leg mirrors the medial architecture of the left, dominated by adductors, femoral shaft, and connective fascia channeling neurovascular supply (Standring, 2016). The Spleen (SP) and Liver (LV) meridians trace this course, regulating metabolic balance, circulation, and musculoskeletal coherence.

Deadman et al. (2007) noted that points such as SP9 and LV8 influence not only local knee pain but also systemic digestive and hepatic functions, demonstrating the interconnectedness of these channels. Langevin and Yandow (2002) highlighted how meridians may correspond to connective tissue planes, reinforcing their clinical palpability and projection.

Symptomatically, disruption may present as medial knee weakness, tension, or systemic metabolic complaint. In emissive mapping, surface imaging reveals longitudinal bands of hypoemission or hyperemission aligned with SP–LV trajectories, reflecting energetic dysregulation superimposed on the anatomical substrate, and confirming the diagnostic value of these fields.

Step 2,3,4: ROI Classification and Interpretive Questions

Hyperemission indicates Qi stagnation or meridian reactivity along the pathway.

- Is there localized tenderness, swelling, or sharp pain?
- Are symptoms worsened by movement or pressure?

Hypoemission suggests Qi deficiency or chronic stagnation, with reduced energy flow and localized oxygenation decline.

- Does the patient report weakness, coldness, numbness, or chronic dull pain?
- Are signs of poor circulation or fatigue present?

Step 5: Confirmatory Evaluations

Test	Purpose & Justification	Relevance to Emissive Pattern
Pulse diagnosis and tongue examination	Traditional TCM diagnostic tools assessing Qi and blood status (Flaws, 2000).	Correlates with emissive findings for refined interpretation.
Biospectral imaging	Detects emissive asymmetries along meridian pathways.	Directly visualizes hyper- or hypoemissive meridian zones.
Patient symptom questionnaire	Evaluates pain patterns, energy levels, and functional status.	Supports differentiation between Qi stagnation and Qi deficiency.

Step 6: Care Strategies and Intervention Pathways

Naturopathic Approach

Acupuncture targeting points such as SP6 and LV3 regulates Qi and blood flow, reduces inflammation, and restores function (Lao et al., 2004). Moxibustion warms hypoemissive meridians. Herbal formulas like *Dang Gui* and *Chuan Xiong* nourish blood and harmonize Qi (Bensky et al., 2004). Nutritional support with Qi-building foods complements therapy.

Standard Medical Approaches

Acupuncture is an adjunct to physical therapy and pain management in musculoskeletal disorders linked to meridian imbalance.

Specialty / Practitioner Care Strategies Table

Specialty Group	Practitioners Included	Hyperemissive Strategies	Hypoemissive Strategies
Biochemistry	Nutritionists, Orthomolecular, Herbalists, Naturopaths	Herbal formulas to regulate Qi and blood, antioxidants	Qi tonics, blood-nourishing supplements
Rehabilitation	Physiotherapists, Massage Therapists, Osteopaths / Chiropractors	Trigger point therapy complementary to acupuncture	Gentle mobilization, warming massage
Energetics	Acupuncturists (TCM), Bioenergetic Therapists	Acupuncture, moxibustion, PEMF	Warming acupuncture, Qi tonics, energy healing
Psychological	GNM practitioners, Psychotherapists, Vibrational therapists, Family constellation facilitators	Mind-body therapies, bioresonance, energy clearing	Psychosomatic conflict resolution, emotional balancing

Educational Pearls & Considerations.

- Precise point selection is vital to balance hyper- and hypoemissive patterns.
- Use moxibustion cautiously in heat-sensitive patients.
- Herbal treatments require professional supervision.
- Combining acupuncture with rehabilitation enhances recovery.

GROUP 1 - ZONE 4 – INTERNAL RIGHT LEG

Category 8: *Energetic*

Step 1: Functional Anatomy and Interpretive Importance

The right medial leg parallels the left, composed of adductor musculature, the femoral shaft, and fascial planes transmitting vascular and neural supply (Standring, 2016). Energetically, this surface reflects balance of circulatory and immune modulation through subtle biofield currents.

Hammerschlag et al. (2015) demonstrated that targeted biofield interventions alter autonomic regulation and pain perception, supporting clinical relevance of medial emissive changes.

In practice, right-sided medial disturbances may manifest as tension, vague discomfort, or reduced recovery following exertion. On spectral imaging, hypoemission signifies energy depletion or blocked conduction, while hyperemission indicates reparative intensification.

The medial right leg thus serves as a surface projection of systemic energy balance, integrating musculoskeletal and subtle field dynamics into a coherent interpretive model.

Step 2,3,4: ROI Classification and Interpretive Questions

Hyperemission indicates localized energy congestion or reactivity.

- Are there sensations of heat, tingling, or discomfort without physical cause?
- Do stress or emotional factors exacerbate symptoms?

Hypoemission reflects energy underexpression or stagnation.

- Does the patient report coldness, fatigue, numbness, or low vitality?
- Are symptoms chronic and resistant to conventional therapies?

Step 5: Confirmatory Evaluations

Test	Purpose & Justification	Relevance to Emissive Pattern
Bioresonance testing	Measures tissue energy frequencies and imbalances.	Correlates with emission patterns.
Electrodermal screening (EDS)	Assesses skin conductance related to energy pathways.	Supports interpretation of energetic dynamics.
Patient emotional and symptom history	Provides clinical context for energetic dysfunction.	Aids differential assessment.

Step 6: Care Strategies and Intervention Pathways

Naturopathic Approach

Use bioresonance, PEMF, and herbal adaptogens to restore energetic balance and support physiological healing (Matsumoto et al., 2010). Nutritional antioxidants and adaptogens improve systemic resilience. Mindfulness and stress reduction techniques complement energetic therapies.

Standard Medical Approaches

Energetic therapies serve as adjuncts to conventional medical and rehabilitative treatments to optimize patient outcomes.

Specialty / Practitioner Care Strategies Table

Specialty Group	Practitioners Included	Hyperemissive Strategies	Hypoemissive Strategies
Biochemistry	Nutritionists, Orthomolecular, Herbalists, Naturopaths	Adaptogens, antioxidants, herbal energetics	Nutritional support for energy deficiency
Rehabilitation	Physiotherapists, Massage Therapists, Osteopaths / Chiropractors	Energy-based manual therapies, PEMF, therapeutic touch	Gentle stimulation, mobilization
Energetics	Acupuncturists (TCM), Bioenergetic Therapists	Bioresonance, PEMF, acupuncture	Warming acupuncture, energy balancing
Psychological	GNM practitioners, Psychotherapists, Vibrational therapists, Family constellation facilitators	Psychotherapy, bioresonance, mindfulness	Emotional balancing, vibrational medicine

Educational Pearls & Considerations.

- Use energetic therapies as complementary, integrated with conventional care.
- Patient response and practitioner skill influence outcomes.
- Monitor clinical changes and adjust therapies accordingly.
- Address psychological and physical factors holistically.

GROUP 1 - ZONE 4 – INTERNAL RIGHT LEG

Category 9: *Metabolic / Endocrine*

Step 1: Functional Anatomy and Interpretive Importance

The internal right leg shares structural parallels with the left, including the distal femur, medial knee stabilizers, and venous conduits supporting postural endurance (Standring, 2016).

Metabolic and endocrine systems directly influence vascular tone, connective tissue turnover, and neurosensory regulation in this region. Brent (2012) outlined the pervasive effects of thyroid hormones on skeletal muscle and vascular physiology, offering a model for interpreting medial leg alterations.

Clinically, patients may present with weakness, instability, or poor recovery after exertion. Spectral surface readings demonstrate diffuse hypoemissive zones aligned with vascular insufficiency or thyroid-linked metabolic suppression, contrasted by localized hyperemissive foci representing reparative activity.

These emissive signatures highlight how systemic hormonal imbalance projects into peripheral surfaces, allowing clinicians to interpret medial leg biosignals as markers of metabolic and endocrine regulation.

Step 2,3,4: ROI Classification and Interpretive Questions

Hyperemission may indicate localized tissue activation, immune response, or metabolic overactivity.

- Is there warmth, redness, or swelling?
- Is the patient's metabolic control suboptimal?

Hypoemission suggests perfusion reduction, neural suppression, or impaired circulation related to metabolic/endocrine regulatory shifts.

- Is there coldness, numbness, chronic wounds, or fatigue?
- Are systemic symptoms such as temperature intolerance present?

Step 5: Confirmatory Evaluations

Test	Purpose & Justification	Relevance to Emissive Pattern
HbA1c, fasting glucose	Monitors glycemic control in diabetes.	Correlates with hypoemissive neuropathic or ischemic zones.
Thyroid function tests (TSH, Free T4)	Detect thyroid disorders affecting metabolism and circulation.	Associated with altered emission regulation.

Lipid profile	Evaluates cardiovascular risk factors impacting tissue perfusion.	Supports metabolic vascular compromise.
Inflammatory markers (CRP, ESR)	Identifies systemic inflammation influencing tissue health.	Correlates with hyperemissive regulatory activation.

Step 6: Care Strategies and Intervention Pathways

Naturopathic Approach

Focus on metabolic optimization with low glycemic diet, antioxidants, and micronutrients improving insulin sensitivity (Alberti et al., 2006). Adaptogenic herbs like *Panax ginseng* and *Gymnema sylvestre* support endocrine balance. Supplement chromium, magnesium, and alpha-lipoic acid to aid glucose metabolism and nerve protection. Regular aerobic exercise improves circulation and metabolism.

Standard Medical Approaches

Strict glycemic and metabolic control via pharmacotherapy and lifestyle modification is vital. Thyroid hormone replacement and lipid management reduce complications.

Specialty / Practitioner Care Strategies Table

Specialty Group	Practitioners Included	Hyperemissive Strategies	Hypoemissive Strategies
Biochemistry	Nutritionists, Orthomolecular, Herbalists, Naturopaths	Antioxidants, adaptogens, insulin sensitizers, micronutrients	Metabolic support, neuroprotective nutrients, dietary management
Rehabilitation	Physiotherapists, Massage Therapists, Osteopaths / Chiropractors	Exercise therapy, circulation enhancement	Neuromuscular re-education, aerobic conditioning
Energetics	Acupuncturists (TCM), Bioenergetic Therapists	Acupuncture supporting metabolic function	Energy balancing, PEMF
Psychological	GNM practitioners, Psychotherapists, Vibrational therapists, Family constellation facilitators	Mind-body therapies supporting metabolic regulation	Stress reduction, emotional balancing

Educational Pearls & Considerations.

- Continuous metabolic monitoring prevents tissue complications.
- Lifestyle and diet changes complement medical management.
- Adaptogens support but do not replace conventional therapies.
- Patient education on foot care is critical to prevent ulcerations.

GROUP 1

ZONE 5 – EXTERNAL LEFT LEG

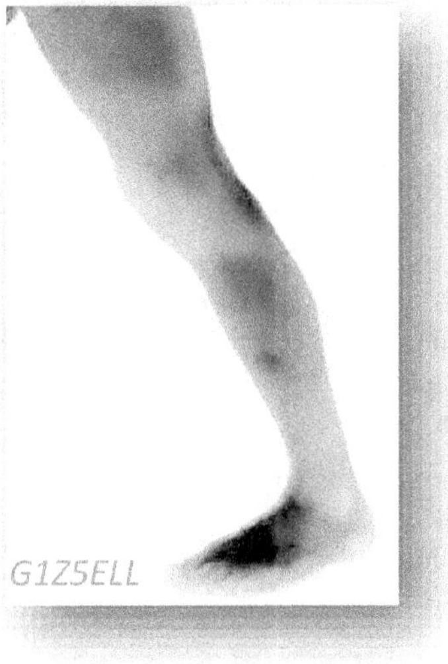

The external left leg, dominated by the iliotibial tract and fibular musculature, is a region where biomechanical tension often manifests as emissive asymmetry. Unlike medial compartments, which reflect visceral or lymphatic influences, the lateral thigh is primarily shaped by musculoskeletal dynamics and fascial continuity. The iliotibial band (ITB), one of the densest fascial structures, transmits force between pelvis and knee, and its limited compliance makes it highly prone to overuse and lateral chain imbalance (Standring, 2016).

Hyperemissive or hypoemissive streaks along this tract generally reflect fascial strain rather than vascular perfusion, refining interpretive analysis. In athletes, ITB syndrome accounts for up to 12% of running-related knee injuries, especially in long-distance runners and cyclists (Fairclough et al., 2006). The lateral thigh also compensates in pelvic deviation or scoliosis, frequently displaying asymmetry when chronically overloaded. Fascial research confirms that altered ITB tension can propagate strain into the lumbar spine and knee, reinforcing the systemic importance of this zone (Wilke et al., 2016).

From a biospectral perspective, lateral asymmetries often indicate postural adaptation rather than isolated pathology. The relative vascular resistance of the ITB corridor further limits subcutaneous blood flow compared with medial compartments, making emissive irregularities here especially sensitive markers of muscular overuse rather than circulatory stress (Benjamin, 2009).

Clinically, patients with lateral thigh deviations frequently report hip discomfort or contralateral strain, underscoring the biomechanical interdependence of this zone. Its interpretive strength lies in revealing fascial imbalance, overuse syndromes, and postural compensation long before imaging confirms structural change, making it a valuable zone for preventive observation in athletes, sedentary individuals, and those with chronic postural strain.

Zone 5 – External Left Leg: Emission-Relevant Structures.

Category	Relevant Structures	Emission Relevance
1. Vascular / Circulatory	- Small saphenous vein (posterolateral leg) - Peroneal veins and perforators - Popliteal tributaries	Hyperemission may reflect venous congestion, reflux, or early varicosities. Hypoemission suggests impaired return, peripheral stagnation, or chronic vasoconstriction.
2. Muscular / Myofascial	- Peroneus longus and brevis - Fibularis muscle group - Lateral gastrocnemius - Soleus fascia - Distal iliotibial band	Local Hyperemission indicates muscular overload, lateral compensation, or fascial restriction. Hypoemission is linked to disuse, atrophy, or fascial rigidity in the lateral leg chain.
3. Skeletal / Articular	- Fibula shaft and head - Lateral tibial plateau - Talocrural (ankle) joint – lateral aspect	Bone-related hyperemission may reflect joint strain, trauma, or enthesopathy. Hypoemissive zones suggest degeneration, lateral instability, or altered joint mechanics.
4. Nervous System / Spine	- Superficial peroneal nerve - Common fibular (peroneal) nerve - L5 dermatome (lateral leg and foot dorsum)	Hyperemission of neuropathic type may result from peroneal nerve irritation or mechanical entrapment. Hypoemission is often associated with L5 root compression or autonomic hypoactivity.
5. Lymphatic / Immune	- Superficial lateral lymphatic channels - Popliteal lymph nodes	Hyperemission can signal lymphatic stasis, toxic load, or local regulatory activation. Hypoemission may reflect low immune tone or inefficient lateral drainage.
6. Organs / GNM	*(Typically excluded for direct mapping in this zone)*	
7. Acupuncture / Meridians	- Gallbladder Meridian (GB) – runs along lateral leg and thigh - Bladder Meridian (BL) – lateral branches	Heat may reflect Gallbladder Qi stagnation, emotional frustration, or meridian overload. Cold often correlates with Yang depletion or weakness in lateral energetic circuits.
8. Energetic / Frequency	- Zone linked to boundary-setting, direction, and decision-making energetics	Hyperemission can indicate performance stress, reactive defense, or unexpressed assertiveness. Hypoemission reflects energetic depletion, insecurity, or weakened lateral polarity.
9. Metabolic / Endocrine	- Reflex pathways for bile metabolism, stress hormones, and detoxification load	Hyperemission signals metabolic strain or detox activity. Hypoemission may suggest bile insufficiency, adrenal hyporegulation, or suppressed lateral metabolic flow.

GROUP 1 - ZONE 5 – EXTERNAL LEFT LEG

Category 1: Vascular / Circulatory

Step 1: Functional Anatomy and Interpretive Importance

The lateral compartment receives inflow from the anterior tibial artery anteriorly and from the fibular artery posteriorly. These vessels supply the fibularis longus and brevis and contribute to cutaneous perfusion along the lateral shin.

Venous return is managed by the anterior tibial veins and superficial tributaries that communicate with the saphenous systems (Standring, 2016). Population-based studies show that the fibular artery often functions as an important collateral channel in peripheral artery disease, reinforcing its clinical significance (Fowkes et al., 2013).

Emissive asymmetries along the lateral shin frequently follow these vascular lines on spectral surface reading. Such findings may indicate mechanical stress, venous retention, or subtle modulation of arterial tone. Because this compartment stabilizes the ankle and supports balance, its emissive profile is a valuable indicator of circulatory load during movement.

Step 2,3,4: ROI Classification and Interpretive Questions

Hyperemission indicates venous congestion, microvascular activation, or vascular reactivity.

- Does the patient experience swell, warmth, or heaviness?
- Are varicosities or skin changes present?

Hypoemission suggests arterial underperfusion, flow restriction, or vasospasm.

- Are there complaints of coldness, numbness, or intermittent claudication?
- Are pulses diminished or delayed wound healing observed?

Step 5: Confirmatory Evaluations

Test	Purpose & Justification	Relevance to Emissive Pattern
Doppler ultrasound	Evaluates arterial and venous blood flow (Brant et al., 2016).	Correlates hyperemissive venous and hypoemissive arterial patterns.
Ankle-Brachial Index (ABI)	Quantifies arterial perfusion; <0.9 suggests peripheral arterial disease (Norgren et al., 2007).	Validates hypoemissive arterial insufficiency.
Capillary refill time	Assesses microcirculatory status.	Supports hypoemissive microvascular compromise.
Blood tests (CBC, CRP, coagulation)	Detect systemic inflammation or thrombophilia.	upports hyperemissive vascular or thrombotic activity.

Step 6: Care Strategies and Intervention Pathways

Naturopathic Approach

Botanical venotonics such as *Aesculus hippocastanum* and *Centella asiatica* improve venous tone (Chrubasik et al., 2011). Hydrotherapy with contrast baths enhances circulation and reduces edema (Sutkowy et al., 2019). An anti-inflammatory diet rich in antioxidants, vitamin C, and omega-3 fatty acids supports vascular health (Calder, 2017). Nitric oxide donors improve arterial perfusion (Moncada & Higgs, 1993). Limb elevation and exercise promote venous return. Supplement iron, B12, and folate to support oxygen transport.

Standard Medical Approaches

Doppler and ABI assessments guide compression therapy, venoactive drugs, NSAIDs, sclerotherapy, or revascularization (Brant et al., 2016; Norgren et al., 2007). Wound care is critical for ischemic ulcers.

Specialty / Practitioner Care Strategies Table

Specialty Group	Practitioners Included	Hyperemissive Strategies	Hypoemissive Strategies
Biochemistry	Nutritionists, Orthomolecular, Herbalists, Naturopaths	Botanical venotonics, anti-inflammatory diet, antioxidants, vitamins C, E, selenium, CoQ10, bioflavonoids, omega-3s	Circulatory stimulants (*Ginkgo*, cayenne), blood-building nutrients (iron, B12, folate), magnesium, arginine, nitrate-rich diet
Rehabilitation	Physiotherapists, Massage Therapists, Osteopaths / Chiropractors	Lymphatic drainage, calf pump exercises, postural retraining, gentle Swedish massage, myofascial release	Graded aerobic exercise, gait training, emission protection, foot care, warming massage, reflexology, ergonomic guidance
Energetics	Acupuncturists (TCM), Bioenergetic Therapists	Acupuncture (SP6, ST36), moxibustion, herbal formulas, Qi and Blood tonics, bioresonance, PEMF	Warming acupuncture, Qi and Blood tonics, PEMF, energy healing
Psychological	GNM practitioners, Psychotherapists, Vibrational therapists, Family constellation facilitators	GNM conflict protocols, psychotherapy, bioresonance, mindfulness, energy clearing	Psychosomatic conflict resolution, vibrational medicine, stress reduction, emotional balancing

Educational Pearls & Considerations.

- Rule out deep vein thrombosis or critical ischemia prior to heat, massage, or exercise.
- Botanical venotonics combined with hydrotherapy synergistically reduce venous congestion.
- Nitric oxide boosters and omega-3 fatty acids improve arterial endothelial function.
- Compression therapy contraindicated in severe arterial disease.
- Early mobilization and limb elevation prevent chronic complications.

GROUP 1 - ZONE 5 – EXTERNAL LEFT LEG

Category 2: Muscular

Step 1: Functional Anatomy and Interpretive Importance

The external compartment contains the fibularis longus and brevis, innervated by the superficial fibular nerve. These muscles perform foot eversion, contribute to ankle stability, and assist in weight transfer across the first ray through the fibularis longus tendon, which passes under the foot to the medial cuneiform (Standring, 2016).

Clinical research identifies the fibularis tendons as frequent sites of pathology in chronic ankle instability, with tendinopathy and tendon subluxation linked to repetitive inversion stress and poor mechanical control (Sobel et al., 1990).

These same mechanical demands are reflected biospectrally as linear emissive gradients tracking the fibularis tendons, particularly evident after instability events or repetitive lateral loading. When evaluated in relation to ankle stability, such asymmetries reveal early adaptation in lateral stabilizers and serve as predictive markers for potential inversion injury or chronic instability syndromes.

Step 2,3,4: ROI Classification and Interpretive Questions

Hyperemission indicates acute muscular overload, myofascial reactivity, or inflammatory response with increased circulatory dynamics.

- Has the patient experienced trauma or repetitive stress?
- Is there localized pain, swelling, or muscle spasm?

Hypoemission uggests chronic perfusion deficit, compartmental flow restriction, or neuromuscular decline associated with reduced metabolic activity.

- Are there numbness, weakness, or muscle wasting?
- Is gait or limb function impaired?

Step 5: Confirmatory Evaluations

Test	Purpose & Justification	Relevance to Emissive Pattern
Creatine kinase (CK), LDH	Detect muscle damage or inflammation (Maffulli et al., 2014).	Elevated in hyperemissive tissue activation.
MRI	Visualizes edema, inflammation, ischemia, or muscle atrophy.	Supports hyper- or hypoemissive findings.

Compartment pressure measurement	Diagnoses compartment syndrome via pressure assessment.	Relevant for hypoemissive ischemic patterns.
Nerve conduction studies (NCS), Electromyography (EMG)	Evaluates neurogenic muscle dysfunction.	Correlates with hypoemissive neurogenic causes.
Blood tests (CBC, inflammatory markers)	Detect systemic inflammation or infection.	Supports hyperemissive regulatory activation.

Step 6: Care Strategies and Intervention Pathways

Naturopathic Approach

Anti-inflammatory botanicals such as *Curcuma longa* and *Boswellia serrata* reduce muscle inflammation (Hewlings & Kalman, 2017). Magnesium supplementation aids muscle relaxation. Hydrotherapy with alternating warm and cold compresses improves circulation (Sutkowy et al., 2019). Gentle stretching and progressive strengthening support functional recovery. Adequate protein and antioxidants promote healing.

Standard Medical Approaches

Rest, NSAIDs, and physical therapy are standard for acute muscle injuries (Maffulli et al., 2014). Compartment syndrome requires urgent surgical intervention. Neurogenic muscle weakness warrants neurological assessment.

Specialty / Practitioner Care Strategies Table

Specialty Group	Practitioners Included	Hyperemissive Strategies	Hypoemissive Strategies
Biochemistry	Nutritionists, Orthomolecular, Herbalists, Naturopaths	Anti-inflammatory botanicals, magnesium, antioxidants, protein	Circulatory support, neurotrophic nutrients, protein support
Rehabilitation	Physiotherapists, Massage Therapists, Osteopaths / Chiropractors	Myofascial release, trigger point therapy, gentle massage	Graded aerobic exercise, neurorehabilitation, ergonomic guidance
Energetics	Acupuncturists (TCM), Bioenergetic Therapists	Acupuncture, moxibustion, PEMF	Warming acupuncture, frequency therapy
Psychological	GNM practitioners, Psychotherapists, Vibrational therapists, Family constellation facilitators	Psychotherapy, bioresonance, mindfulness	Psychosomatic conflict resolution, emotional balancing

Educational Pearls & Considerations.

- Early recognition of compartment syndrome is vital.
- Magnesium helps reduce cramps and spasms.
- Hydrotherapy protocols should be matched to inflammation stages.
- Neurogenic muscle weakness requires thorough evaluation.
- Graded rehabilitation prevents chronic disability.

GROUP 1 - ZONE 5 – EXTERNAL LEFT LEG

Category 3: Skeletal

Step 1: Functional Anatomy and Interpretive Importance

The external left leg contains the shafts of the tibia and fibula as they descend toward the ankle joint, forming the lateral stabilizing framework of the lower limb (Standring, 2016). These bones provide rigid support for load transfer and serve as anchor points for ligamentous and muscular insertions that maintain lateral stability.

Mechanical stress in this zone is often asymmetrical, as lateral loading tends to concentrate during uneven terrain or sports requiring sudden directional changes. Repetitive strain in this region has been associated with localized periosteal stress and ankle joint dysfunction, which can destabilize gait mechanics (Taunton et al., 1984). Such skeletal load imbalance influences surrounding tissue perfusion and regulatory dynamics, producing external signals on spectral surface readings.

Biospectral asymmetries commonly align longitudinally along the tibial shaft or fibular contour, distinguished from broader muscular fields by their sharply confined geometry. These emissive expressions provide early evidence of osseous adaptation, mapping skeletal overload before overt degenerative change becomes clinically evident.

Step 2,3,4: ROI Classification and Interpretive Questions

Hyperemission indicates periosteal activation, osseous remodeling, or joint fluid accumulation associated with increased localized perfusion.

- Is there recent trauma or overuse?
- Are swelling, tenderness, or limited mobility present?

Hypoemission suggests chronic articular remodeling, structural depletion, or perfusion decline related to long-term mechanical imbalance.

- Is there chronic pain, stiffness, or functional limitations?
- Is there history of joint deformity or instability?

Step 5: Confirmatory Evaluations

Test	Purpose & Justification	Relevance to Emissive Pattern
X-ray imaging	Detects fractures, stress injuries, and joint space narrowing.	Confirms hyperemissive acute injuries or hypoemissive chronic pathology.
MRI	Visualizes bone marrow edema, occult fractures, cartilage, and soft tissue.	Supports hyperemissive tissue activation or hypoemissive chronic changes.

Bone scan	Assesses bone metabolism and detects stress fractures or infection.	Correlates with hyperemissive bone involvement.
Blood tests (inflammatory markers)	Detect systemic inflammation related to bone injury or infection.	Supports hyperemissive regulatory activation

Step 6: Care Strategies and Intervention Pathways

Naturopathic Approach

Bone healing supported by calcium, vitamin D, magnesium, and vitamin K intake (Heaney, 2006). Anti-inflammatory botanicals like *Boswellia serrata* reduce inflammation. Therapeutic ultrasound and PEMF stimulate bone repair (Gordon et al., 2016). Immobilization protects injured bones.

Standard Medical Approaches

Imaging guides immobilization or surgery. NSAIDs and physical therapy manage symptoms. Osteoarthritis requires supportive treatment.

Specialty / Practitioner Care Strategies Table

Specialty Group	Practitioners Included	Hyperemissive Strategies	Hypoemissive Strategies
Biochemistry	Nutritionists, Orthomolecular, Herbalists, Naturopaths	Bone-supportive nutrients, anti-inflammatory botanicals	Nutritional support for bone remodeling and joint health
Rehabilitation	Physiotherapists, Massage Therapists, Osteopaths / Chiropractors	Joint mobilization, therapeutic ultrasound, myofascial release	Joint stabilization, graded strengthening, ergonomic guidance
Energetics	Acupuncturists (TCM), Bioenergetic Therapists	Acupuncture, PEMF, herbal formulas for inflammation	Warming acupuncture, energy balancing
Psychological	GNM practitioners, Psychotherapists, Vibrational therapists, Family constellation facilitators	Mind-body therapies supporting pain management and healing	Psychosomatic support, emotional balancing

Educational Pearls & Considerations.

- Immobilize fractures promptly.
- Nutrition accelerates bone repair.
- PEMF requires professional application.
- Chronic hypoemissive joint changes need multidisciplinary care.
- Psychological support aids recovery.

GROUP 1 - ZONE 5 – EXTERNAL LEFT LEG

Category 4: Nervous

Step 1: Functional Anatomy and Interpretive Importance

The external aspect of the lower leg is innervated by branches of the common peroneal nerve, which supply motor control for dorsiflexion and eversion, and sensation to the lateral leg and dorsum of the foot (Standring, 2016).

The nerve's superficial course along the fibular head renders it particularly vulnerable to compression or traction injuries. Stewart (2008) reported that peroneal neuropathy is the most common mononeuropathy of the lower limb, frequently caused by entrapment or external compression. These neural disturbances extend beyond motor deficits, reshaping vascular regulation and fascial recruitment in ways that alter regional biosignals.

On the surface, these changes manifest as sharply defined emissive asymmetries that trace the fibular line or lateral tibial border, distinct from the diffuse fields of muscular activation. The clarity of such signals provides a visual translation of peroneal dysfunction, enabling clinicians to recognize early neuropathic stress in the lateral compartment before overt weakness emerges.

Step 2,3,4: ROI Classification and Interpretive Questions

Hyperemission may reflect nerve irritation or localized neurogenic activation with increased perfusion.

- Are there burning, tingling, or sharp pains along the lateral leg?
- Is there localized hypersensitivity or swelling?

Hypoemission suggests compression, ischemic suppression, or reduced neuro-autonomic regulation affecting emissive output.

- Are numbness, weakness, or muscle wasting present?
- Do symptoms worsen with specific movements or postures?

Step 5: Confirmatory Evaluations

Test	Purpose & Justification	Relevance to Emissive Pattern
Nerve conduction studies (NCS), Electromyography (EMG)	Assess nerve and muscle function (Campbell & Meyer, 2006).	Correlate with hypoemissive neurogenic dysfunction.
Quantitative sensory testing (QST)	Measures sensory thresholds and nerve function.	Supports interpretation of neuropathic patterns.
MRI / Ultrasound	Detects nerve compression or structural abnormalities.	Identifies neurogenic involvement.
Blood tests (glucose, vitamin B12)	Evaluates metabolic causes of neuropathy.	Supports interpretation of metabolic neuropathic patters.

Step 6: Care Strategies and Intervention Pathways

Naturopathic Approach

Support nerve repair with B-complex vitamins, alpha-lipoic acid, and Acetyl-L-carnitine (Papanas & Ziegler, 2014). Herbal anti-inflammatories like *Hypericum perforatum* may alleviate neuropathic pain (Kasper et al., 2010). Neural mobilization and gentle stretching promote recovery. Mind-body therapies and bioresonance modulate pain and neurovascular regulation.

Standard Medical Approaches

Pharmacologic treatments include anticonvulsants, antidepressants, and analgesics. Surgical decompression may be necessary. Metabolic control is essential in systemic neuropathies.

Specialty / Practitioner Care Strategies Table

Specialty Group	Practitioners Included	Hyperemissive Strategies	Hypoemissive Strategies
Biochemistry	Nutritionists, Orthomolecular, Herbalists, Naturopaths	Neurotrophic vitamins, alpha-lipoic acid, anti-inflammatory botanicals	Circulatory stimulants, metabolic support, neuroprotective nutrients
Rehabilitation	Physiotherapists, Massage Therapists, Osteopaths / Chiropractors	Neural mobilization, myofascial release, gentle massage	Neural gliding exercises, ergonomic guidance, neurorehabilitation
Energetics	Acupuncturists (TCM), Bioenergetic Therapists	Acupuncture, moxibustion, PEMF	Warming acupuncture, frequency therapy, energy healing
Psychological	GNM practitioners, Psychotherapists, Vibrational therapists, Family constellation facilitators	Psychotherapy, bioresonance, mindfulness	Psychosomatic conflict resolution, vibrational medicine

Educational Pearls & Considerations.

- Early diagnosis prevents permanent nerve damage.
- Nutritional support complements medical treatment.
- Mind-body and energetic therapies assist pain management.
- Monitor metabolic contributors like diabetes.
- Avoid aggressive treatments during acute inflammation.

GROUP 1 - ZONE 5 – EXTERNAL LEFT LEG

Category 5: Lymphatic

Step 1: Functional Anatomy and Interpretive Importance

The external left leg is served by lymphatic vessels that accompany the superficial veins, particularly the small saphenous, and connect to both popliteal and inguinal lymph nodes (Standring, 2016). These channels maintain equilibrium between interstitial fluid removal and immune surveillance of the lateral leg.

Browse et al. (2003) emphasized that dysfunction in this region often presents as early dermal backflow or localized stasis, which may progress to chronic edema if left untreated. Altered lymphatic transport changes the biomechanical properties of the lateral compartment and modifies adjacent vascular reactivity.

Externally, these shifts often present as biospectral asymmetries that trace the fibular margin or lateral tibial contour, showing greater confinement than muscular patterns. Such emissive signatures provide clinicians with a noninvasive window into lateral leg lymphatic strain, highlighting early dysfunction before visible swelling or tissue induration develops.

Step 2,3,4: ROI Classification and Interpretive Questions

Hyperemission indicates acute lymphatic activation, immune response, or interstitial congestion, often accompanied by increased surface perfusion and soft tissue swelling.

- Is there redness, tenderness, or rapid onset swelling?
- Has the patient had recent injury or infection?

Hypoemission suggests chronic lymphodynamic impairment with tissue fibrosis, drainage restriction, and reduced biosignal expression.

- Is swelling persistent, firm, or accompanied by skin changes?
- Are recurrent infections or slow-healing wounds present?

Step 5: Confirmatory Evaluations

Test	Purpose & Justification	Relevance to Emissive Pattern
Lymphoscintigraphy	Evaluates lymphatic drainage and obstruction.	Confirms lymphatic burden or hypoperfusion.
Doppler ultrasound	Excludes venous insufficiency as cause of swelling.	Differentiates vascular from lymphatic causes.
Blood tests (CBC, inflammatory markers)	Detect infection or systemic inflammation.	Supports hyperemissive regulatory activation.
Physical exam (Stemmer's sign, limb measurements)	Assesses clinical signs of lymphedema.	Correlates with emissive findings.

Step 6: Care Strategies and Intervention Pathways

Naturopathic Approach

Enhance lymphatic flow using herbal lymphagogues such as *Hedera helix* and *Vitis vinifera* (Godoy et al., 2012). Manual lymphatic drainage by trained therapists promotes fluid movement. Compression therapy aids lymph return and should be customized. Nutritional antioxidants and anti-inflammatory agents support tissue health. Hydrotherapy stimulates lymph circulation.

Standard Medical Approaches

Standard treatments include manual lymph drainage, compression garments, physical therapy, and infection management. Surgery may be necessary in advanced cases.

Specialty / Practitioner Care Strategies Table

Specialty Group	Practitioners Included	Hyperemissive Strategies	Hypoemissive Strategies
Biochemistry	Nutritionists, Orthomolecular, Herbalists, Naturopaths	Herbal lymphagogues, antioxidants, anti-inflammatory nutrients	Circulatory support, nutritional tissue repair support
Rehabilitation	Physiotherapists, Massage Therapists, Osteopaths / Chiropractors	Manual lymphatic drainage, gentle massage, postural retraining	Compression therapy, graded exercise, ergonomic guidance
Energetics	Acupuncturists (TCM), Bioenergetic Therapists	Acupuncture, herbal formulas, PEMF	Warming acupuncture, energy balancing
Psychological	GNM practitioners, Psychotherapists, Vibrational therapists, Family constellation facilitators	Mind-body therapies supporting immune function and healing	Psychosomatic conflict resolution, emotional balancing

Educational Pearls & Considerations.

- Early treatment prevents progression to chronic lymphedema.
- Manual lymph drainage should be performed by skilled therapists.
- Compression therapy requires individualized fitting and monitoring.
- Nutritional support enhances lymphatic and tissue health.
- Promptly treat infections to avoid worsening lymphatic dysfunction.

GROUP 1 - ZONE 5 – EXTERNAL LEFT LEG

Category 7: Acupuncture / Meridian

Step 1: Functional Anatomy and Interpretive Importance

The external left leg is supported by the fibula, lateral compartment muscles including peroneus longus and brevis, and associated fascial and vascular structures (Standring, 2016). In meridian mapping, this zone corresponds to the Stomach (ST) and Gallbladder (GB) channels, both of which traverse the lateral surface.

Flaws (2000) emphasized their influence on digestion, balance, and neuromuscular tone, with imbalances often producing lateral leg pain or instability. Deadman et al. (2007) described how ST36 and GB34 are central points for harmonizing systemic energy while relieving local musculoskeletal complaints.

Disturbances along these meridians are reported clinically as weakness, cramping, or proprioceptive dysfunction. On emissive imaging, surface fields emerge as longitudinal strips of hyper- or hypoemission aligned with the meridian pathways, distinct from diffuse muscular exertion. These findings highlight how surface biosignals project energetic imbalance along ST and GB trajectories, bridging anatomical landmarks with subtle regulatory physiology.

Step 2,3,4: ROI Classification and Interpretive Questions

Hyperemission indicates Qi restriction or localized energetic reactivity along the meridian.

- Is there localized tenderness, swelling, or sharp pain?
- Are symptoms worsened by movement or pressure?

Hypoemission suggests Qi depletion or long-standing stagnation, resulting in reduced flow dynamics and tissue underactivation.

- Does the patient report weakness, coldness, numbness, or chronic dull pain?
- Are there signs of poor circulation or fatigue?

Step 5: Confirmatory Evaluations

Test	Purpose & Justification	Relevance to Emissive Pattern
Pulse diagnosis and tongue examination	Traditional TCM diagnostic tools assessing Qi and blood status (Flaws, 2000).	Correlates with emissive findings for refined interpretation.
Biospectral imaging	Detects emissive asymmetries along meridian pathways.	Directly visualizes hyper- or hypoemissive meridian zones.
Patient symptom questionnaire	Evaluates pain patterns, energy levels, and functional status.	Supports differentiation between Qi stagnation and Qi deficiency.

Step 6: Care Strategies and Intervention Pathways

Naturopathic Approach

Acupuncture targeting points such as ST36 and GB34 regulates Qi and blood flow, reduces inflammation, and restores function (Lao et al., 2004). Moxibustion warms hypoemissive meridians. Herbal formulas like *Dang Gui* and *Chuan Xiong* nourish blood and harmonize Qi (Bensky et al., 2004). Nutritional support with Qi-building foods complements therapy.

Standard Medical Approaches

Acupuncture complements physical therapy and pain management for musculoskeletal disorders related to meridian imbalance.

Specialty / Practitioner Care Strategies Table

Specialty Group	Practitioners Included	Hyperemissive Strategies	Hypoemissive Strategies
Biochemistry	Nutritionists, Orthomolecular, Herbalists, Naturopaths	Herbal formulas regulating Qi and blood, antioxidants	Qi tonics, blood nourishing supplements
Rehabilitation	Physiotherapists, Massage Therapists, Osteopaths / Chiropractors	Trigger point therapy complementary to acupuncture	Gentle mobilization, warming massage
Energetics	Acupuncturists (TCM), Bioenergetic Therapists	Acupuncture, moxibustion, PEMF	Warming acupuncture, Qi tonics, energy healing
Psychological	GNM practitioners, Psychotherapists, Vibrational therapists, Family constellation facilitators	Mind-body therapies, bioresonance, energy clearing	Psychosomatic conflict resolution, emotional balancing

Educational Pearls & Considerations.

- Precise point selection is vital to balance hyper- and hypoemissive patterns.
- Moxibustion should be applied cautiously in heat-sensitive patients.
- Herbal treatments require professional supervision.
- Combining acupuncture with rehabilitation improves outcomes.

GROUP 1 - ZONE 5 – EXTERNAL LEFT LEG

Category 8: Energetic

Step 1: Functional Anatomy and Interpretive Importance

The external left leg includes the fibular shaft, peroneal muscles, and fascial layers guiding lateral stability and ankle eversion (Standring, 2016). Energetically, this lateral field is associated with adaptive balance and dynamic load transfer, often reflecting how systemic energy reserves manifest peripherally.

Burr (1936) first described measurable bioelectric fields that varied with physiologic stress, findings that remain relevant for understanding lateral leg disturbances. Clinically, patients may report diffuse weakness, altered proprioception, or episodic tension along the lateral border.

Spectral surface imaging highlights bands of hypoemission suggestive of stagnation or signal depletion, while scattered hyperemissive foci may indicate reparative or compensatory activation.

These emissive dynamics follow fascial currents more than strict anatomic compartments, emphasizing their role as subtle energy expressions rather than local structural pathology. Interpreted within a systemic framework, the external left leg becomes a surface map of broader energetic resilience and adaptability.

Step 2,3,4: ROI Classification and Interpretive Questions

Hyperemission reflects localized energy accumulation or regulatory excitation.

- Does the patient feel heat, tingling, or unexplained discomfort?
- Are stress or emotional factors exacerbating symptoms?

Hypoemission suggests functional depletion or stagnation within the biofield.

- Does the patient experience coldness, fatigue, numbness, or low vitality?
- Are symptoms chronic and resistant to conventional care?

Step 5: Confirmatory Evaluations

Test	Purpose & Justification	Relevance to Emissive Pattern
Bioresonance testing	Measures tissue energy frequencies and imbalances.	Correlates with emission irregularities.
Electrodermal screening (EDS)	Assesses skin conductance linked to energy pathways.	Supports interpretation of energetic dynamics.
Patient emotional and symptom history	Provides clinical context for energetic dysfunction.	Assists differential assessment.

Step 6: Care Strategies and Intervention Pathways

Naturopathic Approach

Employ bioresonance, pulsed electromagnetic fields (PEMF), and herbal adaptogens to restore energetic balance and support healing (Matsumoto et al., 2010). Nutritional antioxidants and adaptogens enhance systemic resilience. Mindfulness and stress-reduction techniques complement energetic therapies.

Standard Medical Approaches

Energetic therapies serve as adjuncts to conventional medical and rehabilitative treatments, enhancing overall patient outcomes.

Specialty / Practitioner Care Strategies Table

Specialty Group	Practitioners Included	Hyperemissive Strategies	Hypoemissive Strategies
Biochemistry	Nutritionists, Orthomolecular, Herbalists, Naturopaths	Adaptogens, antioxidants, herbal energetics	Nutritional support for energy deficiency
Rehabilitation	Physiotherapists, Massage Therapists, Osteopaths / Chiropractors	Energy-based manual therapies, PEMF, therapeutic touch	Gentle stimulation, mobilization
Energetics	Acupuncturists (TCM), Bioenergetic Therapists	Bioresonance, PEMF, acupuncture	Warming acupuncture, energy balancing
Psychological	GNM practitioners, Psychotherapists, Vibrational therapists, Family constellation facilitators	Psychotherapy, bioresonance, mindfulness	Emotional balancing, vibrational medicine

Educational Pearls & Considerations.

- Energetic therapies complement but do not replace conventional care.
- Patient responsiveness and practitioner expertise influence outcomes.
- Monitor clinical progress to adjust therapy accordingly.
- Address psychological and physical aspects holistically.

GROUP 1 - ZONE 5 – EXTERNAL LEFT LEG

Category 9: Metabolic / Endocrine

Step 1: Functional Anatomy and Interpretive Importance

The external left leg comprises the fibula, peroneal musculature, and fascial planes that stabilize gait and ankle eversion (Standring, 2016). This region is metabolically sensitive, as peripheral tissues are among the first to show systemic glycoregulatory or lipid-related disturbances.

Vinik et al. (2003) described how diabetic neuropathy and peripheral arterial compromise manifest in lateral compartments as both vascular and neural dysfunction. Dyslipidemia and impaired fatty acid metabolism also contribute to reduced tissue repair and chronic fatigue in this field.

Clinically, patients may report lateral ankle instability, numbness, or recurrent strain. Spectral surface readings reveal elongated hypoemissive streaks aligned with vascular conduits, signaling perfusion decline or neuropathic suppression, while focal hyperemissive areas appear with reparative or adaptive activity.

These biospectral signatures, when interpreted systemically, position the external left leg as a visible index of metabolic resilience and lipid–glucose regulatory balance.

Step 2,3,4: ROI Classification and Interpretive Questions

Hyperemission may indicate local activation, microbial imbalance, or metabolic overactivity.

- Is there redness, warmth, or swelling?
- Is metabolic control suboptimal?

Hypoemission suggests ischemia, neurogenic dysfunction, or reduced perfusion due to metabolic/endocrine dysfunction.

- Is there coldness, numbness, chronic wounds, or fatigue?
- Are systemic symptoms such as temperature intolerance present?

Step 5: Confirmatory Evaluations

Test	Purpose & Justification	Relevance to Emissive Pattern
HbA1c, fasting glucose	Monitors glycemic control in diabetes.	Correlates with hypoemissive neuropathic or ischemic zones.
Thyroid function tests (TSH, Free T4)	Detect thyroid disorders affecting metabolism and circulation.	Associated with altered regulatory patterns of emission.
Lipid profile	Assesses cardiovascular risk factors impacting tissue perfusion.	Supports metabolic vascular imbalance.
Inflammatory markers (CRP, ESR)	Identifies systemic inflammation influencing tissue health.	Correlates with hyperemissive regulatory activation.

Step 6: Care Strategies and Intervention Pathways

Naturopathic Approach

Optimize metabolic function with low glycemic diet, antioxidants, and micronutrients improving insulin sensitivity (Alberti et al., 2006). Adaptogenic herbs such as *Panax ginseng* and *Gymnema sylvestre* support endocrine balance. Supplement chromium, magnesium, and alpha-lipoic acid to enhance glucose metabolism and nerve protection. Regular aerobic exercise improves circulation and metabolism.

Standard Medical Approaches

Strict metabolic control with pharmacotherapy and lifestyle modification is essential. Thyroid hormone replacement and lipid management reduce complications.

Specialty / Practitioner Care Strategies Table

Specialty Group	Practitioners Included	Hyperemissive Strategies	Hypoemissive Strategies
Biochemistry	Nutritionists, Orthomolecular, Herbalists, Naturopaths	Antioxidants, adaptogens, insulin sensitizers, micronutrients	Metabolic support, neuroprotective nutrients, dietary management
Rehabilitation	Physiotherapists, Massage Therapists, Osteopaths / Chiropractors	Exercise therapy, circulation enhancement	Neuromuscular re-education, aerobic conditioning
Energetics	Acupuncturists (TCM), Bioenergetic Therapists	Acupuncture supporting metabolic function	Energy balancing, PEMF
Psychological	GNM practitioners, Psychotherapists, Vibrational therapists, Family constellation facilitators	Mind-body therapies supporting metabolic regulation	Stress reduction, emotional balancing

Educational Pearls & Considerations.

- Regular metabolic monitoring prevents tissue complications.
- Lifestyle and dietary changes complement clinical management.
- Adaptogens support but do not replace conventional therapies.
- Patient education on foot care is critical to avoid ulcers.

GROUP 1

ZONE 6 – EXTERNAL RIGHT LEG

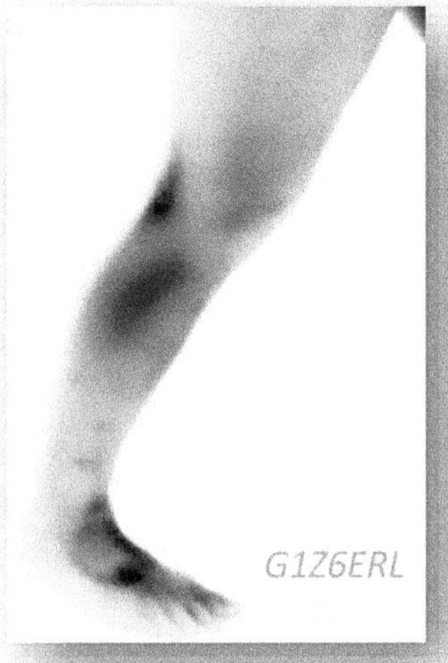

The The external right leg mirrors the biomechanical features of its left counterpart but often carries greater systemic significance due to dominance patterns and reflexive associations. In right-leg dominant individuals, this zone frequently expresses repetitive overuse effects, particularly in locomotion and postural compensation. It includees the iliotibial tract and fibular musculature, yet its interpretive role extends into systemic physiology. Biospectrally, persistent right-sided lateral hyperemission has been associated with compensatory pelvic imbalance, reflecting how the lateral kinetic chain absorbs and redistributes asymmetric load (Standring, 2016).

Clinically, right-sided asymmetry may also correlate with hepatic regulatory stress or gallbladder field sensitivity, links noted in clinical and meridian frameworks (Deadman et al., 2007). Fascial research supports this association, showing that lateral line tension can influence diaphragmatic mechanics and visceral regulation (Myers, 2014).

From a musculoskeletal perspective, iliotibial band friction syndrome, a leading cause of lateral knee pain, affects up to 22% of athletes training with repetitive flexion-extension, and biospectral disturbances in the right lateral thigh often precede overt symptoms (Lavine, 2010). In systemic disease contexts, emissive suppression here may reflect compromised perfusion in early peripheral vascular disease, particularly in diabetes or metabolic syndrome where lateral chain circulation is vulnerable (Criqui & Aboyans, 2015).

Functionally, this zone highlights compensatory adaptations of core stability, as lateral chain hyperactivity often stabilizes weak or misaligned pelvic foundations. Taken together, the external right leg serves as both a biomechanical indicator of muscular dominance and a peripheral marker of systemic states. Its interpretive value lies in revealing the interplay between postural load, hepatic or biliary regulation, and lateral chain overuse, positioning it as a uniquely integrative site for biospectral observation.

Zone 6 – External Right Leg: Emission-Relevant Structures.

Category	Relevant Structures	Emission Relevance
1. Vascular / Circulatory	- Small saphenous vein (posterolateral leg) - Peroneal veins and lateral perforators - Popliteal tributaries	Hyperemission may indicate venous congestion, reflux, or vascular activation along the lateral leg. Hypoemission reflects poor venous return, vascular insufficiency, or lateral flow collapse.
2. Muscular / Myofascial	- Peroneus longus and brevis - Lateral gastrocnemius head - Soleus fascia (lateral portion) - Iliotibial tract insertion	Hyperemissive activity may signal lateral overuse, compensatory gait, or fascial strain. Hypoemissive zones often represent disuse atrophy, lateral inhibition, or fascial fixation.
3. Skeletal / Articular	- Fibula (shaft and head) - Lateral tibial plateau - Lateral ankle joint (talocrural complex)	Bone-related hyperemission may reflect stress reaction, periostitis, or mechanical irritation. Hypoemission is associated with joint degeneration or reduced osseous regulatory activity.
4. Nervous System / Spine	- Superficial peroneal nerve - Common fibular nerve - L5 dermatome (lateral leg and dorsum of foot)	Hyperemission may arise from fibular nerve compression or L5 radiculopathy. Hypoemission may reflect neuropathic weakening, sympathetic tone loss, or neurovascular dysregulation.
5. Lymphatic / Immune	- Superficial lateral lymphatic network - Popliteal lymph nodes	Hyperemission may reflect lymphatic overload, toxic load, or regional regulatory activation. Hypoemission can be a sign of stagnated flow, immune hyporegulation, or localized lymphatic weakness.
6. Organs / GNM	*(Typically excluded from direct structural mapping in this zone)*	
7. Acupuncture / Meridians	- Gallbladder Meridian (GB) – lateral leg - Bladder Meridian (BL) – lateral collateral paths	Hyperemission is common with Gallbladder meridian congestion or decision-related frustration. Hypoemission may indicate Yang deficiency or weakened gallbladder–adrenal axis.
8. Energetic / Frequency	- Lateral energy field for assertiveness, movement, and directional focus	Heat suggests reactive drive, emotional tension, or overextension. Cold is associated with energetic withdrawal, loss of drive, or decision paralysis in right-side polarity.
9. Metabolic / Endocrine	- Reflex areas for adrenal stress, bile flow, and metabolic detox	Hyperemission implies metabolic activation or detox effort. Hypoemission reflects low adrenal output, bile stagnation, or diminished lateral metabolic expression.

GROUP 1 - ZONE 6 – EXTERNAL RIGHT LEG

Category 1: Vascular / Circulatory

Step 1: Functional Anatomy and Interpretive Importance

The external right lower leg is supplied anteriorly by the anterior tibial artery, which runs along the interosseous membrane, and posteriorly by the fibular artery supporting the lateral compartment. These vessels nourish the fibularis longus and brevis and contribute to cutaneous supply over the lateral shin. Venous return follows the anterior tibial veins draining into the popliteal vein, with clearance also through superficial tributaries connected to the saphenous system (Standring, 2016). Vascular studies identify the fibular artery as an important collateral during arterial compromise, underscoring its role in preserving limb perfusion (Fowkes et al., 2013).

On spectral surface reading, the lateral compartment often displays emissive asymmetries following arterial and venous pathways. These patterns may reflect repetitive load, venous pooling, or subtle arterial modulation. As the lateral leg contributes to ankle stabilization and balance, irregularities here are sensitive indicators of circulatory stress during locomotion.

Step 2,3,4: ROI Classification and Interpretive Questions

Hyperemission suggests venous stasis, tissue activation, or microangiopathy with increased blood flow.

- Is there swelling, warmth, or discomfort?
- Are varicose veins or skin changes evident?

Hypoemission indicates arterial insufficiency, vasospasm, or ischemia with reduced spectral surface reading.

- Is coldness, numbness, or intermittent claudication reported?
- Are peripheral pulses diminished?

Step 5: Confirmatory Evaluations

Test	Purpose & Justification	Relevance to Emissive Pattern
Doppler ultrasound	Assesses arterial and venous blood flow (Brant et al., 2016).	Correlates with hyperemissive venous congestion and hypoemissive arterial disease.
Ankle-Brachial Index (ABI)	Quantifies arterial perfusion; ABI <0.9 indicates peripheral arterial disease (Norgren et al., 2007).	Validates hypoemissive arterial insufficiency.
Capillary refill time	Evaluates microcirculation.	Supports hypoemissive microvascular compromise.
Blood tests (CBC, CRP, coagulation)	Detects systemic inflammation or thrombotic risk factors.	Supports vascular regulatory activation.

Step 6: Care Strategies and Intervention Pathways

Naturopathic Approach

Botanical venotonics such as *Aesculus hippocastanum* and *Centella asiatica* improve venous tone (Chrubasik et al., 2011). Hydrotherapy with contrast baths stimulates circulation and reduces edema (Sutkowy et al., 2019). Anti-inflammatory diets rich in antioxidants, vitamin C, and omega-3 fatty acids support vascular health (Calder, 2017). Nitric oxide donors improve arterial perfusion (Moncada & Higgs, 1993). Limb elevation and exercise promote venous return. Supplement iron, B12, and folate to enhance oxygen transport.

Standard Medical Approaches

Imaging guides use of compression stockings, venoactive drugs, NSAIDs, sclerotherapy, or surgical revascularization (Brant et al., 2016; Norgren et al., 2007). Wound care is critical for ischemic ulcers.

Specialty / Practitioner Care Strategies Table

Specialty Group	Practitioners Included	Hyperemissive Strategies	Hypoemissive Strategies
Biochemistry	Nutritionists, Orthomolecular, Herbalists, Naturopaths	Botanical venotonics, anti-inflammatory diet, antioxidants, vitamins C, E, selenium, CoQ10, bioflavonoids, omega-3s	Circulatory stimulants (*Ginkgo biloba*, cayenne), blood-building nutrients (iron, B12, folate), magnesium, arginine, nitrate-rich diet
Rehabilitation	Physiotherapists, Massage Therapists, Osteopaths / Chiropractors	Lymphatic drainage, calf pump exercises, postural retraining, gentle Swedish massage, myofascial release	Graded aerobic exercise, gait training, emission protection, foot care, warming massage, reflexology, ergonomic guidance
Energetics	Acupuncturists (TCM), Bioenergetic Therapists	Acupuncture (SP6, ST36), moxibustion, herbal formulas, Qi and Blood tonics, bioresonance, PEMF	Warming acupuncture, Qi and Blood tonics, PEMF, energy healing
Psychological	GNM practitioners, Psychotherapists, Vibrational therapists, Family constellation facilitators	GNM conflict protocols, psychotherapy, bioresonance, mindfulness, energy clearing	Psychosomatic conflict resolution, vibrational medicine, stress reduction, emotional balancing

Educational Pearls & Considerations.

- Exclude deep vein thrombosis or critical ischemia before applying heat, massage, or exercise.
- Botanical venotonics combined with hydrotherapy effectively reduce venous congestion.
- Nitric oxide boosters and omega-3 fatty acids enhance endothelial function and arterial perfusion.
- Compression therapy is contraindicated in severe arterial insufficiency.
- Early mobilization and limb elevation prevent chronic complications.

GROUP 1 - ZONE 6 – EXTERNAL RIGHT LEG

Category 2: Muscular

Step 1: Functional Anatomy and Interpretive Importance

The lateral compartment of the right leg is composed of the fibularis longus and brevis, supplied by the superficial fibular nerve. These muscles produce foot eversion, contribute to ankle stability, and transmit load through the transverse arch via the fibularis longus tendon, which crosses the sole to insert at the medial cuneiform.

The retinacula around the lateral malleolus secure these tendons during dynamic activity (Standring, 2016). Clinical observations note that peroneal tendon disorders are highly prevalent in individuals with chronic ankle instability, where repetitive inversion episodes create tendinopathy or subluxation (Ferran & Maffulli, 2006).

In functional emissive analysis, this region often reveals linear patterns extending along the fibularis trajectory, with signal irregularities arising from overload or compensatory recruitment. These findings are especially relevant in athletes exposed to multidirectional stress, where subtle biospectral shifts may indicate an evolving imbalance in lateral stabilizers.

Step 2,3,4: ROI Classification and Interpretive Questions

Hyperemission suggests acute muscle strain, myositis, or tissue activation with increased blood flow.

- Has the patient experienced trauma or repetitive stress?
- Is there localized pain, swelling, or muscle spasm?

Hypoemission indicates chronic vascular restriction, compartment adaptation, or neurogenic atrophy with decreased circulatory efficiency.

- Are numbness, weakness, or muscle wasting present?
- Is gait or limb function impaired?

Step 5: Confirmatory Evaluations

Test	Purpose & Justification	Relevance to Emissive Pattern
Creatine kinase (CK), LDH	Detects muscle damage or inflammation (Maffulli et al., 2014).	Elevated in hyperemissive tissue activation
MRI	Visualizes edema, inflammation, ischemia, or muscle atrophy.	Supports hyper- or hypoemissive findings.
Compartment pressure measurement	Diagnoses compartment syndrome by measuring intracompartmental pressure.	Relevant for hypoemissive ischemic patterns.

Nerve conduction studies (NCS), Electromyography (EMG)	Evaluates neurogenic muscle dysfunction.	Correlates with hypoemissive neurogenic causes.
Blood tests (CBC, inflammatory markers)	Detect systemic inflammation or infection.	Supports hyperemissive regulatory activation

Step 6: Care Strategies and Intervention Pathways

Naturopathic Approach

Anti-inflammatory botanicals such as *Curcuma longa* and *Boswellia serrata* reduce muscle inflammation (Hewlings & Kalman, 2017). Magnesium supports muscle relaxation. Hydrotherapy with alternating warm and cold compresses improves circulation (Sutkowy et al., 2019). Gentle stretching and graded strengthening restore function. Protein and antioxidants aid repair.

Standard Medical Approaches

Rest, NSAIDs, and physical therapy are standard for acute muscle injuries (Maffulli et al., 2014). Compartment syndrome requires urgent surgical intervention. Neurogenic muscle weakness warrants neurological assessment.

Specialty / Practitioner Care Strategies Table

Specialty Group	Practitioners Included	Hyperemissive Strategies	Hypoemissive Strategies
Biochemistry	Nutritionists, Orthomolecular, Herbalists, Naturopaths	Anti-inflammatory botanicals, magnesium, antioxidants, protein	Circulatory support, neurotrophic nutrients, protein support
Rehabilitation	Physiotherapists, Massage Therapists, Osteopaths / Chiropractors	Myofascial release, trigger point therapy, gentle massage	Graded aerobic exercise, neurorehabilitation, ergonomic guidance
Energetics	Acupuncturists (TCM), Bioenergetic Therapists	Acupuncture, moxibustion, PEMF	Warming acupuncture, frequency therapy
Psychological	GNM practitioners, Psychotherapists, Vibrational therapists, Family constellation facilitators	Psychotherapy, bioresonance, mindfulness	Psychosomatic conflict resolution, emotional balancing

Educational Pearls & Considerations.

- Early recognition of compartment syndrome is essential.
- Magnesium supports muscle relaxation and reduces cramps.
- Hydrotherapy protocols should be matched to inflammation stages.
- Neurogenic muscle weakness requires thorough evaluation.
- Graded rehabilitation prevents chronic disability.

GROUP 1 - ZONE 6 – EXTERNAL RIGHT LEG

Category 3: Skeletal

Step 1: Functional Anatomy and Interpretive Importance

The external right leg mirrors the skeletal structure of the tibia and fibula, together with the lateral ankle complex that supports locomotion and weight transfer (Standring, 2016). The fibula, though slender, contributes significantly to lateral ankle stability, and its integrity is vital for resisting inversion stresses.

Recurrent strain or repetitive microtrauma in this region has been correlated with stress reactions and degenerative remodeling, particularly in the fibular shaft and tibial metaphysis (Brukner et al., 1996). These processes subtly alter vascular signaling and periosteal responsiveness, creating emissive irregularities that are traceable on spectral surface readings.

Biospectral asymmetries in the lateral leg often manifest as narrow fields overlying the osseous contours, differing from diffuse muscular activation zones. Their precise topography reflects the skeletal origin of the disturbance, illustrating how structural stress translates into external biosignals. This integration enhances clinical interpretation by differentiating articular-ligamentous strain from muscular load, guiding more targeted interventions.

Step 2,3,4: ROI Classification and Interpretive Questions

Hyperemission indicates acute fractures, periosteal reactivity, or joint effusion with increased blood flow.

- Is there recent trauma or overuse?
- Are swelling, tenderness, or joint stiffness present?

Hypoemission suggests chronic joint remodeling, structural degeneration, or vascular compromise with reduced perfusion.

- Are there chronic pain, stiffness, or limited mobility?
- Is there history of deformity or instability?

Step 5: Confirmatory Evaluations

Test	Purpose & Justification	Relevance to Emissive Pattern
X-ray imaging	Detects fractures, stress injuries, and joint space narrowing.	Confirms hyperemissive acute injury or hypoemissive chronic changes.
MRI	Visualizes bone marrow edema, occult fractures, cartilage, and soft tissues.	Supports regulatory activation or degenerative changes.
Bone scan	Assesses bone metabolism and detects stress fractures or infection.	Correlates with hyperemissive bone involvement.
Blood tests (inflammatory markers)	Detects systemic inflammation related to bone injury or infection.	Supports hyperemissive regulatory activation.

Step 6: Care Strategies and Intervention Pathways

Naturopathic Approach

Bone healing is supported by adequate intake of calcium, vitamin D, magnesium, and vitamin K (Heaney, 2006). Anti-inflammatory botanicals like *Boswellia serrata* reduce periosteal inflammation. Therapeutic ultrasound and PEMF stimulate bone repair (Gordon et al., 2016). Immobilization protects injured structures.

Standard Medical Approaches

Imaging guides immobilization or surgery. NSAIDs and physical therapy manage symptoms. Osteoarthritis requires supportive care.

Specialty / Practitioner Care Strategies Table

Specialty Group	Practitioners Included	Hyperemissive Strategies	Hypoemissive Strategies
Biochemistry	Nutritionists, Orthomolecular, Herbalists, Naturopaths	Bone-supportive nutrients, anti-inflammatory botanicals	Nutritional support for bone remodeling and joint health
Rehabilitation	Physiotherapists, Massage Therapists, Osteopaths / Chiropractors	Joint mobilization, therapeutic ultrasound, myofascial release	Joint stabilization, graded strengthening, ergonomic guidance
Energetics	Acupuncturists (TCM), Bioenergetic Therapists	Acupuncture, PEMF, herbal formulas for inflammation	Warming acupuncture, energy balancing
Psychological	GNM practitioners, Psychotherapists, Vibrational therapists, Family constellation facilitators	Mind-body therapies supporting pain management and healing	Psychosomatic support, emotional balancing

Educational Pearls & Considerations.

- Prompt immobilization prevents further injury.
- Adequate nutrition accelerates bone healing.
- PEMF therapy requires skilled application.
- Chronic hypoemissive patterns suggest degenerative disease needing multidisciplinary care.
- Psychological support enhances recovery.

GROUP 1 - ZONE 6 – EXTERNAL RIGHT LEG

Category 4: Nervous

Step 1: Functional Anatomy and Interpretive Importance

The external right leg receives innervation from superficial and deep branches of the common peroneal nerve, coordinating dorsiflexion, toe extension, and eversion while conveying sensation from the lateral leg and dorsum of the foot (Standring, 2016). Compression neuropathies are common in sports and prolonged postures, where loading provokes pain, weakness, or paresthesia; habitual leg crossing is a frequent cause of peroneal palsy, producing acute conduction failure (Katirji, 1999).

These disturbances alter vascular tone and local recruitment, generating emissive profiles externally visible as biospectral asymmetries along the fibular trajectory. Such narrow, linear signals differ from broader muscular fields, reflecting their neurogenic origin. Correlating these emissive patterns with clinical findings allows practitioners to distinguish peroneal compression from muscular strain, supporting earlier intervention and refined localization of neuropathy.

Step 2,3,4: ROI Classification and Interpretive Questions

Hyperemission indicates nerve irritation or neurogenic activation with increased local perfusion.

- Are there burning, tingling, or sharp pain sensations?
- Is there localized hypersensitivity or swelling?

Hypoemission suggests reduced neurovascular signaling due to compression, ischemia, or denervation, contributing to diminished biosignal regulation and lower spectral surface readings.

- Are numbness, weakness, or muscle wasting reported?
- Do symptoms worsen with certain movements or positions?

Step 5: Confirmatory Evaluations

Test	Purpose & Justification	Relevance to Emissive Pattern
Nerve conduction studies (NCS), Electromyography (EMG)	Evaluate nerve and muscle function (Campbell & Meyer, 2006).	Correlate with hypoemissive neurogenic dysfunction.
Quantitative sensory testing (QST)	Assesses sensory nerve function and thresholds.	Supports interpretation of neuropathic signatures.
MRI / Ultrasound	Visualizes nerve compression or structural pathology.	Identifies nerve-related contribution
Blood tests (glucose, vitamin B12)	Assess metabolic causes of neuropathy.	Supports interpretation of neuroregulatory patterns

Step 6: Care Strategies and Intervention Pathways

Naturopathic Approach

Neurotrophic vitamins (B-complex), alpha-lipoic acid, and Acetyl-L-carnitine support nerve regeneration (Papanas & Ziegler, 2014). Herbal anti-inflammatories like *Hypericum perforatum* may alleviate neuropathic pain (Kasper et al., 2010). Neural mobilization and gentle stretching facilitate recovery. Mind-body therapies and bioresonance modulate pain and neurovascular function.

Standard Medical Approaches

Pharmacologic options include anticonvulsants, antidepressants, and analgesics. Surgical decompression may be indicated. Metabolic control is vital for systemic neuropathies.

Specialty / Practitioner Care Strategies Table

Specialty Group	Practitioners Included	Hyperemissive Strategies	Hypoemissive Strategies
Biochemistry	Nutritionists, Orthomolecular, Herbalists, Naturopaths	Neurotrophic vitamins, alpha-lipoic acid, anti-inflammatory botanicals	Circulatory stimulants, metabolic support, neuroprotective nutrients
Rehabilitation	Physiotherapists, Massage Therapists, Osteopaths / Chiropractors	Neural mobilization, myofascial release, gentle massage	Neural gliding exercises, ergonomic guidance, neurorehabilitation
Energetics	Acupuncturists (TCM), Bioenergetic Therapists	Acupuncture, moxibustion, PEMF	Warming acupuncture, frequency therapy, energy healing
Psychological	GNM practitioners, Psychotherapists, Vibrational therapists, Family constellation facilitators	Psychotherapy, bioresonance, mindfulness	Psychosomatic conflict resolution, vibrational medicine

Educational Pearls & Considerations.

- Early detection prevents permanent nerve damage.
- Nutritional support complements medical therapies.
- Mind-body and energetic therapies aid pain management.
- Monitor for metabolic contributors like diabetes.
- Avoid aggressive treatments during acute inflammation.

GROUP 1 - ZONE 6 – EXTERNAL RIGHT LEG

Category 5: Lymphatic

Step 1: Functional Anatomy and Interpretive Importance

The external right leg shares the same lymphatic configuration, with superficial and deep collectors running alongside the small saphenous and peroneal veins before draining into popliteal and inguinal stations (Standring, 2016).

Proper function ensures clearance of immune cells and metabolic byproducts from the lateral compartment. Szuba and Rockson (1998) noted that lymphatic failure in the lower limb contributes significantly to chronic lymphedema, often exacerbated by trauma or venous disease. Functional disruption modifies local compliance and neurovascular regulation, changes that extend outward to the surface field.

Biospectral asymmetries here typically align with the fibular shaft and lateral malleolus, their sharply bounded distribution reflecting the linear course of drainage pathways. These emissive variations represent the externalized footprint of lymphatic congestion, allowing clinicians to separate neurovascular imbalance from lymphatic transport failure in the lateral leg.

Step 2,3,4: ROI Classification and Interpretive Questions

Hyperemission indicates acute lymphangitis, infection, or lymphatic congestion with warmth and swelling.

- Is there redness, tenderness, or rapid swelling?
- Has the patient experienced recent trauma or infection?

Hypoemission suggests chronic lymphedema with fibrosis and reduced drainage causing diminished perfusion.

- Is swelling persistent and firm?
- Are recurrent infections or slow-healing wounds present?

Step 5: Confirmatory Evaluations

Test	Purpose & Justification	Relevance to Emissive Pattern
Lymphoscintigraphy	Assesses lymphatic drainage and detects obstruction.	Confirms lymphatic stasis or hypoperfusion.
Doppler ultrasound	Excludes venous insufficiency contributing to swelling.	Differentiates vascular from lymphatic causes.
Blood tests (CBC, inflammatory markers)	Detect infection or systemic inflammation.	Supports hyperemissive functional activation
Physical exam (Stemmer's sign, limb measurements)	Identifies clinical signs of lymphedema.	Correlates with biospectral observations.

Step 6: Care Strategies and Intervention Pathways

Naturopathic Approach

Stimulate lymphatic flow with herbal lymphagogues such as *Hedera helix* and *Vitis vinifera* (Godoy et al., 2012). Manual lymphatic drainage by trained therapists facilitates fluid movement. Compression therapy supports lymph return and should be individualized. Nutritional antioxidants and anti-inflammatory nutrients promote tissue repair. Hydrotherapy with alternating warm and cold stimulation enhances lymphatic circulation.

Standard Medical Approaches

Standard treatments include manual lymphatic drainage, compression garments, physical therapy, and infection control. Surgery is reserved for advanced cases.

Specialty / Practitioner Care Strategies Table

Specialty Group	Practitioners Included	Hyperemissive Strategies	Hypoemissive Strategies
Biochemistry	Nutritionists, Orthomolecular, Herbalists, Naturopaths	Herbal lymphagogues, antioxidants, anti-inflammatory nutrients	Circulatory support, nutritional tissue repair support
Rehabilitation	Physiotherapists, Massage Therapists, Osteopaths / Chiropractors	Manual lymphatic drainage, gentle massage, postural retraining	Compression therapy, graded exercise, ergonomic guidance
Energetics	Acupuncturists (TCM), Bioenergetic Therapists	Acupuncture, herbal formulas, PEMF	Warming acupuncture, energy balancing
Psychological	GNM practitioners, Psychotherapists, Vibrational therapists, Family constellation facilitators	Mind-body therapies supporting immune function and healing	Psychosomatic conflict resolution, emotional balancing

Educational Pearls & Considerations.

- Early intervention prevents progression to chronic lymphedema.
- Manual lymph drainage should be performed by certified therapists.
- Compression therapy requires proper fitting and monitoring.
- Nutritional support enhances lymphatic function and tissue repair.
- Prompt infection treatment is essential to avoid worsening.

GROUP 1 - ZONE 6 – EXTERNAL RIGHT LEG

Category 7: Acupuncture / Meridian

Step 1: Functional Anatomy and Interpretive Importance

The external right leg contains the fibula, lateral muscles of dorsiflexion and eversion, and supportive fascial planes (Standring, 2016). This surface is aligned with the Stomach (ST) and Gallbladder (GB) meridians, which regulate balance, circulation, and energy distribution in the lower extremity.

Maciocia (2015) noted that the Gallbladder channel governs decision-making energetics and lateral body stability, linking musculoskeletal and emotional states. Cheng (1987) reinforced classical associations of lateral leg weakness with disruptions of GB flow. Clinically, dysfunction presents as tension, fatigue, or sensory disturbance in the lateral leg.

On emissive evaluation, biosignal mapping reveals asymmetrical fields that follow GB and ST trajectories, their clear linearity differentiating them from vascular insufficiency. These patterns illustrate the translation of Qi stagnation or deficiency into observable emissive fields, validating the diagnostic convergence of meridian theory and spectral surface assessment.

Step 2,3,4: ROI Classification and Interpretive Questions

Hyperemission indicates Qi stagnation or local emissive activity along the meridian.

- Is there localized tenderness, swelling, or sharp pain?
- Do symptoms worsen with movement or pressure?

Hypoemission suggests Qi deficiency or chronic energetic stagnation with reduced energy flow and tissue oxygenation.

- Does the patient report weakness, coldness, numbness, or chronic dull pain?
- Are poor circulation or fatigue evident?

Step 5: Confirmatory Evaluations

Test	Purpose & Justification	Relevance to Emissive Pattern
Pulse diagnosis and tongue examination	Traditional TCM tools assessing Qi and blood status (Flaws, 2000).	Correlates with biospectral observations for interpretation.
Biospectral imaging	Detects emissive asymmetries along meridians.	Visualizes hyper- or hypoemissive meridian zones.
Patient symptom questionnaire	Evaluates pain patterns, energy levels, and functional status.	Supports differentiation between stagnation and deficiency.

Step 6: **Care Strategies and Intervention Pathways**

Naturopathic Approach

Acupuncture at points such as ST36 and GB34 regulates Qi and blood flow, reducing inflammation and restoring function (Lao et al., 2004). Moxibustion warms hypoemissive meridians. Herbal formulas like *Dang Gui* and *Chuan Xiong* nourish blood and harmonize Qi (Bensky et al., 2004). Nutritional support with Qi-building foods complements therapy.

Standard Medical Approaches

Acupuncture is an adjunct to physical therapy and pain management for musculoskeletal conditions related to meridian imbalance.

Specialty / Practitioner Care Strategies Table

Specialty Group	Practitioners Included	Hyperemissive Strategies	Hypoemissive Strategies
Biochemistry	Nutritionists, Orthomolecular, Herbalists, Naturopaths	Herbal formulas regulating Qi and blood, antioxidants	Qi tonics, blood-nourishing supplements
Rehabilitation	Physiotherapists, Massage Therapists, Osteopaths / Chiropractors	Trigger point therapy complementary to acupuncture	Gentle mobilization, warming massage
Energetics	Acupuncturists (TCM), Bioenergetic Therapists	Acupuncture, moxibustion, PEMF	Warming acupuncture, Qi tonics, energy healing
Psychological	GNM practitioners, Psychotherapists, Vibrational therapists, Family constellation facilitators	Mind-body therapies, bioresonance, energy clearing	Psychosomatic conflict resolution, emotional balancing

Educational Pearls & Considerations.

- Precise acupuncture point selection is essential to balance thermal patterns.
- Use moxibustion cautiously in heat-sensitive patients.
- Herbal treatments should be supervised by qualified practitioners.
- Combining acupuncture with rehabilitation improves therapeutic outcomes.

GROUP 1 - ZONE 6 – EXTERNAL RIGHT LEG

Category 8: Energetic

Step 1: Functional Anatomy and Interpretive Importance

The external right leg mirrors its left counterpart, including the fibula, peroneal group, and lateral fascial expansions, functioning to stabilize gait and absorb rotational loads (Standring, 2016). Energetically, this field has been linked to resilience and systemic regulation, often revealing subtle dysfunctions not captured by structural examination alone.

Motoyama (1977) demonstrated correlations between lateral limb energy flow and electrophysiological meridian measurements, supporting the notion that peripheral emissive signals can indicate systemic imbalance. Clinically, disturbances manifest as lateral instability, recurrent strain, or unexplained fatigue.

Biospectral imaging often reveals hypoemissive streaks marking under-conduction or diffuse hyperemissive arcs consistent with compensatory activation. These emissive dynamics point to subtle disruptions of systemic coherence, integrating local findings with an understanding of energy network behavior across the body.

Step 2,3,4: ROI Classification and Interpretive Questions

Hyperemission indicates localized energy congestion or elevated emissive activity.

- Does the patient feel heat, tingling, or unexplained discomfort?
- Are stress or emotional factors worsening symptoms?

Hypoemission suggests Qi deficiency or chronic energetic stagnation with reduced energy flow and tissue oxygenation.

- Does the patient experience fatigue, coldness, numbness, or low vitality?
- Are symptoms chronic or resistant to conventional therapies?

Step 5: Confirmatory Evaluations

Test	Purpose & Justification	Relevance to Emissive Pattern
Bioresonance testing	Measures tissue energy frequencies and imbalances.	Correlates with emission variations.
Electrodermal screening (EDS)	Assesses skin conductance related to energy pathways.	Supports interpretation of energetic patterns.
Patient emotional and symptom history	Provides clinical context for energetic dysfunction.	Assists in differential assessment.

Step 6: **Care Strategies and Intervention Pathways**

Naturopathic Approach

Utilize bioresonance, pulsed electromagnetic fields (PEMF), and adaptogenic herbs to restore energetic balance and support healing (Matsumoto et al., 2010). Nutritional antioxidants and adaptogens enhance systemic resilience. Mindfulness and stress-reduction techniques complement energetic therapies.

Standard Medical Approaches

Energetic therapies serve as adjuncts to conventional medical and rehabilitative treatments to optimize patient outcomes.

Specialty / Practitioner Care Strategies Table

Specialty Group	Practitioners Included	Hyperemissive Strategies	Hypoemissive Strategies
Biochemistry	Nutritionists, Orthomolecular, Herbalists, Naturopaths	Adaptogens, antioxidants, herbal energetics	Nutritional support for energy deficiency
Rehabilitation	Physiotherapists, Massage Therapists, Osteopaths / Chiropractors	Energy-based manual therapies, PEMF, therapeutic touch	Gentle stimulation, mobilization
Energetics	Acupuncturists (TCM), Bioenergetic Therapists	Bioresonance, PEMF, acupuncture	Warming acupuncture, energy balancing
Psychological	GNM practitioners, Psychotherapists, Vibrational therapists, Family constellation facilitators	Psychotherapy, bioresonance, mindfulness	Emotional balancing, vibrational medicine

Educational Pearls & Considerations.

- Energetic therapies complement but do not replace conventional care.
- Patient response and practitioner skill influence outcomes.
- Monitor clinical progress and adjust therapies accordingly.
- Address psychological and physical factors holistically.

GROUP 1 - ZONE 6 – EXTERNAL RIGHT LEG

Category 9: Metabolic / Endocrine

Step 1: Functional Anatomy and Interpretive Importance

The external right leg parallels the left anatomically, incorporating the fibula, peroneal group, and lateral fascial tracts that mediate rotational stability (Standring, 2016). Endocrine and metabolic regulation strongly modulates this surface, particularly through thyroidal influences on muscle tone and mitochondrial energy production.

Brent (2012) emphasized the broad effects of thyroid hormone on skeletal muscle, linking thyroid imbalance to fatigue and weakness often expressed peripherally. Clinically, patients may present with recurrent strain, diffuse aching, or neuropathic tingling exacerbated by exertion.

Biospectral imaging reveals hypoemissive zones corresponding to reduced metabolic drive and perfusion decline, along with hyperemissive bands reflecting compensatory repair. These signals map onto fascial currents more than isolated structures, reinforcing the systemic origin of local expression. The external right leg thereby reflects the interaction between thyroidal dynamics, metabolic stability, and peripheral tissue integrity.

Step 2,3,4: ROI Classification and Interpretive Questions

Hyperemission suggests localized biosignal activation, immune burden, or metabolic overactivity.

- Is there redness, warmth, or swelling?
- Is metabolic control suboptimal?

Hypoemission indicates vascular restriction, neuropathy, or autonomic inefficiency due to metabolic/endocrine imbalance.

- Is there coldness, numbness, chronic wounds, or fatigue?
- Are systemic symptoms such as temperature intolerance present?

Step 5: Confirmatory Evaluations

Test	Purpose & Justification	Relevance to Emissive Pattern
HbA1c, fasting glucose	Monitors glycemic control in diabetes.	Correlates with hypoemissive neuropathic or ischemic zones.
Thyroid function tests (TSH, Free T4)	Detects thyroid dysfunction affecting metabolism and circulation.	Associated with altered emissive regulation.
Lipid profile	Evaluates cardiovascular risk factors impacting tissue perfusion.	Supports metabolic vascular imbalance.
Inflammatory markers (CRP, ESR)	Identifies systemic inflammation influencing tissue health.	Correlates with hyperemissive regulatory activity.

Step 6: Care Strategies and Intervention Pathways

Naturopathic Approach

Optimize metabolic function with a low glycemic diet, antioxidants, and micronutrients improving insulin sensitivity (Alberti et al., 2006). Adaptogenic herbs such as *Panax ginseng* and *Gymnema sylvestre* support endocrine balance. Supplement chromium, magnesium, and alpha-lipoic acid to enhance glucose metabolism and nerve protection. Regular aerobic exercise improves circulation and metabolism.

Standard Medical Approaches

Pharmacotherapy and lifestyle modification for glycemic and metabolic control are essential. Thyroid hormone replacement and lipid management reduce complications.

Specialty / Practitioner Care Strategies Table

Specialty Group	Practitioners Included	Hyperemissive Strategies	Hypoemissive Strategies
Biochemistry	Nutritionists, Orthomolecular, Herbalists, Naturopaths	Antioxidants, adaptogens, insulin sensitizers, micronutrients	Metabolic support, neuroprotective nutrients, dietary management
Rehabilitation	Physiotherapists, Massage Therapists, Osteopaths / Chiropractors	Exercise therapy, circulation enhancement	Neuromuscular re-education, aerobic conditioning
Energetics	Acupuncturists (TCM), Bioenergetic Therapists	Acupuncture supporting metabolic function	Energy balancing, PEMF
Psychological	GNM practitioners, Psychotherapists, Vibrational therapists, Family constellation facilitators	Mind-body therapies supporting metabolic regulation	Stress reduction, emotional balancing

Educational Pearls & Considerations.

- Continuous metabolic monitoring prevents tissue complications.
- Lifestyle and diet changes complement clinical management.
- Adaptogens support but do not replace conventional therapies.
- Patient education on foot care is critical to prevent ulcerations.

GROUP 1

ZONE 7 – FRONTAL UPPER LEG

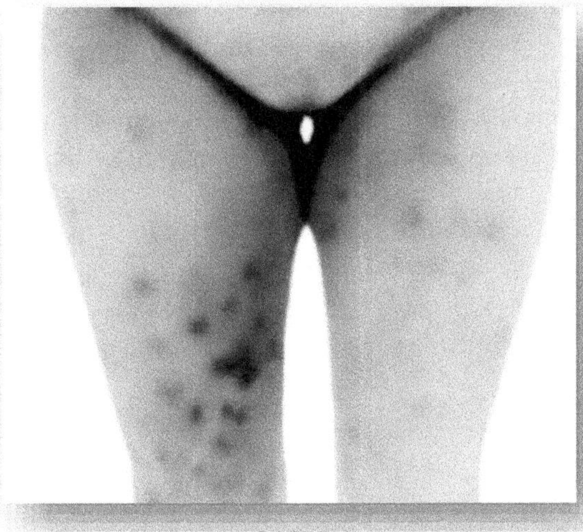

G1Z7FUL

The frontal upper thighs function as emissive integrators between lower limb circulation and abdominal regulation, reflecting both vascular load and muscular dynamics. This region includes the quadriceps group, superficial inguinal nodes, and major venous pathways such as the femoral vein (Standring, 2016). Because of this proximity, emissive variations often correspond with metabolic or circulatory load, offering a reliable surface for early interpretive analysis.

Symmetrical hypoemissive zones along the anterior thigh have been linked to systemic stress states such as adrenal dysregulation or digestive burden, where reduced perfusion reflects regulatory withdrawal rather than localized dysfunction.

Conversely, focal hyperemissive ROIs often indicate quadriceps overload or pelvic strain, particularly in athletes, dancers, or those with postural imbalance. Quadriceps injuries account for up to 20% of acute thigh injuries in professional athletes, often showing regulatory changes before rupture (Ekstrand et al., 2011). The femoral vein, one of the body's main venous return channels, also traverses this zone, making it sensitive to circulatory irregularities.

Deep vein thrombosis occurs most often in proximal thigh veins, and emissive asymmetry may reveal venous strain before swelling or pain develops (Kakkos et al., 2016). The inguinal nodes likewise drain both lower limb and pelvic viscera, and asymmetry here may reflect immune or drainage burdens (Mortimer & Rockson, 2014). In patients with systemic metabolic load, persistent hypoactivity of the anterior thighs may correlate with fatigue or endocrine strain.

Functionally, the strength of this zone lies in integrating musculoskeletal dynamics with systemic vascular and lymphatic influences. Its emissive patterns provide insight into quadriceps activity and into the hidden balance of circulation, metabolism, and immune regulation.

Zone 7 – Frontal Upper Legs: Emission-Relevant Structures.

Category	Relevant Structures	Emission Relevance
1. Vascular / Circulatory	- Femoral artery and vein (superficial and deep branches) - Lateral circumflex femoral vessels - Capillary beds of anterior thigh	Hyperemission may signal vascular dilation, arterial activation, or early varicosity. Hypoemission suggests vascular insufficiency, flow redistribution, or local sympathetic dominance.
2. Muscular / Myofascial	- Rectus femoris - Vastus lateralis and medialis - Sartorius (medially) - Tensor fasciae latae (laterally) - Anterior thigh fascia	Hyperemissive activity often reflects muscular compensation, pelvic imbalance, or fascial overstrain. Hypoemission may indicate quadriceps inhibition, hip flexor weakness, or fascial tension affecting circulation.
3. Skeletal / Articular	- Anterior femur shaft - Hip joint (anterior aspect) - Iliac crest (superiorly)	Hyperemission may result from joint overload, tendinopathy, or regulatory strain near the acetabulum. Hypoemission is seen with degenerative hip mechanics or anterior pelvic rotation.
4. Nervous System / Spine	- Femoral nerve and branches - L2–L4 dermatomes (anterior thigh distribution)	Hyperemissive signals may be due to femoral nerve tension or plexus irritation. Hypoemissive fields may reflect root-level compression, motor inhibition, or reduced spinal outflow.
5. Lymphatic / Immune	- Inguinal lymph nodes - Superficial anterior thigh lymphatic drainage	Hyperemission typically indicates lymphatic congestion, toxic load, or hormonal drainage overload. Hypoemission may suggest immune hyporegulation or localized lymphatic drainage failure.
6. Organs / GNM	*(Viscera not mapped directly here, but nearby pelvic reflexes may apply)*	
7. Acupuncture / Meridians	- Stomach Meridian (ST) – runs down anterior thigh - Spleen Meridian (SP) – medial upper leg - Liver Meridian (LR) – medial–anterior transition zone	Heat often relates to Stomach/Spleen Qi stasis or Liver constraint in the pelvic region. Cold zones may indicate Yin depletion or meridian exhaustion linked to digestive or pelvic strain.
8. Energetic / Frequency	- Zones linked to movement, sexuality, and personal expression through legs	Hyperemission may reflect emotional overload, drive tension, or expressive frustration. Cold zones suggest blocked creative flow, self-suppression, or pelvic-energy disconnection.
9. Metabolic / Endocrine	- Reflexes of glucose regulation (quadriceps metabolism) - Sex hormone activity (estrogen/androgen distribution)	Heat suggests hormonal fluctuation, muscular insulin demand, or detox response. Hypoemission indicates metabolic slowdown, testosterone/estrogen imbalance, or pelvic endocrine suppression.

GROUP 1 - ZONE 7 – FRONTAL UPPER LEGS

Category 1: Vascular / Circulatory

Step 1: Functional Anatomy and Interpretive Importance

The anterior thigh is perfused primarily by the femoral artery and its profunda femoris branches, which supply the quadriceps, sartorius, and anterior fascial layers. Venous return occurs through the femoral vein, augmented by the great saphenous vein draining superficial territories (Standring, 2016).

Clinical vascular reviews emphasise the femoral system's centrality in revascularization and bypass procedures, confirming its status as a critical inflow pathway for the lower limb (Rutherford, 2009).

Emissive asymmetries across the anterior thigh often align with these vascular lines. They may represent venous pooling in the superficial system or increased circulatory demand in the quadriceps during exertion. As one of the primary locomotor zones, the anterior thigh frequently demonstrates spectral variations that reflect both regional and systemic circulatory adaptation.

Step 2,3,4: ROI Classification and Interpretive Questions

Hyperemission suggests venous congestion, microvascular stasis, or reactive tissue activation.

- Is there localized warmth, swelling, or pain?
- Are varicosities or skin changes present?

Hypoemission indicates reduced arterial flow or tissue underperfusion.

- Are there complaints of coldness, numbness, or claudication?
- Is there diminished pulse or delayed wound healing?

Step 5: Confirmatory Evaluations

Test	Purpose & Justification	Relevance to Emissive Pattern
Doppler ultrasound	Evaluates arterial and venous blood flow (Brant et al., 2016).	Correlates hyperemissive venous congestion and hypoemissive arterial disease.
Ankle-Brachial Index (ABI)	Assesses arterial perfusion; ABI < 0.9 indicates PAD (Norgren et al., 2007).	Validates hypoemissive arterial insufficiency.
Venography / MR Venography	Detects venous obstruction or thrombosis.	Confirms venous activation corresponding to Hyperemission.
Blood tests (CBC, CRP, D-dimer)	Identifies infection, inflammation, or thrombotic risk.	Supports hyperemissive vascular or thrombotic activity.

Step 6: Care Strategies and Intervention Pathways

Naturopathic Approach

Botanical venotonics such as *Aesculus hippocastanum* and *Centella asiatica* improve venous tone and reduce edema (Chrubasik et al., 2011). Contrast hydrotherapy enhances circulation and lymphatic drainage (Sutkowy et al., 2019). An anti-inflammatory diet rich in antioxidants, vitamin C, and omega-3 fatty acids supports vascular integrity (Calder, 2017). Nitric oxide donors improve endothelial function (Moncada & Higgs, 1993). Limb elevation and exercise promote venous return. Supplementation with iron, B12, and folate supports oxygen transport.

Standard Medical Approaches

Doppler and imaging guide compression therapy, pharmacologic interventions (venoactive drugs, anticoagulants), or surgical procedures in venous or arterial disease (Brant et al., 2016; Norgren et al., 2007). Wound care is essential for ischemic ulcers.

Specialty / Practitioner Care Strategies Table

Specialty Group	Practitioners Included	Hyperemissive Strategies	Hypoemissive Strategies
Biochemistry	Nutritionists, Orthomolecular, Herbalists, Naturopaths	Botanical venotonics, anti-inflammatory diet, antioxidants, vitamins C, E, selenium, CoQ10, bioflavonoids, omega-3s	Circulatory stimulants (*Ginkgo biloba*, cayenne), blood-building nutrients (iron, B12, folate), magnesium, arginine, nitrate-rich diet
Rehabilitation	Physiotherapists, Massage Therapists, Osteopaths / Chiropractors	Lymphatic drainage, calf pump exercises, postural retraining, gentle Swedish massage, myofascial release	Graded aerobic exercise, gait training, emission protection, foot care, warming massage, reflexology, ergonomic guidance
Energetics	Acupuncturists (TCM), Bioenergetic Therapists	Acupuncture (SP6, ST36), moxibustion, herbal formulas, Qi and Blood tonics, bioresonance, PEMF	Warming acupuncture, Qi and Blood tonics, PEMF, energy healing
Psychological	GNM practitioners, Psychotherapists, Vibrational therapists, Family constellation facilitators	GNM conflict protocols, psychotherapy, bioresonance, mindfulness, energy clearing	Psychosomatic conflict resolution, vibrational medicine, stress reduction, emotional balancing

Educational Pearls & Considerations.

- Exclude deep vein thrombosis urgently if suspected.
- Botanical venotonics combined with hydrotherapy reduce venous congestion.
- Nitric oxide boosters and omega-3 fatty acids enhance arterial function.
- Compression therapy contraindicated in severe arterial insufficiency.
- Early mobilization and limb elevation prevent chronic sequelae.

GROUP 1 - ZONE 7 – FRONTAL UPPER LEGS

Category 2: Muscular

Step 1: Functional Anatomy and Interpretive Importance

The anterior thigh contains the quadriceps femoris group, rectus femoris, vastus lateralis, vastus medialis, and vastus intermedius, all innervated by the femoral nerve. Together, they extend the knee and assist in hip flexion, providing essential force for walking, running, and maintaining upright posture.

The rectus femoris, being biarticular, is particularly vulnerable to eccentric loading, while the vastus medialis stabilizes the patella (Standring, 2016). Sports medicine reviews identify quadriceps injuries as frequent in sprinting and kicking disciplines, with rectus femoris tears among the most recurrent muscle injuries in athletes (Cross et al., 2004).

Biospectral readings in this region frequently present as broad anterior gradients or focal signals near the rectus femoris origin, corresponding to localized strain or fascial rigidity. Such patterns allow clinicians to distinguish between superficial fatigue and deeper myotendinous overload, thereby situating the quadriceps as a key biosignal source for performance monitoring.

Step 2,3,4: ROI Classification and Interpretive Questions

Hyperemission suggests acute muscle strain, myositis, or localized tissue activation.

- Has the patient experienced trauma or repetitive strain?
- Is there localized pain, swelling, or muscle spasm?

Hypoemission indicates chronic ischemia, compartment syndrome, or neurogenic muscle atrophy.

- Are numbness, weakness, or muscle wasting present?
- Is there impaired gait or functional limitation?

Step 5: Confirmatory Evaluations

Test	Purpose & Justification	Relevance to Emissive Pattern
Creatine kinase (CK), LDH	Detects muscle injury or inflammation (Maffulli et al., 2014).	Elevated in hyperemissive tissue activation
MRI	Visualizes edema, inflammation, ischemia, or muscle atrophy.	Supports hyper- or hypoemissive findings.
Compartment pressure measurement	Diagnoses compartment syndrome through pressure monitoring.	Relevant to hypoemissive ischemic presentations.

Nerve conduction studies (NCS), Electromyography (EMG)	Evaluates neurogenic muscle dysfunction.	Correlates with hypoemissive neurogenic causes.
Blood tests (CBC, inflammatory markers)	Detects systemic inflammation or infection.	Supports hyperemissive regulatory activation

Step 6: Care Strategies and Intervention Pathways

Naturopathic Approach

Use anti-inflammatory botanicals such as *Curcuma longa* and *Boswellia serrata* to reduce muscle inflammation (Hewlings & Kalman, 2017). Magnesium supplementation supports muscle relaxation. Hydrotherapy with alternating warm and cold compresses enhances circulation (Sutkowy et al., 2019). Gentle stretching and progressive strengthening promote recovery. Adequate protein and antioxidants support healing.

Standard Medical Approaches

Rest, NSAIDs, and physical therapy are standard treatments for acute muscle injuries (Maffulli et al., 2014). Compartment syndrome requires urgent surgical intervention. Neurogenic muscle weakness warrants neurological evaluation.

Specialty / Practitioner Care Strategies Table

Specialty Group	Practitioners Included	Hyperemissive Strategies	Hypoemissive Strategies
Biochemistry	Nutritionists, Orthomolecular, Herbalists, Naturopaths	Anti-inflammatory botanicals, magnesium, antioxidants, protein	Circulatory support, neurotrophic nutrients, protein support
Rehabilitation	Physiotherapists, Massage Therapists, Osteopaths / Chiropractors	Myofascial release, trigger point therapy, gentle massage	Graded aerobic exercise, neurorehabilitation, ergonomic guidance
Energetics	Acupuncturists (TCM), Bioenergetic Therapists	Acupuncture, moxibustion, PEMF	Warming acupuncture, frequency therapy
Psychological	GNM practitioners, Psychotherapists, Vibrational therapists, Family constellation facilitators	Psychotherapy, bioresonance, mindfulness	Psychosomatic conflict resolution, emotional balancing

Educational Pearls & Considerations.

- Early recognition of compartment syndrome is critical.
- Magnesium assists in reducing cramps and spasms.
- Hydrotherapy should be adjusted to the inflammation stage.
- Neurogenic weakness requires thorough assessment.
- Gradual rehabilitation prevents chronic impairment.

GROUP 1 - ZONE 7 – FRONTAL UPPER LEGS

Category 3: Skeletal

Step 1: Functional Anatomy and Interpretive Importance

The frontal upper leg zone is defined by the femoral shaft and the anterior aspect of the knee joint complex, essential for weight-bearing and forward propulsion (Standring, 2016). The femur acts as the longest lever in the body, transmitting high compressive and rotational loads during ambulation.

Clinical observations confirm the vulnerability of the anterior femur to stress syndromes, particularly in long-distance runners where cortical thickening and microfractures may develop (Milgrom et al., 1985). Such skeletal responses influence periosteal regulation and fascial connectivity, creating emissive signatures that emerge externally.

On spectral surface readings, biospectral asymmetries are often localized to the anterior femoral shaft or peripatellar region, presenting as linear or focal intensifications distinct from surrounding muscular activity.

These signals provide noninvasive markers of early osseous adaptation, translating deep skeletal strain into observable surface biosignals. In this way, the emissive profile of the anterior thigh contributes valuable insight into the interaction of load distribution, skeletal stress, and articular integrity.

Step 2,3,4: ROI Classification and Interpretive Questions

Hyperemission indicates acute fractures, periosteal biosignal activation, or joint effusion with increased blood flow.

- Is there recent trauma or repetitive overuse?
- Are swelling, tenderness, or joint stiffness present?

Hypoemission suggests chronic structural degeneration, joint wear, or vascular compromise with reduced perfusion.

- Are chronic pain, stiffness, or functional limitation reported?
- Is there history of deformity or joint instability?

Step 5: Confirmatory Evaluations

Test	Purpose & Justification	Relevance to Emissive Pattern
X-ray imaging	Detects fractures, stress injuries, and joint space narrowing.	Confirms hyperemissive acute injury or hypoemissive chronic changes.

MRI	Visualizes bone marrow edema, occult fractures, cartilage, and soft tissues.	Supports regulatory activation or degenerative findings.
Bone scan	Assesses bone metabolism and detects stress fractures or infection.	Correlates with hyperemissive bone involvement.
Blood tests (inflammatory markers)	Detects systemic inflammation related to bone injury or infection.	Supports hyperemissive functional activation.

Step 6: Care Strategies and Intervention Pathways

Naturopathic Approach

Support bone healing with calcium, vitamin D, magnesium, and vitamin K (Heaney, 2006). Use anti-inflammatory botanicals like *Boswellia serrata* to reduce periosteal inflammation. Therapeutic ultrasound and PEMF promote bone repair (Gordon et al., 2016). Immobilization protects injured bones.

Standard Medical Approaches

Imaging guides immobilization or surgical intervention. NSAIDs and physical therapy manage symptoms. Osteoarthritis requires supportive care.

Specialty / Practitioner Care Strategies Table

Specialty Group	Practitioners Included	Hyperemissive Strategies	Hypoemissive Strategies
Biochemistry	Nutritionists, Orthomolecular, Herbalists, Naturopaths	Bone-supportive nutrients, anti-inflammatory botanicals	Nutritional support for bone remodeling and joint health
Rehabilitation	Physiotherapists, Massage Therapists, Osteopaths / Chiropractors	Joint mobilization, therapeutic ultrasound, myofascial release	Joint stabilization, graded strengthening, ergonomic guidance
Energetics	Acupuncturists (TCM), Bioenergetic Therapists	Acupuncture, PEMF, herbal formulas for inflammation	Warming acupuncture, energy balancing
Psychological	GNM practitioners, Psychotherapists, Vibrational therapists, Family constellation facilitators	Mind-body therapies supporting pain management and healing	Psychosomatic support, emotional balancing

Educational Pearls & Considerations.

- Prompt immobilization prevents further injury.
- Adequate nutrition accelerates bone healing.
- PEMF requires professional administration.
- Chronic hypoemissive patterns suggest degenerative disease needing multidisciplinary management.
- Psychological support enhances recovery.

GROUP 1 - ZONE 7 – FRONTAL UPPER LEGS

Category 4: Nervous

Step 1: Functional Anatomy and Interpretive Importance

The frontal upper legs are supplied by the femoral nerve, which provides motor control to the quadriceps and sensory innervation to the anterior thigh (Standring, 2016). This large nerve is vulnerable to compression in the pelvis or thigh, and femoral neuropathy often presents with quadriceps weakness and anterior thigh sensory loss.

Khalil and Sundaram (2009) emphasized that iatrogenic femoral nerve injury, particularly after pelvic or abdominal surgery, remains an important cause of functional impairment. Neural dysfunction in this distribution alters the coordination of muscular activation and disrupts autonomic balance, leading to surface emissive changes.

These appear as biospectral asymmetries localized to the anterior femoral shaft or peripatellar region, whose confined geometry reflects the nerve's distribution. By translating femoral nerve compromise into a visible biosignal, emissive analysis provides clinicians with an external indicator of early neurogenic disturbance, allowing differentiation from myofascial pain syndromes of the anterior thigh.

Step 2,3,4: ROI Classification and Interpretive Questions

Hyperemission may indicate nerve irritation or neurogenic activation.

- Are there burning, tingling, or sharp pains?
- Is there localized hypersensitivity or swelling?

Hypoemission suggests nerve ischemia, compression, or denervation leading to reduced autonomic regulation.

- Are numbness, weakness, or muscle wasting present?
- Do symptoms worsen with certain movements or positions?

Step 5: Confirmatory Evaluations

Test	Purpose & Justification	Relevance to Emissive Pattern
Nerve conduction studies (NCS), Electromyography (EMG)	Assess nerve and muscle function (Campbell & Meyer, 2006).	Correlate with hypoemissive neurogenic dysfunction.
Quantitative sensory testing (QST)	Measures sensory thresholds and nerve function.	Supports interpretation of neuropathic expressions.
MRI / Ultrasound	Detects nerve compression or structural pathology.	Identifies neurogenic contribution.
Blood tests (glucose, vitamin B12)	Evaluates metabolic causes of neuropathy.	Supports interpretation of patterns consistent with metabolic neuroregulatory changes.

Step 6: Care Strategies and Intervention Pathways

Naturopathic Approach

Use B-complex vitamins, alpha-lipoic acid, and Acetyl-L-carnitine to support nerve regeneration (Papanas & Ziegler, 2014). Herbal anti-inflammatories such as *Hypericum perforatum* may reduce neuropathic pain (Kasper et al., 2010). Neural mobilization and gentle stretching facilitate recovery. Mind-body therapies and bioresonance modulate neurovascular function.

Standard Medical Approaches

Pharmacotherapy includes anticonvulsants, antidepressants, and analgesics. Surgical decompression may be necessary. Metabolic control is essential in systemic neuropathies.

Specialty / Practitioner Care Strategies Table

Specialty Group	**Practitioners Included**	**Hyperemissive Strategies**	**Hypoemissive Strategies**
Biochemistry	Nutritionists, Orthomolecular, Herbalists, Naturopaths	Neurotrophic vitamins, alpha-lipoic acid, anti-inflammatory botanicals	Circulatory stimulants, metabolic support, neuroprotective nutrients
Rehabilitation	Physiotherapists, Massage Therapists, Osteopaths / Chiropractors	Neural mobilization, myofascial release, gentle massage	Neural gliding exercises, ergonomic guidance, neurorehabilitation
Energetics	Acupuncturists (TCM), Bioenergetic Therapists	Acupuncture, moxibustion, PEMF	Warming acupuncture, frequency therapy, energy healing
Psychological	GNM practitioners, Psychotherapists, Vibrational therapists, Family constellation facilitators	Psychotherapy, bioresonance, mindfulness	Psychosomatic conflict resolution, vibrational medicine

Educational Pearls & Considerations.

- Early diagnosis prevents permanent nerve damage.
- Nutritional support complements medical therapies.
- Mind-body and energetic therapies assist pain management.
- Monitor metabolic contributors such as diabetes.
- Avoid aggressive interventions during acute inflammation.

GROUP 1 - ZONE 7 – FRONTAL UPPER LEGS

Category 5: Lymphatic

Step 1: Functional Anatomy and Interpretive Importance

The The frontal upper legs contain lymphatic vessels that converge medially with the great saphenous system and drain toward superficial inguinal lymph nodes (Standring, 2016). This drainage is central to immune surveillance of the thigh and anterior pelvic region.

Stanton et al. (2009) described how impaired lymphatic return in the proximal thigh leads to functional overload, often presenting as heaviness or fatigue before overt swelling occurs. Such dysfunction influences fluid transport, fascial dynamics, and vascular dynamics, producing characteristic surface signatures.

Biospectral asymmetries in the anterior thigh often appear as localized emissive zones around the femoral shaft or peripatellar region, distinguished by their containment compared with broader muscular emissions. These visible patterns provide an external correlate of early lymphatic strain in the anterior compartment, bridging anatomy, clinical presentation, and emissive analysis.

Step 2,3,4: ROI Classification and Interpretive Questions

Hyperemission indicates acute lymphangitis, infection, or lymphatic stasis with warmth and swelling.

- Is there redness, tenderness, or rapid swelling?
- Has the patient experienced recent trauma or infection?

Hypoemission suggests chronic lymphedema with fibrosis, reduced flow, and reduced perfusion.

- Is swelling persistent and firm?
- Are recurrent infections or slow-healing wounds present?

Step 5: Confirmatory Evaluations

Test	Purpose & Justification	Relevance to Emissive Pattern
Lymphoscintigraphy	Assesses lymphatic drainage and obstruction.	Confirms lymphatic stasis or hypoperfusion.
Doppler ultrasound	Excludes venous insufficiency as cause of swelling.	Differentiates vascular from lymphatic causes.
Blood tests (CBC, inflammatory markers)	Detect infection or systemic inflammation.	Supports hyperemissive regulatory activation
Physical exam (Stemmer's sign, limb measurements)	Identifies clinical signs of lymphedema.	Correlates with biospectral findings.

Step 6: Care Strategies and Intervention Pathways

Naturopathic Approach

Stimulate lymphatic flow using herbal lymphagogues such as *Hedera helix* and *Vitis vinifera* (Godoy et al., 2012). Manual lymphatic drainage by trained therapists enhances fluid movement. Compression therapy supports lymph return and must be personalized. Nutritional antioxidants and anti-inflammatory nutrients promote tissue repair. Hydrotherapy with alternating warm and cold stimulation improves lymphatic circulation.

Standard Medical Approaches

Standard care includes manual lymphatic drainage, compression garments, physical therapy, and infection management. Surgery is reserved for advanced cases.

Specialty / Practitioner Care Strategies Table

Specialty Group	Practitioners Included	Hyperemissive Strategies	Hypoemissive Strategies
Biochemistry	Nutritionists, Orthomolecular, Herbalists, Naturopaths	Herbal lymphagogues, antioxidants, anti-inflammatory nutrients	Circulatory support, nutritional tissue repair support
Rehabilitation	Physiotherapists, Massage Therapists, Osteopaths / Chiropractors	Manual lymphatic drainage, gentle massage, postural retraining	Compression therapy, graded exercise, ergonomic guidance
Energetics	Acupuncturists (TCM), Bioenergetic Therapists	Acupuncture, herbal formulas, PEMF	Warming acupuncture, energy balancing
Psychological	GNM practitioners, Psychotherapists, Vibrational therapists, Family constellation facilitators	Mind-body therapies supporting immune function and healing	Psychosomatic conflict resolution, emotional balancing

Educational Pearls & Considerations.

- Early intervention prevents progression to chronic lymphedema.
- Manual lymphatic drainage requires skilled therapists.
- Compression therapy must be individualized and regularly monitored.
- Nutritional support enhances lymphatic and tissue health.
- Prompt treatment of infections prevents worsening lymphatic dysfunction.

GROUP 1 - ZONE 7 – FRONTAL UPPER LEGS

Category 7: Acupuncture / Meridian

Step 1: Functional Anatomy and Interpretive Importance

The anterior thigh is dominated by the quadriceps femoris, femoral shaft, and associated vascular structures, forming the primary weight-bearing surface of the upper leg (Standring, 2016). This zone corresponds to the Stomach (ST) and Spleen (SP) meridians, which ascend through the anterior thigh toward the trunk.

Flaws (2000) described their role in digestive and circulatory regulation, while Deadman et al. (2007) emphasized points such as ST31 and SP10 in influencing systemic blood circulation and leg vitality. Kaptchuk (2000) linked SP channel balance with both muscular endurance and metabolic stability.

Clinically, blockages manifest as thigh weakness, edema, or heaviness. In biosignal imaging, emissive asymmetries appear as vertical fields paralleling the femoral shaft, distinguishable from diffuse muscular exertion patterns. These variations reflect how systemic imbalances in digestion or blood coherence are externalized in anterior thigh fields, linking classical meridian mapping with biospectral evidence.

Step 2,3,4: ROI Classification and Interpretive Questions

Hyperemission indicates Qi stagnation or congestive activation along the meridian.

- Is there localized tenderness, swelling, or sharp pain?
- Do symptoms worsen with movement or pressure?

Hypoemission suggests Qi deficiency or chronic stagnation with reduced energy flow and tissue underoxygenation.

- Does the patient report weakness, coldness, numbness, or dull chronic pain?
- Are signs of poor circulation or fatigue present?

Step 5: Confirmatory Evaluations

Test	Purpose & Justification	Relevance to Emissive Pattern
Pulse diagnosis and tongue examination	Traditional TCM diagnostic tools assessing Qi and blood status (Flaws, 2000).	Correlates with emissive findings to refine interpretation.
Biospectral imaging	Detects emissive asymmetries along meridian pathways.	Traces hyper- or hypoemissive meridian zones.
Patient symptom questionnaire	Assesses pain patterns, energy levels, and functional status.	Supports differentiation between Qi stagnation and Qi deficiency.

Step 6: **Care Strategies and Intervention Pathways**

Naturopathic Approach

Acupuncture points such as ST36 and SP6 regulate Qi and blood flow, reduce inflammation, and restore function (Lao et al., 2004). Moxibustion warms hypoemissive meridians. Herbal formulas including *Dang Gui* and *Bai Zhu* nourish blood and strengthen Qi (Bensky et al., 2004). Dietary support with Qi-building foods complements therapy.

Standard Medical Approaches

Acupuncture serves as an adjunct to physical rehabilitation and pain management for musculoskeletal and circulatory dysfunction related to meridian imbalances.

Specialty / Practitioner Care Strategies Table

Specialty Group	Practitioners Included	Hyperemissive Strategies	Hypoemissive Strategies
Biochemistry	Nutritionists, Orthomolecular, Herbalists, Naturopaths	Herbal formulas regulating Qi and blood, antioxidants	Qi tonics, blood nourishing supplements
Rehabilitation	Physiotherapists, Massage Therapists, Osteopaths / Chiropractors	Trigger point therapy complementary to acupuncture	Gentle mobilization, warming massage
Energetics	Acupuncturists (TCM), Bioenergetic Therapists	Acupuncture, moxibustion, PEMF	Warming acupuncture, Qi tonics, energy healing
Psychological	GNM practitioners, Psychotherapists, Vibrational therapists, Family constellation facilitators	Mind-body therapies, bioresonance, energy clearing	Psychosomatic conflict resolution, emotional balancing

Educational Pearls & Considerations.

- Precise acupuncture point selection is essential to balance hyper- and hypoemissive areas.
- Moxibustion should be used cautiously in patient's sensitive to heat.
- Herbal therapies require professional guidance.
- Combining acupuncture with physical therapy enhances clinical outcomes.

GROUP 1 - ZONE 7 – FRONTAL UPPER LEGS

Category 8: Energetic

Step 1: Functional Anatomy and Interpretive Importance

The anterior thigh incorporatees the quadriceps group, femoral neurovascular bundle, and fascial interfaces linking pelvis and knee (Standring, 2016). From an energetic perspective, this surface represents fields of strength, propulsion, and systemic vitality.

Rein (1992) highlighted that exposure to coherent energy fields modulates cellular physiology, suggesting a plausible basis for anterior thigh emissive changes observed in clinical practice. Symptomatically, patients may describe fatigue, tension, or reduced recovery capacity following exertion.

Spectral surface readings frequently reveal diffuse hypoemissive depressions reflecting depleted systemic drive or sharply demarcated hyperemissive foci associated with reparative intensification. These findings extend beyond musculoskeletal interpretation, situating the anterior thighs as major conductors of systemic vitality and coherence.

Integrating these emissive signatures provides a refined lens through which clinicians assess both local strength capacity and global energetic adaptation.

Step 2,3,4: ROI Classification and Interpretive Questions

Hyperemission indicates localized energetic congestion or tissue reactivity.

- Does the patient report heat, tingling, or unexplained discomfort?
- Are emotional or stress factors exacerbating symptoms?

Hypoemission suggests energy deficiency or biofield stagnation.

- Does the patient experience fatigue, coldness, numbness, or reduced vitality?
- Are symptoms chronic or resistant to conventional therapies?

Step 5: Confirmatory Evaluations

Test	Purpose & Justification	Relevance to Emissive Pattern
Bioresonance testing	Assesses tissue energy frequencies and imbalances.	Correlates with emissive anomalies.
Electrodermal screening (EDS)	Measures skin conductance linked to energy pathways.	Supports interpretation of energetic dynamics.
Patient emotional and symptom history	Provides clinical context for energetic dysfunction.	Aids differential assessment.

Step 6: Care Strategies and Intervention Pathways

Naturopathic Approach

Utilize bioresonance, pulsed electromagnetic fields (PEMF), and adaptogenic herbs to restore energetic balance and promote healing (Matsumoto et al., 2010). Nutritional antioxidants and adaptogens enhance systemic resilience. Mindfulness and stress reduction complement energetic therapies.

Standard Medical Approaches

Energetic therapies function as adjuncts to conventional medical and rehabilitative treatments to optimize patient outcomes.

Specialty / Practitioner Care Strategies Table

Specialty Group	Practitioners Included	Hyperemissive Strategies	Hypoemissive Strategies
Biochemistry	Nutritionists, Orthomolecular, Herbalists, Naturopaths	Adaptogens, antioxidants, herbal energetics	Nutritional support for energy deficiency
Rehabilitation	Physiotherapists, Massage Therapists, Osteopaths / Chiropractors	Energy-based manual therapies, PEMF, therapeutic touch	Gentle stimulation, mobilization
Energetics	Acupuncturists (TCM), Bioenergetic Therapists	Bioresonance, PEMF, acupuncture	Warming acupuncture, energy balancing
Psychological	GNM practitioners, Psychotherapists, Vibrational therapists, Family constellation facilitators	Psychotherapy, bioresonance, mindfulness	Emotional balancing, vibrational medicine

Educational Pearls & Considerations.

- Energetic therapies complement but do not replace conventional treatments.
- Patient responsiveness and practitioner expertise influence effectiveness.
- Regular monitoring is needed to adjust therapies appropriately.
- Address both psychological and physical aspects holistically.

GROUP 1 - ZONE 7 – FRONTAL UPPER LEGS

Category 9: Metabolic / Endocrine

Step 1: Functional Anatomy and Interpretive Importance

The frontal upper legs include the quadriceps group, femoral vessels, and fascial continuities essential for propulsion and systemic venous return (Standring, 2016). This region is closely tied to metabolic and endocrine status, as it demands high energy turnover during locomotion.

DeFronzo & Ferrannini (1991) linked insulin resistance with impaired glucose uptake in skeletal muscle, directly impacting anterior thigh physiology. Patients often describe exertional fatigue, delayed recovery, or aching localized to quadriceps.

Spectral surface readings highlight broad hypoemissive depressions consistent with suppressed glycoregulatory efficiency and focal hyperemissive arcs linked with reparative or compensatory activation.

These emissive dynamics illustrate how systemic metabolic dysfunction manifests in high-demand muscle groups, positioning the anterior thighs as early detectors of insulin resistance and endocrine imbalance. Clinically, interpreting these signals expands assessment beyond structural load, integrating metabolic function into biospectral reading.

Step 2,3,4: ROI Classification and Interpretive Questions

Hyperemission may reflect local tissue activation, bioaccumulation, or metabolic overactivity.

- Is redness, warmth, or swelling present?
- Is metabolic control suboptimal?

Hypoemission suggests reduced perfusion, neurogenic changes, or stagnation due to metabolic/endocrine imbalance.

- Is there coldness, numbness, chronic wounds, or fatigue?
- Are systemic symptoms such as temperature intolerance reported?

Step 5: Confirmatory Evaluations

Test	Purpose & Justification	Relevance to Emissive Pattern
HbA1c, fasting glucose	Monitors glycemic control in diabetes.	Correlates with hypoemissive neuropathic or ischemic zones.
Thyroid function tests (TSH, Free T4)	Detects thyroid dysfunction affecting metabolism and circulation.	Associated with altered regulatory emission patterns.
Lipid profile	Assesses cardiovascular risk impacting tissue perfusion.	Supports metabolic vascular imbalance.
Inflammatory markers (CRP, ESR)	Identifies systemic inflammation influencing tissue health.	Correlates with hyperemissive regulatory activation.

Step 6: Care Strategies and Intervention Pathways

Naturopathic Approach

Optimize metabolic health with a low glycemic diet, antioxidants, and micronutrients improving insulin sensitivity (Alberti et al., 2006). Adaptogenic herbs like *Panax ginseng* and *Gymnema sylvestre* support endocrine balance. Supplement chromium, magnesium, and alpha-lipoic acid to enhance glucose metabolism and nerve protection. Regular aerobic exercise improves circulation and metabolism.

Standard Medical Approaches

Pharmacologic and lifestyle interventions aim for strict metabolic control. Thyroid hormone replacement and lipid management reduce complications.

Specialty / Practitioner Care Strategies Table

Specialty Group	Practitioners Included	Hyperemissive Strategies	Hypoemissive Strategies
Biochemistry	Nutritionists, Orthomolecular, Herbalists, Naturopaths	Antioxidants, adaptogens, insulin sensitizers, micronutrients	Metabolic support, neuroprotective nutrients, dietary management
Rehabilitation	Physiotherapists, Massage Therapists, Osteopaths / Chiropractors	Exercise therapy, circulation enhancement	Neuromuscular re-education, aerobic conditioning
Energetics	Acupuncturists (TCM), Bioenergetic Therapists	Acupuncture supporting metabolic function	Energy balancing, PEMF
Psychological	GNM practitioners, Psychotherapists, Vibrational therapists, Family constellation facilitators	Mind-body therapies supporting metabolic regulation	Stress reduction, emotional balancing

Educational Pearls & Considerations.

- Regular metabolic monitoring prevents tissue complications.
- Lifestyle and dietary modifications are essential adjuncts to treatment.
- Adaptogens complement but do not replace conventional therapies.
- Patient education on foot care is crucial to prevent ulcers.

GROUP 1

ZONE 8 – DORSAL UPPER LEG

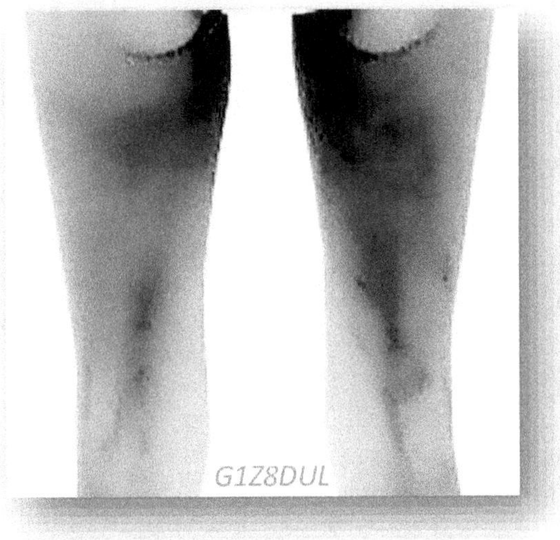

TThe dorsal upper legs, covering the hamstrings, gluteal attachments, and posterior venous networks, are among the most diagnostically revealing surfaces of the lower body. This region includes the semitendinosus, semimembranosus, and biceps femoris, along with perforating branches of the deep femoral vein and extensive lymphatic pathways (Standring, 2016).

Functionally, the hamstrings are prone to strain and chronic overload due to their dual role in hip extension and knee flexion. Sports medicine identifies hamstring injuries as the most common lower limb soft-tissue injury, with recurrence rates up to 30% (Opar et al., 2012). Emissively, sedentary individuals often show persistent hypoactivity from reduced activation, venous pooling, or lymphatic stagnation, whereas athletes more frequently display localized hyperemissive streaks from fascial overload or postural imbalance.

The posterior thigh also compensates for spinal mechanics, with asymmetry correlated to pelvic tilt, scoliosis, and lumbar dysfunction (Schache et al., 2012). Importantly, emissive suppression here can occur even under systemic regulatory load, highlighting that global circulation does not ensure balanced perfusion in dependent venous zones.

Venous studies confirm that posterior thigh reflux often remains subclinical despite measurable strain (Labropoulos et al., 2005). From a lymphatic perspective, posterior thigh emissive retention may indicate early stagnation, especially in prolonged standing or obesity where lymphatic efficiency is reduced (Greene & Goss, 2018).

Clinically, this makes the dorsal upper leg a sensitive surface for observing musculoskeletal imbalance and circulatory burden. Its interpretive power lies in revealing the intersection of hamstring dynamics, venous return, and spinal compensation, often highlighting regulatory imbalance before clinical pain or dysfunction is reported.

Zone 8 – Dorsal Upper Legs: Emission-Relevant Structures.

Category	Relevant Structures	Emission Relevance
1. Vascular / Circulatory	- Posterior femoral vein - Deep femoral artery and perforating branches - Gluteal venous plexus (superior and inferior)	Hyperemission may reflect vascular congestion, venous pooling, or gluteal overload. Hypoemission often indicates reduced circulation due to inactivity, compression, or chronic stasis.
2. Muscular / Myofascial	- Biceps femoris (long and short head) - Semitendinosus and semimembranosus - Gluteus maximus insertion - Posterior fascial chain	Hyperemissive patterns suggest muscular tension, overload from posture or gait imbalance, or fascial strain in the posterior chain. Hypoemission may reflect muscular inhibition, atrophy, or gluteal underuse.
3. Skeletal / Articular	- Ischial tuberosity - Femoral shaft (posterior) - Sacroiliac joint margin (upper border)	Hyperemission may point to tendinopathy (e.g., proximal hamstring), ischial bursitis, or posterior pelvic misalignment. Hypoemissive zones often suggest degenerative hip or sacroiliac dysfunction.
4. Nervous System / Spine	- Sciatic nerve (posterior thigh trajectory) - Inferior gluteal nerve - S1–S2 dermatomes (posterior thigh)	Hyperemissive activity may indicate sciatic nerve irritation, neural entrapment, or root-level strain. Hypoemission can reflect chronic radiculopathy, nerve dysfunction, or low sacral tone.
5. Lymphatic / Immune	- Gluteal lymphatic drainage - Posterior thigh superficial pathways	Hyperemission is often tied to toxic load, hormonal overflow, or regulatory retention. Hypoemission may reflect stagnant lymph, immune hyporegulation, or gluteal-area detox inefficiency.
6. Organs / GNM	*(Organs not directly projected here; reflex patterns may involve pelvic structures)*	
7. Acupuncture / Meridians	- Bladder Meridian (BL) – descends through posterior thigh - Gallbladder Meridian (GB) – lateral posterior leg	Heat suggests meridian congestion, fear tension (Bladder), or frustration (Gallbladder). Cold indicates Qi deficiency, energetic exhaustion, or blocked pelvic meridian flow.
8. Energetic / Frequency	- Biofield zone for foundational support, drive, and instinctual response	Hyperemission can indicate primal survival tension, suppressed drive, or overcompensation patterns. Hypoemission reflects depleted instinctual energy, fatigue, or loss of internal grounding.
9. Metabolic / Endocrine	- Reflex zones for testosterone balance, gluteal metabolism, and adrenal reserves	Hyperemission may reflect detox activity, hormonal shifts, or posterior chain recruitment. Hypoemission often indicates adrenal hyporegulation, hormonal suppression, or reduced posterior metabolic activation.

GROUP 1 - ZONE 8 – DORSAL UPPER LEGS

Category 1: Vascular / Circulatory

Step 1: Functional Anatomy and Interpretive Importance

The posterior thigh receives arterial supply mainly from perforating branches of the profunda femoris artery, which pass through the adductor magnus to nourish the hamstrings and posterior fascia.

Venous return occurs via perforator veins into the profunda femoris vein, with communication to the great saphenous and popliteal systems (Standring, 2016). Surgical and imaging studies highlight the profunda femoris as a crucial collateral channel, particularly when the superficial femoral artery is compromised (Cina & Safar, 2002).

On spectral surface reading, emissive asymmetries are often observed along the hamstring compartment and posterior thigh fascia. These may reflect venous retention, circulatory load, or adaptive arterial redistribution. Because this region plays a major role in propulsion and postural support, its emissive signals are clinically relevant for assessing functional vascular performance.

Step 2,3,4: ROI Classification and Interpretive Questions

Hyperemission indicates venous congestion, vasoregulatory dysfunction, or circulatory disturbance with increased local biospectral emission.

- Is there swelling, warmth, or pain in the posterior thigh?
- Are varicosities or skin changes present?

Hypoemission suggests circulatory restriction, vasospasm, or perfusion deficit with decreased biospectral emission.

- Does the patient report coldness, numbness, or claudication?
- Are peripheral pulses diminished or delayed?

Step 5: Confirmatory Evaluations

Test	Purpose & Justification	Relevance to Emissive Pattern
Doppler ultrasound	Assesses arterial and venous flow (Brant et al., 2016).	Correlates hyperemissive venous congestion and hypoemissive arterial disease.
Ankle-Brachial Index (ABI)	Measures arterial perfusion; ABI < 0.9 indicates peripheral arterial disease (Norgren et al., 2007).	Confirms hypoemissive arterial insufficiency.
Venography / MR Venography	Detects venous obstruction or thrombosis.	Confirms venous activation associated with Hyperemission.
Blood tests (CBC, CRP, D-dimer)	Detects infection, inflammation, or thrombotic risk.	Supports hyperemissive vascular or thrombotic activity.

Step 6: Care Strategies and Intervention Pathways

Naturopathic Approach

Botanical venotonics such as *Aesculus hippocastanum* and *Centella asiatica* improve venous tone and reduce edema (Chrubasik et al., 2011). Contrast hydrotherapy stimulates circulation and lymphatic flow (Sutkowy et al., 2019). An anti-inflammatory diet rich in antioxidants, vitamins C and E, and omega-3 fatty acids supports vascular integrity (Calder, 2017). Nitric oxide donors improve endothelial function (Moncada & Higgs, 1993). Limb elevation and exercise enhance venous return. Supplement iron, B12, and folate for oxygen transport.

Standard Medical Approaches

Doppler imaging guides use of compression stockings, venoactive drugs, anticoagulants, or surgical interventions in vascular disease (Brant et al., 2016; Norgren et al., 2007). Wound care is vital for ischemic ulcers.

Specialty / Practitioner Care Strategies Table

Specialty Group	Practitioners Included	Hyperemissive Strategies	Hypoemissive Strategies
Biochemistry	Nutritionists, Orthomolecular, Herbalists, Naturopaths	Botanical venotonics, anti-inflammatory diet, antioxidants, vitamins C, E, selenium, CoQ10, bioflavonoids, omega-3s	Circulatory stimulants (*Ginkgo biloba*, cayenne), blood-building nutrients (iron, B12, folate), magnesium, arginine, nitrate-rich diet
Rehabilitation	Physiotherapists, Massage Therapists, Osteopaths / Chiropractors	Lymphatic drainage, calf pump exercises, postural retraining, gentle Swedish massage, myofascial release	Graded aerobic exercise, gait training, emission protection, foot care, warming massage, reflexology, ergonomic guidance
Energetics	Acupuncturists (TCM), Bioenergetic Therapists	Acupuncture (SP6, ST36), moxibustion, herbal formulas, Qi and Blood tonics, bioresonance, PEMF	Warming acupuncture, Qi and Blood tonics, PEMF, energy healing
Psychological	GNM practitioners, Psychotherapists, Vibrational therapists, Family constellation facilitators	GNM conflict protocols, psychotherapy, bioresonance, mindfulness, energy clearing	Psychosomatic conflict resolution, vibrational medicine, stress reduction, emotional balancing

Educational Pearls & Considerations.

- Promptly exclude deep vein thrombosis when Hyperemission and swelling occur.
- Botanical venotonics combined with hydrotherapy reduce venous congestion effectively.
- Nitric oxide boosters and omega-3 fatty acids enhance endothelial function and arterial perfusion.
- Compression therapy is contraindicated in severe arterial insufficiency.
- Early mobilization and limb elevation prevent chronic complications.

GROUP 1 - ZONE 8 – DORSAL UPPER LEGS

Category 2: Muscular

Step 1: Functional Anatomy and Interpretive Importance

The posterior thigh musculature is formed by the hamstring group: biceps femoris, semitendinosus, and semimembranosus, supplied by the sciatic nerve. These muscles extend the hip, flex the knee, and contribute to pelvic stabilization during running and gait deceleration.

Their proximal ischial origin and long fascicles make them prone to high-tension strain, especially in sprinting (Standring, 2016). Epidemiological studies consistently highlight hamstring strains as one of the most frequent athletic injuries, with biceps femoris involvement being dominant due to its dual function and length (Orchard, 2015).

Spectral evaluation often demonstrates emissive irregularities tracing the hamstring lines, with localized hotspots indicating myotendinous stress or uneven fascial load distribution. Because of their central role in propulsion, these signals are clinically valuable for distinguishing adaptive tension from pathological overload, and they frequently serve as early predictors of injury recurrence.

Step 2,3,4: ROI Classification and Interpretive Questions

Hyperemission indicates acute muscle strain, myofascial reactivity, or localized congestion.

- Has the patient experienced trauma or repetitive stress?
- Is there localized pain, swelling, or muscle spasm?

Hypoemission suggests chronic ischemia, compartment syndrome, or neurogenic muscle atrophy.

- Are numbness, weakness, or muscle wasting present?
- Is there impaired mobility or gait dysfunction?

Step 5: Confirmatory Evaluations

Test	Purpose & Justification	Relevance to Emissive Pattern
Creatine kinase (CK), LDH	Detects muscle injury or inflammation (Maffulli et al., 2014).	Elevated in hyperemissive tissue activation
MRI	Visualizes edema, inflammation, ischemia, or muscle atrophy.	Supports hyper- or hypoemissive findings.
Compartment pressure measurement	Diagnoses compartment syndrome via pressure monitoring.	Relevant for hypoemissive ischemic presentations.
Nerve conduction studies (NCS), Electromyography (EMG)	Assesses neurogenic muscle dysfunction.	Correlates with hypoemissive neurogenic causes.
Blood tests (CBC, inflammatory markers)	Detect systemic inflammation or infection.	Supports hyperemissive regulatory activation

Step 6: Care Strategies and Intervention Pathways

Naturopathic Approach

Anti-inflammatory botanicals such as *Curcuma longa* and *Boswellia serrata* reduce muscle inflammation (Hewlings & Kalman, 2017). Magnesium supplementation supports muscle relaxation. Hydrotherapy with alternating warm and cold compresses enhances circulation (Sutkowy et al., 2019). Gentle stretching and graded strengthening promote recovery. Adequate protein and antioxidants aid tissue repair.

Standard Medical Approaches

Rest, NSAIDs, and physical therapy are standard for acute muscle injuries (Maffulli et al., 2014). Compartment syndrome requires urgent surgical intervention. Neurogenic muscle weakness demands neurological evaluation.

Specialty / Practitioner Care Strategies Table

Specialty Group	Practitioners Included	Hyperemissive Strategies	Hypoemissive Strategies
Biochemistry	Nutritionists, Orthomolecular, Herbalists, Naturopaths	Anti-inflammatory botanicals, magnesium, antioxidants, protein	Circulatory support, neurotrophic nutrients, protein support
Rehabilitation	Physiotherapists, Massage Therapists, Osteopaths / Chiropractors	Myofascial release, trigger point therapy, gentle massage	Graded aerobic exercise, neurorehabilitation, ergonomic guidance
Energetics	Acupuncturists (TCM), Bioenergetic Therapists	Acupuncture, moxibustion, PEMF	Warming acupuncture, frequency therapy
Psychological	GNM practitioners, Psychotherapists, Vibrational therapists, Family constellation facilitators	Psychotherapy, bioresonance, mindfulness	Psychosomatic conflict resolution, emotional balancing

Educational Pearls & Considerations.

- Early diagnosis of compartment syndrome is critical.
- Magnesium assists muscle relaxation and reduces cramps.
- Hydrotherapy should be adapted to inflammation phases.
- Neurogenic muscle weakness requires comprehensive assessment.
- Gradual rehabilitation prevents chronic dysfunction.

GROUP 1 - ZONE 8 – DORSAL UPPER LEGS

Category 3: Skeletal

Step 1: Functional Anatomy and Interpretive Importance

The dorsal upper leg involvees the posterior femoral shaft and knee joint surfaces, forming a structural pillar that sustains weight and coordinates locomotion (Standring, 2016). The posterior femur and articular surfaces experience high compressive loads during sitting, squatting, and activities involving hip extension.

Clinical literature notes that posterior femoral stress injuries and degenerative remodeling frequently occur in athletes and manual laborers exposed to prolonged load cycles (Biedert & Warnke, 2001). These skeletal processes shape periosteal reactivity and influence surrounding vascular regulation, leading to emissive modifications detectable on the body surface.

Spectral surface readings of this zone often reveal biospectral asymmetries that follow the posterior femoral line, contrasting with the diffuse emissions of adjacent hamstring musculature.

Their contained geometry signals a skeletal-articular basis, offering external visualization of deep joint loading dynamics. Such emissive patterns thus bridge the clinical gap between subclinical bone stress and its externalized regulatory imprint, enhancing early recognition of posterior skeletal adaptation.

Step 2,3,4: ROI Classification and Interpretive Questions

Hyperemission indicates acute fractures, periosteal activity, or joint fluid accumulation with increased blood flow.

- Is there recent trauma or repetitive overuse?
- Are swelling, tenderness, or joint stiffness present?

Hypoemission suggests chronic structural degeneration, osteoarthritis, or bone tissue compromise with reduced perfusion.

- Are chronic pain, stiffness, or functional limitation reported?
- Is there a history of deformity or instability?

Step 5: Confirmatory Evaluations

Test	Purpose & Justification	Relevance to Emissive Pattern
X-ray imaging	Detects fractures, stress injuries, and joint space narrowing.	Confirms hyperemissive acute injury or hypoemissive chronic changes.
MRI	Visualizes bone marrow edema, occult fractures, cartilage, and soft tissues.	Supports regulatory activation or degenerative findings.

Bone scan	Assesses bone metabolism, stress fractures, or infection.	Correlates with hyperemissive bone involvement.
Blood tests (inflammatory markers)	Detects systemic inflammation related to bone injury or infection.	Supports hyperemissive functional activation.

Step 6: Care Strategies and Intervention Pathways

Naturopathic Approach

Support bone healing with calcium, vitamin D, magnesium, and vitamin K (Heaney, 2006). Anti-inflammatory botanicals such as *Boswellia serrata* reduce periosteal inflammation. Therapeutic ultrasound and PEMF stimulate bone repair (Gordon et al., 2016). Immobilization protects injured bones.

Standard Medical Approaches

Imaging guides immobilization or surgery. NSAIDs and physical therapy manage symptoms. Osteoarthritis requires supportive care.

Specialty / Practitioner Care Strategies Table

Specialty Group	Practitioners Included	Hyperemissive Strategies	Hypoemissive Strategies
Biochemistry	Nutritionists, Orthomolecular, Herbalists, Naturopaths	Bone-supportive nutrients, anti-inflammatory botanicals	Nutritional support for bone remodeling and joint health
Rehabilitation	Physiotherapists, Massage Therapists, Osteopaths / Chiropractors	Joint mobilization, therapeutic ultrasound, myofascial release	Joint stabilization, graded strengthening, ergonomic guidance
Energetics	Acupuncturists (TCM), Bioenergetic Therapists	Acupuncture, PEMF, herbal formulas for inflammation	Warming acupuncture, energy balancing
Psychological	GNM practitioners, Psychotherapists, Vibrational therapists, Family constellation facilitators	Mind-body therapies supporting pain management and healing	Psychosomatic support, emotional balancing

Educational Pearls & Considerations.

- Prompt immobilization prevents further injury.
- Adequate nutrition accelerates bone healing.
- PEMF requires professional administration.
- Chronic hypoemissive patterns suggest degenerative disease needing multidisciplinary care.
- Psychological support enhances recovery.

GROUP 1 - ZONE 8 – DORSAL UPPER LEGS

Category 4: Nervous

Step 1: Functional Anatomy and Interpretive Importance

The dorsal upper legs are innervated primarily by the sciatic nerve and its tibial and common peroneal divisions, which supply both motor and sensory functions essential for hip extension, knee flexion, and lower limb sensation (Standring, 2016).

The length and superficial course of the sciatic nerve predispose it to compression, trauma, or irritation from adjacent structures. Stafford et al. (2007) noted that sciatic neuropathy can produce a broad spectrum of pain and weakness, often mimicking lumbosacral radiculopathy.

These neural disturbances impair conduction and disrupt neurovascular regulation in the posterior thigh, producing emissive signatures on the body surface. Such biospectral asymmetries commonly appear as elongated fields paralleling the femoral shaft, distinguished from the diffuse activation of hamstring musculature.

Their linear, nerve-oriented distribution externalizes the hidden stress of sciatic compromise, giving clinicians a valuable visual marker for neurogenic contributions to posterior thigh dysfunction.

Step 2,3,4: ROI Classification and Interpretive Questions

Hyperemission indicates nerve irritation or neurogenic stimulation with increased local circulatory activity.

- Are there burning, tingling, or sharp pain sensations?
- Is there localized hypersensitivity or swelling?

Hypoemission suggests nerve suppression, compression, or denervation leading to decreased autonomic regulation and reduced surface emission.

- Are numbness, weakness, or muscle wasting present?
- Do symptoms worsen with certain movements or positions?

Step 5: Confirmatory Evaluations

Test	Purpose & Justification	Relevance to Emissive Pattern
Nerve conduction studies (NCS), Electromyography (EMG)	Assess nerve and muscle function (Campbell & Meyer, 2006).	Correlate with hypoemissive neurogenic dysfunction.
Quantitative sensory testing (QST)	Measures sensory nerve function and thresholds.	Supports interpretation of neuropathic signatures.

MRI / Ultrasound	Visualizes nerve compression or structural pathology.	Identifies neurogenic contribution
Blood tests (glucose, vitamin B12)	Assesses metabolic causes of neuropathy.	Supports interpretation of metabolic neuroregulatory patterns

Step 6: Care Strategies and Intervention Pathways

Naturopathic Approach

Use neurotrophic vitamins (B-complex), alpha-lipoic acid, and Acetyl-L-carnitine to support nerve regeneration (Papanas & Ziegler, 2014). Herbal anti-inflammatories such as *Hypericum perforatum* may alleviate neuropathic pain (Kasper et al., 2010). Neural mobilization and gentle stretching facilitate recovery. Mind-body therapies and bioresonance modulate neurovascular function.

Standard Medical Approaches

Pharmacologic treatments include anticonvulsants, antidepressants, and analgesics. Surgical decompression may be necessary. Metabolic control is essential for systemic neuropathies.

Specialty / Practitioner Care Strategies Table

Specialty Group	Practitioners Included	Hyperemissive Strategies	Hypoemissive Strategies
Biochemistry	Nutritionists, Orthomolecular, Herbalists, Naturopaths	Neurotrophic vitamins, alpha-lipoic acid, anti-inflammatory botanicals	Circulatory stimulants, metabolic support, neuroprotective nutrients
Rehabilitation	Physiotherapists, Massage Therapists, Osteopaths / Chiropractors	Neural mobilization, myofascial release, gentle massage	Neural gliding exercises, ergonomic guidance, neurorehabilitation
Energetics	Acupuncturists (TCM), Bioenergetic Therapists	Acupuncture, moxibustion, PEMF	Warming acupuncture, frequency therapy, energy healing
Psychological	GNM practitioners, Psychotherapists, Vibrational therapists, Family constellation facilitators	Psychotherapy, bioresonance, mindfulness	Psychosomatic conflict resolution, vibrational medicine

Educational Pearls & Considerations.

- Early diagnosis prevents permanent nerve damage.
- Nutritional support complements medical therapies.
- Mind-body and energetic therapies aid pain management.
- Monitor metabolic contributors like diabetes.
- Avoid aggressive treatments during acute inflammation.

GROUP 1 - ZONE 8 – DORSAL UPPER LEGS

Category 5: Lymphatic

Step 1: Functional Anatomy and Interpretive Importance

The dorsal upper leg lymphatics accompany the deep venous system and connect to both superficial and deep inguinal nodes, ensuring clearance from the posterior thigh and gluteal interface (Standring, 2016). This region's drainage is particularly important in maintaining immune defense and preventing tissue congestion under prolonged load.

Modi et al. (2007) observed that posterior thigh involvement is common in patients with lower limb lymphedema, often manifesting as subtle dermal thickening and reduced compliance. These functional alterations extend to regulatory dynamics, with their imprint emerging on surface assessment.

Biospectral asymmetries here frequently follow the femoral shaft posteriorly, their elongated, contained geometry contrasting with diffuse hamstring activity. Such emissive fields serve as noninvasive indicators of posterior thigh lymphatic compromise, enhancing early recognition of immune drainage dysfunction in a zone prone to hidden accumulation.

Step 2,3,4: ROI Classification and Interpretive Questions

Hyperemission indicates acute lymphangitis, infection, or lymphatic congestion with swelling and elevated spectral emission.

- Is there redness, tenderness, or rapid swelling?
- Has the patient experienced recent infection or injury?

Hypoemission suggests chronic lymphedema with fibrosis and reduced drainage causing diminished perfusion.

- Is swelling persistent and firm?
- Are recurrent infections or slow wound healing reported?

Step 5: Confirmatory Evaluations

Test	Purpose & Justification	Relevance to Emissive Pattern
Lymphoscintigraphy	Assesses lymphatic flow and detects obstructions.	Confirms lymphatic stasis or hypoperfusion.
Doppler ultrasound	Excludes venous insufficiency contributing to swelling.	Differentiates vascular from lymphatic causes.
Blood tests (CBC, inflammatory markers)	Detect infection or systemic inflammation.	Supports hyperemissive regulatory activity
Physical exam (Stemmer's sign, limb measurements)	Identifies clinical signs of lymphedema.	Correlates with emissive observations

Step 6: Care Strategies and Intervention Pathways

Naturopathic Approach

Stimulate lymphatic drainage with herbal lymphagogues like *Hedera helix* and *Vitis vinifera* (Godoy et al., 2012). Manual lymphatic drainage by trained therapists enhances fluid movement. Compression therapy supports lymph return and requires customization. Nutritional antioxidants and anti-inflammatory nutrients promote tissue repair. Hydrotherapy with alternating warm and cold stimulation improves lymphatic circulation.

Standard Medical Approaches

Standard care involves manual lymphatic drainage, compression garments, physical therapy, and infection control. Surgery is considered in advanced cases.

Specialty / Practitioner Care Strategies Table

Specialty Group	Practitioners Included	Hyperemissive Strategies	Hypoemissive Strategies
Biochemistry	Nutritionists, Orthomolecular, Herbalists, Naturopaths	Herbal lymphagogues, antioxidants, anti-inflammatory nutrients	Circulatory support, nutritional tissue repair support
Rehabilitation	Physiotherapists, Massage Therapists, Osteopaths / Chiropractors	Manual lymphatic drainage, gentle massage, postural retraining	Compression therapy, graded exercise, ergonomic guidance
Energetics	Acupuncturists (TCM), Bioenergetic Therapists	Acupuncture, herbal formulas, PEMF	Warming acupuncture, energy balancing
Psychological	GNM practitioners, Psychotherapists, Vibrational therapists, Family constellation facilitators	Mind-body therapies supporting immune function and healing	Psychosomatic conflict resolution, emotional balancing

Educational Pearls & Considerations.

- Early treatment prevents progression to chronic lymphedema.
- Manual lymphatic drainage should be performed by certified therapists.
- Compression therapy requires proper fitting and monitoring.
- Nutritional support enhances lymphatic function and tissue repair.
- Prompt infection treatment prevents worsening.

GROUP 1 - ZONE 8 – DORSAL UPPER LEGS

Category 7: Acupuncture / Meridian

Step 1: Functional Anatomy and Interpretive Importance

The posterior thigh includes the hamstring muscles, sciatic nerve pathways, and vascular structures framed by fascial septa (Standring, 2016). In TCM, this zone corresponds primarily to the Bladder (BL) and Gallbladder (GB) meridians, which run longitudinally along the posterior thigh.

Maciocia (2015) highlighted the Bladder channel's role in regulating autonomic function, fluid balance, and spinal coherence. Langevin and Yandow (2002) suggested meridians correspond to connective tissue planes, offering a structural rationale for the BL–GB trajectories observed clinically.

Dysfunction is often expressed as hamstring tension, posterior thigh pain, or fatigue. In emissive imaging, surface fields appear as sharply delineated bands of hyper- or hypoemission along BL–GB lines, distinct from nonspecific muscular activation.

These emissive signatures demonstrate how disruptions in energy flow along posterior meridians become visible externally, reinforcing the link between channel physiology and biosignal expression.

Step 2,3,4: ROI Classification and Interpretive Questions

Hyperemission indicates Qi stagnation or localized energetic congestion along the meridian.

- Is there localized tenderness, swelling, or sharp pain?
- Do symptoms worsen with movement or pressure?

Hypoemission suggests Qi deficiency or chronic stagnation with reduced energy flow and tissue oxygenation.

- Does the patient report weakness, coldness, numbness, or dull chronic pain?
- Are there signs of poor circulation or fatigue?

Step 5: Confirmatory Evaluations

Test	Purpose & Justification	Relevance to Emissive Pattern
Pulse diagnosis and tongue examination	Traditional TCM diagnostic tools assessing Qi and blood status (Flaws, 2000).	Correlates with emissive findings to refine interpretation.
Biospectral imaging	Detects emissive asymmetries along meridian pathways.	Identifies hyper- or hypoemissive meridian zones.
Patient symptom questionnaire	Assesses pain patterns, energy levels, and functional status.	Supports differentiation between Qi stagnation and Qi deficiency.

Step 6: Care Strategies and Intervention Pathways

Naturopathic Approach

Acupuncture points such as BL40 and GB34 regulate Qi and blood flow, reduce inflammation, and restore function (Lao et al., 2004). Moxibustion warms hypoemissive meridians. Herbal formulas including *Du Huo* and *Qiang Huo* alleviate pain and promote circulation (Bensky et al., 2004). Dietary support with Qi-building foods complements therapy.

Standard Medical Approaches

Acupuncture serves as an adjunct to physical rehabilitation and pain management for musculoskeletal and circulatory dysfunction related to meridian imbalances.

Specialty / Practitioner Care Strategies Table

Specialty Group	Practitioners Included	Hyperemissive Strategies	Hypoemissive Strategies
Biochemistry	Nutritionists, Orthomolecular, Herbalists, Naturopaths	Herbal formulas regulating Qi and blood, antioxidants	Qi tonics, blood nourishing supplements
Rehabilitation	Physiotherapists, Massage Therapists, Osteopaths / Chiropractors	Trigger point therapy complementary to acupuncture	Gentle mobilization, warming massage
Energetics	Acupuncturists (TCM), Bioenergetic Therapists	Acupuncture, moxibustion, PEMF	Warming acupuncture, Qi tonics, energy healing
Psychological	GNM practitioners, Psychotherapists, Vibrational therapists, Family constellation facilitators	Mind-body therapies, bioresonance, energy clearing	Psychosomatic conflict resolution, emotional balancing

Educational Pearls & Considerations.

- Accurate acupuncture point selection is key to balancing hyper- and hypoemissive areas.
- Moxibustion should be applied cautiously in heat-sensitive patients.
- Herbal treatments require professional supervision.
- Combining acupuncture with rehabilitation enhances outcomes.

GROUP 1 - ZONE 8 – DORSAL UPPER LEGS

Category 8: Energetic

Step 1: Functional Anatomy and Interpretive Importance

The posterior thighs are defined by the hamstring complex, gluteal insertions, and fascial planes that couple hip extension to postural stability (Standring, 2016). Energetically, this region is associated with grounding forces and integrative systemic flow, often acting as a stabilizing field in locomotor coherence.

Rubik (2002) proposed that the human biofield regulates physiologic signaling, offering an interpretive basis for emissive changes commonly observed in posterior thighs.

Clinically, patients may experience diffuse aching, tension during prolonged sitting, or recurrent hamstring tightness. Biospectral imaging reveals broad hypoemissive fields reflecting stagnation or depletion, contrasted with narrow hyperemissive lines indicative of localized reparative activation.

These emissive dynamics consistently align with fascial currents and energy conduction pathways rather than isolated muscular compartments. As such, the dorsal upper legs provide insight into systemic energetic anchoring, highlighting the relationship between surface biosignals and integrative physiologic stability.

Step 2,3,4: ROI Classification and Interpretive Questions

Hyperemission suggests localized energy congestion or overactivity.

- Does the patient experience heat, tingling, or unexplained discomfort?
- Are emotional or stress factors aggravating symptoms?

Hypoemission indicates energy deficiency or stagnation.

- Does the patient report fatigue, coldness, numbness, or low vitality?
- Are symptoms chronic or refractory to conventional treatments?

Step 5: Confirmatory Evaluations

Test	Purpose & Justification	Relevance to Emissive Pattern
Bioresonance testing	Measures tissue energy frequencies and imbalances.	Correlates with emission variations.
Electrodermal screening (EDS)	Assesses skin conductance linked to energy pathways.	Supports interpretation of energetic patterns.
Patient emotional and symptom history	Provides clinical context for energetic dysfunction.	Assists in differential assessment.

Step 6: Care Strategies and Intervention Pathways

Naturopathic Approach

Employ bioresonance, pulsed electromagnetic fields (PEMF), and adaptogenic herbs to restore energetic balance and promote healing (Matsumoto et al., 2010). Nutritional antioxidants and adaptogens enhance systemic resilience. Mindfulness and stress reduction complement energetic therapies.

Standard Medical Approaches

Energetic therapies complement conventional and rehabilitative treatments, optimizing patient outcomes.

Specialty / Practitioner Care Strategies Table

Specialty Group	Practitioners Included	Hyperemissive Strategies	Hypoemissive Strategies
Biochemistry	Nutritionists, Orthomolecular, Herbalists, Naturopaths	Adaptogens, antioxidants, herbal energetics	Nutritional support for energy deficiency
Rehabilitation	Physiotherapists, Massage Therapists, Osteopaths / Chiropractors	Energy-based manual therapies, PEMF, therapeutic touch	Gentle stimulation, mobilization
Energetics	Acupuncturists (TCM), Bioenergetic Therapists	Bioresonance, PEMF, acupuncture	Warming acupuncture, energy balancing
Psychological	GNM practitioners, Psychotherapists, Vibrational therapists, Family constellation facilitators	Psychotherapy, bioresonance, mindfulness	Emotional balancing, vibrational medicine

Educational Pearls & Considerations.

- Energetic therapies support but do not replace conventional care.
- Patient response and practitioner skill influence outcomes.
- Regular assessment guides therapeutic adjustments.
- Address psychological and physical factors holistically.

GROUP 1 - ZONE 8 – DORSAL UPPER LEGS

Category 9: Metabolic / Endocrine

Step 1: Functional Anatomy and Interpretive Importance

The dorsal upper legs contain the hamstring complex, gluteal insertions, and vascular pathways critical for locomotion and postural stability (Standring, 2016). Endocrine and metabolic disorders influence these tissues through alterations in energy metabolism, vascular supply, and neurosensory regulation.

Chrousos (2009) highlighted the central role of the stress system in modulating endocrine and metabolic activity, with peripheral manifestations often observed in posterior musculature.

Patients may present with persistent tightness, fatigue during sitting or walking, or unexplained weakness. Spectral surface readings show broad hypoemissive fields reflecting systemic depletion or adrenal dysregulation, contrasted with localized hyperemissive streaks linked to reparative or compensatory responses.

These emissive expressions align with fascial and vascular continuity, underscoring how systemic endocrine stress and metabolic dysfunction imprint visibly on posterior thigh surfaces. Clinically, this region provides biospectral insight into stress-mediated endocrine imbalance and systemic energy reserve.

Step 2,3,4: ROI Classification and Interpretive Questions

Hyperemission indicates localized congestion, imbalance, or metabolic overactivity.

- Is there redness, warmth, or swelling?
- Is metabolic control suboptimal?

Hypoemission suggests hypoperfusion, neurogenic dysfunction, or impaired perfusion due to metabolic or endocrine causes.

- Is coldness, numbness, chronic wounds, or fatigue present?
- Are systemic symptoms such as sensitivity to ambient temperatures reported?

Step 5: Confirmatory Evaluations

Test	Purpose & Justification	Relevance to Emissive Pattern
HbA1c, fasting glucose	Monitors glycemic control in diabetes.	Correlates with hypoemissive neuropathic or ischemic zones.
Thyroid function tests (TSH, Free T4)	Detects thyroid dysfunction affecting metabolism and circulation.	Associated with regulatory emission patters

Lipid profile	Assesses cardiovascular risk impacting tissue perfusion.	Supports metabolic vascular imbalance.
Inflammatory markers (CRP, ESR)	Identifies systemic inflammation influencing tissue health.	Correlates with hyperemissive regulatory activation

Step 6: Care Strategies and Intervention Pathways

Naturopathic Approach

Promote metabolic health with a low glycemic diet, antioxidants, and micronutrients enhancing insulin sensitivity (Alberti et al., 2006). Adaptogenic herbs such as *Panax ginseng* and *Gymnema sylvestre* support endocrine balance. Supplement chromium, magnesium, and alpha-lipoic acid for glucose metabolism and neuroprotection. Regular aerobic exercise improves circulation.

Standard Medical Approaches

Pharmacological and lifestyle interventions aim for metabolic control. Thyroid hormone replacement and lipid management reduce complications.

Specialty / Practitioner Care Strategies Table

Specialty Group	Practitioners Included	Hyperemissive Strategies	Hypoemissive Strategies
Biochemistry	Nutritionists, Orthomolecular, Herbalists, Naturopaths	Antioxidants, adaptogens, insulin sensitizers, micronutrients	Metabolic support, neuroprotective nutrients, dietary management
Rehabilitation	Physiotherapists, Massage Therapists, Osteopaths / Chiropractors	Exercise therapy, circulation enhancement	Neuromuscular re-education, aerobic conditioning
Energetics	Acupuncturists (TCM), Bioenergetic Therapists	Acupuncture supporting metabolic function	Energy balancing, PEMF
Psychological	GNM practitioners, Psychotherapists, Vibrational therapists, Family constellation facilitators	Mind-body therapies supporting metabolic regulation	Stress reduction, emotional balancing

Educational Pearls & Considerations.

- Regular metabolic monitoring prevents complications.
- Lifestyle and dietary changes complement clinical management.
- Adaptogens support but do not replace conventional therapy.
- Patient education on foot care prevents ulcerations.

GROUP 2

ABDOMINAL AND LUMBAR ZONES

The abdominal and lumbar regions represent a coordinated integration of visceral, musculoskeletal, and neurovascular structures, offering a detailed emissive landscape that reflects both localized influences and systemic regulatory states. Imaging of these zones often shows patterns of emissive asymmetry, segmental hyperactivity, and emissive suppression that correspond with organ-related function, fascial tension, and autonomic modulation.

From an interpretive perspective, these zones are important for recognizing visceral reflex expressions together with musculoskeletal compensations that may precede clinical presentations. The lumbar area, in particular, acts as a hub for neurovascular convergence and postural adaptation, often displaying profiles consistent with long-standing myofascial strain or autonomic dysregulation. Emissive variations in the abdominal region may also signal changes in digestive motility, regulatory activity, or lymphatic flow, making these zones valuable for monitoring both short-term changes and persistent systemic tendencies.

The interaction between visceral reflexes and somatic tissues in these areas highlights the need for integrated interpretation, where biospectral analysis maps localized irregularities and demonstrates functional interdependence. Practitioners will find that the emissive profiles of this group support early recognition of terrain load and provide markers for tracking regulatory adaptation over time.

Zones 9 to 12: Abdominal and Lumbar – Frontal and Lateral Regions

Emissive imaging of the abdominal and lumbar regions provides a detailed view of visceral function, musculoskeletal stability, autonomic regulation, and systemic adaptation. These zones include the abdominal wall musculature, lumbar spine and paraspinal structures, visceral organs such as the kidneys, intestines, and urinary bladder, as well as neurovascular pathways involved in both somatic and visceral regulation. Their central position within the trunk makes them sensitive to localized strain while also reflecting broader systemic dynamics.

From a biomechanical perspective, the lumbar region sustains significant postural load and functions as a convergence point for neurovascular structures. It often displays emissive asymmetries, focal hyperemission, or areas of suppression that correspond with musculoskeletal strain, nerve root involvement, or autonomic modulation. Ring and Ammer (2012) describe how sympathetic activity can influence emissive distribution in the lumbar spine, where altered regulatory tone produces patterns indicative of neurovascular stress.

The abdominal zones also present dynamic emissive responses associated with visceral motility, fascial tension, and lymphatic drainage. Lahiri et al. (2012) emphasize that visceral states frequently generate emissive changes through viscerosomatic reflex pathways, observable with high-resolution imaging. Such patterns may provide early interpretive signals of digestive variation, reative activity, or lymphatic load before overt clinical signs appear. Reitz (2024) further notes that metabolic and energetic regulation shape the emissive profiles of this region, with shifts in oxidative stress or systemic overload frequently

expressed in these zones.

Collectively, the abdominal and lumbar zones function as a physiologic and emissive hub, integrating somatic, visceral, and autonomic inputs. The interaction of these systems generates diverse emissive patterns, requiring a structured, systems-based approach to interpretation. This group includes four zones:

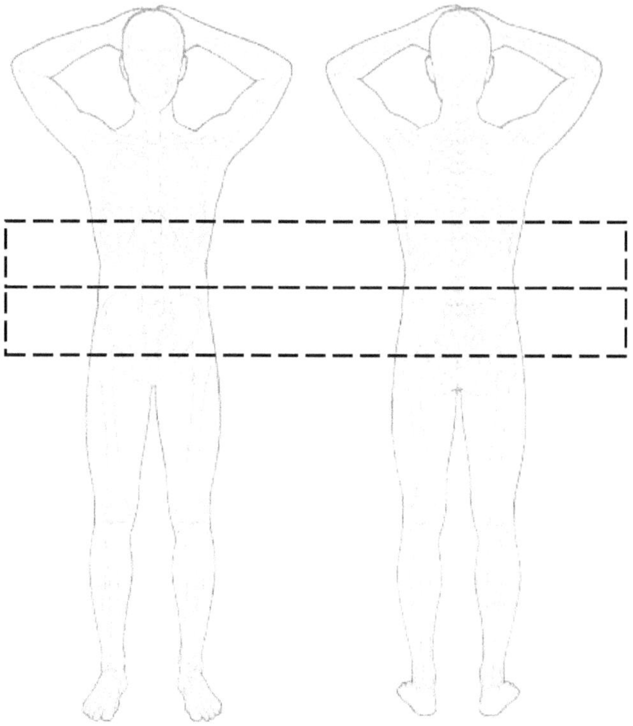

9. Frontal Abdomen
10. Lateral Right Abdomen
11. Lateral Left Abdomen
12. Lumbar Region

Each zone corresponds to a distinct anatomical compartment with specific interpretive significance. The frontal abdomen reflects visceral organ activity and abdominal wall tone, while the lateral zones capture asymmetries in muscular tension and visceral influence. The lumbar region, in contrast, provides information on neurovascular regulation and postural adaptations essential for trunk stability and function.

Recognizing the integrated emissive patterns within these zones allows practitioners to identify early regulatory changes such as visceral stress, musculoskeletal overload, lymphatic stagnation, or autonomic imbalance. Myers (2014) highlights the role of fascial continuity in shaping emissive distribution, noting that altered fascial tension can create regional emissive variations even in the absence of clear structural findings. This supports the interpretive value of emissive imaging as an investigative method, complementing anatomical perspectives by demonstrating the dynamic relationships between structure and function in this region.

GROUP 2

ZONE 9 – FRONTAL ABDOMEN

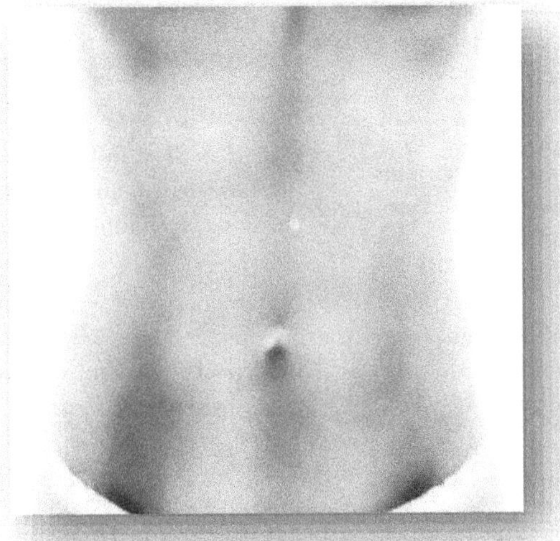

G2Z9FA

The frontal abdomen comprehendes the anterior abdominal wall and underlying visceral structures, forming one of the most emissively active surfaces of the body. It includes the rectus abdominis, transversalis fascia, superficial vasculature, and lies in proximity to metabolically dynamic organs such as the stomach, intestines, and liver (Standring, 2016). Because the abdominal wall is relatively thin, emissive patterns are highly responsive to visceral activity, digestive motility, and fascial tone.

Even small focal asymmetries may provide cues, with hyperemissive fields often aligning with gastrointestinal regulation or fascial strain. Disorders of gastrointestinal motility affect up to 30% of the population, and functional changes may be observed before structural abnormalities become evident (Camilleri, 2001). Biospectrally, this makes the frontal abdomen an early observation field for stress linked to digestion, intestinal permeability, or abdominal wall fatigue.

Regulatory influences extend to autonomic balance, as the abdomen is richly innervated by the enteric nervous system and vagal pathways, making it sensitive to sympathetic–parasympathetic shifts (Furness, 2012). Metabolic load adds another dimension: abdominal adipose tissue is metabolically active, and increased central fat has been associated with altered mediators and perfusion changes detectable at the surface (Després, 2012).

From a lymphatic perspective, irregularities may reflect impaired drainage along superficial epigastric pathways, particularly in sedentary individuals. Clinically, early emissive variations here often correlate with subtle hepatic or gastric burdens, sometimes preceding laboratory confirmation of digestive or metabolic stress. For integrative analysis, the frontal abdomen thus serves as a central diagnostic landscape where organ function, systemic metabolism, and neuroautonomic regulation converge, making it indispensable for terrain-level interpretation.

Zone 9 – Frontal Abdomen: Emission-Relevant Structures.

Category	Relevant Structures	Emission Relevance
1. Vascular / Circulatory	- Superior and inferior epigastric arteries and veins - Superficial abdominal veins - Capillary plexuses in skin and fascia	Hyperemission suggests visceral intensification, wall reactivity, or focal activation. Hypoemission indicates reduced perfusion or autonomic downregulation.
2. Muscular / Myofascial	- Rectus abdominis - External and internal obliques - Transversus abdominis - Fascia transversalis and linea alba	Hyperemission reflects overload, strain, or acute fascial response. Hypoemission signals underuse, restriction, or chronic fascial limitation.
3. Skeletal / Articular	- Costal cartilages (lower ribs) - Xiphoid process - Lumbar vertebrae anteriorly - Pubic symphysis (inferior boundary)	Hyperemission may show periosteal stress, costal overload, or vertebral signal activation. Hypoemission reflects chronic suppression or long-term osseous downregulation.
4. Nervous System / Spine	- Thoracoabdominal nerves (T7-T12) - Sympathetic chain ganglia - Phrenic nerve	Hyperemission indicates neurostress, radicular amplification, or segmental irritation. Hypoemission reflects chronic dampening, autonomic underregulation, or disrupted somatic–visceral integration.
5. Lymphatic / Immune	- Superficial lymphatic vessels of anterior abdominal wall - Axillary and inguinal lymphatic drainage pathways	Local Hyperemission often correlates with drainage field signal buildup or lymphodynamic stagnation, while hypoemissive zones may reveal signal immobility, interstitial rigidity, or suppressed immunoregulatory resonance.
6. Organs / GNM (German New Medicine)	- Stomach, liver, pancreas, intestines (small and large bowel) - Urinary bladder - Reproductive organs (anterior pelvis)	High-emission patterns may suggest visceral stress response or internal zone activation consistent with adaptive conflict processing, while Hypoemission may correspond to resolution-phase signal withdrawal or reflexively mediated biosignal dormancy.
7. Acupuncture / Meridians	- Stomach Meridian (runs midline over abdomen) - Liver and Gallbladder Meridians (right abdomen) - Spleen Meridian (left side)	Elevated biosignal patterns may suggest visceral stress response or internal zone activation consistent with adaptive conflict processing, while Hypoemission may correspond to resolution-phase signal withdrawal or reflexively mediated biosignal dormancy.
8. Energetic / Frequency	- Energetic reflex zones related to digestion, detoxification, and metabolic energy - Abdominal Qi flow centers	Hyperemission may relate to energetic hyperactivity, stress responses, or metabolic overload, while Hypoemission suggests regulatory depletion, adrenal underperformance, or impaired autonomic regulation of visceral functions.
9. Metabolic / Endocrine	- Reflex zones for liver metabolism, pancreatic endocrine function, adrenal glands, and thyroid influence	Hypoemissive patterns can suggest thyroid downregulation, adrenal hypofunction, or systemic metabolic suppression. Hyperemission may be present in accelerated regulatory states, excretory mobilization, or terrain activation processes.

GROUP 2 - ZONE 9 – FRONTAL ABDOMEN

Category 1: *Vascular / Circulatory*

Step 1: Functional Anatomy and Interpretive Importance

The anterior abdominal wall is vascularized by the superior and inferior epigastric arteries, which form a vertical anastomotic arcade within the rectus sheath. These vessels supply the rectus abdominis and adjacent fascia. Venous return occurs through the superior and inferior epigastric veins, supported by the superficial epigastric vein that drains into the femoral system (Standring, 2016).

Clinical reports describe this arcade as a key landmark in reconstructive surgery, confirming its importance in maintaining abdominal wall integrity (Moon & Taylor, 1988).

Spectral surface readings frequently reveal emissive asymmetries along the vertical midline of the abdomen. These may indicate increased muscular demand, abdominal wall strain, or adaptive circulatory changes influenced by visceral function.

Because of its central location, the frontal abdomen often provides early signs of regulatory adjustment in both somatic and visceral systems.

Step 2,3,4: ROI Classification and Interpretive Questions

Hyperemission suggests circulatory field intensification, signal retention, or localized emissive overload possibly linked to tissue reactivity.

- Is there localized redness, tenderness, or swelling?
- Are systemic signs such as fever or chills present?

Hypoemission indicates hypoperfusion, circulatory insufficiency, or compromised vascular delivery.

- Are there complaints of coldness, pallor, or delayed wound healing?
- Is there a history of vascular disease or claudication?

Step 5: Confirmatory Evaluations

Test	Purpose & Justification	Relevance to Emissive Pattern
Doppler ultrasound	Assesses arterial and venous flow in abdominal wall vessels.	Correlates hyperemissive signal activation and hypoemissive circulatory underexpression.
CT or MRI Angiography	Visualizes vessel patency and detects occlusions or thrombosis.	Confirms flow disruption or tissue-level signal intensification.

Blood tests (CBC, CRP, coagulation profile)	Detect infection, inflammation, or coagulopathies.	Supports emissive patterns suggestive of retention or vascular overload.
Physical exam (inspection, palpation)	Evaluates local signs of vascular compromise or inflammation.	Complements biospectral field analysis.

Step 6: Care Strategies and Intervention Pathways

Naturopathic Approach

Botanical venotonics such as *Aesculus hippocastanum* and *Ruscus aculeatus* improve microcirculation and reduce edema (Chrubasik et al., 2011). Anti-inflammatory diets rich in antioxidants and omega-3 fatty acids support vascular health (Calder, 2017). Contrast hydrotherapy with alternating warm and cold applications stimulates circulation (Sutkowy et al., 2019). Nutritional support with vitamins C, E, and bioflavonoids enhances endothelial function. Limb elevation and gentle massage promote venous return.

Standard Medical Approaches

Imaging guides anticoagulation, anti-inflammatory medication, or surgical intervention. Management of systemic causes such as coagulopathies is critical.

Specialty / Practitioner Care Strategies Table

Specialty Group	Practitioners Included	Hyperemissive Strategies	Hypoemissive Strategies
Biochemistry	Nutritionists, Orthomolecular, Herbalists, Naturopaths	Botanical venotonics, antioxidants, anti-inflammatory diet	Circulatory stimulants, nutritional endothelial support
Rehabilitation	Physiotherapists, Massage Therapists, Osteopaths / Chiropractors	Gentle massage, lymphatic drainage, postural correction	Graded exercise, circulatory enhancement
Energetics	Acupuncturists (TCM), Bioenergetic Therapists	Acupuncture, moxibustion, herbal formulas	Warming acupuncture, energy balancing
Psychological	GNM practitioners, Psychotherapists, Vibrational therapists, Family constellation facilitators	Psychotherapy, bioresonance, mindfulness	Stress reduction, emotional balancing

Educational Pearls & Considerations.

- Promptly exclude abdominal wall thrombophlebitis or infection.
- Botanical venotonics combined with diet and hydrotherapy support vascular health.
- Monitor for systemic signs of inflammation or coagulopathy.
- Avoid vigorous massage if acute inflammation is present.
- Elevation and gentle mobilization improve venous return.

GROUP 2 - ZONE 9 – FRONTAL ABDOMEN

Category 2: *Muscular*

Step 1: Functional Anatomy and Interpretive Importance

The frontal abdominal wall is composed of the rectus abdominis, supported laterally by the external and internal obliques and the transversus abdominis. These muscles, innervated by the thoracoabdominal nerves, generate trunk flexion, maintain intra-abdominal pressure, and link the rib cage to the pelvis via the linea alba (Standring, 2016).

Surgical literature emphasizes the importance of balanced abdominal wall integrity, noting that fascial weakness or rectus diastasis predisposes to hernias and chronic dysfunction (Rath et al., 1997).

Biospectral mapping of this region often reveals vertical emissive bands along the rectus sheath or diffuse gradients reflecting myofascial load. Such signals correspond to changes in tension distribution, providing interpreters with functional markers that integrate trunk support with visceral regulation.

This makes the anterior abdomen a sensitive region for detecting both localized strain and systemic stress adaptation.

Step 2,3,4: ROI Classification and Interpretive Questions

Hyperemission indicates acute muscle strain, myositis, or trigger point activation with increased local spectral emission.

- Has the patient experienced overuse or trauma?
- Are there localized pain, tenderness, or muscle tightness?

Hypoemission suggests chronic muscle hypoperfusion, fibrosis, or neurogenic atrophy.

- Are there complaints of weakness, stiffness, or reduced range of motion?
- Is muscle wasting or altered sensation present?

Step 5: Confirmatory Evaluations

Test	Purpose & Justification	Relevance to Emissive Pattern
Creatine kinase (CK), LDH	Detects muscle injury or inflammation (Simons et al., 1999).	Elevated in hyperemissive biosignal activation patterns.
MRI	Visualizes muscle edema, inflammation, or fibrosis.	Supports hyper- or hypoemissive zone expression.
Electromyography (EMG)	Assesses muscle and nerve function.	Correlates with hypoemissive neuroregulatory influence.
Blood tests (CBC, inflammatory markers)	Detects systemic inflammation or infection.	Supports hyperemissive terrain excitation states.

Step 6: Care Strategies and Intervention Pathways

Naturopathic Approach

Anti-inflammatory botanicals such as *Curcuma longa* and *Boswellia serrata* reduce muscle inflammation (Hewlings & Kalman, 2017). Magnesium supports muscle relaxation. Hydrotherapy with alternating warm and cold applications enhances circulation (Sutkowy et al., 2019). Gentle stretching and progressive strengthening promote recovery. Adequate protein and antioxidants support tissue repair.

Standard Medical Approaches

Rest, NSAIDs, and physical therapy are standard treatments for muscle injuries (Simons et al., 1999). Neurogenic muscle weakness requires neurological assessment.

Specialty / Practitioner Care Strategies Table

Specialty Group	Practitioners Included	Hyperemissive Strategies	Hypoemissive Strategies
Biochemistry	Nutritionists, Orthomolecular, Herbalists, Naturopaths	Anti-inflammatory botanicals, magnesium, antioxidants, protein	Circulatory support, neurotrophic nutrients, protein support
Rehabilitation	Physiotherapists, Massage Therapists, Osteopaths / Chiropractors	Myofascial release, trigger point therapy, gentle massage	Graded aerobic exercise, neurorehabilitation, ergonomic guidance
Energetics	Acupuncturists (TCM), Bioenergetic Therapists	Acupuncture, moxibustion, PEMF	Warming acupuncture, frequency therapy
Psychological	GNM practitioners, Psychotherapists, Vibrational therapists, Family constellation facilitators	Psychotherapy, bioresonance, mindfulness	Psychosomatic conflict resolution, emotional balancing

Educational Pearls & Considerations.

- Early identification of myofascial trigger points improves outcomes.
- Magnesium aids in reducing muscle cramps and spasms.
- Hydrotherapy should be adapted according to inflammation phase.
- Neurological evaluation is essential when weakness is present.
- Gradual rehabilitation prevents chronic dysfunction.

GROUP 2 - ZONE 9 – FRONTAL ABDOMEN

Category 4: *Nervous*

Step 1: Functional Anatomy and Interpretive Importance

The frontal abdominal wall is innervated by thoracoabdominal nerves (T7–T12) and branches of the iliohypogastric and ilioinguinal nerves, providing sensory input to skin and musculature and coordinating abdominal wall reflexes (Standring, 2016).

These nerves are subject to entrapment in fascial planes or surgical scars, leading to pain syndromes that are frequently misattributed to visceral disease. Janis et al. (2010) reported that abdominal cutaneous nerve entrapment is a recognized source of chronic abdominal pain, often overlooked in routine assessment. Neural stress of this kind alters motor recruitment and autonomic regulation, creating irregularities in regional control.

These regulatory shifts leave a surface imprint, with biospectral asymmetries often appearing as localized emissive variations across the abdominal wall, distinct from diffuse visceral influences.

Their sharply confined nature reflects the neural origin of the disturbance, allowing clinicians to visualize abdominal wall neuropathies externally and to distinguish them from deeper intra-abdominal pathology.

Step 2,3,4: ROI Classification and Interpretive Questions

Hyperemission suggests nerve irritation, neurogenic reactivity, or neuropathic pain.

- Is there burning, tingling, or sharp pain in the abdominal wall?
- Are there localized hypersensitivity or swelling?

Hypoemission indicates nerve hypoperfusion, compression, or denervation with decreased autonomic activity.

- Are numbness, weakness, or muscle atrophy present?
- Do symptoms worsen with certain positions or movements?

Step 5: Confirmatory Evaluations

Test	Purpose & Justification	Relevance to Emissive Pattern
Nerve conduction studies (NCS), Electromyography (EMG)	Assess nerve and muscle function (Janis et al., 2010).	Correlates with hypoemissive neurofunctional suppression.
Quantitative sensory testing (QST)	Measures sensory nerve function and thresholds.	Supports interpretation of neurofunctional patterns.
Ultrasound / MRI	Detects nerve entrapment or structural abnormalities.	Identifies contributors to nerve field dysfunction.
Blood tests (glucose, vitamin B12)	Evaluates metabolic causes of neuropathy.	Supports interpretation of metabolic neuroregulatory imbalances.

Step 6: **Care Strategies and Intervention Pathways**

Naturopathic Approach

B-complex vitamins, alpha-lipoic acid, and Acetyl-L-carnitine support nerve repair (Papanas & Ziegler, 2014). Herbal anti-inflammatories like *Hypericum perforatum* may reduce neuropathic pain (Kasper et al., 2010). Neural mobilization, gentle stretching, and bioresonance modulate neurovascular function.

Standard Medical Approaches

Pharmacologic treatments include anticonvulsants, antidepressants, and analgesics. Surgical decompression may be required. Metabolic optimization is critical in systemic neuropathies.

Specialty / Practitioner Care Strategies Table

Specialty Group	Practitioners Included	Hyperemissive Strategies	Hypoemissive Strategies
Biochemistry	Nutritionists, Orthomolecular, Herbalists, Naturopaths	Neurotrophic vitamins, alpha-lipoic acid, anti-inflammatory botanicals	Circulatory stimulants, metabolic support, neuroprotective nutrients
Rehabilitation	Physiotherapists, Massage Therapists, Osteopaths / Chiropractors	Neural mobilization, myofascial release, gentle massage	Neural gliding exercises, ergonomic guidance, neurorehabilitation
Energetics	Acupuncturists (TCM), Bioenergetic Therapists	Acupuncture, moxibustion, PEMF	Warming acupuncture, frequency therapy, energy healing
Psychological	GNM practitioners, Psychotherapists, Vibrational therapists, Family constellation facilitators	Psychotherapy, bioresonance, mindfulness	Psychosomatic conflict resolution, vibrational medicine

Educational Pearls & Considerations.

- Early detection prevents chronic nerve damage.
- Nutritional and energetic support enhances nerve repair.
- Monitor for metabolic contributors such as diabetes.
- Avoid aggressive treatments during acute inflammation.
- Tailor neural mobilization to patient tolerance.

GROUP 2 - ZONE 9 – FRONTAL ABDOMEN

Category 5: *Lymphatic*

Step 1: Functional Anatomy and Interpretive Importance

The frontal abdominal wall is supplied by superficial lymphatics that drain superiorly toward axillary nodes and inferiorly into the inguinal chain, while deeper vessels accompany the inferior epigastric and iliac routes (Standring, 2016).

This dual system regulates tissue fluid balance and contributes to immune surveillance of abdominal structures. Al-Hadithy and Khan (2012) observed that abdominal wall lymphedema often complicates prior surgery or obesity, producing persistent swelling and discomfort that are commonly misattributed to visceral disorders. When drainage is impaired, fascial compliance and neurovascular regulation are altered, reshaping the functional landscape of the abdominal wall.

These shifts imprint themselves externally, where clinicians may observe focal emissive variations confined to the anterior midline or periumbilical zone. Their distinct geometry contrasts with diffuse visceral patterns, highlighting their lymphatic origin. In this way, spectral surface interpretation provides a window into the early burden of abdominal lymphatic strain, refining differential assessment of anterior wall dysfunction.

Step 2,3,4: ROI Classification and Interpretive Questions

Hyperemission indicates acute lymphatic reactivity, microbial activity, or congestion with spectral intensification and swelling.

- Is there redness, tenderness, or rapid swelling?
- Has the patient experienced recent infection or trauma?

Hypoemission suggests chronic lymphatic stasis with fibrosis and impaired drainage causing reduced biosignal.

- Is swelling persistent and firm?
- Are recurrent infections or delayed wound healing present?

Step 5: Confirmatory Evaluations

Test	Purpose & Justification	Relevance to Emissive Pattern
Lymphoscintigraphy	Evaluates lymphatic flow and obstruction.	Confirms lymphatic field retention or reduced perfusion.
Doppler ultrasound	Excludes venous insufficiency contributing to swelling.	Differentiates vascular from lymphatic signal patterns.

Blood tests (CBC, inflammatory markers)	Detect infection or systemic inflammation.	Supports hyperemissive tissue activation states.
Physical exam (Stemmer's sign, limb measurements)	Identifies clinical signs of lymphedema.	Correlates with biospectral field findings.

Step 6: Care Strategies and Intervention Pathways

Naturopathic Approach

Stimulate lymphatic drainage with herbal lymphagogues such as *Hedera helix* and *Vitis vinifera* (Godoy et al., 2012). Manual lymphatic drainage by trained therapists improves fluid movement. Compression therapy supports lymph return and must be individualized. Nutritional antioxidants and anti-inflammatory nutrients promote tissue repair. Hydrotherapy with alternating warm and cold applications enhances lymphatic circulation.

Standard Medical Approaches

Standard treatments include manual lymphatic drainage, compression garments, physical therapy, and infection control. Surgical intervention is reserved for refractory cases.

Specialty / Practitioner Care Strategies Table

Specialty Group	Practitioners Included	Hyperemissive Strategies	Hypoemissive Strategies
Biochemistry	Nutritionists, Orthomolecular, Herbalists, Naturopaths	Herbal lymphagogues, antioxidants, anti-inflammatory nutrients	Circulatory support, nutritional tissue repair support
Rehabilitation	Physiotherapists, Massage Therapists, Osteopaths / Chiropractors	Manual lymphatic drainage, gentle massage, postural retraining	Compression therapy, graded exercise, ergonomic guidance
Energetics	Acupuncturists (TCM), Bioenergetic Therapists	Acupuncture, herbal formulas, PEMF	Warming acupuncture, energy balancing
Psychological	GNM practitioners, Psychotherapists, Vibrational therapists, Family constellation facilitators	Mind-body therapies supporting immune function and healing	Psychosomatic conflict resolution, emotional balancing

Educational Pearls & Considerations.

- Early intervention prevents chronic lymphedema progression.
- Manual lymphatic drainage should be performed by certified therapists.
- Compression therapy requires proper fitting and monitoring.
- Nutritional support enhances lymphatic and tissue health.
- Prompt infection treatment is essential to prevent worsening.

GROUP 2 - ZONE 9 – FRONTAL ABDOMEN

Category 6: *Organ-related (GNM)*

Step 1: Functional Anatomy and Interpretive Importance

The anterior abdominal wall overlies key visceral structures including the stomach, intestines, liver, and pancreas, supported by multiple muscular layers and fascia (Standring, 2016). In German New Medicine (GNM), conflicts involving nourishment, survival, or processing activate biological programs in these organs, producing phase-dependent emissive responses.

Hamer (2012) described that during conflict-active states, biosignal suppression appears as hypoemission, while in healing, tissue repair drives hyperemissive intensification.

These surface manifestations can be misinterpreted as nonspecific unless their psychosomatic origin is considered. Pert (1997) highlighted that neuropeptides and emotional states are closely integrated with gut physiology, underscoring the validity of mind–body connections in abdominal function.

On emissive assessment, sharply localized surface variations over the abdomen may represent muscular and vascular influences as well as deeper visceral programs linked to unresolved psychosomatic conflicts.

Step 2,3,4: ROI Classification and Interpretive Questions

Hyperemission often corresponds to the "healing" or tissue recovery phase of an organ conflict, with increased metabolic activity and tissue regeneration.

- Is the patient experiencing pain or swelling in the abdomen?
- Are there symptoms of inflammation or infection?

Hypoemission relates to the "conflict active" phase, often involving tissue loss or functional reduction.

- Are there functional deficits, fatigue, or diminished organ function?
- Is there a history of psychological stress or trauma correlating with symptoms?

Step 5: Confirmatory Evaluations

Test	Purpose & Justification	Relevance to Emissive Pattern
Ultrasound / CT / MRI imaging	Visualizes organ morphology and detects structural changes.	Correlates with emissive anomalies suggesting organ field engagement.
Liver function tests (ALT, AST, bilirubin)	Assess hepatic cellular injury or dysfunction.	Supports hyperemissive tissue activity in hepatic terrain.

Pancreatic enzymes (amylase, lipase)	Detect pancreatic inflammation or damage.	Correlates with biospectral patterns in the pancreatic zone.
Complete blood count (CBC), inflammatory markers	Detect systemic inflammation or infection.	Supports hyperemissive expression linked to conflict phases.
Psychological assessment	Identifies underlying biological conflicts and stressors.	Complements GNM-based interpretive mapping.

Step 6: Care Strategies and Intervention Pathways

Naturopathic Approach

Support organ healing with hepatoprotective botanicals such as *Silybum marianum* (milk thistle) and *Curcuma longa* (turmeric) (Friedman et al., 2017). Promote digestive health with probiotics and digestive enzymes. Stress management and psychotherapy assist conflict resolution. Nutritional support with antioxidants and anti-inflammatory nutrients enhances repair.

Standard Medical Approaches

Imaging and labs guide medical management of organ-specific pathology. Pharmacologic and surgical interventions are used as indicated.

Specialty / Practitioner Care Strategies Table

Specialty Group	Practitioners Included	Hyperemissive Strategies	Hypoemissive Strategies
Biochemistry	Nutritionists, Orthomolecular, Herbalists, Naturopaths	Hepatoprotective herbs, antioxidants, digestive enzymes	Nutritional support for organ function
Rehabilitation	Physiotherapists, Massage Therapists, Osteopaths / Chiropractors	Supportive therapies promoting relaxation and circulation	Gentle mobilization and relaxation techniques
Energetics	Acupuncturists (TCM), Bioenergetic Therapists	Acupuncture for organ function and inflammation	Energy balancing and harmonization
Psychological	GNM practitioners, Psychotherapists, Vibrational therapists, Family constellation facilitators	Psychotherapy, bioresonance, conflict resolution	Emotional balancing and stress reduction

Educational Pearls & Considerations.

- Recognize the psychosomatic origin of organ pathology per GNM principles.
- Support both physical healing and psychological conflict resolution.
- Monitor organ function carefully with appropriate testing.
- Coordinate multidisciplinary care for optimal outcomes.

GROUP 2 - ZONE 9 – FRONTAL ABDOMEN

Category 7: *Acupuncture / Meridian*

Step 1: Functional Anatomy and Interpretive Importance

The anterior abdominal wall includes rectus abdominis, oblique musculature, and fascial layers protecting the digestive viscera such as stomach, intestines, and pancreas (Standring, 2016). In Traditional Chinese Medicine (TCM), this zone aligns with the Conception Vessel (Ren Mai) and the Stomach (ST) meridian.

Flaws (2000) noted their significance for digestive strength, reproductive health, and abdominal circulation. Deadman et al. (2007) highlighted points such as Ren12 and ST25 as central regulators of gastrointestinal balance and systemic Qi distribution.

Disturbance in these pathways often manifests clinically as digestive discomfort, bloating, or weakness of abdominal tone. In emissive assessment, biosignal fields are seen as circular or linear variations localized to the midline or lateral abdomen, reflecting the course of Ren Mai and ST trajectories.

These findings suggest that abdominal biospectral asymmetries may represent surface correlates of meridian disruption, offering visible markers of digestive imbalance.

Step 2,3,4: ROI Classification and Interpretive Questions

Hyperemission suggests Qi stagnation or energetic reactivity along the meridian pathways.

- Is there localized pain, tenderness, or distension?
- Do symptoms worsen with stress or certain foods?

Hypoemission indicates Qi deficiency or chronic stagnation causing poor circulation and cold sensations.

- Does the patient experience fatigue, coldness, or digestive sluggishness?
- Are there chronic digestive complaints or weakness?

Step 5: Confirmatory Evaluations

Test	Purpose & Justification	Relevance to Emissive Pattern
Pulse diagnosis and tongue examination	Traditional TCM tools assessing Qi and blood status (Flaws, 2000).	Correlates with emissive zone patterns to refine interpretation.
Biospectral imaging	Detects emissive asymmetries along meridian pathways.	Visualizes hyper- or hypoemissive meridian expressions.
Patient symptom questionnaire	Assesses digestive symptoms, energy levels, and pain patterns.	Supports differentiation of Qi stagnation versus Qi deficiency.

Step 6: Care Strategies and Intervention Pathways

Naturopathic Approach

Acupuncture points such as Ren12, ST25, and ST36 regulate digestive function and promote Qi flow (Lao et al., 2004). Moxibustion warms hypoemissive areas. Herbal formulas including *Bao He Wan* and *Xiao Yao San* harmonize digestion and relieve stagnation (Bensky et al., 2004). Dietary modifications with Qi-building foods complement treatment.

Standard Medical Approaches

Acupuncture supports symptom management alongside medical and nutritional therapies for digestive and abdominal conditions.

Specialty / Practitioner Care Strategies Table

Specialty Group	Practitioners Included	Hyperemissive Strategies	Hypoemissive Strategies
Biochemistry	Nutritionists, Orthomolecular, Herbalists, Naturopaths	Herbal formulas for digestive harmonization, antioxidants	Qi tonics, digestive support supplements
Rehabilitation	Physiotherapists, Massage Therapists, Osteopaths / Chiropractors	Abdominal massage, myofascial release	Gentle mobilization, warming massage
Energetics	Acupuncturists (TCM), Bioenergetic Therapists	Acupuncture, moxibustion, PEMF	Warming acupuncture, energy balancing
Psychological	GNM practitioners, Psychotherapists, Vibrational therapists, Family constellation facilitators	Mind-body therapies, bioresonance, energy clearing	Psychosomatic conflict resolution, emotional balancing

Educational Pearls & Considerations.

- Careful point selection tailors treatment to hyper- or hypoemissive patterns.
- Moxibustion should be cautiously applied in heat-sensitive patients.
- Herbal treatments require professional guidance.
- Combining acupuncture with physical and nutritional therapy optimizes results.

GROUP 2 - ZONE 9 – FRONTAL ABDOMEN

Category 8: *Energetic*

Step 1: Functional Anatomy and Interpretive Importance

The frontal abdomen contains the rectus abdominis, abdominal wall fascia, and visceral overlay including stomach, intestines, and associated vessels (Standring, 2016). Energetically, this surface is tied to regulation of digestion and central vitality, functioning as a hub of systemic coherence.

Oschman (2016) emphasized the connective tissue matrix as a conductor of subtle energy and information, a framework that helps explain emissive irregularities in this region. Clinically, disturbances may present as digestive discomfort, bloating, or reduced vitality.

Biospectral imaging often reveals broad hypoemissive zones signaling stagnation or under-conduction, while patchy hyperemissive clusters indicate reparative activity or heightened autonomic regulation.

These emissive signatures can extend across fascial lines, aligning more with energy pathways than organ boundaries. By interpreting these signals within the energetic model, the frontal abdomen is understood as a central biospectral map of systemic balance and digestive coherence.

Step 2,3,4: ROI Classification and Interpretive Questions

Hyperemission suggests localized energy congestion or field reactivity.

- Does the patient report sensations of heat, tension, or discomfort?
- Are stress or emotional factors contributing?

Hypoemission indicates energy deficiency or stagnation.

- Does the patient experience fatigue, coldness, or digestive sluggishness?
- Are symptoms chronic or resistant to conventional therapies?

Step 5: Confirmatory Evaluations

Test	Purpose & Justification	Relevance to Emissive Pattern
Bioresonance testing	Measures tissue energy frequencies and imbalances.	Correlates with emissive anomalies.
Electrodermal screening (EDS)	Assesses skin conductance linked to energy pathways.	Supports interpretation of bioenergetic imbalances.
Patient emotional and symptom history	Provides clinical context for energetic dysfunction.	Assists differential biospectral interpretation.

Step 6: Care Strategies and Intervention Pathways

Naturopathic Approach

Use bioresonance, pulsed electromagnetic fields (PEMF), and adaptogenic herbs to restore energetic balance and promote healing (Matsumoto et al., 2010). Nutritional antioxidants and adaptogens enhance systemic resilience. Mindfulness and stress reduction complement energetic therapies.

Standard Medical Approaches

Energetic therapies complement conventional medical and rehabilitative treatments to optimize patient outcomes.

Specialty / Practitioner Care Strategies Table

Specialty Group	Practitioners Included	Hyperemissive Strategies	Hypoemissive Strategies
Biochemistry	Nutritionists, Orthomolecular, Herbalists, Naturopaths	Adaptogens, antioxidants, herbal energetics	Nutritional support for energy deficiency
Rehabilitation	Physiotherapists, Massage Therapists, Osteopaths / Chiropractors	Energy-based manual therapies, PEMF, therapeutic touch	Gentle stimulation, mobilization
Energetics	Acupuncturists (TCM), Bioenergetic Therapists	Bioresonance, PEMF, acupuncture	Warming acupuncture, energy balancing
Psychological	GNM practitioners, Psychotherapists, Vibrational therapists, Family constellation facilitators	Psychotherapy, bioresonance, mindfulness	Emotional balancing, vibrational medicine

Educational Pearls & Considerations.

- Energetic therapies support but do not replace conventional care.
- Patient responsiveness and practitioner skill influence outcomes.
- Regular assessment guides therapeutic adjustments.
- Address psychological and physical factors holistically.

GROUP 2 - ZONE 9 – FRONTAL ABDOMEN

Category 9: Metabolic / *Endocrine*

Step 1: Functional Anatomy and Interpretive Importance

The frontal abdomen contains the rectus abdominis, abdominal fascia, and visceral overlay including the stomach, intestines, liver, and pancreas (Standring, 2016). Metabolically, this region is central to glycoregulation, lipid storage, and endocrine signaling, making it highly reflective of systemic dysfunction.

DeFronzo & Ferrannini (1991) described insulin resistance as a defining feature of metabolic syndrome, with abdominal tissues acting as both contributors and responders. Patients frequently present with central adiposity, digestive discomfort, or systemic fatigue.

Biospectral imaging reveals diffuse hypoemissive fields in states of suppressed metabolic efficiency, while hyperemissive foci emerge during reparative or inflammatory activation.

These emissive patterns often follow fascial planes rather than organ borders, underscoring systemic endocrine influence over local expression. Clinically, the frontal abdomen is an external map of metabolic stability, reflecting early signs of insulin resistance, glycoregulatory imbalance, and visceral stress.

Step 2,3,4: ROI Classification and Interpretive Questions

Hyperemission may reflect local metabolic reactivity, microbial activity, or biosignal intensification.

- Is there warmth, redness, or swelling in the abdominal area?
- Is metabolic control suboptimal?

Hypoemission indicates hypoperfusion, neuropathy, or impaired circulation from metabolic or endocrine causes.

- Are there cold sensations, numbness, or chronic wounds?
- Are systemic symptoms such as fatigue or temperature intolerance present?

Step 5: Confirmatory Evaluations

Test	Purpose & Justification	Relevance to Emissive Pattern
HbA1c, fasting glucose	Assesses glycemic control in diabetes.	Correlates with hypoemissive neurofunctional or perfusion-restricted zones.

Thyroid function tests (TSH, Free T4)	Evaluates thyroid disorders affecting metabolism and circulation.	Linked to altered emissive regulation.
Lipid profile	Assesses cardiovascular risk impacting tissue perfusion.	Supports metabolic circulatory adaptation.
Inflammatory markers (CRP, ESR)	Detects systemic inflammation influencing tissue health.	Correlates with hyperemissive tissue activation states.

Step 6: Care Strategies and Intervention Pathways

Naturopathic Approach

Promote metabolic balance with low glycemic diet, antioxidants, and adaptogens (Alberti et al., 2006). Herbs such as *Panax ginseng* and *Gymnema sylvestre* support endocrine function. Supplement chromium, magnesium, and alpha-lipoic acid to enhance glucose metabolism and neuroprotection. Regular aerobic exercise improves circulation and metabolism.

Standard Medical Approaches

Pharmacologic and lifestyle interventions target metabolic control. Thyroid hormone replacement and lipid management reduce complications.

Specialty / Practitioner Care Strategies Table

Specialty Group	Practitioners Included	Hyperemissive Strategies	Hypoemissive Strategies
Biochemistry	Nutritionists, Orthomolecular, Herbalists, Naturopaths	Antioxidants, adaptogens, insulin sensitizers, micronutrients	Metabolic support, neuroprotective nutrients, dietary management
Rehabilitation	Physiotherapists, Massage Therapists, Osteopaths / Chiropractors	Exercise therapy, circulation enhancement	Neuromuscular re-education, aerobic conditioning
Energetics	Acupuncturists (TCM), Bioenergetic Therapists	Acupuncture supporting metabolic function	Energy balancing, PEMF
Psychological	GNM practitioners, Psychotherapists, Vibrational therapists, Family constellation facilitators	Mind-body therapies supporting metabolic regulation	Stress reduction, emotional balancing

Educational Pearls & Considerations.

- Regular monitoring of metabolic parameters is essential.
- Lifestyle changes significantly complement medical treatment.
- Adaptogens support but do not replace conventional therapy.
- Patient education on skin and wound care prevents complications.

GROUP 2

ZONE 10 – LATERAL RIGHT ABDOMEN

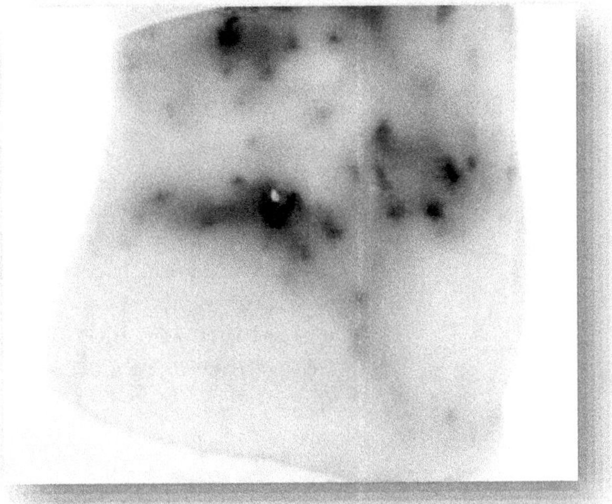

G2Z10LRA

The lateral right abdomen integrates muscular layers, superficial vascular networks, and visceral structures such as the liver, gallbladder, and ascending colon, making it a clinically significant zone. It includes the external and internal oblique muscles, the transversus abdominis, and their fascial connections, overlying a segment dominated by hepatic and biliary influence (Standring, 2016).

Because of the liver's metabolic centrality, emissive asymmetries here often carry systemic meaning, with subtle hyper- or hypoemissive fields revealing early hepatic stress, sometimes preceding changes in serum tests. Hepatic steatosis, for example, affects over 25% of the global population, and peripheral markers of altered microvascular reactivity have been observed before ultrasound confirmation (Younossi et al., 2016).

The gallbladder further adds diagnostic value, as biliary dysmotility or stone formation often generates localized field changes. Musculoskeletal strain in the lateral wall may also create emissive irregularities, especially in postural imbalance or core instability. Neurovascular interactions enrich interpretation, since hepatic innervation via sympathetic and vagal pathways leaves systemic regulatory imprints (Berthoud, 2004).

Clinically, emissive asymmetry here has been associated with right-sided lymphatic retention linked to hepatic or portal burden, aligning with evidence that hepatic congestion can impair systemic lymphatic flow (Witte et al., 2001). Right-sided abdominal wall hernias and strain injuries, which account for nearly 60% of lateral wall defects, may likewise present first as emissive anomalies before structural confirmation (Novitsky et al., 2006).

From a biospectral perspective, the lateral right abdomen thus reflects both somatic strain and deeper metabolic, digestive, and lymphatic coherence, serving as a sensitive site for early terrain imbalance detection.

Zone 10 – Lateral Right Abdomen: Emission-Relevant Structures

Category	Relevant Structures	Emission Relevance
1. Vascular / Circulatory	- Right hepatic artery and portal vein branches - Superior mesenteric artery (right branch) - Superficial abdominal veins	Hyperemission may indicate visceral biosignal intensification, including hepatic or biliary field retention. Hypoemission can reflect vascular narrowing, signal suppression, or autonomic modulation reducing abdominal wall biosignal flow.
2. Muscular / Myofascial	- External oblique (right side) - Internal oblique (right side) - Transversus abdominis (right side)	Hyperemission usually corresponds to muscular strain, fascial activation, or postural overload. Hypoemission may reflect disuse-related signal reduction, fascial restriction, or myofascial adaptation limiting local expression.
3. Skeletal / Articular	- Lower ribs (right side) - Costal cartilages - Lumbar vertebrae (right lateral aspect)	Hyperemission may signal periosteal field activation, costal interface stress, or vertebral zone excitation. Hypoemission may be associated with chronic biosignal decline or reduced expression in osseous metabolic fields.
4. Nervous System / Spine	- Intercostal nerves (right T8-T12) - Sympathetic ganglia - Lumbar plexus branches	Hyperemissive zones suggest neural field excitation; Hypoemission may indicate neurofunctional suppression, nerve field inhibition, or autonomic underregulation affecting somatic and visceral integration.
5. Lymphatic / Immune	- Superficial lymphatic vessels draining right abdomen - Right inguinal and axillary lymph nodes	Hyperemission often correlates with immune-regulatory field activation or lymphatic signal buildup; Hypoemissive zones may reflect stagnation, tissue density, or reduced immunoregulatory dynamics in the drainage pathways.
6. Organs / GNM (German New Medicine)	- Liver (right lobe) - Gallbladder - Right colon (hepatic flexure) - Part of the kidney (upper pole, right side)	Elevated biosignal expression may indicate active visceral conflict, terrain activation, or hepatobiliary retention. Hypoemission can correspond to resolution phases or functional suppression mediated by reflexive mechanisms.
7. Acupuncture / Meridians	- Gallbladder Meridian (lateral right abdomen) - Liver Meridian - Small Intestine Meridian	High-expression patterns may indicate Qi retention or meridian signal excess in hepatobiliary zones; Low-emission regions often reflect Qi deficiency, fluid-phase retention, or diminished meridian flow affecting digestive and hepatic zones.
8. Energetic / Frequency	- Reflex zones linked to hepatobiliary energetics and detoxification pathways - Localized frequency disruptions	Hyperemission may relate to bioenergetic excitation or emotional regulation impacting hepatobiliary terrain; Hypoemission may indicate regulatory depletion or impaired excretory mobilization.
9. Metabolic / Endocrine	- Reflex zones for liver metabolism and adrenal function influencing right abdominal energetics	Hypoemissive expression patterns may suggest metabolic signal suppression, adrenal underregulation, or hepatic terrain inhibition. Persistent Hyperemission may represent metabolic overload or regulatory stress in the right abdominal field.

GROUP 2 - ZONE 10 – LATERAL RIGHT ABDOMEN

Category 1: *Vascular / Circulatory*

Step 1: Functional Anatomy and Interpretive Importance

The lateral right abdominal wall is supplied by segmental branches of the intercostal, subcostal, and lumbar arteries, together with tributaries from the inferior epigastric system. These vessels nourish the oblique and transversus abdominis muscles and their fascial planes.

Venous return follows the intercostal and lumbar veins, with connections to the azygos and femoral systems (Standring, 2016). Anatomical mapping of angiosomes has emphasized the role of these segmental vessels in abdominal wall perfusion and surgical flap design (Taylor & Palmer, 1987).

On spectral surface reading, emissive asymmetries in this zone often appear as horizontal or oblique bands corresponding to the course of intercostal or lumbar vessels. These patterns may reflect localized strain, circulatory modulation, or regulatory tension in the lateral abdominal wall, where musculoskeletal and visceral influences converge.

Step 2,3,4: ROI Classification and Interpretive Questions

Hyperemission suggests vascular reactivity, venous congestion, or thrombophlebitis with increased local spectral emission.

- Is there localized redness, tenderness, or swelling?
- Are systemic symptoms such as fever present?

Hypoemission indicates hypoperfusion or vascular insufficiency with reduced circulation.

- Are there complaints of coldness, pallor, or delayed healing?
- Is there a history of vascular disease?

Step 5: Confirmatory Evaluations

Test	Purpose & Justification	Relevance to Emissive Pattern
Doppler ultrasound	Evaluates arterial and venous flow in abdominal wall vessels.	Correlates hyperemissive tissue activation and hypoemissive perfusion decline.
CT or MRI angiography	Visualizes vessel patency and identifies occlusions or thrombosis.	Confirms vascular signal disruption or localized field intensification.
Blood tests (CBC, CRP, coagulation profile)	Detect infection, inflammation, or coagulation disorders.	Supports hyperemissive retention or circulatory impedance states.
Physical exam	Inspects and palpates for local signs of vascular compromise.	Complements biospectral imaging findings.

Step 6: Care Strategies and Intervention Pathways

Naturopathic Approach

Use botanical venotonics such as *Aesculus hippocastanum* and *Ruscus aculeatus* to improve microcirculation and reduce edema (Chrubasik et al., 2011). An anti-inflammatory diet rich in antioxidants and omega-3 fatty acids supports vascular health (Calder, 2017). Contrast hydrotherapy with warm and cold applications stimulates circulation (Sutkowy et al., 2019). Vitamins C, E, and bioflavonoids enhance endothelial function. Limb elevation and gentle massage promote venous return.

Standard Medical Approaches

Imaging guides anticoagulation, anti-inflammatory medication, or surgical intervention as needed. Managing systemic contributors such as coagulopathies is critical.

Specialty / Practitioner Care Strategies Table

Specialty Group	Practitioners Included	Hyperemissive Strategies	Hypoemissive Strategies
Biochemistry	Nutritionists, Orthomolecular, Herbalists, Naturopaths	Botanical venotonics, antioxidants, anti-inflammatory diet	Circulatory stimulants, nutritional endothelial support
Rehabilitation	Physiotherapists, Massage Therapists, Osteopaths / Chiropractors	Gentle massage, lymphatic drainage, postural correction	Graded exercise, circulatory enhancement
Energetics	Acupuncturists (TCM), Bioenergetic Therapists	Acupuncture, moxibustion, herbal formulas	Warming acupuncture, energy balancing
Psychological	GNM practitioners, Psychotherapists, Vibrational therapists, Family constellation facilitators	Psychotherapy, bioresonance, mindfulness	Stress reduction, emotional balancing

Educational Pearls & Considerations.

- Exclude thrombophlebitis promptly in cases of Hyperemission and swelling.
- Botanical venotonics combined with diet and hydrotherapy support vascular health effectively.
- Nitric oxide donors and omega-3 fatty acids enhance endothelial function and perfusion.
- Compression therapy is contraindicated in severe arterial insufficiency.
- Early mobilization and limb elevation prevent chronic complications.

GROUP 2 - ZONE 10 – LATERAL RIGHT ABDOMEN

Category 2: *Muscular*

Step 1: Functional Anatomy and Interpretive Importance

The right lateral abdominal wall comprises the external oblique, internal oblique, and transversus abdominis, which overlap to provide trunk rotation, lateral flexion, and spinal stability. These layers are innervated by thoracoabdominal and subcostal nerves, with fascial continuity into the thoracolumbar system (Standring, 2016).

Clinical evidence demonstrates that dysfunction or delayed activation of the obliques is associated with low-back pain and compromised trunk stability, underscoring their importance in lumbopelvic control (Koumantakis et al., 2005).

Spectral surface readings of this region often display diagonal emissive bands aligned with oblique fibers, revealing muscular overuse, myofascial restriction, or asymmetric stabilization during spinal loading.

Because the obliques connect thoracic and pelvic mechanics, these emissive signals provide insight into the integrative regulation of the trunk and its compensatory responses to daily postural demands.

Step 2,3,4: ROI Classification and Interpretive Questions

Hyperemission indicates acute muscle strain, muscular reactivity, or active trigger points with increased local spectral emission.

- Has the patient experienced trauma, overuse, or sudden twisting?
- Are there localized pain, tenderness, or muscle tightness?

Hypoemission suggests chronic muscle hypoperfusion, fibrosis, or neurogenic atrophy.

- Are there complaints of weakness, stiffness, or limited range of motion?
- Is muscle wasting or altered sensation present?

Step 5: Confirmatory Evaluations

Test	Purpose & Justification	Relevance to Emissive Pattern
Creatine kinase (CK), LDH	Detects muscle injury or inflammation (Simons et al., 1999).	Elevated in hyperemissive tissue activation states.
MRI	Visualizes muscle edema, inflammation, or fibrosis.	Supports hyper- or hypoemissive zone expressions.
Electromyography (EMG)	Assesses muscle and nerve function.	Correlates with hypoemissive neurofunctional patterns.
Blood tests (CBC, inflammatory markers)	Detects systemic inflammation or infection.	Supports hyperemissive regulatory field activity.

Step 6: Care Strategies and Intervention Pathways

Naturopathic Approach

Anti-inflammatory botanicals such as *Curcuma longa* and *Boswellia serrata* reduce muscle inflammation (Hewlings & Kalman, 2017). Magnesium supports muscle relaxation. Hydrotherapy with alternating warm and cold applications enhances circulation (Sutkowy et al., 2019). Gentle stretching and progressive strengthening promote recovery. Adequate protein and antioxidants support tissue repair.

Standard Medical Approaches

Rest, NSAIDs, and physical therapy are standard treatments for muscle injuries (Simons et al., 1999). Neurological evaluation is recommended if weakness is present.

Specialty / Practitioner Care Strategies Table

Specialty Group	Practitioners Included	Hyperemissive Strategies	Hypoemissive Strategies
Biochemistry	Nutritionists, Orthomolecular, Herbalists, Naturopaths	Anti-inflammatory botanicals, magnesium, antioxidants, protein	Circulatory support, neurotrophic nutrients, protein support
Rehabilitation	Physiotherapists, Massage Therapists, Osteopaths / Chiropractors	Myofascial release, trigger point therapy, gentle massage	Graded aerobic exercise, neurorehabilitation, ergonomic guidance
Energetics	Acupuncturists (TCM), Bioenergetic Therapists	Acupuncture, moxibustion, PEMF	Warming acupuncture, frequency therapy
Psychological	GNM practitioners, Psychotherapists, Vibrational therapists, Family constellation facilitators	Psychotherapy, bioresonance, mindfulness	Psychosomatic conflict resolution, emotional balancing

Educational Pearls & Considerations.

- Early identification of myofascial trigger points improves prognosis.
- Magnesium aids muscle relaxation and reduces spasms.
- Hydrotherapy should be tailored to inflammation phases.
- Neurological assessment is essential when weakness or sensory changes occur.
- Gradual rehabilitation prevents chronic dysfunction.

GROUP 2 - ZONE 10 – LATERAL RIGHT ABDOMEN

Category 4: *Nervous*

Step 1: Functional Anatomy and Interpretive Importance

The lateral right abdominal wall receives innervation from lower thoracic nerves (T7–T12) together with the iliohypogastric and ilioinguinal nerves, which supply motor control to the lateral abdominal muscles and sensory input to overlying skin (Standring, 2016).

These nerves are frequently involved in postoperative entrapments or radiculopathic syndromes that radiate pain along the abdominal flank. Hershfield (1992) described chronic abdominal wall pain as a common yet underdiagnosed condition often caused by nerve entrapment in this distribution. Such disturbances affect sensation and autonomic regulation, modifying perfusion and fascial tone in the lateral wall.

The altered regulatory state is reflected externally, with biospectral asymmetries appearing as focal fields tracking obliquely along the abdominal contour. Unlike the broad emissions associated with muscular overload, these signals align with nerve pathways, providing clinicians with a visible marker of neurogenic disturbance in the flank region.

Step 2,3,4: ROI Classification and Interpretive Questions

Hyperemission suggests nerve irritation or neurogenic reactivity.

- Are there burning, tingling, or sharp pains?
- Is localized hypersensitivity or swelling noted?

Hypoemission indicates nerve hypoperfusion, compression, or denervation leading to reduced autonomic function.

- Are numbness, weakness, or muscle wasting present?
- Do symptoms worsen with movement or certain positions?

Step 5: Confirmatory Evaluations

Test	Purpose & Justification	Relevance to Emissive Pattern
Nerve conduction studies (NCS), Electromyography (EMG)	Evaluate nerve and muscle function (Janis et al., 2010).	Correlates with hypoemissive neurofunctional suppression.
Quantitative sensory testing (QST)	Measures sensory nerve thresholds.	Supports interpretation of neurofunctional patterns.
Ultrasound / MRI	Detects nerve entrapment or structural abnormalities.	Identifies nerve field restriction or signal disruption.
Blood tests (glucose, vitamin B12)	Assesses metabolic causes of neuropathy.	Supports interpretation of patterns consistent with metabolic neuroregulation.

Step 6: Care Strategies and Intervention Pathways

Naturopathic Approach

Use B-complex vitamins, alpha-lipoic acid, and Acetyl-L-carnitine to support nerve regeneration (Papanas & Ziegler, 2014). Herbal anti-inflammatories such as *Hypericum perforatum* may reduce neuropathic pain (Kasper et al., 2010). Neural mobilization and bioresonance aid recovery. Mind-body therapies modulate neurovascular function.

Standard Medical Approaches

Pharmacological treatment includes anticonvulsants, antidepressants, and analgesics. Surgical decompression may be necessary. Metabolic control is essential in systemic neuropathies.

Specialty / Practitioner Care Strategies Table

Specialty Group	Practitioners Included	Hyperemissive Strategies	Hypoemissive Strategies
Biochemistry	Nutritionists, Orthomolecular, Herbalists, Naturopaths	Neurotrophic vitamins, alpha-lipoic acid, anti-inflammatory botanicals	Circulatory stimulants, metabolic support, neuroprotective nutrients
Rehabilitation	Physiotherapists, Massage Therapists, Osteopaths / Chiropractors	Neural mobilization, myofascial release, gentle massage	Neural gliding exercises, ergonomic guidance, neurorehabilitation
Energetics	Acupuncturists (TCM), Bioenergetic Therapists	Acupuncture, moxibustion, PEMF	Warming acupuncture, frequency therapy, energy healing
Psychological	GNM practitioners, Psychotherapists, Vibrational therapists, Family constellation facilitators	Psychotherapy, bioresonance, mindfulness	Psychosomatic conflict resolution, vibrational medicine

Educational Pearls & Considerations.

- Early diagnosis reduces risk of chronic nerve damage.
- Nutritional and energetic support enhances nerve repair.
- Monitor metabolic contributors such as diabetes.
- Avoid aggressive treatment during acute inflammation.
- Tailor neural mobilization to patient tolerance.

GROUP 2 - ZONE 10 – LATERAL RIGHT ABDOMEN

Category 5: *Lymphatic*

Step 1: Functional Anatomy and Interpretive Importance

The lateral abdominal wall is drained by superficial lymphatics running with cutaneous vessels and deeper channels accompanying the intercostal and lumbar vasculature, converging toward both axillary and inguinal stations (Standring, 2016).

This network ensures balance of interstitial fluid and maintains immune integrity of the flank. Mehrara and Zampell (2008) described truncal lymphedema as a frequent sequela of oncologic procedures, often first presenting with localized fullness or tension in the lateral abdomen. Functional compromise in this region alters both fascial dynamics and perfusion tone, producing a signature that extends outward to the surface.

Externally, these disturbances appear as oblique emissive fields tracing the contour of the abdominal wall, sharper in outline than the broader activations of oblique musculature. The visibility of such patterns helps clinicians identify lymphatic involvement in cases of chronic flank discomfort or unresolved edema, clarifying when immune drainage dysfunction is a primary driver.

Step 2,3,4: ROI Classification and Interpretive Questions

Hyperemission indicates acute lymphatic reactivity, microbial activity, or congestion with swelling and spectral intensification.

- Is there redness, tenderness, or rapid swelling?
- Has the patient experienced recent infection or injury?

Hypoemission suggests chronic lymphatic stasis with fibrosis and impaired drainage causing reduced biosignal.

- Is swelling persistent and firm?
- Are recurrent infections or delayed wound healing present?

Step 5: Confirmatory Evaluations

Test	Purpose & Justification	Relevance to Emissive Pattern
Lymphoscintigraphy	Evaluates lymphatic flow and obstruction.	Confirms lymphatic retention or reduced perfusion.
Doppler ultrasound	Excludes venous insufficiency contributing to swelling.	Differentiates vascular from lymphatic signal behavior.
Blood tests (CBC, inflammatory markers)	Detect infection or systemic inflammation.	Supports hyperemissive tissue activation states.
Physical exam (Stemmer's sign, limb measurements)	Identifies clinical signs of lymphedema.	Correlates with biospectral imaging patterns.

Step 6: Care Strategies and Intervention Pathways

Naturopathic Approach

Stimulate lymphatic drainage with herbal lymphagogues such as *Hedera helix* and *Vitis vinifera* (Godoy et al., 2012). Manual lymphatic drainage by trained therapists improves fluid movement. Compression therapy supports lymph return and must be individualized. Nutritional antioxidants and anti-inflammatory nutrients promote tissue repair. Hydrotherapy with alternating warm and cold applications enhances lymphatic circulation.

Standard Medical Approaches

Standard treatments include manual lymphatic drainage, compression garments, physical therapy, and infection control. Surgery is considered in refractory cases.

Specialty / Practitioner Care Strategies Table

Specialty Group	Practitioners Included	Hyperemissive Strategies	Hypoemissive Strategies
Biochemistry	Nutritionists, Orthomolecular, Herbalists, Naturopaths	Herbal lymphagogues, antioxidants, anti-inflammatory nutrients	Circulatory support, nutritional tissue repair support
Rehabilitation	Physiotherapists, Massage Therapists, Osteopaths / Chiropractors	Manual lymphatic drainage, gentle massage, postural retraining	Compression therapy, graded exercise, ergonomic guidance
Energetics	Acupuncturists (TCM), Bioenergetic Therapists	Acupuncture, herbal formulas, PEMF	Warming acupuncture, energy balancing
Psychological	GNM practitioners, Psychotherapists, Vibrational therapists, Family constellation facilitators	Mind-body therapies supporting immune function and healing	Psychosomatic conflict resolution, emotional balancing

Educational Pearls & Considerations.

- Early treatment prevents chronic lymphedema progression.
- Manual lymphatic drainage should be performed by certified therapists.
- Compression therapy requires proper fitting and monitoring.
- Nutritional support enhances lymphatic and tissue health.
- Prompt infection treatment is essential to prevent worsening.

GROUP 2 - ZONE 10 – LATERAL RIGHT ABDOMEN

Category 6: *Organ-related (GNM)*

Step 1: **Functional Anatomy and Interpretive Importance**

The lateral right abdominal wall covers hepatic and biliary structures, including portions of the liver, gallbladder, and ascending colon, framed by the oblique musculature (Standring, 2016).

Within GNM, conflicts tied to territorial control or survival often engage these organs, producing distinct biosignal phases. Hamer (2012) explained that active conflicts correspond to hypoemissive suppression, while resolution and repair are characterized by hyperemissive fields.

These external patterns align with visceral rather than muscular geometry, often appearing oblique along the right flank. Ader (2007) expanded on how psychoneuroimmunology links psychosocial stressors to immune regulation and organ adaptation, reinforcing that stress-induced hepatic and biliary changes can manifest peripherally.

Observed emissive variations in this region therefore serve as visible correlates of psychosomatic conflicts, guiding interpretation of right-sided abdominal dysfunction beyond purely structural causes.

Step 2,3,4: **ROI Classification and Interpretive Questions**

Hyperemission reflects the reactive or post-conflict repair phase of an organ conflict, associated with increased metabolic activity.

- Are there symptoms such as localized pain, swelling, or functional disturbance?
- Is there evidence of inflammation or infection?

Hypoemission corresponds to the conflict-active phase involving tissue loss or functional suppression.

- Are there chronic symptoms, fatigue, or reduced organ function?
- Is psychological stress or unresolved conflict present?

Step 5: **Confirmatory Evaluations**

Test	Purpose & Justification	Relevance to Emissive Pattern
Ultrasound / CT / MRI imaging	Visualizes organ structure, inflammation, or lesions.	Correlates with emissive anomalies suggesting organ field engagement.
Liver function tests (ALT, AST, bilirubin)	Assesses hepatic injury or dysfunction.	Supports hyperemissive activation in hepatic terrain.
Gallbladder imaging (ultrasound)	Detects cholelithiasis or inflammation.	Correlates with localized biospectral changes.

Complete blood count (CBC), inflammatory markers	Detects systemic inflammation or infection.	Supports hyperemissive expression during conflict-related phases.
Psychological assessment	Evaluates underlying biological conflicts and stressors.	Complements the GNM interpretive framework.

Step 6: Care Strategies and Intervention Pathways

Naturopathic Approach

Use hepatoprotective botanicals such as *Silybum marianum* (milk thistle) and *Curcuma longa* (turmeric) to support liver and gallbladder function (Friedman et al., 2017). Promote digestive health with probiotics and bile-supportive nutrients. Psychotherapy and stress management facilitate conflict resolution. Nutritional antioxidants and anti-inflammatory compounds aid tissue repair.

Standard Medical Approaches

Imaging and labs guide medical or surgical management of organ pathology. Pharmacological treatments and lifestyle modifications are utilized as needed.

Specialty / Practitioner Care Strategies Table

Specialty Group	Practitioners Included	Hyperemissive Strategies	Hypoemissive Strategies
Biochemistry	Nutritionists, Orthomolecular, Herbalists, Naturopaths	Hepatoprotective herbs, antioxidants, digestive support	Nutritional support for organ function
Rehabilitation	Physiotherapists, Massage Therapists, Osteopaths / Chiropractors	Supportive therapies promoting relaxation and circulation	Gentle mobilization and relaxation techniques
Energetics	Acupuncturists (TCM), Bioenergetic Therapists	Acupuncture for organ function and inflammation	Energy balancing and harmonization
Psychological	GNM practitioners, Psychotherapists, Vibrational therapists, Family constellation facilitators	Psychotherapy, bioresonance, conflict resolution	Emotional balancing and stress reduction

Educational Pearls & Considerations.

- Address the psychosomatic root per GNM principles alongside physical treatment.
- Monitor organ function closely with appropriate testing.
- Support both psychological and physiological healing.
- Coordinate multidisciplinary care for best outcomes.

GROUP 2 - ZONE 10 – LATERAL RIGHT ABDOMEN

Category 7: *Acupuncture / Meridian*

Step 1: Functional Anatomy and Interpretive Importance

The right lateral abdomen integrates oblique musculature with fascial planes overlying the liver and gallbladder (Standring, 2016). In acupuncture theory, this zone is traversed by the Gallbladder (GB) and Triple Burner (San Jiao, SJ) meridians.

Maciocia (2015) emphasized the GB channel's role in decision-making, bile regulation, and muscular tone along the lateral trunk. Cheng (1987) described the SJ meridian as critical for fluid transformation and coordination between upper and lower body systems.

Clinically, disruptions are associated with flank pain, digestive complaints, or impaired energy flow. On emissive imaging, asymmetrical patterns emerge obliquely across the lateral trunk, mapping closely to GB and SJ trajectories. T

heir sharp alignment distinguishes them from diffuse muscular activation, supporting the view that biospectral variations along the right flank may externalize functional imbalance in gallbladder or hepatobiliary regulation.

Step 2,3,4: ROI Classification and Interpretive Questions

Hyperemission indicates Qi stagnation or energetic reactivity along the meridians.

- Is there localized tenderness, distension, or sharp pain?
- Are symptoms worsened by stress or diet?

Hypoemission suggests Qi deficiency or chronic stagnation causing poor circulation and cold sensations.

- Does the patient report fatigue, coldness, or digestive sluggishness?
- Are symptoms persistent or chronic?

Step 5: Confirmatory Evaluations

Test	Purpose & Justification	Relevance to Emissive Pattern
Pulse diagnosis and tongue examination	Traditional TCM diagnostic tools assessing Qi and blood status (Flaws, 2000).	Correlates with emissive patterns to refine interpretation.
Biospectral imaging	Detects emissive asymmetries along meridian pathways.	Visualizes hyper- or hypoemissive meridian zones.
Patient symptom questionnaire	Assesses digestive symptoms, energy levels, and pain patterns.	Supports differentiation of Qi stagnation vs Qi deficiency.

Step 6: Care Strategies and Intervention Pathways

Naturopathic Approach

Acupuncture points such as GB34, GB41, and SJ6 regulate meridian flow and relieve stagnation (Lao et al., 2004). Moxibustion warms hypoemissive meridians. Herbal formulas including *Xiao Yao San* and *Chai Hu Shu Gan San* harmonize liver and gallbladder Qi (Bensky et al., 2004). Dietary adjustments complement therapy.

Standard Medical Approaches

Acupuncture is used adjunctively for symptom relief in digestive and musculoskeletal disorders affecting this region.

Specialty / Practitioner Care Strategies Table

Specialty Group	Practitioners Included	Hyperemissive Strategies	Hypoemissive Strategies
Biochemistry	Nutritionists, Orthomolecular, Herbalists, Naturopaths	Herbal formulas for Qi regulation, antioxidants	Qi tonics, digestive support supplements
Rehabilitation	Physiotherapists, Massage Therapists, Osteopaths / Chiropractors	Abdominal massage, myofascial release	Gentle mobilization, warming massage
Energetics	Acupuncturists (TCM), Bioenergetic Therapists	Acupuncture, moxibustion, PEMF	Warming acupuncture, energy balancing
Psychological	GNM practitioners, Psychotherapists, Vibrational therapists, Family constellation facilitators	Mind-body therapies, bioresonance, energy clearing	Psychosomatic conflict resolution, emotional balancing

Educational Pearls & Considerations.

- Accurate point selection tailors treatment to biospectral pattern.
- Moxibustion requires caution in heat-sensitive patients.
- Herbal treatments should be supervised by qualified professionals.
- Combine acupuncture with dietary and physical therapies for best outcomes.

GROUP 2 - ZONE 10 – LATERAL RIGHT ABDOMEN

Category 8: *Energetic*

Step 1: Functional Anatomy and Interpretive Importance

The lateral right abdomen overlays the oblique musculature, fascial layers, and visceral fields related to the liver and ascending colon (Standring, 2016). Energetically, this area reflects themes of processing, detoxification, and directional flow.

Popp and Beloussov (2003) described biophoton emissions as markers of cellular communication, offering a plausible foundation for spectral surface signals in this zone. Patients often describe localized discomfort, tension, or diffuse fatigue linked to digestive irregularities.

Spectral imaging may reveal hypoemissive fields along oblique fascial lines consistent with slowed energetic processing, or focal hyperemissive bursts corresponding to adaptive repair.

These emissive variations integrate both local fascial currents and systemic energy dynamics, enabling a layered interpretation that surpasses structural explanation. The lateral right abdomen thus serves as an emissive indicator of systemic processing, where biofield irregularities often parallel visceral and metabolic stress.

Step 2,3,4: ROI Classification and Interpretive Questions

Hyperemission indicates localized energy congestion or field reactivity.

- Does the patient experience sensations of heat, tension, or discomfort?
- Are stress or emotional factors exacerbating symptoms?

Hypoemission suggests energy deficiency or stagnation.

- Does the patient report fatigue, coldness, or decreased vitality?
- Are symptoms chronic or refractory to conventional treatments?

Step 5: Confirmatory Evaluations

Test	Purpose & Justification	Relevance to Emissive Pattern
Bioresonance testing	Measures tissue energy frequencies and imbalances.	Correlates with emissive anomalies.
Electrodermal screening (EDS)	Assesses skin conductance linked to energy pathways.	Supports interpretation of energetic imbalances.
Patient emotional and symptom history	Provides clinical context for energetic dysfunction.	Assists in differential interpretation.

Step 6: Care Strategies and Intervention Pathways

Naturopathic Approach

Employ bioresonance, pulsed electromagnetic fields (PEMF), and adaptogenic herbs to restore energetic balance and promote healing (Matsumoto et al., 2010). Nutritional antioxidants and adaptogens support systemic resilience. Mindfulness and stress reduction techniques complement energetic therapies.

Standard Medical Approaches

Energetic therapies serve as adjuncts to conventional and rehabilitative treatments to optimize patient outcomes.

Specialty / Practitioner Care Strategies Table

Specialty Group	Practitioners Included	Hyperemissive Strategies	Hypoemissive Strategies
Biochemistry	Nutritionists, Orthomolecular, Herbalists, Naturopaths	Adaptogens, antioxidants, herbal energetics	Nutritional support for energy deficiency
Rehabilitation	Physiotherapists, Massage Therapists, Osteopaths / Chiropractors	Energy-based manual therapies, PEMF, therapeutic touch	Gentle stimulation, mobilization
Energetics	Acupuncturists (TCM), Bioenergetic Therapists	Bioresonance, PEMF, acupuncture	Warming acupuncture, energy balancing
Psychological	GNM practitioners, Psychotherapists, Vibrational therapists, Family constellation facilitators	Psychotherapy, bioresonance, mindfulness	Emotional balancing, vibrational medicine

Educational Pearls & Considerations.

- Energetic therapies complement but do not replace conventional care.
- Patient responsiveness and practitioner expertise influence outcomes.
- Regular reassessment ensures therapy adapts to clinical changes.
- Address psychological and physical factors holistically.

GROUP 2 - ZONE 10 – LATERAL RIGHT ABDOMEN

Category 9: *Metabolic / Endocrine*

Step 1: Functional Anatomy and Interpretive Importance

The lateral right abdomen overlies the oblique musculature, hepatic field, and ascending colon (Standring, 2016). Endocrine and metabolic disturbances such as diabetes, dyslipidemia, or thyroid dysfunction often manifest here through vascular and reparative irregularities.

Vinik et al. (2003) emphasized the link between metabolic disease and peripheral neuropathy, which extends to abdominal fascial signaling. Clinically, patients may report right-sided tension, digestive irregularities, or unexplained fatigue.

Spectral surface readings highlight hypoemissive streaks consistent with perfusion decline and neural suppression, while patchy hyperemissive zones suggest adaptive hepatic or metabolic activation.

These emissive signatures extend across fascial lines, illustrating how systemic endocrine dysfunction translates into peripheral surface irregularities. The lateral right abdomen thus provides biospectral insight into systemic glycoregulatory burden and hepatic-metabolic integration.

Step 2,3,4: ROI Classification and Interpretive Questions

Hyperemission reflects localized reactivity, microbial activity, or metabolic overactivity.

- Is there warmth, redness, or swelling?
- Is metabolic control adequate?

Hypoemission indicates hypoperfusion, neuropathy, or impaired perfusion due to metabolic/endocrine causes.

- Are cold sensations, numbness, or chronic wounds present?
- Are systemic symptoms such as fatigue or temperature intolerance reported?

Step 5: Confirmatory Evaluations

Test	Purpose & Justification	Relevance to Emissive Pattern
HbA1c, fasting glucose	Assesses glycemic control in diabetes.	Correlates with hypoemissive neurofunctional or perfusion-restricted zones.
Thyroid function tests (TSH, Free T4)	Evaluates thyroid disorders affecting metabolism and circulation.	Associated with altered emissive regulation.

Lipid profile	Assesses cardiovascular risk impacting tissue perfusion.	Supports metabolic vascular adaptation.
Inflammatory markers (CRP, ESR)	Detects systemic inflammation influencing tissue health.	Correlates with hyperemissive tissue activation states.

Step 6: Care Strategies and Intervention Pathways

Naturopathic Approach

Promote metabolic health with a low glycemic diet, antioxidants, and adaptogens (Alberti et al., 2006). Herbs such as *Panax ginseng* and *Gymnema sylvestre* support endocrine function. Supplement chromium, magnesium, and alpha-lipoic acid to enhance glucose metabolism and neuroprotection. Regular aerobic exercise improves circulation.

Standard Medical Approaches

Pharmacologic and lifestyle interventions target metabolic control. Thyroid hormone replacement and lipid management reduce complications.

Specialty / Practitioner Care Strategies Table

Specialty Group	Practitioners Included	Hyperemissive Strategies	Hypoemissive Strategies
Biochemistry	Nutritionists, Orthomolecular, Herbalists, Naturopaths	Antioxidants, adaptogens, insulin sensitizers, micronutrients	Metabolic support, neuroprotective nutrients, dietary management
Rehabilitation	Physiotherapists, Massage Therapists, Osteopaths / Chiropractors	Exercise therapy, circulation enhancement	Neuromuscular re-education, aerobic conditioning
Energetics	Acupuncturists (TCM), Bioenergetic Therapists	Acupuncture supporting metabolic function	Energy balancing, PEMF
Psychological	GNM practitioners, Psychotherapists, Vibrational therapists, Family constellation facilitators	Mind-body therapies supporting metabolic regulation	Stress reduction, emotional balancing

Educational Pearls & Considerations.

- Regular metabolic monitoring prevents complications.
- Lifestyle and dietary modifications complement clinical treatment.
- Adaptogens support but do not replace conventional therapies.
- Patient education on skin and wound care is critical.

GROUP 2

ZONE 11 – LATERAL LEFT ABDOMEN

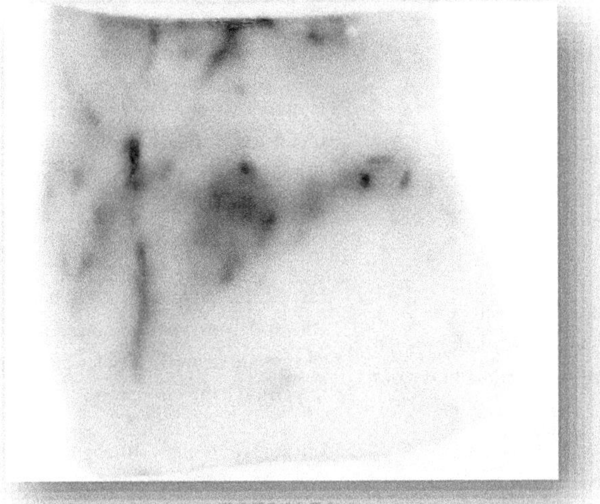

G2Z11LFA

The lateral left abdomen comprisees the oblique musculature, fascial layers, and superficial vasculature, overlying the spleen, portions of the pancreas, the descending colon, and the upper pole of the left kidney. This region represents a dense convergence of metabolic and immune-related structures, making it one of the most emissively responsive abdominal surfaces (Standring, 2016).

Clinically, emissive asymmetries here often correspond to splenic congestion or pancreatic activation, both of which may precede structural or biochemical signs. The spleen, as a major lymphoid organ, enlarges with infectious or hematologic stress, present in up to 30–50% of chronic conditions (Broudy, 2004), while pancreatic microcirculatory changes have been shown to precede detectable tissue damage in metabolic disease (Ishikawa et al., 2009).

Fascial mechanics reinforce the significance of this region: the lateral abdominal wall integrates into the thoracolumbar fascia, and strain may manifest as emissive disturbances reflecting systemic postural compensation (Willard et al., 2012). Lymphatic pathways here also drain both pelvic and lower limb territories, making localized retention patterns systemically relevant.

Gastrointestinal regulation adds another layer, as left-sided colonic stasis in constipation has been linked to altered microperfusion (Camilleri, 2001). In metabolic contexts, asymmetries may accompany splenic enlargement from portal hypertension, offering a non-invasive marker of visceral adaptation (D'Amico et al., 2006).

Taken together, the lateral left abdomen functions as a sensitive diagnostic surface linking immune surveillance, digestive motility, fascial tension, and vascular balance. Its strength lies in revealing immune and metabolic strain early, providing terrain-level markers of adaptation that complement anatomical imaging and support timely clinical intervention.

Zone 11 – Lateral Left Abdomen: Emission-Relevant Structures

Category	Relevant Structures	Emission Relevance
1. Vascular / Circulatory	- Splenic artery and vein - Left renal artery branches - Inferior mesenteric artery (left branch) - Superficial abdominal veins	Hyperemission may indicate visceral signal intensification or tissue activation, including splenic congestion or left colonic irritation. Hypoemission may suggest vascular spasm or sympathetic vasoconstriction limiting perfusion.
2. Muscular / Myofascial	- External oblique (left side) - Internal oblique (left side) - Transversus abdominis (left side)	Hyperemissive patterns often relate to muscular overuse, fascial activation, or postural compensations. Hypoemission may be due to chronic disuse, fascial adhesions, or myofascial restrictions impairing local circulation.
3. Skeletal / Articular	- Left lower ribs - Costal cartilages - Lumbar vertebrae (left lateral aspect)	Local Hyperemission may reflect periosteal signal activation or field changes in ribs or vertebrae. Hypoemission may suggest chronic degenerative changes or reduced bone metabolism in these areas.
4. Nervous System / Spine	- Intercostal nerves (left T8-T12) - Sympathetic ganglia - Lumbar plexus branches	Hyperemissive zones may signal neural field irritation or tissue-level activation; Hypoemission can indicate nerve compression, neurofunctional suppression, or autonomic dysfunction affecting left-sided somatic and visceral innervation.
5. Lymphatic / Immune	- Superficial lymphatic vessels draining left abdomen - Left inguinal and axillary lymph nodes	Hyperemission often correlates with immune-related tissue activity or lymphatic field reactivity; Hypoemission may reflect lymphatic congestion, fibrosis, or immune suppression in drainage pathways.
6. Organs / GNM (German New Medicine)	- Spleen - Pancreas (body and tail) - Left colon (splenic flexure) - Left kidney (upper pole)	Elevated emissive activity may indicate active visceral conflict, immune field stress, or regulatory disturbance. Hypoemission corresponds to healing phases or functional suppression mediated by viscerosomatic reflex mechanisms.
7. Acupuncture / Meridians	- Spleen Meridian (left abdomen) - Pancreas influence - Kidney Meridian	Emissive patterns suggest Qi stagnation or excess; low-emission zones may indicate Qi deficiency, dampness, or blood stasis affecting digestive, pancreatic, and renal functions.
8. Energetic / Frequency	- Reflex zones associated with pancreatic and splenic energetics and detoxification pathways	Hyperemission may be related to bioenergetic activation or stress responses; Hypoemission may reflect regulatory depletion or impaired excretory mobilization.
9. Metabolic / Endocrine	- Reflex zones for pancreatic endocrine function, adrenal influence, and metabolic regulation	Hypoemissive emissive patterns may indicate metabolic regulation decline, adrenal underperformance, or pancreatic signal suppression. Persistent Hyperemission may represent metabolic overload or regulatory stress in the left abdominal organs.

GROUP 2 - ZONE 11 – LATERAL LEFT ABDOMEN

Category 1: *Vascular / Circulatory*

Step 1: Functional Anatomy and Interpretive Importance

The lateral left abdominal wall receives arterial supply from branches of the intercostal, subcostal, and lumbar arteries, in combination with tributaries from the inferior epigastric system. These vessels perfuse the oblique and transversus abdominis muscles as well as the associated fascial layers.

Venous return follows intercostal and lumbar veins, which communicate with the azygos and femoral systems (Standring, 2016). Anatomical studies of abdominal angiosomes emphasize the importance of these segmental vessels in flap surgery and reconstructive planning (Taylor & Palmer, 1987).

Spectral surface readings of the left lateral abdomen often reveal band-like emissive patterns aligned with these vascular territories. Such findings may represent localized strain within the oblique musculature, adaptive circulatory changes from visceral pressure, or venous stasis in segmental tributaries.

This zone therefore provides a functional window into how lateral abdominal circulation responds to mechanical and visceral demands.

Step 2,3,4: ROI Classification and Interpretive Questions

Hyperemission indicates vascular reactivity, venous congestion, or thrombophlebitis.

- Are there localized swelling, redness, or tenderness?
- Are systemic symptoms such as fever present?

Hypoemission suggests hypoperfusion or vascular compromise.

- Are there complaints of coldness, pallor, or delayed healing?
- Is there a history of vascular disease?

Step 5: Confirmatory Evaluations

Test	Purpose & Justification	Relevance to Emissive Pattern
Doppler ultrasound	Evaluates arterial and venous flow in abdominal wall vessels.	Correlates hyperemissive tissue activation and hypoemissive perfusion decline.
CT or MRI angiography	Visualizes vessel patency and identifies occlusions or thrombosis.	Confirms vascular flow disruption or signal intensification.
Blood tests (CBC, CRP, coagulation profile)	Detect infection, inflammation, or coagulation disorders.	Supports hyperemissive retention or circulatory impedance states.
Physical exam	Inspects and palpates for local signs of vascular compromise.	Complements biospectral findings.

Step 6: Care Strategies and Intervention Pathways

Naturopathic Approach

Botanical venotonics such as *Aesculus hippocastanum* and *Ruscus aculeatus* improve microcirculation and reduce edema (Chrubasik et al., 2011). An anti-inflammatory diet rich in antioxidants and omega-3 fatty acids supports vascular health (Calder, 2017). Contrast hydrotherapy with warm and cold applications stimulates circulation (Sutkowy et al., 2019). Vitamins C, E, and bioflavonoids enhance endothelial function. Limb elevation and gentle massage promote venous return.

Standard Medical Approaches

Imaging guides anticoagulation, anti-inflammatory medication, or surgical intervention as needed. Managing systemic contributors such as coagulopathies is critical.

Specialty / Practitioner Care Strategies Table

Specialty Group	Practitioners Included	Hyperemissive Strategies	Hypoemissive Strategies
Biochemistry	Nutritionists, Orthomolecular, Herbalists, Naturopaths	Botanical venotonics, antioxidants, anti-inflammatory diet	Circulatory stimulants, nutritional endothelial support
Rehabilitation	Physiotherapists, Massage Therapists, Osteopaths / Chiropractors	Gentle massage, lymphatic drainage, postural correction	Graded exercise, circulatory enhancement
Energetics	Acupuncturists (TCM), Bioenergetic Therapists	Acupuncture, moxibustion, herbal formulas	Warming acupuncture, energy balancing
Psychological	GNM practitioners, Psychotherapists, Vibrational therapists, Family constellation facilitators	Psychotherapy, bioresonance, mindfulness	Stress reduction, emotional balancing

Educational Pearls & Considerations.

- Prompt diagnosis of thrombophlebitis or vascular inflammation is critical.
- Botanical venotonics combined with diet and hydrotherapy support vascular health effectively.
- Nitric oxide donors and omega-3 fatty acids enhance endothelial function and perfusion.
- Compression therapy is contraindicated in severe arterial insufficiency.
- Early mobilization and limb elevation prevent chronic complications.

GROUP 2 - ZONE 11 – LATERAL LEFT ABDOMEN

Category 2: *Muscular*

Step 1: Functional Anatomy and Interpretive Importance

The left lateral abdominal wall is structured by the external and internal obliques together with the transversus abdominis, each contributing to trunk rotation, lateral flexion, and abdominal wall stability.

These layers, innervated by thoracoabdominal nerves, interlace through aponeurotic connections that converge at the linea alba, ensuring force transfer between the thorax and pelvis (Standring, 2016).

Electromyographic studies confirm that delayed or asymmetric activation of the oblique system is strongly associated with recurrent low-back pain and reduced spinal control (Hodges & Richardson, 1997).

In spectral assessment, the oblique fiber direction often appears as diagonal emissive gradients, reflecting altered tension or adaptive stabilization during asymmetric load. These irregularities frequently coincide with clinical reports of trunk imbalance, offering a biosignal correlate of compromised lumbopelvic mechanics.

Step 2,3,4: ROI Classification and Interpretive Questions

Hyperemission suggests acute muscle strain, muscular reactivity, or active trigger points with increased local spectral emission.

- Has the patient had recent overuse or trauma?
- Are there localized pain, tenderness, or muscle tightness?

Hypoemission indicates chronic muscle hypoperfusion, fibrosis, or neurogenic atrophy.

- Are symptoms of weakness, stiffness, or reduced mobility present?
- Is muscle wasting or altered sensation noted?

Step 5: Confirmatory Evaluations

Test	Purpose & Justification	Relevance to Emissive Pattern
Creatine kinase (CK), LDH	Detects muscle injury or inflammation (Simons et al., 1999).	Elevated in hyperemissive tissue activation states.
MRI	Visualizes muscle edema, fibrosis, or inflammation.	Supports hyper- or hypoemissive findings.
Electromyography (EMG)	Assesses muscle and nerve function.	Correlates with hypoemissive neurofunctional causes.
Blood tests (CBC, inflammatory markers)	Detects systemic inflammation or infection.	Supports hyperemissive regulatory field conditions.

Step 6: Care Strategies and Intervention Pathways

Naturopathic Approach

Use anti-inflammatory botanicals such as *Curcuma longa* and *Boswellia serrata* to reduce muscle inflammation (Hewlings & Kalman, 2017). Magnesium supplementation supports muscle relaxation. Hydrotherapy with alternating warm and cold applications enhances circulation (Sutkowy et al., 2019). Progressive stretching and strengthening promote recovery. Adequate protein and antioxidants support tissue repair.

Standard Medical Approaches

Rest, NSAIDs, and physical therapy are standard treatments for muscle injuries (Simons et al., 1999). Neurological assessment is recommended if weakness or sensory changes occur.

Specialty / Practitioner Care Strategies Table

Specialty Group	Practitioners Included	Hyperemissive Strategies	Hypoemissive Strategies
Biochemistry	Nutritionists, Orthomolecular, Herbalists, Naturopaths	Anti-inflammatory botanicals, magnesium, antioxidants, protein	Circulatory support, neurotrophic nutrients, protein support
Rehabilitation	Physiotherapists, Massage Therapists, Osteopaths / Chiropractors	Myofascial release, trigger point therapy, gentle massage	Graded aerobic exercise, neurorehabilitation, ergonomic guidance
Energetics	Acupuncturists (TCM), Bioenergetic Therapists	Acupuncture, moxibustion, PEMF	Warming acupuncture, frequency therapy
Psychological	GNM practitioners, Psychotherapists, Vibrational therapists, Family constellation facilitators	Psychotherapy, bioresonance, mindfulness	Psychosomatic conflict resolution, emotional balancing

Educational Pearls & Considerations.

- Early identification of myofascial trigger points improves prognosis.
- Magnesium supports muscle relaxation and reduces spasms.
- Hydrotherapy should be tailored to inflammation phases.
- Neurological evaluation is essential when weakness or sensory changes are present.
- Gradual rehabilitation prevents chronic dysfunction.

GROUP 2 - ZONE 11 – LATERAL LEFT ABDOMEN

Category 4: *Nervous*

Step 1: Functional Anatomy and Interpretive Importance

The lateral left abdominal wall mirrors the right, receiving innervation from thoracic spinal nerves (T7–T12) and the iliohypogastric and ilioinguinal branches that supply both muscular and cutaneous territories (Standring, 2016).

Compression or entrapment of these nerves is a recognized source of chronic flank pain, often mistaken for visceral pathology. Greenbaum et al. (1994) emphasized that flank pain of neural origin is underdiagnosed and can mimic renal or gastrointestinal disorders. These neuropathic disturbances alter local recruitment and sympathetic regulation, projecting their effects to the surface as distinctive emissive signals.

On spectral surface analysis, biospectral asymmetries in this region often trace oblique lines consistent with nerve pathways, appearing sharper than diffuse muscular fields. Such patterns provide clinicians with an externalized marker of neural compromise, helping to separate abdominal wall neuropathies from visceral causes of lateral abdominal pain.

Step 2,3,4: ROI Classification and Interpretive Questions

Hyperemission indicates nerve irritation or neurogenic reactivity.

- Are there burning, tingling, or sharp pains?
- Is localized hypersensitivity or swelling noted?

Hypoemission suggests nerve hypoperfusion, compression, or denervation with reduced autonomic activity.

- Are numbness, weakness, or muscle atrophy present?
- Do symptoms worsen with movement or certain postures?

Step 5: Confirmatory Evaluations

Test	Purpose & Justification	Relevance to Emissive Pattern
Nerve conduction studies (NCS), Electromyography (EMG)	Assess nerve and muscle function (Janis et al., 2010).	Correlates with hypoemissive neurofunctional dysfunction.
Quantitative sensory testing (QST)	Measures sensory nerve thresholds.	Supports interpretation of neurofunctional patterns.
Ultrasound / MRI	Detects nerve entrapment or structural abnormalities.	Identifies nerve field compression or signal disruption.
Blood tests (glucose, vitamin B12)	Evaluates metabolic causes of neuropathy.	Supports interpretation of patterns consistent with metabolic neuroregulation.

Step 6: Care Strategies and Intervention Pathways

Naturopathic Approach

B-complex vitamins, alpha-lipoic acid, and Acetyl-L-carnitine support nerve regeneration (Papanas & Ziegler, 2014). Herbal anti-inflammatories like *Hypericum perforatum* may reduce neuropathic pain (Kasper et al., 2010). Neural mobilization and bioresonance aid recovery. Mind-body therapies modulate neurovascular function.

Standard Medical Approaches

Pharmacological treatment includes anticonvulsants, antidepressants, and analgesics. Surgical decompression may be required. Metabolic control is essential in systemic neuropathies.

Specialty / Practitioner Care Strategies Table

Specialty Group	Practitioners Included	Hyperemissive Strategies	Hypoemissive Strategies
Biochemistry	Nutritionists, Orthomolecular, Herbalists, Naturopaths	Neurotrophic vitamins, alpha-lipoic acid, anti-inflammatory botanicals	Circulatory stimulants, metabolic support, neuroprotective nutrients
Rehabilitation	Physiotherapists, Massage Therapists, Osteopaths / Chiropractors	Neural mobilization, myofascial release, gentle massage	Neural gliding exercises, ergonomic guidance, neurorehabilitation
Energetics	Acupuncturists (TCM), Bioenergetic Therapists	Acupuncture, moxibustion, PEMF	Warming acupuncture, frequency therapy, energy healing
Psychological	GNM practitioners, Psychotherapists, Vibrational therapists, Family constellation facilitators	Psychotherapy, bioresonance, mindfulness	Psychosomatic conflict resolution, vibrational medicine

Educational Pearls & Considerations.

- Early diagnosis reduces risk of chronic nerve damage.
- Nutritional and energetic support enhances nerve repair.
- Monitor metabolic contributors such as diabetes.
- Avoid aggressive treatment during acute inflammation.
- Tailor neural mobilization to patient tolerance.

GROUP 2 - ZONE 11 – LATERAL LEFT ABDOMEN

Category 5: *Lymphatic*

Step 1: Functional Anatomy and Interpretive Importance

The lateral left abdomen mirrors the right, with superficial collectors draining cutaneous and fascial tissues toward axillary and inguinal nodes, and deeper vessels linked with iliac channels (Standring, 2016). This bilateral arrangement plays a decisive role in maintaining trunk immune defense.

Slavin et al. (2009) reported that truncal lymphedema frequently follows oncologic surgery, presenting with asymmetrical flank thickening that may persist for years. Even in subclinical states, stagnation of lymphatic flow modifies fascial elasticity and alters vascular response, changes that can be visualized externally.

On spectral surface analysis, characteristic emissive patterns often align obliquely across the lateral torso, reflecting the geometry of the underlying drainage routes. These signals are more contained and sharply bounded than diffuse muscular fields, allowing clinicians to recognize the lymphatic contribution to left-sided flank dysfunction and distinguish it from visceral or myofascial origins.

Step 2,3,4: ROI Classification and Interpretive Questions

Hyperemission indicates acute lymphatic reactivity, microbial activity, or lymphatic congestion with warmth and swelling.

- Is there redness, tenderness, or rapid swelling?
- Has the patient experienced recent infection or trauma?

Hypoemission suggests chronic lymphatic stasis with fibrosis and impaired drainage causing reduced biosignal

- Is swelling persistent and firm?
- Are recurrent infections or slow wound healing present?

Step 5: Confirmatory Evaluations

Test	Purpose & Justification	Relevance to Emissive Pattern
Lymphoscintigraphy	Assesses lymphatic flow and detects obstructions.	Confirms lymphatic retention or reduced perfusion.
Doppler ultrasound	Excludes venous insufficiency contributing to swelling.	Differentiates vascular from lymphatic causes.

Blood tests (CBC, inflammatory markers)	Detect infection or systemic inflammation.	Supports hyperemissive tissue activation states.
Physical exam (Stemmer's sign, limb measurements)	Identifies clinical signs of lymphedema.	Correlates with biospectral findings.

Step 6: Care Strategies and Intervention Pathways

Naturopathic Approach

Stimulate lymphatic drainage with herbal lymphagogues like *Hedera helix* and *Vitis vinifera* (Godoy et al., 2012). Manual lymphatic drainage by certified therapists enhances fluid movement. Compression therapy supports lymph return and requires customization. Nutritional antioxidants and anti-inflammatory nutrients promote tissue repair. Hydrotherapy with alternating warm and cold applications improves lymphatic circulation.

Standard Medical Approaches

Standard treatment includes manual lymphatic drainage, compression garments, physical therapy, and infection management. Surgery is reserved for refractory cases.

Specialty / Practitioner Care Strategies Table

Specialty Group	Practitioners Included	Hyperemissive Strategies	Hypoemissive Strategies
Biochemistry	Nutritionists, Orthomolecular, Herbalists, Naturopaths	Herbal lymphagogues, antioxidants, anti-inflammatory nutrients	Circulatory support, nutritional tissue repair support
Rehabilitation	Physiotherapists, Massage Therapists, Osteopaths / Chiropractors	Manual lymphatic drainage, gentle massage, postural retraining	Compression therapy, graded exercise, ergonomic guidance
Energetics	Acupuncturists (TCM), Bioenergetic Therapists	Acupuncture, herbal formulas, PEMF	Warming acupuncture, energy balancing
Psychological	GNM practitioners, Psychotherapists, Vibrational therapists, Family constellation facilitators	Mind-body therapies supporting immune function and healing	Psychosomatic conflict resolution, emotional balancing

Educational Pearls & Considerations.

- Early treatment prevents progression to chronic lymphedema.
- Manual lymphatic drainage requires trained therapists.
- Compression therapy must be properly fitted and monitored.
- Nutritional support enhances lymphatic function and tissue repair.
- Prompt infection control is essential.

GROUP 2 - ZONE 11 – LATERAL LEFT ABDOMEN

Category 6: *Organ-Related (GNM)*

Step 1: Functional Anatomy and Interpretive Importance

The lateral left abdomen overlies the spleen, descending colon, and portions of the abdominal musculature, forming an interface between visceral and parietal structures (Standring, 2016). In GNM, conflicts concerning protection, assimilation, or filtration may activate organ programs in this region.

Hamer (2012) described that conflict-active phases suppress biosignals, producing hypoemission, while healing phases express increased activity, seen as hyperemission.

These fields can be externally traced along the flank, sharply distinguished from muscular patterns. Kiecolt-Glaser et al. (2002) showed that chronic stress alters immune surveillance and inflammatory signaling, supporting the idea that unresolved psychological states can visibly affect peripheral tissues.

By connecting emissive asymmetries with visceral programs of the spleen and colon, clinicians can better differentiate psychosomatic conflict responses from musculoskeletal activations in the lateral abdomen.

Step 2,3,4: ROI Classification and Interpretive Questions

Hyperemission indicates the healing or reactive phase with increased metabolic activity and tissue regeneration.

- Is there localized pain, swelling, or digestive symptoms?
- Is inflammation or infection present?

Hypoemission reflects the conflict-active phase, often with tissue loss or functional reduction.

- Are there chronic symptoms, fatigue, or diminished organ function?
- Is psychological stress or unresolved conflict reported?

Step 5: Confirmatory Evaluations

Test	Purpose & Justification	Relevance to Emissive Pattern
Ultrasound / CT / MRI imaging	Visualizes organ morphology, inflammation, or lesions.	Correlates with emissive anomalies indicating organ involvement.
Spleen function tests (CBC, peripheral smear)	Detects splenic enlargement or dysfunction.	Supports hyperemissive tissue activation in splenic terrain.

Colonoscopy / imaging	Evaluates colon pathology such as inflammation or lesions.	Correlates with biospectral findings.
Complete blood count (CBC), inflammatory markers	Detects systemic inflammation or infection.	Supports hyperemissive phases of conflict.
Psychological assessment	Identifies biological conflicts and stressors relevant to GNM.	Complements the GNM interpretive framework.

Step 6: Care Strategies and Intervention Pathways

Naturopathic Approach

Use immunomodulatory and anti-inflammatory botanicals such as *Echinacea purpurea* and *Curcuma longa* to support spleen and colon health (Ulbricht et al., 2013). Promote gut microbiota balance with probiotics and prebiotics. Stress management and psychotherapy facilitate conflict resolution. Nutritional antioxidants and anti-inflammatory nutrients support tissue repair.

Standard Medical Approaches

Diagnostic imaging and labs guide medical and surgical management of organ pathology. Pharmacological treatments and lifestyle interventions are used as indicated.

Specialty / Practitioner Care Strategies Table

Specialty Group	Practitioners Included	Hyperemissive Strategies	Hypoemissive Strategies
Biochemistry	Nutritionists, Orthomolecular, Herbalists, Naturopaths	Immunomodulatory herbs, antioxidants, digestive support	Nutritional support for organ function
Rehabilitation	Physiotherapists, Massage Therapists, Osteopaths / Chiropractors	Supportive therapies promoting relaxation and circulation	Gentle mobilization and relaxation techniques
Energetics	Acupuncturists (TCM), Bioenergetic Therapists	Acupuncture for immune and digestive function	Energy balancing and harmonization
Psychological	GNM practitioners, Psychotherapists, Vibrational therapists, Family constellation facilitators	Psychotherapy, bioresonance, conflict resolution	Emotional balancing and stress reduction

Educational Pearls & Considerations.

- Recognize the psychosomatic origin of organ pathology per GNM.
- Support physical and psychological healing simultaneously.
- Monitor organ function closely with appropriate testing.
- Multidisciplinary approach optimizes outcomes.

GROUP 2 - ZONE 11 – LATERAL LEFT ABDOMEN

Category 7: *Acupuncture / Meridian*

Step 1: Functional Anatomy and Interpretive Importance

The left lateral abdomen covers the oblique musculature and fascia overlying the spleen and descending colon (Standring, 2016). TCM identifies this area with the Gallbladder (GB) and Triple Burner (SJ) meridians, which regulate digestion, fluid metabolism, and systemic coordination.

Flaws (2000) emphasized how imbalances in these channels can lead to flank pain, digestive weakness, or localized tension. Deadman et al. (2007) noted the therapeutic use of GB26 and SJ6 in treating lateral abdominal pain and bloating, linking clinical effects with meridian theory.

Disruptions manifest on biosignal imaging as sharply defined emissive variations following oblique trajectories across the flank, distinct from diffuse muscular or vascular signals.

Such findings provide a bridge between traditional meridian mapping and emissive analysis, where localized biospectral asymmetries offer external correlates of Qi stagnation or deficiency in left-sided abdominal channels.

Step 2,3,4: ROI Classification and Interpretive Questions

Hyperemission indicates Qi stagnation or energetic reactivity along the meridians.

- Is there localized pain, distension, or tenderness?
- Are symptoms worsened by stress or diet?

Hypoemission suggests Qi deficiency or chronic stagnation leading to poor circulation and cold sensations.

- Does the patient experience fatigue, coldness, or digestive sluggishness?
- Are symptoms chronic or persistent?

Step 5: Confirmatory Evaluations

Test	Purpose & Justification	Relevance to Emissive Pattern
Pulse diagnosis and tongue examination	Traditional TCM diagnostic methods assessing Qi and blood flow (Flaws, 2000).	Supports differentiation of hyper- and hypoemissive patterns.
Biospectral imaging	Detects emissive asymmetries along meridian pathways.	Visualizes areas of Qi imbalance.
Patient symptom questionnaire	Assesses digestive symptoms, energy levels, and pain patterns.	Assists in clinical differentiation of meridian signal disruption.

Step 6: Care Strategies and Intervention Pathways

Naturopathic Approach

Target acupuncture points such as GB34, GB41, and SJ6 to regulate meridian flow and alleviate stagnation (Lao et al., 2004). Use moxibustion to warm hypoemissive meridian areas. Herbal formulas like *Xiao Yao San* and *Chai Hu Shu Gan San* harmonize liver and gallbladder Qi (Bensky et al., 2004). Dietary modifications support treatment goals.

Standard Medical Approaches

Acupuncture complements medical and nutritional therapies to improve symptoms related to digestive and musculoskeletal dysfunction.

Specialty / Practitioner Care Strategies Table

Specialty Group	Practitioners Included	Hyperemissive Strategies	Hypoemissive Strategies
Biochemistry	Nutritionists, Orthomolecular, Herbalists, Naturopaths	Herbal formulas for Qi regulation, antioxidants	Qi tonics, digestive support supplements
Rehabilitation	Physiotherapists, Massage Therapists, Osteopaths / Chiropractors	Abdominal massage, myofascial release	Gentle mobilization, warming massage
Energetics	Acupuncturists (TCM), Bioenergetic Therapists	Acupuncture, moxibustion, PEMF	Warming acupuncture, energy balancing
Psychological	GNM practitioners, Psychotherapists, Vibrational therapists, Family constellation facilitators	Mind-body therapies, bioresonance, energy clearing	Psychosomatic conflict resolution, emotional balancing

Educational Pearls & Considerations.

- Precise acupuncture point selection enhances therapeutic efficacy.
- Moxibustion must be used cautiously in patients sensitive to heat.
- Herbal treatments require professional oversight.
- Integrating acupuncture with dietary and rehabilitative therapies optimizes outcomes.

GROUP 2 - ZONE 11 – LATERAL LEFT ABDOMEN

Category 8: *Energetic*

Step 1: Functional Anatomy and Interpretive Importance

The lateral left abdomen includes the oblique musculature, descending colon overlay, and fascial expansions linking trunk and pelvis (Standring, 2016).

Energetically, this zone reflects regulation of elimination and systemic adaptability, often mirroring left-sided energy distribution patterns. Van Wijk (2014) documented that ultraweak photon emission fluctuates with physiologic states, aligning with emissive changes observed here.

Clinically, patients may present with altered elimination patterns, lateral abdominal tension, or fatigue during exertion. Biospectral readings reveal diffuse hypoemissive streaks associated with reduced energy flow or punctate hyperemissive foci linked with reparative signaling.

These emissive features often follow fascial vectors rather than organ outlines, reflecting how energy distribution adapts under systemic strain. Interpretation of this zone provides insight into the integration of elimination, adaptation, and energy conservation mechanisms within the biofield context.

Step 2,3,4: ROI Classification and Interpretive Questions

Hyperemission suggests localized energy congestion or field reactivity.

- Does the patient feel heat, tension, or discomfort in this area?
- Are emotional or stress factors contributing?

Hypoemission indicates energy deficiency or stagnation.

- Does the patient experience fatigue, coldness, or sluggish digestion?
- Are symptoms chronic or resistant to conventional treatments?

Step 5: Confirmatory Evaluations

Test	Purpose & Justification	Relevance to Emissive Pattern
Bioresonance testing	Measures tissue energy frequencies and imbalances.	Correlates with emissive anomalies.
Electrodermal screening (EDS)	Assesses skin conductance linked to energy pathways.	Supports interpretation of energetic imbalances.
Patient emotional and symptom history	Provides clinical context for energetic dysfunction.	Assists differential interpretation.

Step 6: **Care Strategies and Intervention Pathways**

Naturopathic Approach

Utilize bioresonance, pulsed electromagnetic fields (PEMF), and adaptogenic botanicals to restore energetic balance and enhance healing (Matsumoto et al., 2010). Nutritional antioxidants and adaptogens support systemic resilience. Mindfulness and stress management complement energetic interventions.

Standard Medical Approaches

Energetic therapies are adjuncts to conventional medical and rehabilitative treatments, aiming to optimize patient outcomes.

Specialty / Practitioner Care Strategies Table

Specialty Group	Practitioners Included	Hyperemissive Strategies	Hypoemissive Strategies
Biochemistry	Nutritionists, Orthomolecular, Herbalists, Naturopaths	Adaptogens, antioxidants, herbal energetics	Nutritional support for energy deficiency
Rehabilitation	Physiotherapists, Massage Therapists, Osteopaths / Chiropractors	Energy-based manual therapies, PEMF, therapeutic touch	Gentle stimulation, mobilization
Energetics	Acupuncturists (TCM), Bioenergetic Therapists	Bioresonance, PEMF, acupuncture	Warming acupuncture, energy balancing
Psychological	GNM practitioners, Psychotherapists, Vibrational therapists, Family constellation facilitators	Psychotherapy, bioresonance, mindfulness	Emotional balancing, vibrational medicine

Educational Pearls & Considerations.

- Energetic therapies complement but do not replace standard care.
- Patient response and practitioner skill are key to effective treatment.
- Regular monitoring allows for treatment adjustments.
- Address both psychological and physical aspects for holistic care.

GROUP 2 - ZONE 11 – LATERAL LEFT ABDOMEN

Category 9: *Metabolic / Endocrine*

Step 1: Functional Anatomy and Interpretive Importance

The lateral left abdomen includes the oblique muscles, fascial expansions, and visceral overlay of the spleen and descending colon (Standring, 2016). Metabolically, this zone reflects elimination and immune–endocrine interaction, as systemic imbalance often alters local circulation and tissue repair.

Reaven (1988) introduced the concept of Syndrome X, later metabolic syndrome, describing patterns of insulin resistance, dyslipidemia, and hypertension that influence peripheral tissues such as this field.

Patients often describe heaviness, left-sided abdominal tension, or irregular elimination patterns. Spectral surface readings reveal diffuse hypoemissive depressions consistent with suppressed metabolic flow, while narrow hyperemissive arcs signal compensatory activity.

These emissive expressions trace fascial lines rather than organ boundaries, reinforcing their systemic interpretation. Clinically, the lateral left abdomen provides biospectral access to the integration of elimination, immune, and endocrine regulation under metabolic strain.

Step 2,3,4: ROI Classification and Interpretive Questions

Hyperemission suggests localized reactivity, microbial activity, or metabolic overactivity.

- Is there warmth, redness, or swelling?
- Is metabolic control suboptimal?

Hypoemission indicates hypoperfusion, neuropathy, or impaired perfusion from metabolic or endocrine causes.

- Are there cold sensations, numbness, or chronic wounds?
- Are systemic symptoms such as fatigue or temperature intolerance present?

Step 5: Confirmatory Evaluations

Test	Purpose & Justification	Relevance to Emissive Pattern
HbA1c, fasting glucose	Assesses glycemic control in diabetes.	Correlates with hypoemissive neurofunctional or perfusion-restricted zones.
Thyroid function tests (TSH, Free T4)	Evaluates thyroid disorders affecting metabolism and circulation.	Associated with altered emissive regulation.

Lipid profile	Assesses cardiovascular risk impacting tissue perfusion.	Supports metabolic vascular adaptation.
Inflammatory markers (CRP, ESR)	Detects systemic inflammation influencing tissue health.	Correlates with hyperemissive tissue activation states.

Step 6: Care Strategies and Intervention Pathways

Naturopathic Approach

Promote metabolic health with low glycemic diet, antioxidants, and adaptogens (Alberti et al., 2006). Herbs such as *Panax ginseng* and *Gymnema sylvestre* support endocrine function. Supplement chromium, magnesium, and alpha-lipoic acid to enhance glucose metabolism and neuroprotection. Regular aerobic exercise improves circulation.

Standard Medical Approaches

Pharmacologic and lifestyle interventions target metabolic control. Thyroid hormone replacement and lipid management reduce complications.

Specialty / Practitioner Care Strategies Table

Specialty Group	Practitioners Included	Hyperemissive Strategies	Hypoemissive Strategies
Biochemistry	Nutritionists, Orthomolecular, Herbalists, Naturopaths	Antioxidants, adaptogens, insulin sensitizers, micronutrients	Metabolic support, neuroprotective nutrients, dietary management
Rehabilitation	Physiotherapists, Massage Therapists, Osteopaths / Chiropractors	Exercise therapy, circulation enhancement	Neuromuscular re-education, aerobic conditioning
Energetics	Acupuncturists (TCM), Bioenergetic Therapists	Acupuncture supporting metabolic function	Energy balancing, PEMF
Psychological	GNM practitioners, Psychotherapists, Vibrational therapists, Family constellation facilitators	Mind-body therapies supporting metabolic regulation	Stress reduction, emotional balancing

Educational Pearls & Considerations.

- Regular monitoring prevents complications.
- Lifestyle and dietary modifications complement clinical treatment.
- Adaptogens support but do not replace conventional therapies.
- Patient education on skin and wound care is essential.

GROUP 2

ZONE 12 – LUMBAR REGION

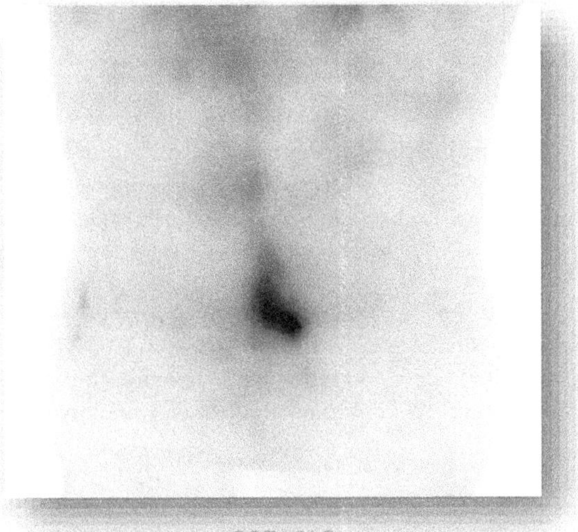

G2Z12LR

The lumbar region covers the lower spinal vertebrae (L1–L5), paraspinal musculature, and thoracolumbar fascia, forming a biomechanical and regulatory hub for the trunk. It bears the highest axial load of the spine and transmits both muscular and visceral forces, explaining its frequent involvement in musculoskeletal complaints (Standring, 2016).

Emissive asymmetries here often reflect interactions between musculoskeletal strain, neurofunctional regulation, and circulatory restriction. Low back pain affects up to 80% of adults worldwide (Hoy et al., 2014), and emissive changes may precede radiological signs of disc degeneration or narrowing, revealing tissue activation or autonomic modulation before structural alteration.

The thoracolumbar fascia influences trunk stability and is implicated in chronic pain through altered tension and perfusion (Willard et al., 2012). Emissive suppression along the paraspinals correlates with postural fatigue in sedentary individuals or those exposed to asymmetric load.

Neurovascular dynamics add systemic relevance: sympathetic fibers of the lumbar plexus regulate limb tone and visceral activity, making local asymmetries indicators of autonomic imbalance (Baron et al., 2013). In diabetes, lumbar microvascular dysfunction has been observed before neuropathic symptoms emerge (Vincent et al., 2004). Compensatory mechanics such as pelvic tilt or leg length discrepancy also generate asymmetric fields through altered load distribution.

Taken together, the lumbar zone serves as a central interpretive surface for biomechanical, vascular, and neuroautonomic dynamics. Its diagnostic strength lies in revealing preclinical dysfunction in one of the body's most common and clinically stressed regions.

Zone 12 – Lumbar Region: Emission-Relevant Structures

Category	Relevant Structures	Emission Relevance
1. Vascular / Circulatory	- Lumbar arteries and veins - Iliolumbar vessels - Paravertebral venous plexus	Hyperemission may reflect localized signal intensification from tissue activation or vascular field retention. Hypoemission can indicate perfusion decline, vascular spasm, or sympathetic vasoconstriction reducing lumbar tissue perfusion.
2. Muscular / Myofascial	- Erector spinae group (iliocostalis, longissimus, spinalis) - Multifidus - Quadratus lumborum	Hyperemission corresponds with muscular spasm, fascial activation, or overuse. Hypoemission is typically associated with muscle atrophy, chronic disuse, or fascial restrictions impacting lumbar mobility and perfusion.
3. Skeletal / Articular	- Lumbar vertebrae (L1-L5) - Sacroiliac joints - Facet joints	Hyperemission may indicate periosteal field reactivity, facet signal excitation, or vertebral zone activation. Hypoemission can be seen in chronic degenerative changes or impaired bone metabolism.
4. Nervous System / Spine	- Lumbar nerve roots (L1-L5) - Cauda equina - Sympathetic chain ganglia	Hyperemission may reflect nerve root signal irritation or neurofield excitation; Hypoemission suggests chronic nerve compression, neurofunctional suppression, or autonomic dysregulation affecting lumbar and lower limb innervation.
5. Lymphatic / Immune	- Lumbar lymphatic channels - Inguinal lymph nodes	Hyperemissive regions may reflect immune-related activation or lymphatic signal buildup; Hypoemission may indicate lymphatic congestion, fibrosis, or immune suppression in drainage pathways.
6. Organs / GNM (German New Medicine)	- Kidney reflex zones - Adrenal gland influence - Pelvic viscera (bladder, reproductive organs)	Elevated biosignal activity may correspond with active visceral conflict or regulatory tension; Hypoemission may represent healing phases or functional suppression through viscerosomatic reflexes involving lumbar spinal segments.
7. Acupuncture / Meridians	- Kidney Meridian - Bladder Meridian - Governing Vessel (Du Mai) along spine	Hyperemission may indicate Qi stagnation or excess; low-emission zones often suggest Qi deficiency, blood stasis, or damp accumulation affecting lumbar and pelvic function.
8. Energetic / Frequency	- Lumbar energetic centers - Reflex zones related to autonomic regulation of lower trunk and pelvis	Hyperemission may reflect sympathetic signal overexpression, bioenergetic load, or emotional stress; Hypoemission indicates regulatory depletion or impaired autonomic balance in lumbar-pelvic regions.
9. Metabolic / Endocrine	- Reflex zones for adrenal function, renal metabolism, and pelvic endocrine influence	Hypoemissive patterns suggest adrenal underregulation, metabolic downshift, or pelvic endocrine modulation; Persistent Hyperemission may indicate regulatory field activation or increased signal demand in lumbar visceral reflex zones.

GROUP 2 - ZONE 12 – LUMBAR REGION

Category 1: *Vascular / Circulatory*

Step 1: Functional Anatomy and Interpretive Importance

The lumbar region is supplied by paired lumbar arteries branching directly from the abdominal aorta, which provide inflow to the quadratus lumborum, psoas major, and paraspinal musculature. Venous return occurs through lumbar veins draining into the ascending lumbar and inferior vena cava pathways (Standring, 2016).

Vascular research has documented the significance of lumbar arteries and veins in spinal and abdominal wall perfusion, particularly in surgical and imaging contexts (Matsumoto et al., 1999).

On spectral surface reading, emissive asymmetries in the lumbar zone often appear as vertical or paramedian bands. These may indicate venous congestion in the paraspinal plexuses, circulatory strain in postural musculature, or adaptive arterial adjustments during trunk stabilization.

Because of its link to spinal support, this region is particularly informative for interpreting circulatory adaptation in integrative assessment.

Step 2,3,4: ROI Classification and Interpretive Questions

Hyperemission indicates vascular reactivity, thrombophlebitis, or vascular congestion.

- Is there localized swelling, redness, or tenderness?
- Are systemic symptoms such as fever or chills present?

Hypoemission suggests hypoperfusion or compromised perfusion.

- Are there complaints of coldness, pallor, or delayed healing?
- Is there a history of vascular disease?

Step 5: Confirmatory Evaluations

Test	Purpose & Justification	Relevance to Emissive Pattern
Doppler ultrasound	Assesses arterial and venous flow in lumbar vessels.	Correlates hyperemissive tissue activation and hypoemissive perfusion decline.
CT or MRI angiography	Visualizes vessel patency and detects occlusions or thrombosis.	Confirms vascular flow restriction or localized signal intensification.
Blood tests (CBC, CRP, coagulation profile)	Detect infection, inflammation, or coagulation disorders.	Supports hyperemissive retention or circulatory impedance states.
Physical exam	Inspects and palpates for local signs of vascular compromise.	Complements biospectral findings.

Step 6: Care Strategies and Intervention Pathways

Naturopathic Approach

Botanical venotonics such as *Aesculus hippocastanum* and *Ruscus aculeatus* improve microcirculation and reduce edema (Chrubasik et al., 2011). An anti-inflammatory diet rich in antioxidants and omega-3 fatty acids supports vascular health (Calder, 2017). Contrast hydrotherapy with warm and cold applications stimulates circulation (Sutkowy et al., 2019). Vitamins C, E, and bioflavonoids enhance endothelial function. Limb elevation and gentle massage promote venous return.

Standard Medical Approaches

Imaging guides anticoagulation, anti-inflammatory medication, or surgical intervention as needed. Managing systemic contributors such as coagulopathies is critical.

Specialty / Practitioner Care Strategies Table

Specialty Group	Practitioners Included	Hyperemissive Strategies	Hypoemissive Strategies
Biochemistry	Nutritionists, Orthomolecular, Herbalists, Naturopaths	Botanical venotonics, antioxidants, anti-inflammatory diet	Circulatory stimulants, nutritional endothelial support
Rehabilitation	Physiotherapists, Massage Therapists, Osteopaths / Chiropractors	Gentle massage, lymphatic drainage, postural correction	Graded exercise, circulatory enhancement
Energetics	Acupuncturists (TCM), Bioenergetic Therapists	Acupuncture, moxibustion, herbal formulas	Warming acupuncture, energy balancing
Psychological	GNM practitioners, Psychotherapists, Vibrational therapists, Family constellation facilitators	Psychotherapy, bioresonance, mindfulness	Stress reduction, emotional balancing

Educational Pearls & Considerations.

- Early diagnosis of thrombophlebitis or vascular inflammation is crucial.
- Botanical venotonics combined with diet and hydrotherapy effectively support vascular health.
- Nitric oxide boosters and omega-3 fatty acids enhance endothelial function and perfusion.
- Compression therapy contraindicated in severe arterial insufficiency.
- Encourage early mobilization and limb elevation to prevent chronic issues.

GROUP 2 - ZONE 12 – LUMBAR REGION

Category 2: *Muscular*

Step 1: Functional Anatomy and Interpretive Importance

The lumbar region contains the erector spinae, quadratus lumborum, and multifidus, which together maintain spinal extension, lateral bending, and segmental stabilization. These muscles, innervated by dorsal rami of spinal nerves, are crucial for upright posture and protect the lumbar spine during load-bearing tasks (Standring, 2016).

Clinical research highlights the multifidus as particularly vulnerable to inhibition following low-back injury, leading to chronic dysfunction and recurrent pain if not reactivated (Hides et al., 2001).

Spectral analysis of the lumbar surface often reveals band-like or focal emissive changes corresponding to paraspinal muscle activity, with asymmetries indicating neuromuscular inhibition or compensatory hypertonicity. This zone therefore provides valuable biospectral insight into the balance between structural support and adaptive dysfunction across the lower spine.

Step 2,3,4: ROI Classification and Interpretive Questions

Hyperemission suggests acute muscle strain, muscular reactivity, or active trigger points with increased local spectral emission.

- Has the patient experienced recent trauma, heavy lifting, or overuse?
- Are there localized pain, tenderness, or muscle tightness?

Hypoemission indicates chronic muscle hypoperfusion, fibrosis, or neurogenic atrophy.

- Are symptoms of weakness, stiffness, or limited range of motion present?
- Is muscle wasting or altered sensation observed?

Step 5: Confirmatory Evaluations

Test	Purpose & Justification	Relevance to Emissive Pattern
Creatine kinase (CK), LDH	Detects muscle injury or inflammation (Simons et al., 1999).	Elevated in **hyperemissive tissue activation states**.
MRI	Visualizes muscle edema, inflammation, or fibrosis.	Supports hyper- or hypoemissive findings.
Electromyography (EMG)	Assesses muscle and nerve function.	Correlates with **hypoemissive neurofunctional causes**.
Blood tests (CBC, inflammatory markers)	Detects systemic inflammation or infection.	Supports **hyperemissive regulatory field conditions**.

Step 6: Care Strategies and Intervention Pathways

Naturopathic Approach

Utilize anti-inflammatory botanicals such as *Curcuma longa* and *Boswellia serrata* to reduce muscle inflammation (Hewlings & Kalman, 2017). Magnesium supports muscle relaxation. Hydrotherapy with alternating warm and cold applications enhances circulation (Sutkowy et al., 2019). Gentle stretching and progressive strengthening promote recovery. Adequate protein and antioxidants support tissue repair.

Standard Medical Approaches

Rest, NSAIDs, and physical therapy are standard treatments for muscle injuries (Simons et al., 1999). Neurological evaluation is advised if weakness or sensory changes occur.

Specialty / Practitioner Care Strategies Table

Specialty Group	Practitioners Included	Hyperemissive Strategies	Hypoemissive Strategies
Biochemistry	Nutritionists, Orthomolecular, Herbalists, Naturopaths	Anti-inflammatory botanicals, magnesium, antioxidants, protein	Circulatory support, neurotrophic nutrients, protein support
Rehabilitation	Physiotherapists, Massage Therapists, Osteopaths / Chiropractors	Myofascial release, trigger point therapy, gentle massage	Graded aerobic exercise, neurorehabilitation, ergonomic guidance
Energetics	Acupuncturists (TCM), Bioenergetic Therapists	Acupuncture, moxibustion, PEMF	Warming acupuncture, frequency therapy
Psychological	GNM practitioners, Psychotherapists, Vibrational therapists, Family constellation facilitators	Psychotherapy, bioresonance, mindfulness	Psychosomatic conflict resolution, emotional balancing

Educational Pearls & Considerations.

- Early identification of myofascial trigger points improves outcomes.
- Magnesium helps reduce muscle spasms and supports relaxation.
- Hydrotherapy should be adapted to the phase of inflammation.
- Neurological assessment is essential when weakness or sensory deficits are present.
- Progressive rehabilitation prevents chronic dysfunction.

GROUP 2 - ZONE 12 – LUMBAR REGION

Category 3: *Skeletal*

Step 1: Functional Anatomy and Interpretive Importance

The lumbar spine is composed of five vertebrae (L1–L5), which provide the principal structural support for the trunk and house the spinal cord and nerve roots within the vertebral canal (Standring, 2016).

These vertebrae sustain axial loading, transmit forces between the upper body and pelvis, and permit a balance between stability and mobility. Degenerative remodeling, facet arthropathy, and disc-related skeletal changes are frequent in this region, with Adams and Dolan (2012) emphasizing their contribution to chronic low back pain syndromes.

Such structural alterations alter the biomechanics of paraspinal musculature and vascular signaling, producing emissive irregularities that extend across the lumbar surface. Spectral surface readings often capture biospectral asymmetries as vertically oriented fields aligned with vertebral levels, differing from the broader, less geometric expressions of muscular activation.

These externalized signals highlight the interplay of vertebral load-bearing and compensatory tissue regulation, offering a noninvasive view of skeletal stress before advanced deformity develops.

Step 2,3,4: ROI Classification and Interpretive Questions

Hyperemission suggests active tissue reactivity from vertebral or joint pathology.

- Is there localized tenderness, swelling, or increased warmth?
- Are pain and stiffness present, worsened by movement?

Hypoemission indicates chronic degeneration, hypoperfusion, or nerve root compromise.

- Are there symptoms of numbness, weakness, or reduced mobility?
- Is there a history of chronic back pain or spinal deformity?

Step 5: Confirmatory Evaluations

Test	Purpose & Justification	Relevance to Emissive Pattern
X-ray	Evaluates bone structure, alignment, and degenerative changes.	Supports interpretation of chronic skeletal adaptation.
MRI	Visualizes soft tissues, discs, nerve roots, and inflammation.	Correlates with hyper- and hypoemissive zones.
CT scan	Provides detailed bony anatomy and detection of fractures.	Confirms structural signal alterations.
Physical examination	Assesses range of motion, tenderness, and neurological signs.	Complements emissive analysis and structural imaging.

Step 6: Care Strategies and Intervention Pathways

Naturopathic Approach

Support skeletal health with bone-strengthening nutrients like calcium, magnesium, vitamin D, and collagen peptides (Kruger & Kruger, 2019). Anti-inflammatory botanicals such as *Boswellia serrata* reduce joint inflammation. Physiotherapy focusing on postural correction and spinal mobilization improves function. Acupuncture and bioresonance support pain relief and inflammation modulation.

Standard Medical Approaches

Pharmacologic treatments include NSAIDs and muscle relaxants. Surgical intervention may be necessary in severe cases. Physical therapy is integral to rehabilitation.

Specialty / Practitioner Care Strategies Table

Specialty Group	**Practitioners Included**	**Hyperemissive Strategies**	**Hypoemissive Strategies**
Biochemistry	Nutritionists, Orthomolecular, Herbalists, Naturopaths	Bone-supportive nutrients, anti-inflammatory herbs	Nutritional support for bone regeneration
Rehabilitation	Physiotherapists, Osteopaths / Chiropractors, Massage Therapists	Spinal mobilization, myofascial release, pain management	Postural correction, ergonomic training
Energetics	Acupuncturists (TCM), Bioenergetic Therapists	Acupuncture, PEMF, energy healing	Energy balancing and stimulation
Psychological	GNM practitioners, Psychotherapists, Vibrational therapists, Family constellation facilitators	Psychotherapy, bioresonance, stress management	Emotional balancing and pain coping strategies

Educational Pearls & Considerations.

- Early intervention improves long-term spinal health.
- Nutritional support enhances bone and joint repair.
- Combine manual therapies with rehabilitative exercises for optimal outcomes.
- Monitor for neurological signs indicating urgent referral.
- Tailor treatment to patient tolerance and progression.

GROUP 2 - ZONE 12 – LUMBAR REGION

Category 4: *Nervous*

Step 1: Functional Anatomy and Interpretive Importance

The lumbar region houses the lumbar plexus and nerve roots (L1–L5), which supply motor and sensory innervation to the trunk, pelvis, and lower limb (Standring, 2016). These neural structures are vulnerable to compression from degenerative spinal changes or disc herniation, often leading to radiculopathy with pain radiating into the lower limb.

Dillingham (1995) highlighted that lumbosacral radiculopathy is one of the most frequent causes of lower back and leg pain, frequently associated with neurological deficits. Such nerve root compromise alters local autonomic balance, reshaping vascular and muscular responses.

These modifications appear externally as vertical biospectral asymmetries aligned with lumbar vertebral levels, differing from diffuse paraspinal muscular fields.

By projecting neural root stress into visible emissive patterns, surface analysis allows early recognition of radiculopathic involvement and refines the interpretation of chronic lumbar pain.

Step 2,3,4: ROI Classification and Interpretive Questions

Hyperemission indicates nerve irritation or neurogenic reactivity.

- Are there symptoms of burning, tingling, or sharp pain?
- Is localized hypersensitivity or swelling present?

Hypoemission suggests nerve hypoperfusion, compression, or denervation causing decreased autonomic activity.

- Are numbness, weakness, or muscle atrophy observed?
- Do symptoms worsen with posture or movement?

Step 5: Confirmatory Evaluations

Test	Purpose & Justification	Relevance to Emissive Pattern
Nerve conduction studies (NCS), Electromyography (EMG)	Assess nerve and muscle function (Janis et al., 2010).	Correlates with hypoemissive neurofunctional disruption.
Quantitative sensory testing (QST)	Measures sensory nerve thresholds.	Supports interpretation of neuroregulatory patterns.
MRI	Detects nerve root compression or structural abnormalities.	Identifies origin of neural field symptoms.
Blood tests (glucose, vitamin B12)	Evaluate metabolic causes of neuropathy.	Supports systemic neurofunctional assessment.

Step 6: Care Strategies and Intervention Pathways

Naturopathic Approach

Support nerve health with B-complex vitamins, alpha-lipoic acid, and Acetyl-L-carnitine (Papanas & Ziegler, 2014). Use herbal anti-inflammatories such as *Hypericum perforatum* for neuropathic pain (Kasper et al., 2010). Neural mobilization and bioresonance therapies support nerve regeneration. Mind-body approaches modulate neurovascular function.

Standard Medical Approaches

Pharmacologic agents include anticonvulsants, antidepressants, and analgesics. Surgical decompression may be indicated. Metabolic control is essential for systemic neuropathies.

Specialty / Practitioner Care Strategies Table

Specialty Group	Practitioners Included	Hyperemissive Strategies	Hypoemissive Strategies
Biochemistry	Nutritionists, Orthomolecular, Herbalists, Naturopaths	Neurotrophic vitamins, alpha-lipoic acid, anti-inflammatory botanicals	Circulatory stimulants, metabolic support, neuroprotective nutrients
Rehabilitation	Physiotherapists, Massage Therapists, Osteopaths / Chiropractors	Neural mobilization, myofascial release, gentle massage	Neural gliding exercises, ergonomic guidance, neurorehabilitation
Energetics	Acupuncturists (TCM), Bioenergetic Therapists	Acupuncture, moxibustion, PEMF	Warming acupuncture, frequency therapy, energy healing
Psychological	GNM practitioners, Psychotherapists, Vibrational therapists, Family constellation facilitators	Psychotherapy, bioresonance, mindfulness	Psychosomatic conflict resolution, vibrational medicine

Educational Pearls & Considerations.

- Early diagnosis prevents chronic nerve damage.
- Nutritional and energetic therapies enhance nerve repair.
- Monitor for metabolic contributors such as diabetes.
- Avoid aggressive therapy during acute inflammation.
- Tailor neural mobilization to patient tolerance.

GROUP 2 - ZONE 12 – LUMBAR REGION

Category 5: *Lymphatic*

Step 1: Functional Anatomy and Interpretive Importance

The lumbar lymphatics drain the posterior abdominal wall and lower trunk into the iliac nodes and ultimately the thoracic duct, a major pathway for systemic immune traffic (Standring, 2016). This drainage is crucial for maintaining both local fluid balance and global immune regulation.

Brorson (2003) documented lumbar lymphedema as a secondary complication after pelvic or retroperitoneal surgery, often manifesting with tissue heaviness and pain. Even prior to overt swelling, functional impairment reshapes paraspinal tension and modifies perfusion in the lumbar fascia.

Externally, these changes appear as vertical emissive fields along the paravertebral column or iliac crest, differing from the broader signals of muscular overload.

Their clear alignment with drainage routes provides an externalized correlate of lumbar lymphatic compromise, offering a visual dimension that supports early recognition of immune stagnation and informs the clinical approach to persistent lower back dysfunction.

Step 2,3,4: ROI Classification and Interpretive Questions

Hyperemission reflects acute lymphatic reactivity, microbial activity, or lymphatic congestion with swelling and spectral intensification.

- Is there redness, tenderness, or rapid swelling?
- Has the patient experienced recent trauma or infection?

Hypoemission indicates chronic lymphatic stasis with fibrosis and impaired lymph flow.

- Is swelling persistent and firm?
- Are recurrent infections or delayed wound healing present?

Step 5: Confirmatory Evaluations

Test	Purpose & Justification	Relevance to Emissive Pattern
Lymphoscintigraphy	Assesses lymphatic flow and detects obstructions.	Confirms lymphatic retention or reduced perfusion.
Doppler ultrasound	Excludes venous insufficiency contributing to swelling.	Differentiates vascular from lymphatic causes.
Blood tests (CBC, inflammatory markers)	Detect infection or systemic inflammation.	Supports hyperemissive tissue activation states.
Physical exam (Stemmer's sign, limb measurements)	Identifies clinical signs of lymphedema.	Correlates with biospectral imaging patterns.

Step 6: Care Strategies and Intervention Pathways

Naturopathic Approach

Use herbal lymphagogues such as *Hedera helix* and *Vitis vinifera* to stimulate lymphatic drainage (Godoy et al., 2012). Manual lymphatic drainage performed by trained therapists promotes fluid movement. Compression therapy supports lymph return and requires proper fitting. Nutritional antioxidants and anti-inflammatory nutrients enhance tissue repair. Hydrotherapy with alternating warm and cold applications aids lymphatic circulation.

Standard Medical Approaches

Standard treatments include manual lymphatic drainage, compression garments, physical therapy, and infection management. Surgery is reserved for refractory cases.

Specialty / Practitioner Care Strategies Table

Specialty Group	Practitioners Included	Hyperemissive Strategies	Hypoemissive Strategies
Biochemistry	Nutritionists, Orthomolecular, Herbalists, Naturopaths	Herbal lymphagogues, antioxidants, anti-inflammatory nutrients	Circulatory support, nutritional tissue repair support
Rehabilitation	Physiotherapists, Massage Therapists, Osteopaths / Chiropractors	Manual lymphatic drainage, gentle massage, postural retraining	Compression therapy, graded exercise, ergonomic guidance
Energetics	Acupuncturists (TCM), Bioenergetic Therapists	Acupuncture, herbal formulas, PEMF	Warming acupuncture, energy balancing
Psychological	GNM practitioners, Psychotherapists, Vibrational therapists, Family constellation facilitators	Mind-body therapies supporting immune function and healing	Psychosomatic conflict resolution, emotional balancing

Educational Pearls & Considerations.

- Early intervention prevents progression to chronic lymphedema.
- Manual lymphatic drainage should be performed by certified therapists.
- Compression therapy must be correctly fitted and monitored.
- Nutritional support enhances lymphatic function and tissue repair.
- Prompt infection control is essential.

GROUP 2 - ZONE 12 – LUMBAR REGION

Category 6: *Organ-Related (GNM)*

Step 1: Functional Anatomy and Interpretive Importance

The lumbar region overlies retroperitoneal structures including kidneys, adrenal glands, and segments of the colon, together with vertebral and paraspinal elements (Standring, 2016). In GNM, conflicts tied to water balance, existential threat, or survival activate adaptive responses in renal and adrenal tissues.

Hamer (2012) described that hypoemissive suppression marks the conflict-active state, while hyperemissive intensification characterizes repair.

On the surface, these phase-dependent adaptations appear as vertically oriented emissive fields adjacent to the spine or iliac crest, distinct from diffuse paraspinal muscular activity. Chrousos (2009) explained how chronic stress disrupts hypothalamic–pituitary–adrenal regulation, altering both endocrine and immune function.

This reinforces the observation that lumbar emissive signals may represent mechanical and vascular imbalance as well as systemic responses to psychobiological conflict, projected outward through surface biosignal variations.

Step 2,3,4: ROI Classification and Interpretive Questions

Hyperemission indicates the reactive or healing phase with increased metabolic activity.

- Are there symptoms such as localized pain, swelling, or urinary or digestive complaints?
- Is inflammation or infection present?

Hypoemission reflects the active conflict phase involving tissue loss or functional suppression.

- Are there chronic symptoms, fatigue, or reduced organ function?
- Is psychological stress or unresolved conflict evident?

Step 5: Confirmatory Evaluations

Test	Purpose & Justification	Relevance to Emissive Pattern
Ultrasound / CT / MRI imaging	Visualizes kidney, adrenal, and colon morphology and pathology.	Correlates with emissive anomalies indicating organ involvement.
Renal function tests (creatinine, BUN)	Assesses kidney function and injury.	Supports hyperemissive activation in renal terrain.
Urinalysis	Detects urinary tract infections or abnormalities.	Correlates with tissue-level reactivity or immune field response.

Complete blood count (CBC), inflammatory markers	Detects systemic inflammation or infection.	Supports hyperemissive phases of conflict.
Psychological assessment	Evaluates biological conflicts and psychosomatic factors.	Complements GNM interpretive approach.

Step 6: Care Strategies and Intervention Pathways

Naturopathic Approach

Use nephroprotective herbs such as *Cornus officinalis* and *Orthosiphon stamineus* to support kidney function (Chan et al., 2017). Promote adrenal health with adaptogens like *Withania somnifera.* Encourage hydration and urinary tract support with cranberry extract. Psychotherapy and stress management facilitate conflict resolution. Nutritional antioxidants aid tissue repair.

Standard Medical Approaches

Medical and surgical interventions guided by imaging and labs. Pharmacological treatment of infections and inflammation as needed.

Specialty / Practitioner Care Strategies Table

Specialty Group	Practitioners Included	Hyperemissive Strategies	Hypoemissive Strategies
Biochemistry	Nutritionists, Orthomolecular, Herbalists, Naturopaths	Nephroprotective herbs, antioxidants, adaptogens	Nutritional support for organ and adrenal function
Rehabilitation	Physiotherapists, Massage Therapists, Osteopaths / Chiropractors	Supportive therapies promoting circulation and relaxation	Gentle mobilization, relaxation techniques
Energetics	Acupuncturists (TCM), Bioenergetic Therapists	Acupuncture for renal and adrenal support	Energy balancing and harmonization
Psychological	GNM practitioners, Psychotherapists, Vibrational therapists, Family constellation facilitators	Psychotherapy, bioresonance, conflict resolution	Emotional balancing and stress reduction

Educational Pearls & Considerations.

- Address psychosomatic root causes per GNM while managing physical symptoms.
- Monitor renal and adrenal function regularly.
- Multidisciplinary approach improves outcomes.
- Hydration and urinary tract health are essential components.

GROUP 2 - ZONE 12 – LUMBAR REGION

Category 7: *Acupuncture / Meridian*

Step 1: **Functional Anatomy and Interpretive Importance**

The lumbar region houses vertebral bodies, erector spinae muscles, and fascial planes, with retroperitoneal structures including kidneys and ureters beneath (Standring, 2016). Acupuncture mapping associates this zone primarily with the Bladder (BL) and Kidney (KI) meridians.

Deadman et al. (2007) described points such as BL23 (Shenshu) and KI3 as essential for urinary regulation, spinal vitality, and systemic energy balance. Langevin and Yandow (2002) suggested meridians may follow connective tissue planes, explaining their anatomical palpability along paraspinal pathways.

Clinically, dysfunction is expressed as lumbar stiffness, kidney-related complaints, or systemic fatigue. In biosignal assessment, emissive fields are observed as vertical bands parallel to the spine or iliac crest, their linear orientation aligning with BL–KI trajectories.

These patterns illustrate how lumbar biospectral signals provide a visible window into meridian coherence, complementing anatomical and physiological evaluation.

Step 2,3,4: **ROI Classification and Interpretive Questions**

Hyperemission indicates Qi stagnation or energetic reactivity along the meridians.

- Are there localized pain, tension, or sensitivity?
- Are symptoms exacerbated by physical activity or stress?

Hypoemission suggests Qi deficiency or chronic stagnation causing poor circulation and cold sensations.

- Does the patient report fatigue, coldness, or weakness?
- Are symptoms chronic or worsening?

Step 5: **Confirmatory Evaluations**

Test	Purpose & Justification	Relevance to Emissive Pattern
Pulse diagnosis and tongue examination	Traditional TCM assessment of meridian Qi and Blood status (Flaws, 2000).	Supports differentiation of emissive patterns.
Biospectral imaging	Visualizes thermal asymmetries along meridian pathways.	Correlates with Qi imbalances in lumbar region.
Patient symptom questionnaire	Assesses lumbar pain, urinary symptoms, and energy levels.	Assists clinical differentiation of meridian signal disruption.

Step 6: Care Strategies and Intervention Pathways

Naturopathic Approach

Acupuncture points such as BL23 (Kidney Shu), BL40 (Lumbar Shu), and KI3 support meridian flow and alleviate stagnation (Lao et al., 2004). Moxibustion warms hypoemissive areas. Herbal formulas like *Shen Qi Wan* and *Du Huo Ji Sheng Tang* nourish Kidney and Bladder meridians (Bensky et al., 2004). Dietary adjustments and lifestyle modifications complement treatment.

Standard Medical Approaches

Acupuncture is utilized adjunctively for lumbar pain relief and urinary function support.

Specialty / Practitioner Care Strategies Table

Specialty Group	Practitioners Included	Hyperemissive Strategies	Hypoemissive Strategies
Biochemistry	Nutritionists, Orthomolecular, Herbalists, Naturopaths	Herbal formulas nourishing Kidney and Bladder meridians	Qi tonics and nutritional support
Rehabilitation	Physiotherapists, Massage Therapists, Osteopaths / Chiropractors	Lumbar mobilization, myofascial release	Gentle mobilization, warming massage
Energetics	Acupuncturists (TCM), Bioenergetic Therapists	Acupuncture, moxibustion, PEMF	Warming acupuncture, energy balancing
Psychological	GNM practitioners, Psychotherapists, Vibrational therapists, Family constellation facilitators	Mind-body therapies, bioresonance, energy clearing	Psychosomatic conflict resolution, emotional balancing

Educational Pearls & Considerations.

- Correct point selection tailored to thermal findings enhances efficacy.
- Moxibustion requires caution in heat-sensitive patients.
- Herbal prescriptions should be supervised by qualified practitioners.
- Integrate acupuncture with physical therapies for optimal results.

GROUP 2 - ZONE 12 – LUMBAR REGION

Category 8: *Energetic*

Step 1: **Functional Anatomy and Interpretive Importance**

The lumbar region contains the paraspinal musculature, vertebral structures, and overlay of retroperitoneal organs such as kidneys and adrenals (Standring, 2016). Energetically, this surface field is tied to systemic grounding, vitality, and stress adaptation.

Becker and Selden (1985) demonstrated that electrical signaling is integral to tissue regulation and repair, highlighting the importance of bioelectric coherence in lumbar fields. Patients often present with chronic tension, reduced endurance, or non-specific pain in this region.

Spectral surface readings reveal hypoemissive depressions correlating with systemic depletion and hyperemissive arcs aligned with adaptive repair or heightened regulatory demand.

These emissive dynamics follow spinal and fascial planes, underscoring the lumbar region's role as both a mechanical and energetic anchor. By integrating biospectral findings with energetic physiology, this zone is recognized as a pivotal field of systemic resilience and neuroenergetic regulation.

Step 2,3,4: **ROI Classification and Interpretive Questions**

Hyperemission indicates localized energy congestion or field reactivity.

- Does the patient report sensations of heat, tension, or discomfort in the lumbar area?
- Are emotional or stress factors contributing?

Hypoemission suggests energy deficiency or stagnation.

- Does the patient experience fatigue, coldness, or low vitality?
- Are symptoms chronic or resistant to conventional treatments?

Step 5: **Confirmatory Evaluations**

Test	Purpose & Justification	Relevance to Emissive Pattern
Bioresonance testing	Measures tissue energy imbalances and frequencies.	Correlates with emissive anomalies.
Electrodermal screening (EDS)	Assesses skin conductance reflecting energetic pathway status.	Supports interpretation of energetic imbalances.
Patient symptom and emotional history	Provides context for energetic dysfunction and stress factors.	Assists biospectral differentiation.

Step 6: Care Strategies and Intervention Pathways

Naturopathic Approach

Use bioresonance, pulsed electromagnetic fields (PEMF), and adaptogenic botanicals to restore energetic balance and promote healing (Matsumoto et al., 2010). Nutritional antioxidants and adaptogens enhance systemic resilience. Mindfulness and stress reduction techniques complement energetic therapies.

Standard Medical Approaches

Energetic modalities serve as adjuncts to conventional and rehabilitative therapies to optimize patient outcomes.

Specialty / Practitioner Care Strategies Table

Specialty Group	Practitioners Included	Hyperemissive Strategies	Hypoemissive Strategies
Biochemistry	Nutritionists, Orthomolecular, Herbalists, Naturopaths	Adaptogens, antioxidants, herbal energetics	Nutritional support for energy deficiency
Rehabilitation	Physiotherapists, Massage Therapists, Osteopaths / Chiropractors	Energy-based manual therapies, PEMF, therapeutic touch	Gentle stimulation, mobilization
Energetics	Acupuncturists (TCM), Bioenergetic Therapists	Bioresonance, PEMF, acupuncture	Warming acupuncture, energy balancing
Psychological	GNM practitioners, Psychotherapists, Vibrational therapists, Family constellation facilitators	Psychotherapy, bioresonance, mindfulness	Emotional balancing, vibrational medicine

Educational Pearls & Considerations.

- Energetic therapies complement but do not replace conventional medical care.
- Patient response and practitioner expertise influence treatment success.
- Regular reassessment is essential to adapt therapy to clinical changes.
- Address psychological and physical factors holistically for best outcomes.

GROUP 2 - ZONE 12 – LUMBAR REGION

Category 9: *Metabolic / Endocrine*

Step 1: Functional Anatomy and Interpretive Importance

The lumbar region includes the paraspinal musculature, vertebral column, and retroperitoneal fields containing the kidneys and adrenal glands (Standring, 2016). Endocrine and metabolic systems converge here, as adrenal function regulates stress adaptation and renal physiology reflects vascular–endocrine balance.

Chrousos (2009) emphasized the impact of chronic stress on the hypothalamic–pituitary–adrenal axis, linking systemic endocrine dysregulation with musculoskeletal and vascular dysfunction in the lumbar field. Patients often present with chronic fatigue, low back discomfort, or systemic exhaustion.

Spectral surface readings reveal broad hypoemissive depressions indicating adrenal depletion or vascular insufficiency, while hyperemissive bands align with compensatory activation or heightened regulatory demand.

These emissive dynamics follow spinal and fascial continuities, underscoring the lumbar field as both a mechanical support and an energetic-metabolic anchor. Clinically, it serves as a biospectral map of systemic stress, endocrine adaptation, and metabolic reserve.

Step 2,3,4: ROI Classification and Interpretive Questions

Hyperemission reflects localized reactivity, microbial activity, or metabolic overactivity.

- Is there warmth, redness, or swelling in the lumbar area?
- Is metabolic control adequate?

Hypoemission indicates hypoperfusion, neuropathy, or impaired perfusion due to metabolic or endocrine dysfunction.

- Are there cold sensations, numbness, or chronic wounds?
- Are systemic symptoms such as fatigue or temperature intolerance present?

Step 5: Confirmatory Evaluations

Test	Purpose & Justification	Relevance to Emissive Pattern
HbA1c, fasting glucose	Assesses glycemic control in diabetes.	Correlates with hypoemissive neurofunctional or perfusion-restricted areas.
Thyroid function tests (TSH, Free T4)	Evaluates thyroid disorders affecting metabolism and circulation.	Associated with altered emissive regulation.

Lipid profile	Assesses cardiovascular risk impacting tissue perfusion.	Supports metabolic vascular adaptation.
Inflammatory markers (CRP, ESR)	Detects systemic inflammation influencing tissue health.	Correlates with hyperemissive tissue activation states.

Step 6: Care Strategies and Intervention Pathways

Naturopathic Approach

Support metabolic health with low glycemic diet, antioxidants, and adaptogens (Alberti et al., 2006). Use herbs like *Panax ginseng* and *Gymnema sylvestre* to support endocrine function. Supplement chromium, magnesium, and alpha-lipoic acid for glucose metabolism and neuroprotection. Encourage regular aerobic exercise to improve circulation.

Standard Medical Approaches

Pharmacologic and lifestyle interventions focus on metabolic control. Thyroid hormone replacement and lipid management reduce complications.

Specialty / Practitioner Care Strategies Table

Specialty Group	Practitioners Included	Hyperemissive Strategies	Hypoemissive Strategies
Biochemistry	Nutritionists, Orthomolecular, Herbalists, Naturopaths	Antioxidants, adaptogens, insulin sensitizers, micronutrients	Metabolic support, neuroprotective nutrients, dietary management
Rehabilitation	Physiotherapists, Massage Therapists, Osteopaths / Chiropractors	Exercise therapy, circulation enhancement	Neuromuscular re-education, aerobic conditioning
Energetics	Acupuncturists (TCM), Bioenergetic Therapists	Acupuncture supporting metabolic function	Energy balancing, PEMF
Psychological	GNM practitioners, Psychotherapists, Vibrational therapists, Family constellation facilitators	Mind-body therapies supporting metabolic regulation	Stress reduction, emotional balancing

Educational Pearls & Considerations.

- Regular metabolic monitoring is essential to prevent complications.
- Lifestyle and dietary changes complement clinical treatment.
- Adaptogens support but do not replace conventional therapies.
- Patient education on skin and wound care is critical.

GROUP 3

THORAX AND AXILLARY REGIONS

The thorax and axillary zones represent a critical intersection of respiratory, cardiovascular, lymphatic, and neuro-musculoskeletal systems, offering an emissive view into both central and peripheral functional dynamics. These areas frequently reveal nuanced biospectral patterns reflecting the interplay between deep visceral activity and superficial musculoskeletal tension, which often precedes or accompanies clinical symptom expression.

Emissive imaging here allows early recognition of vascular field alterations such as angiospasm or retention, tissue activation within thoracic musculature, and lymphatic stasis that may contribute to or result from systemic regulatory imbalance. The axillary regions, rich in lymph nodes and neural plexuses, serve as sentinel zones for immunological status and neurovascular coherence, with biospectral asymmetries often signaling subtle but clinically relevant dysfunctions.

Thermal responses in these zones are particularly responsive to respiratory mechanics and postural adaptations, which may manifest as localized hyper- or hypoemissive areas indicative of underlying regulation shifts or compensatory activity. This group's emissive findings contribute meaningfully to the early detection of patterns consistent with thoracic outlet compression, lymphatic retention, breast terrain alterations, and cardiopulmonary field stress.

Integrative interpretation in these zones aids clinicians in distinguishing regulatory disturbances from structural adaptations, guiding targeted investigation and tailored intervention with a precision seldom achievable by conventional imaging alone.

Zones 13 to 16: Thorax and Upper back - Axillary Regions

The thorax and axillary regions represent a critical convergence point of several vital physiological systems, including the respiratory, cardiovascular, lymphatic, and neuromuscular networks. These zones include complex anatomical structures such as the ribs, sternum, intercostal muscles, thoracic spine, large vessels including the subclavian and axillary arteries and veins, and dense lymphatic clusters within the axillae.

The functional integration within these regions makes them particularly responsive to a wide spectrum of regulatory and structural variations, which are clearly visualized through emissive imaging.

Biospectrally, the thoracic and axillary zones often exhibit intricate emissive patterns that reflect the balance between deep visceral activity and superficial musculoskeletal and circulatory dynamics.

The chest wall's biomechanical role in respiration and postural control contributes to characteristic zone expressions, including segmental hyperemission associated with muscular strain, tissue activation, or vascular retention, as well as hypoemissive areas indicative of circulatory reduction or underregulated tissue fields.

Ring and Ammer (2012) highlight the interpretive value of these emissive profiles in distinguishing between vasoregulatory, immune, and neurofunctional phenomena in the thoracic region.

The axillary zones, rich in lymph nodes and critical neurovascular plexuses, function as sentinel sites for immune field status and neurovascular coherence. Early lymphatic retention or neurovascular compression patterns, such as those associated with thoracic outlet-related mechanisms, can present with distinct biospectral asymmetries well before clinical manifestations become evident.

Lahiri et al. (2012) describe how emissive assessment of these zones supports early recognition of lymphatic field stress, vascular modulation, and neural tissue excitation, all of which are relevant for terrain-based intervention.

The emissive profile of these regions is also highly responsive to respiratory mechanics and autonomic regulation, as changes in breathing dynamics, sympathetic tone, or cardiopulmonary field demand modulate local biosignal expression.

Myers (2014) describes the influence of fascial continuity and respiration-induced muscular behavior on emissive variability, reinforcing the need for integrative interpretation that includes both visceral and somatic regulatory components.

This group includes four specific zones:
13. Chest and Sternum
14. Left Axillary
15. Right Axillary
16. Upper Back

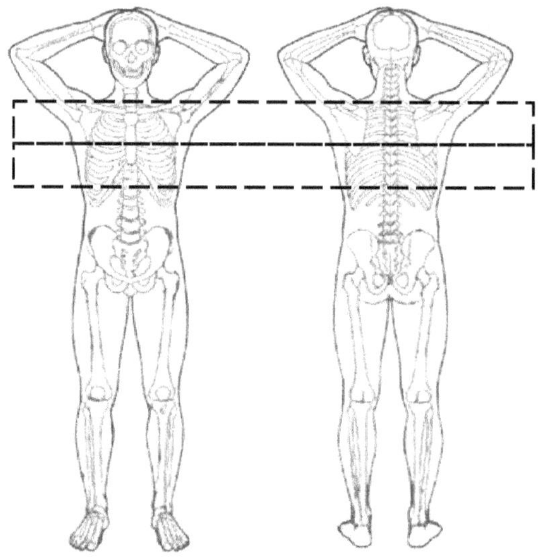

Each zone presents unique anatomical and physiological characteristics, contributing to the group's overall interpretive depth. The chest and sternum zones reflect thoracic organ function and musculoskeletal balance; the axillary zones provide insight into lymphatic and neurovascular status; while the upper back captures the interplay of postural musculature, spinal alignment, and autonomic tone.

The integration of these zones within a biospectral atlas enhances the practitioner's ability to discern subtle emissive patterns, supporting targeted interpretive evaluation and individualized care strategies. This comprehensive approach leverages the modality's strength in emissive interpretation, complementing traditional anatomical studies with dynamic physiological insights essential for holistic understanding.

GROUP 3

ZONE 13 – CHEST AND STERNUM

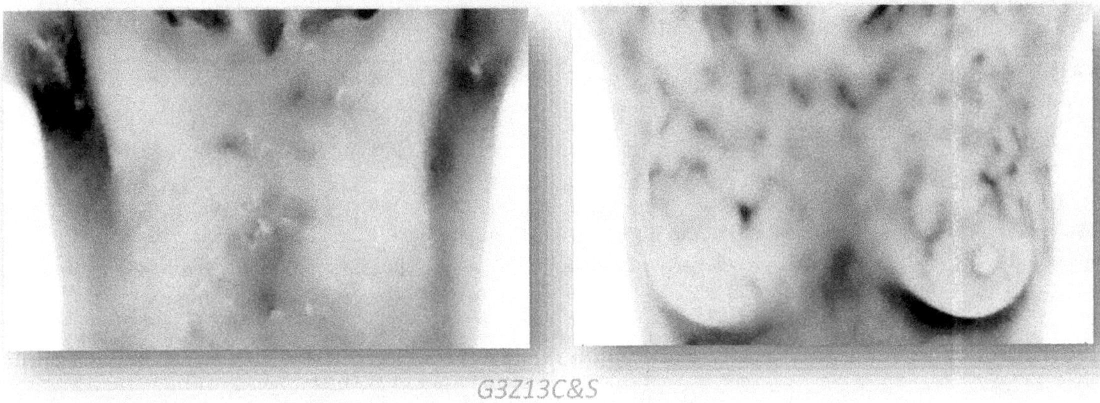

G3Z13C&S

The chest and sternum form a structurally and functionally complex region integrating musculoskeletal, respiratory, and cardiovascular influences. It includes the sternum, costal cartilages, intercostal musculature, and underlying viscera such as the lungs and heart (Standring, 2016). Because of the thinness of the soft tissues and the density of vascular and neural pathways, this is one of the most emissively dynamic thoracic zones. Biospectrally, it often reveals early regulatory changes linked to costosternal tension, respiratory demand, or cardiac load.

Clinically, subtle asymmetries here may precede overt cardiovascular or pulmonary symptoms; chest wall microvascular reactivity alters even in early cardiopulmonary stress (Cheng et al., 2012). Emissive sensitivity also reflects autonomic innervation, where sympathetic and parasympathetic fibers converge, producing functional signatures of stress or imbalance (Nishi, 2018).

Vascular remodeling adds further significance: abnormal angiogenesis within the thorax has been linked to tumor development, and emissive irregularities along the sternum or costal margins may act as non-invasive indicators (Hanahan & Weinberg, 2011).

Musculoskeletal strain is equally relevant, as costochondritis and sternal overload, conditions affecting up to 10% of the population, often present as focal hyperactivity before pain localizes (Disla et al., 1994). The sternum also resonates systemic states, with immune activation in the mediastinum, thymus, or upper lymphatic chains projecting emissive asymmetries before conventional tests detect change.

Taken together, the chest and sternum represent a highly sensitive diagnostic surface where musculoskeletal, vascular, respiratory, and immune influences converge. Its interpretive strength lies in revealing subtle regulatory signatures of systemic significance, offering clinicians an early functional window across multiple physiological systems.

Zone 13 – Chest and Sternum: Emission-Relevant Structures

Category	Relevant Structures	Emission Relevance
1. Vascular / Circulatory	- Internal mammary arteries and veins - Thoracic aorta branches - Intercostal vessels	Hyperemission may indicate vascular field retention, tissue activation, or vasoregulatory expansion; Hypoemission may suggest perfusion decline or restricted circulatory flow to chest wall tissues.
2. Muscular / Myofascial	- Pectoralis major and minor - Intercostal muscles - Subclavius	Hyperemission reflects muscular overuse, fascial activation, or load-related strain; Hypoemission may signal muscle disuse or fascial adhesions affecting thoracic mobility.
3. Skeletal / Articular	- Sternum - Costal cartilages - Ribs (anterior segments)	Local Hyperemission may be due to periosteal activation or costosternal signal excitation; Hypoemission may be linked to chronic degenerative changes or reduced perfusion in bony structures.
4. Nervous System / Spine	- Intercostal nerves - Sympathetic fibers of thoracic chain	Hyperemissive zones can indicate nerve field irritation or segmental signal tension; Hypoemission may represent neurofunctional suppression or autonomic dysregulation impacting thoracic innervation.
5. Lymphatic / Immune	- Parasternal lymph nodes - Superficial lymphatic vessels of anterior thorax	Hyperemission often correlates with immune field activation or lymphatic signal buildup; Hypoemission may reflect lymphatic retention or drainage inefficiency.
6. Organs / GNM (German New Medicine)	- Heart, lungs, thymus	Hyperemissive signals may reflect active visceral conflict or cardiopulmonary field reactivity; Hypoemission may suggest functional suppression or resolution phases in cardiopulmonary terrain.
7. Acupuncture / Meridians	- Heart Meridian - Lung Meridian - Pericardium Meridian	Emissive patterns suggest Qi stagnation or excess; low-emission areas indicate deficiency or dampness affecting cardiopulmonary meridians.
8. Energetic / Frequency	- Reflex energetic centers for cardiopulmonary function	Hyperemission may reflect sympathetic field excitation or emotional stress; Hypoemission may indicate regulatory depletion or reduced autonomic tone.
9. Metabolic / Endocrine	- Cardiac metabolic zones - Pulmonary reflex areas	Hypoemissive patterns may indicate metabolic downregulation; Hyperemission may be present in cardiopulmonary signal amplification or terrain-level activation states.

GROUP 3 - ZONE 13 – CHEST AND STERNUM

Category 1: *Vascular / Circulatory*

Step 1: Functional Anatomy and Interpretive Importance

The sternum and anterior thoracic wall are supplied primarily by the internal thoracic artery and its anterior intercostal branches, with additional inflow from the posterior intercostal arteries. Venous drainage occurs through the internal thoracic and intercostal veins, which connect into the brachiocephalic venous system (Standring, 2016).

Clinical imaging has underlined the reliability of the internal thoracic system in coronary artery bypass grafting, reflecting its robust vascular profile (Barner, 2002).

Emissive asymmetries across the anterior chest often trace the parasternal line, corresponding to the internal thoracic arcade. These irregularities may reflect increased circulatory demand during respiration, localized overload in intercostal spaces, or shifts in venous return.

Because of its structural and clinical significance, this zone frequently displays spectral signals that provide early orientation to thoracic circulatory dynamics.

Step 2,3,4: ROI Classification and Interpretive Questions

Hyperemission may suggest vascular reactivity, venous congestion, or patterns consistent with possible thrombotic involvement.

- Is there localized redness, swelling, or tenderness?
- Are systemic symptoms like fever present?

Hypoemission suggests hypoperfusion or vascular compromise.

- Are there complaints of coldness, pallor, or delayed wound healing?
- Is there a history of vascular disease?

Step 5: Confirmatory Evaluations

Test	Purpose & Justification	Relevance to Emissive Pattern
Doppler ultrasound	Evaluates arterial and venous flow in thoracic vessels.	Correlates hyperemissive tissue activation and hypoemissive perfusion decline.
CT or MRI angiography	Visualizes vessel patency and detects occlusions or thrombosis.	Confirms vascular flow restriction or signal intensification.
Blood tests (CBC, CRP, coagulation profile)	Detect infection, inflammation, or coagulation disorders.	Supports hyperemissive retention or circulatory impedance states.
Physical exam	Inspects and palpates for signs of vascular compromise.	Complements biospectral findings.

Step 6: Care Strategies and Intervention Pathways

Naturopathic Approach

Botanical venotonics such as *Aesculus hippocastanum* and *Ruscus aculeatus* improve microcirculation and reduce edema (Chrubasik et al., 2011). Anti-inflammatory diets rich in antioxidants and omega-3 fatty acids support vascular health (Calder, 2017). Contrast hydrotherapy with warm and cold applications stimulates circulation (Sutkowy et al., 2019). Vitamins C, E, and bioflavonoids enhance endothelial function. Limb elevation and gentle massage promote venous return.

Standard Medical Approaches

Imaging guides anticoagulation, anti-inflammatory medication, or surgical intervention as needed. Managing systemic contributors such as coagulopathies is critical.

Specialty / Practitioner Care Strategies Table

Specialty Group	Practitioners Included	Hyperemissive Strategies	Hypoemissive Strategies
Biochemistry	Nutritionists, Orthomolecular, Herbalists, Naturopaths	Botanical venotonics, antioxidants, anti-inflammatory diet	Circulatory stimulants, nutritional endothelial support
Rehabilitation	Physiotherapists, Massage Therapists, Osteopaths / Chiropractors	Gentle massage, lymphatic drainage, postural correction	Graded exercise, circulatory enhancement
Energetics	Acupuncturists (TCM), Bioenergetic Therapists	Acupuncture, moxibustion, herbal formulas	Warming acupuncture, energy balancing
Psychological	GNM practitioners, Psychotherapists, Vibrational therapists, Family constellation facilitators	Psychotherapy, bioresonance, mindfulness	Stress reduction, emotional balancing

Educational Pearls & Considerations.

- Early diagnosis of thrombophlebitis or vascular inflammation is critical.
- Botanical venotonics combined with diet and hydrotherapy support vascular health effectively.
- Nitric oxide boosters and omega-3 fatty acids enhance endothelial function and perfusion.
- Compression therapy is contraindicated in severe arterial insufficiency.
- Early mobilization and limb elevation prevent chronic complications.

GROUP 3 - ZONE 13 – CHEST AND STERNUM

Category 2: *Muscular*

Step 1: Functional Anatomy and Interpretive Importance

The anterior thoracic wall is supported by the pectoralis major, pectoralis minor, subclavius, and intercostal muscles, all of which contribute to respiration, shoulder motion, and thoracic stability.

These muscles receive innervation from the pectoral nerves and intercostals, integrating upper limb mobility with breathing mechanics (Standring, 2016). Clinical studies show that pectoralis major tears are relatively common in strength athletes, while chronic intercostal strain may result from repetitive coughing or postural loading (ElMaraghy & Devereaux, 2012).

Spectral surface findings in this region often present as transverse or fan-shaped emissive asymmetries reflecting tension at the sternocostal junction or along the pectoral fascial planes.

These signatures highlight muscular overload or adaptive recruitment that bridges respiratory and postural demands, linking thoracic integrity to systemic functional patterns.

Step 2,3,4: ROI Classification and Interpretive Questions

Hyperemission suggests acute muscle strain, muscular reactivity, or active trigger points.

- Has the patient had recent trauma, heavy lifting, or coughing?
- Is there localized tenderness, swelling, or muscle tightness?

Hypoemission indicates chronic muscle hypoperfusion, fibrosis, or neurogenic atrophy.

- Are symptoms of weakness, stiffness, or limited range of motion present?
- Is muscle wasting or altered sensation observed?

Step 5: Confirmatory Evaluations

Test	Purpose & Justification	Relevance to Emissive Pattern
Creatine kinase (CK), LDH	Detects muscle injury or inflammation (Simons et al., 1999).	Elevated in hyperemissive tissue activation states.
MRI	Visualizes muscle edema, inflammation, or fibrosis.	Supports hyper- or hypoemissive findings.
Electromyography (EMG)	Assesses muscle and nerve function.	Correlates with hypoemissive neurofunctional causes.
Blood tests (CBC, inflammatory markers)	Detects systemic inflammation or infection.	Supports hyperemissive regulatory field conditions.

Step 6: Care Strategies and Intervention Pathways

Naturopathic Approach

Use anti-inflammatory botanicals such as *Curcuma longa* and *Boswellia serrata* to reduce muscle inflammation (Hewlings & Kalman, 2017). Magnesium supports muscle relaxation. Hydrotherapy with alternating warm and cold applications enhances circulation (Sutkowy et al., 2019). Progressive stretching and strengthening promote recovery. Adequate protein and antioxidants support tissue repair.

Standard Medical Approaches

Rest, NSAIDs, and physical therapy are standard treatments for muscle injuries (Simons et al., 1999). Neurological evaluation is recommended if weakness or sensory changes occur.

Specialty / Practitioner Care Strategies Table

Specialty Group	Practitioners Included	Hyperemissive Strategies	Hypoemissive Strategies
Biochemistry	Nutritionists, Orthomolecular, Herbalists, Naturopaths	Anti-inflammatory botanicals, magnesium, antioxidants, protein	Circulatory support, neurotrophic nutrients, protein support
Rehabilitation	Physiotherapists, Massage Therapists, Osteopaths / Chiropractors	Myofascial release, trigger point therapy, gentle massage	Graded aerobic exercise, neurorehabilitation, ergonomic guidance
Energetics	Acupuncturists (TCM), Bioenergetic Therapists	Acupuncture, moxibustion, PEMF	Warming acupuncture, frequency therapy
Psychological	GNM practitioners, Psychotherapists, Vibrational therapists, Family constellation facilitators	Psychotherapy, bioresonance, mindfulness	Psychosomatic conflict resolution, emotional balancing

Educational Pearls & Considerations.

- Early identification of myofascial trigger points improves prognosis.
- Magnesium supports muscle relaxation and reduces spasms.
- Hydrotherapy should be tailored to inflammatory phases.
- Neurological evaluation is essential if weakness or sensory deficits appear.
- Gradual rehabilitation prevents chronic dysfunction.

GROUP 3 - ZONE 13 – CHEST AND STERNUM

Category 3: *Skeletal*

Step 1: Functional Anatomy and Interpretive Importance

The skeletal architecture of the thorax includes the sternum, ribs, and costal cartilages, which shield vital organs while serving as anchors for respiratory musculature (Standring, 2016). The sternocostal joints and rib articulations are frequently subjected to mechanical strain, particularly in occupations or activities requiring repetitive upper body effort.

Miller et al. (2014) describe costosternal and rib joint irritation as underrecognized causes of anterior chest discomfort, often misattributed to cardiopulmonary origins. These subtle skeletal irritations provoke localized regulatory responses that become externally perceptible.

On spectral surface readings, biospectral asymmetries typically appear as focal emissive variations across the sternum or along costal margins, presenting with sharper contours than muscular contributions.

Such patterns capture the skeletal component of thoracic stress, illustrating how articular micro-irritation projects into observable emissive fields. By mapping these external signals, clinicians gain a window into chest wall skeletal adaptation, enhancing differentiation between musculoskeletal and visceral contributors to anterior thoracic pain.

Step 2,3,4: ROI Classification and Interpretive Questions

Hyperemission suggests tissue reactivity or acute injury consistent with costal joint irritation or fracture.

- Is there localized tenderness, swelling, or warmth?
- Are symptoms worsened by movement or respiration?

Hypoemission indicates chronic degeneration or hypoperfusion in skeletal tissues.

- Are there persistent dull pain or stiffness?
- Is there a history of trauma or repetitive stress?

Step 5: Confirmatory Evaluations

Test	Purpose & Justification	Relevance to Emissive Pattern
X-ray	Detects fractures, degenerative changes, or deformities.	Supports interpretive understanding of acute or chronic skeletal adaptations.
MRI	Visualizes soft tissue involvement and bone marrow edema.	Correlates with activation and structural modification patterns.

Bone scan	Assesses bone metabolism and detects occult lesions.	Confirms skeletal field activity or remodeling dynamics.
Physical exam	Evaluates tenderness, mobility, and neurological signs.	Complements imaging and emissive findings.

Step 6: Care Strategies and Intervention Pathways

Naturopathic Approach

Provide bone-supportive nutrients such as calcium, magnesium, vitamin D, and collagen peptides (Kruger & Kruger, 2019). Use anti-inflammatory herbs like *Boswellia serrata* to reduce joint inflammation. Physical therapy focusing on posture and mobility aids recovery. Acupuncture and bioresonance support pain relief and inflammation modulation.

Standard Medical Approaches

Treatment includes analgesics, anti-inflammatory medications, and physical rehabilitation. Surgical intervention may be considered in severe cases.

Specialty / Practitioner Care Strategies Table

Specialty Group	Practitioners Included	Hyperemissive Strategies	Hypoemissive Strategies
Biochemistry	Nutritionists, Orthomolecular, Herbalists, Naturopaths	Bone-supportive nutrients, anti-inflammatory herbs	Nutritional support for bone repair
Rehabilitation	Physiotherapists, Osteopaths / Chiropractors, Massage Therapists	Manual therapy, posture correction, pain management	Ergonomic training, spinal mobilization
Energetics	Acupuncturists (TCM), Bioenergetic Therapists	Acupuncture, PEMF, energy healing	Energy balancing and stimulation
Psychological	GNM practitioners, Psychotherapists, Vibrational therapists, Family constellation facilitators	Psychotherapy, bioresonance, stress management	Emotional balancing and coping strategies

Educational Pearls & Considerations.

- Early diagnosis and management prevent chronic skeletal dysfunction.
- Nutritional support is vital for bone health and repair.
- Integrate manual therapies with rehabilitation for best outcomes.
- Monitor for complications requiring specialist referral.

GROUP 3 - ZONE 13 – CHEST AND STERNUM

Category 4: *Nervous*

Step 1: Functional Anatomy and Interpretive Importance

The chest wall and sternum receive innervation from intercostal nerves (T1–T11), which supply both motor control to intercostal muscles and sensory input from the overlying thoracic skin (Standring, 2016).

These nerves may be affected by trauma, rib dysfunction, or radiculopathy, resulting in pain syndromes that can mimic cardiopulmonary disease. Kuntz and Ricci (1996) noted that intercostal neuralgia often presents with localized chest pain exacerbated by movement or respiration, creating diagnostic confusion.

Neural irritation modifies autonomic signaling within the thoracic wall, producing emissive irregularities that are detectable at the surface.

Biospectral asymmetries typically present as linear fields across costal margins or localized variations near the sternum, their distribution reflecting intercostal nerve pathways. These emissive signals provide clinicians with a noninvasive means of differentiating chest wall neuropathy from visceral cardiopulmonary causes of anterior thoracic pain.

Step 2,3,4: ROI Classification and Interpretive Questions

Hyperemission indicates nerve irritation or neurogenic reactivity.

- Are there burning, tingling, or sharp pains?
- Is there localized hypersensitivity or swelling?

Hypoemission suggests nerve hypoperfusion, compression, or denervation with decreased autonomic activity.

- Are numbness, weakness, or muscle atrophy present?
- Do symptoms worsen with posture or movement?

Step 5: Confirmatory Evaluations

Test	Purpose & Justification	Relevance to Emissive Pattern
Nerve conduction studies (NCS), Electromyography (EMG)	Assess nerve and muscle function (Janis et al., 2010).	Correlates with hypoemissive neurofunctional disruption.
Quantitative sensory testing (QST)	Measures sensory nerve thresholds.	Supports interpretation of neurofunctional patterns.

MRI	Detects nerve root compression or structural abnormalities.	Identifies origin of neural signal disturbance.
Blood tests (glucose, vitamin B12)	Evaluates metabolic causes of neuropathy.	Supports interpretive understanding of systemic neuroregulatory involvement.

Step 6: Care Strategies and Intervention Pathways

Naturopathic Approach

Support nerve regeneration with B-complex vitamins, alpha-lipoic acid, and Acetyl-L-carnitine (Papanas & Ziegler, 2014). Use *Hypericum perforatum* to alleviate neuropathic pain (Kasper et al., 2010). Neural mobilization and bioresonance aid recovery. Mind-body therapies modulate neurovascular function.

Standard Medical Approaches

Pharmacological treatments include anticonvulsants, antidepressants, and analgesics. Surgical decompression may be indicated. Metabolic control is essential in systemic neuropathies.

Specialty / Practitioner Care Strategies Table

Specialty Group	Practitioners Included	Hyperemissive Strategies	Hypoemissive Strategies
Biochemistry	Nutritionists, Orthomolecular, Herbalists, Naturopaths	Neurotrophic vitamins, alpha-lipoic acid, anti-inflammatory botanicals	Circulatory stimulants, metabolic support, neuroprotective nutrients
Rehabilitation	Physiotherapists, Massage Therapists, Osteopaths / Chiropractors	Neural mobilization, myofascial release, gentle massage	Neural gliding exercises, ergonomic guidance, neurorehabilitation
Energetics	Acupuncturists (TCM), Bioenergetic Therapists	Acupuncture, moxibustion, PEMF	Warming acupuncture, frequency therapy, energy healing
Psychological	GNM practitioners, Psychotherapists, Vibrational therapists, Family constellation facilitators	Psychotherapy, bioresonance, mindfulness	Psychosomatic conflict resolution, vibrational medicine

Educational Pearls & Considerations.

- Early diagnosis prevents chronic nerve damage.
- Nutritional and energetic therapies support nerve repair.
- Monitor metabolic contributors such as diabetes.
- Avoid aggressive therapy during acute inflammation.
- Tailor neural mobilization to patient tolerance.

GROUP 3 - ZONE 13 – CHEST AND STERNUM

Category 5: *Lymphatic*

Step 1: Functional Anatomy and Interpretive Importance

The chest wall and sternum are drained by superficial lymphatics leading to axillary and parasternal nodes, while deeper channels follow the internal thoracic vessels (Standring, 2016).

These networks secure immune surveillance of the anterior thorax and play a role in maintaining respiratory wall compliance. Clodius et al. (1988) noted that chest wall lymphedema is a common complication of breast and thoracic surgery, associated with heaviness, discomfort, and visible tissue changes.

Functional compromise reshapes vascular dynamics and modifies local tissue compliance, effects that become visible on emissive assessment.

At the surface, these alterations may appear as localized signals bordering the sternum or following costal margins, whose linear geometry mirrors lymphatic drainage routes.

The distinction from diffuse muscular activity allows clinicians to identify lymphatic burden in the anterior chest, refining interpretation of thoracic wall dysfunction and clarifying its immune-mediated contribution.

Step 2,3,4: ROI Classification and Interpretive Questions

Hyperemission indicates acute lymphatic reactivity, microbial activity, or lymphatic congestion characterized by swelling and spectral intensification.

- Is there redness, tenderness, or rapid swelling?
- Is there a history of trauma or infection?

Hypoemission suggests chronic lymphatic stasis with fibrosis and impaired drainage causing reduced biosignal.

- Is swelling persistent and firm?
- Are recurrent infections or delayed wound healing present?

Step 5: Confirmatory Evaluations

Test	Purpose & Justification	Relevance to Emissive Pattern
Lymphoscintigraphy	Assesses lymphatic flow and detects obstructions.	Confirms lymphatic retention or reduced perfusion.
Doppler ultrasound	Excludes venous insufficiency contributing to swelling.	Differentiates vascular from lymphatic causes.

Blood tests (CBC, inflammatory markers)	Detect infection or systemic inflammation.	Supports hyperemissive tissue activation states.
Physical exam (Stemmer's sign, limb measurements)	Identifies clinical signs of lymphedema.	Correlates with biospectral findings.

Step 6: Care Strategies and Intervention Pathways

Naturopathic Approach

Use herbal lymphagogues such as *Hedera helix* and *Vitis vinifera* to stimulate lymphatic drainage (Godoy et al., 2012). Manual lymphatic drainage by certified therapists promotes fluid movement. Compression therapy supports lymph return and requires proper fitting. Nutritional antioxidants and anti-inflammatory nutrients enhance tissue repair. Hydrotherapy with alternating warm and cold applications improves lymphatic circulation.

Standard Medical Approaches

Standard treatment includes manual lymphatic drainage, compression garments, physical therapy, and infection management. Surgery is reserved for refractory cases.

Specialty / Practitioner Care Strategies Table

Specialty Group	Practitioners Included	Hyperemissive Strategies	Hypoemissive Strategies
Biochemistry	Nutritionists, Orthomolecular, Herbalists, Naturopaths	Herbal lymphagogues, antioxidants, anti-inflammatory nutrients	Circulatory support, nutritional tissue repair support
Rehabilitation	Physiotherapists, Massage Therapists, Osteopaths / Chiropractors	Manual lymphatic drainage, gentle massage, postural retraining	Compression therapy, graded exercise, ergonomic guidance
Energetics	Acupuncturists (TCM), Bioenergetic Therapists	Acupuncture, herbal formulas, PEMF	Warming acupuncture, energy balancing
Psychological	GNM practitioners, Psychotherapists, Vibrational therapists, Family constellation facilitators	Mind-body therapies supporting immune function and healing	Psychosomatic conflict resolution, emotional balancing

Educational Pearls & Considerations.

- Early intervention prevents progression to chronic lymphedema.
- Manual lymphatic drainage requires certified therapists.
- Compression therapy must be properly fitted and monitored.
- Nutritional support enhances lymphatic function and tissue repair.
- Prompt infection control is essential.

GROUP 3 - ZONE 13 – CHEST AND STERNUM

Category 6: *Organ-Related (GNM)*

Step 1: **Functional Anatomy and Interpretive Importance**

The chest and sternum cover vital thoracic organs, including the heart, lungs, and mediastinal structures, protected by the rib cage and associated musculature (Standring, 2016). In German New Medicine (GNM), conflicts involving respiration, survival, or relational loss are mapped to pulmonary and cardiac tissues.

Hamer (2012) emphasized that active conflict phases suppress biosignals, leading to hypoemissive fields, while reparative phases heighten activity, visible as localized hyperemission.

These emissive shifts often appear externally near the sternum or along costal margins, their geometry reflecting visceral projection rather than muscular activity. Sapolsky (2004) detailed how chronic stress influences cardiovascular and respiratory physiology, aligning with GNM's premise that unresolved conflict imprints itself through organ-level adaptation.

Observed surface variations in the chest can therefore serve as externalized correlates of heart- and lung-related psychosomatic programs, aiding interpretation of thoracic dysfunction in integrative assessment.

Step 2,3,4: **ROI Classification and Interpretive Questions**

Hyperemission indicates reactive or healing phases with increased metabolic activity.

- Are there symptoms such as localized chest pain, dyspnea, or palpitations?
- Is there evidence of infection or inflammation?

Hypoemission corresponds to conflict-active phases with tissue loss or functional suppression.

- Are symptoms chronic, with fatigue or decreased organ function?
- Is psychological stress or unresolved conflict present?

Step 5: **Confirmatory Evaluations**

Test	Purpose & Justification	Relevance to Emissive Pattern
Chest X-ray, CT, MRI	Visualizes cardiac and pulmonary structures and pathology.	Correlates with emissive anomalies indicating organ involvement.
ECG, Echocardiogram	Assesses cardiac function and detects abnormalities.	Supports interpretive understanding of cardiac field dynamics..
Pulmonary function tests	Evaluates respiratory capacity and lung function.	Correlates with pulmonary zone activity.

Inflammatory markers, CBC	Detects systemic inflammation or infection.	Supports hyperemissive phases of conflict.
Psychological assessment	Identifies psychosomatic conflicts and stressors.	Complements GNM framework.

Step 6: Care Strategies and Intervention Pathways

Naturopathic Approach

Use anti-inflammatory and cardioprotective botanicals such as *Crataegus monogyna* and *Curcuma longa* (Tattelman, 2001). Support respiratory health with expectorants and antioxidants. Stress reduction and psychotherapy facilitate conflict resolution. Nutritional antioxidants aid tissue repair.

Standard Medical Approaches

Medical management guided by imaging and functional tests. Pharmacological therapies address cardiac and pulmonary conditions. Lifestyle modification and rehabilitation support recovery.

Specialty / Practitioner Care Strategies Table

Specialty Group	Practitioners Included	Hyperemissive Strategies	Hypoemissive Strategies
Biochemistry	Nutritionists, Orthomolecular, Herbalists, Naturopaths	Cardioprotective herbs, antioxidants, anti-inflammatories	Nutritional support for organ function and repair
Rehabilitation	Physiotherapists, Massage Therapists, Osteopaths / Chiropractors	Respiratory therapy, circulation enhancement	Gentle mobilization and relaxation techniques
Energetics	Acupuncturists (TCM), Bioenergetic Therapists	Acupuncture for cardiac and pulmonary support	Energy balancing and harmonization
Psychological	GNM practitioners, Psychotherapists, Vibrational therapists, Family constellation facilitators	Psychotherapy, bioresonance, conflict resolution	Emotional balancing and stress management

Educational Pearls & Considerations.

- Recognize psychosomatic influences on thoracic organ pathology per GNM.
- Combine physical and psychological therapies for optimal healing.
- Regular monitoring of cardiac and pulmonary function is essential.
- Multidisciplinary approach enhances patient outcomes.

GROUP 3 - ZONE 13 – CHEST AND STERNUM

Category 7: *Acupuncture / Meridian*

Step 1: Functional Anatomy and Interpretive Importance

The thoracic cage includes the sternum, ribs, and intercostal musculature protecting the heart and lungs (Standring, 2016). In TCM, this region corresponds to the Heart (HT) and Pericardium (PC) meridians, which regulate circulation, emotional stability, and respiratory coherence.

Flaws (2000) highlighted the significance of PC6 and HT7 for balancing emotional distress and thoracic discomfort. Kaptchuk (2000) described how these channels integrate psychological stress with somatic symptoms, bridging cardiovascular and emotional domains.

Clinically, disruptions may present as palpitations, chest tightness, or anxiety-linked somatic complaints. On biosignal imaging, thoracic emissive fields appear as central or lateralized variations, their geometry reflecting HT–PC trajectories.

These patterns provide a visual correlate of Qi disturbance in thoracic meridians, situating biospectral analysis within both cardiovascular and psychosomatic frameworks.

Step 2,3,4: ROI Classification and Interpretive Questions

Hyperemission suggests Qi stagnation or energetic reactivity along the meridians.

- Is there chest discomfort, tightness, or localized pain?
- Are symptoms aggravated by stress or emotional distress?

Hypoemission indicates Qi deficiency or chronic stagnation causing poor circulation and cold sensations.

- Does the patient experience fatigue, coldness, or palpitations?
- Are symptoms persistent or worsening?

Step 5: Confirmatory Evaluations

Test	Purpose & Justification	Relevance to Emissive Pattern
Pulse diagnosis and tongue examination	Traditional TCM diagnostic methods assessing Heart and Pericardium meridian status (Flaws, 2000).	Helps differentiate hyper- and hypoemissive patterns.
Biospectral imaging	Visualizes thermal asymmetries along meridian pathways.	Correlates with Qi imbalances in the thoracic region.
Patient symptom questionnaire	Assesses chest symptoms, palpitations, and emotional state.	Assists clinical differentiation of meridian signal disruption.

Step 6: Care Strategies and Intervention Pathways

Naturopathic Approach

Acupuncture points such as HT7, PC6, and Ren17 regulate Heart and Pericardium meridian flow and relieve stagnation (Lao et al., 2004). Moxibustion warms hypoemissive meridian areas. Herbal formulas like *Tian Wang Bu Xin Dan* and *Bao Yuan Tang* support cardiovascular and emotional health (Bensky et al., 2004). Lifestyle modifications including stress reduction complement treatment.

Standard Medical Approaches

Acupuncture is utilized adjunctively to manage chest discomfort and improve cardiovascular function.

Specialty / Practitioner Care Strategies Table

Specialty Group	Practitioners Included	Hyperemissive Strategies	Hypoemissive Strategies
Biochemistry	Nutritionists, Orthomolecular, Herbalists, Naturopaths	Cardiovascular herbs, antioxidants, adaptogens	Qi tonics and nutritional support
Rehabilitation	Physiotherapists, Massage Therapists, Osteopaths / Chiropractors	Thoracic mobilization, myofascial release	Gentle mobilization, warming massage
Energetics	Acupuncturists (TCM), Bioenergetic Therapists	Acupuncture, moxibustion, PEMF	Warming acupuncture, energy balancing
Psychological	GNM practitioners, Psychotherapists, Vibrational therapists, Family constellation facilitators	Psychotherapy, bioresonance, energy clearing	Psychosomatic conflict resolution, emotional balancing

Educational Pearls & Considerations.

- Accurate acupuncture point selection is vital for effective treatment.
- Moxibustion must be used carefully in patients sensitive to heat.
- Herbal therapies should be prescribed by qualified practitioners.
- Integration with rehabilitative therapies enhances outcomes.

GROUP 3 - ZONE 13 – CHEST AND STERNUM

Category 8: *Energetic*

Step 1: Functional Anatomy and Interpretive Importance

The chest and sternum form the anterior thoracic wall, protecting the heart and lungs and providing muscular attachment for respiration and posture (Standring, 2016). Energetically, this region is a key conductor of systemic regulation, reflecting both cardiopulmonary and emotional coherence.

Hunt (1996) demonstrated measurable electromagnetic fluctuations around the thorax associated with stress and respiratory patterns, providing experimental grounding for biospectral findings here.

Patients may report sensations of tightness, palpitations, or diffuse thoracic heaviness, often without clear structural origin. Spectral surface readings frequently reveal hypoemissive depressions consistent with inhibited energy flow or autonomic restriction, while hyperemissive focal zones reflect adaptive release or reparative activation.

These emissive patterns often cross costal margins and fascial continuities rather than adhering to organ outlines, reinforcing their systemic interpretive significance. Clinically, the chest and sternum function as a biospectral barometer of cardiopulmonary vitality, emotional stability, and systemic integration, where surface signals anticipate deeper regulatory shifts.

Step 2,3,4: ROI Classification and Interpretive Questions

Hyperemission indicates localized energy congestion or field reactivity.

- Does the patient feel heat, tension, or discomfort in the chest area?
- Are stress or emotional factors prominent?

Hypoemission suggests energy deficiency or stagnation.

- Does the patient experience fatigue, coldness, or low vitality?
- Are symptoms chronic or resistant to conventional therapies?

Step 5: Confirmatory Evaluations

Test	Purpose & Justification	Relevance to Emissive Pattern
Bioresonance testing	Measures tissue energy frequencies and imbalances.	Correlates with emissive anomalies.
Electrodermal screening (EDS)	Assesses skin conductance linked to energy pathways.	Supports interpretation of energetic imbalances.
Patient emotional and symptom history	Provides context for energetic dysfunction and stress factors.	Assists biospectral differentiation.

Step 6: Care Strategies and Intervention Pathways

Naturopathic Approach

Employ bioresonance, pulsed electromagnetic fields (PEMF), and adaptogenic botanicals to restore energetic balance and support healing (Matsumoto et al., 2010). Nutritional antioxidants and adaptogens enhance systemic resilience. Mindfulness and stress reduction techniques complement energetic treatments.

Standard Medical Approaches

Energetic therapies serve as adjuncts to conventional medical and rehabilitative interventions to optimize patient outcomes.

Specialty / Practitioner Care Strategies Table

Specialty Group	Practitioners Included	Hyperemissive Strategies	Hypoemissive Strategies
Biochemistry	Nutritionists, Orthomolecular, Herbalists, Naturopaths	Adaptogens, antioxidants, herbal energetics	Nutritional support for energy deficiency
Rehabilitation	Physiotherapists, Massage Therapists, Osteopaths / Chiropractors	Energy-based manual therapies, PEMF, therapeutic touch	Gentle stimulation, mobilization
Energetics	Acupuncturists (TCM), Bioenergetic Therapists	Bioresonance, PEMF, acupuncture	Warming acupuncture, energy balancing
Psychological	GNM practitioners, Psychotherapists, Vibrational therapists, Family constellation facilitators	Psychotherapy, bioresonance, mindfulness	Emotional balancing, vibrational medicine

Educational Pearls & Considerations.

- Energetic therapies complement but do not replace standard medical care.
- Practitioner skill and patient response influence effectiveness.
- Regular monitoring and adjustment optimize outcomes.
- Address psychological and physical factors holistically.

GROUP 3 - ZONE 13 – CHEST AND STERNUM

Category 9: *Metabolic / Endocrine*

Step 1: Functional Anatomy and Interpretive Importance

The chest and sternum protect the thoracic cavity while supporting respiratory musculature and vascular networks (Standring, 2016). Metabolic and endocrine dysfunctions often express here, as systemic conditions such as diabetes, dyslipidemia, and thyroid imbalance alter cardiovascular and muscular performance.

Larsen et al. (2016) emphasized that endocrine regulation directly modulates cardiac contractility and metabolic substrate use, underscoring the systemic vulnerability of thoracic tissues. Patients may report palpitations, diffuse chest tension, or reduced stamina.

Spectral surface readings highlight hypoemissive depressions consistent with impaired metabolic drive and perfusion irregularities, alongside hyperemissive arcs reflecting compensatory repair or endocrine overactivation.

These emissive dynamics often extend across costal and fascial continuities, mapping systemic dysfunction more than localized lesions. Clinically, the chest and sternum serve as a biospectral window into cardiometabolic balance, linking surface findings with systemic regulatory integrity.

Step 2,3,4: ROI Classification and Interpretive Questions

Hyperemission suggests localized reactivity, microbial activity, or metabolic overactivity.

- Is there warmth, redness, or swelling in the chest area?
- Is metabolic control optimal?

Hypoemission indicates hypoperfusion, neuropathy, or impaired perfusion from metabolic or endocrine dysfunction.

- Are there cold sensations, numbness, or chronic wounds?
- Are systemic symptoms like fatigue or temperature intolerance present?

Step 5: Confirmatory Evaluations

Test	Purpose & Justification	Relevance to Emissive Pattern
HbA1c, fasting glucose	Assesses glycemic control in diabetes.	Correlates with hypoemissive neurofunctional or perfusion-restricted zones.
Thyroid function tests (TSH, Free T4)	Evaluates thyroid disorders affecting metabolism and circulation.	Associated with altered emissive regulation.

Lipid profile	Assesses cardiovascular risk impacting tissue perfusion.	Supports metabolic vascular adaptation.
Inflammatory markers (CRP, ESR)	Detects systemic inflammation influencing tissue health.	Correlates with hyperemissive tissue activation states.

Step 6: Care Strategies and Intervention Pathways

Naturopathic Approach

Support metabolic health with low glycemic diet, antioxidants, and adaptogens (Alberti et al., 2006). Herbs such as *Panax ginseng* and *Gymnema sylvestre* support endocrine function. Supplement chromium, magnesium, and alpha-lipoic acid to enhance glucose metabolism and neuroprotection. Encourage regular aerobic exercise to improve circulation.

Standard Medical Approaches

Pharmacologic and lifestyle interventions focus on metabolic control. Thyroid hormone replacement and lipid management reduce complications.

Specialty / Practitioner Care Strategies Table

Specialty Group	Practitioners Included	Hyperemissive Strategies	Hypoemissive Strategies
Biochemistry	Nutritionists, Orthomolecular, Herbalists, Naturopaths	Antioxidants, adaptogens, insulin sensitizers, micronutrients	Metabolic support, neuroprotective nutrients, dietary management
Rehabilitation	Physiotherapists, Massage Therapists, Osteopaths / Chiropractors	Exercise therapy, circulation enhancement	Neuromuscular re-education, aerobic conditioning
Energetics	Acupuncturists (TCM), Bioenergetic Therapists	Acupuncture supporting metabolic function	Energy balancing, PEMF
Psychological	GNM practitioners, Psychotherapists, Vibrational therapists, Family constellation facilitators	Mind-body therapies supporting metabolic regulation	Stress reduction, emotional balancing

Educational Pearls & Considerations.

- Regular metabolic monitoring is essential to prevent complications.
- Lifestyle and dietary modifications complement clinical treatment.
- Adaptogens support but do not replace conventional therapies.
- Patient education on skin and wound care is critical.

GROUP 3

ZONE 14 – LEFT AXILLARY

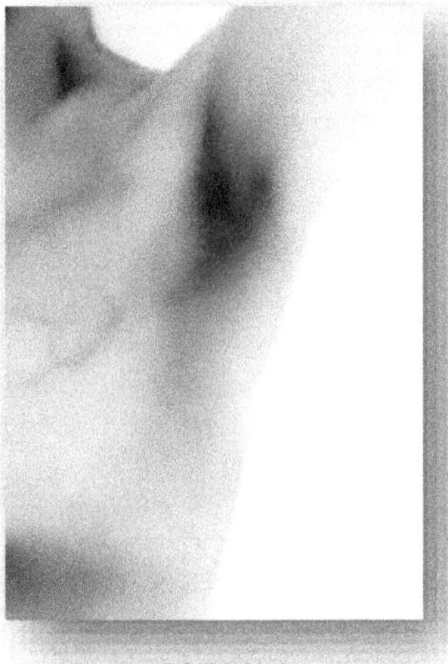

G3Z14LA

The left axillary region is one of the most anatomically dense and clinically relevant surfaces for biospectral analysis. It contains the axillary lymph nodes, brachial plexus, and axillary vessels, making it a convergence of immune, neurovascular, and muscular influences (Standring, 2016).

Functionally, it is highly sensitive to lymphatic retention, and emissive asymmetries often provide early clues of immune strain. Breast cancer remains the most common cancer in women worldwide, with axillary lymph nodes as the primary site of early metastasis (Giuliano et al., 2017), underscoring the clinical importance of subtle irregularities where angiogenesis or lymphatic remodeling may be occurring.

Biospectrally, hyperemission is also noted in neurovascular compression, as in thoracic outlet syndrome, where up to 8% of cases involve vascular or neural compromise detectable before imaging (Sanders & Hammond, 2002).

Muscular factors add to this complexity: tension in the pectoralis major, subscapularis, or serratus anterior can generate persistent irregularities reflecting postural or functional imbalance. Axillary nodes also drain the upper limb, thoracic wall, and breast, making asymmetries markers of regional immune activation (Mortimer & Rockson, 2014). In metabolic contexts, axillary disturbances may correlate with toxic load or altered hormonal regulation, demonstrating the zone's ability to capture systemic burden.

Clinically, the left axilla reveals early immune activation, vascular stress, or muscular overload through subtle biospectral changes. As a non-invasive observation field, it offers insight into processes ranging from localized strain to systemic immune or oncologic adaptation, making it a zone of both preventive and diagnostic value.

Zone 14 – Left Axillary: Emission-Relevant Structures

Category	Relevant Structures	Emission Relevance
1. Vascular / Circulatory	- Axillary artery and vein - Branches of the subclavian vessels	Hyperemission may indicate vascular retention, tissue activation, or vasoregulatory expansion; Hypoemission may suggest perfusion decline or impaired flow due to compression or vasospasm.
2. Muscular / Myofascial	- Pectoralis minor and major (proximal insertions) - Serratus anterior - Subscapularis	Hyperemission often reflects muscular overuse, strain, or fascial activation; Hypoemission may signal chronic disuse, atrophy, or fascial restriction affecting shoulder mechanics.
3. Skeletal / Articular	- Clavicle (medial third) - Scapula (coracoid process) - Ribs (first and second)	Local Hyperemission may indicate periosteal field activity or joint signal irritation; Hypoemission can reflect degenerative changes or reduced bone perfusion.
4. Nervous System / Spine	- Brachial plexus trunks and cords - Sympathetic cervical and thoracic ganglia	Hyperemission may indicate neural field irritation or thoracic outlet compression patterns; Hypoemission may reflect nerve compression or autonomic dysfunction affecting upper limb innervation.
5. Lymphatic / Immune	- Axillary lymph nodes (central, lateral, posterior groups) - Superficial lymphatic vessels	Hyperemissive zones often correspond with lymphatic signal activation, immune field response, or regulatory tension; Hypoemission may indicate lymphatic congestion or fibrosis.
6. Organs / GNM (German New Medicine)	- Lymphatic drainage pathways from upper limb and thorax	Elevated emissive expression may suggest active immune field stress; Hypoemission may represent healing phases or impaired lymphatic drainage in associated organ systems.
7. Acupuncture / Meridians	- Large Intestine Meridian - Lung Meridian - Heart Meridian (axillary branch points)	Hyperemission reflects Qi stagnation or excess; low-emission zones suggest Qi deficiency or dampness affecting immune and respiratory function.
8. Energetic / Frequency	- Energetic reflex zones related to immune and neurovascular function	Hyperemission may be linked to bioenergetic overactivation or emotional stress; Hypoemission indicates regulatory depletion or impaired autonomic regulation.
9. Metabolic / Endocrine	- Reflex zones influencing systemic immune and metabolic activity	Hypoemissive patterns may indicate metabolic downregulation or adrenal underperformance; Hyperemission may be present in terrain-level activation or regulatory stress affecting this zone.

GROUP 3 - ZONE 14 – LEFT AXILLARY

Category 1: *Vascular / Circulatory*

Step 1: Functional Anatomy and Interpretive Importance

The axillary artery, a continuation of the subclavian, supplies the left axillary region and upper limb. Its branches include the superior thoracic, thoracoacromial, lateral thoracic, subscapular, and circumflex humeral arteries.

Venous return occurs through the axillary vein, which receives tributaries paralleling these branches before continuing as the subclavian vein (Standring, 2016). Surgical and anatomical literature highlights the axillary vessels as essential reference points in lymphatic dissection and breast surgery, underlining their clinical importance (Clough et al., 2010).

Spectral surface readings of the axilla often reveal emissive irregularities concentrated near vascular branching zones. These may represent venous stasis, vascular reactivity, or localized circulatory stress. Because the axilla integrates thoracic and upper-limb circulation, emissive signals here carry interpretive value for systemic vascular dynamics.

Step 2,3,4: ROI Classification and Interpretive Questions

Hyperemission indicates vascular reactivity, venous congestion, or patterns suggestive of thrombotic involvement.

- Is there localized swelling, redness, or tenderness?
- Are systemic signs such as fever present?

Hypoemission suggests hypoperfusion or impaired perfusion.

- Are there cold sensations, pallor, or delayed healing?
- Is there a history of vascular or lymphatic disorders?

Step 5: Confirmatory Evaluations

Test	Purpose & Justification	Relevance to Emissive Pattern
Doppler ultrasound	Assesses arterial and venous flow in axillary vessels.	Correlates hyperemissive tissue activation and hypoemissive perfusion decline.
CT or MRI angiography	Visualizes vessel patency and detects occlusions or thrombosis.	Confirms vascular flow restriction or signal intensification.
Blood tests (CBC, CRP, coagulation profile)	Detect infection, inflammation, or coagulation disorders.	Supports hyperemissive retention or circulatory impedance states.
Physical exam	Inspects and palpates for vascular compromise signs.	Complements biospectral findings.

Step 6: Care Strategies and Intervention Pathways

Naturopathic Approach

Use botanical venotonics like *Aesculus hippocastanum* and *Ruscus aculeatus* to improve microcirculation and reduce edema (Chrubasik et al., 2011). Implement anti-inflammatory diet rich in antioxidants and omega-3 fatty acids (Calder, 2017). Contrast hydrotherapy with warm and cold applications stimulates circulation (Sutkowy et al., 2019). Supplement vitamins C, E, and bioflavonoids to enhance endothelial function. Encourage limb elevation and gentle massage to promote venous return.

Standard Medical Approaches

Imaging guides anticoagulation, anti-inflammatory medication, or surgical interventions if necessary. Managing systemic factors such as coagulopathies is vital.

Specialty / Practitioner Care Strategies Table

Specialty Group	Practitioners Included	Hyperemissive Strategies	Hypoemissive Strategies
Biochemistry	Nutritionists, Orthomolecular, Herbalists, Naturopaths	Botanical venotonics, antioxidants, anti-inflammatory diet	Circulatory stimulants, endothelial support nutrients
Rehabilitation	Physiotherapists, Massage Therapists, Osteopaths / Chiropractors	Gentle massage, lymphatic drainage, postural correction	Graded exercise, circulatory enhancement
Energetics	Acupuncturists (TCM), Bioenergetic Therapists	Acupuncture, moxibustion, herbal formulas	Warming acupuncture, energy balancing
Psychological	GNM practitioners, Psychotherapists, Vibrational therapists, Family constellation facilitators	Psychotherapy, bioresonance, mindfulness	Stress reduction, emotional balancing

Educational Pearls & Considerations.

- Prompt identification of thrombophlebitis or vascular inflammation is critical.
- Botanical venotonics, diet, and hydrotherapy support vascular health effectively.
- Nitric oxide boosters and omega-3 fatty acids enhance endothelial function and perfusion.
- Compression therapy is contraindicated in severe arterial insufficiency.
- Early mobilization and limb elevation help prevent chronic complications.

GROUP 3 - ZONE 14 – LEFT AXILLARY

Category 2: *Muscular*

Step 1: Functional Anatomy and Interpretive Importance

The left axilla contains muscular elements of the pectoralis major and minor, subscapularis, latissimus dorsi, and serratus anterior, all contributing to shoulder motion and stabilization. This muscular complex, innervated by brachial plexus branches, facilitates abduction, internal rotation, and scapular positioning (Standring, 2016).

Biomechanical studies confirm that dysfunction in the serratus anterior, such as reduced activation or fatigue, predisposes to scapular winging and shoulder impingement (Ludewig & Cook, 2000).

In spectral analysis, the axillary region often demonstrates emissive changes along the anterior or posterior folds, reflecting altered load transfer across the shoulder girdle. These patterns frequently align with clinical observations of asymmetrical shoulder mechanics, providing a biosignal correlate of impaired scapulothoracic integration.

Step 2,3,4: ROI Classification and Interpretive Questions

Hyperemission indicates acute muscle strain, muscular reactivity, or active trigger points.

- Has the patient experienced trauma, repetitive motion, or overuse?
- Is there localized tenderness, swelling, or muscle tightness?

Hypoemission suggests chronic hypoperfusion, fibrosis, or neurogenic muscle atrophy.

- Are there symptoms of weakness, stiffness, or reduced range of motion?
- Is muscle wasting or sensory alteration noted?

Step 5: Confirmatory Evaluations

Test	Purpose & Justification	Relevance to Emissive Pattern
Creatine kinase (CK), LDH	Detects muscle injury or inflammation (Simons et al., 1999).	Elevated in hyperemissive tissue activation states.
MRI	Visualizes muscle edema, inflammation, or fibrosis.	Supports hyper- or hypoemissive findings.
Electromyography (EMG)	Assesses muscle and nerve function.	Correlates with hypoemissive neurofunctional causes.
Blood tests (CBC, inflammatory markers)	Detects systemic inflammation or infection.	Supports hyperemissive regulatory field conditions.

Step 6: Care Strategies and Intervention Pathways

Naturopathic Approach

Employ anti-inflammatory botanicals such as *Curcuma longa* and *Boswellia serrata* to reduce muscle inflammation (Hewlings & Kalman, 2017). Magnesium supplementation supports muscle relaxation. Hydrotherapy with alternating warm and cold applications improves circulation (Sutkowy et al., 2019). Progressive stretching and strengthening facilitate recovery. Adequate protein and antioxidants support tissue repair.

Standard Medical Approaches

Rest, NSAIDs, and physical therapy remain standard treatments for muscle injury (Simons et al., 1999). Neurological evaluation is advised if weakness or sensory changes are present.

Specialty / Practitioner Care Strategies Table

Specialty Group	Practitioners Included	Hyperemissive Strategies	Hypoemissive Strategies
Biochemistry	Nutritionists, Orthomolecular, Herbalists, Naturopaths	Anti-inflammatory botanicals, magnesium, antioxidants, protein	Circulatory support, neurotrophic nutrients, protein support
Rehabilitation	Physiotherapists, Massage Therapists, Osteopaths / Chiropractors	Myofascial release, trigger point therapy, gentle massage	Graded aerobic exercise, neurorehabilitation, ergonomic guidance
Energetics	Acupuncturists (TCM), Bioenergetic Therapists	Acupuncture, moxibustion, PEMF	Warming acupuncture, frequency therapy
Psychological	GNM practitioners, Psychotherapists, Vibrational therapists, Family constellation facilitators	Psychotherapy, bioresonance, mindfulness	Psychosomatic conflict resolution, emotional balancing

Educational Pearls & Considerations.

- Early identification and treatment of myofascial trigger points improves prognosis.
- Magnesium supports muscle relaxation and reduces spasms.
- Hydrotherapy protocols should align with inflammation phases.
- Neurological assessment is necessary for weakness or sensory deficits.
- Gradual rehabilitation prevents chronic dysfunction.

GROUP 3 - ZONE 14 – LEFT AXILLARY

Category 3: *Skeletal*

Step 1: Functional Anatomy and Interpretive Importance

The skeletal foundation of the left axillary region consists of the clavicle, scapula, and upper ribs, which together form the bony framework of the shoulder girdle (Standring, 2016). These structures support arm mobility, protect neurovascular bundles, and transmit forces between trunk and upper limb.

Fractures, degenerative remodeling, or subluxations in this region may produce mechanical pain and postural asymmetries. Miller et al. (2014) report that scapulothoracic and costoclavicular joint dysfunction frequently manifests with regional discomfort that mimics soft tissue syndromes.

Such skeletal disturbances alter fascial and vascular regulation, and their biospectral imprint becomes visible as emissive asymmetries in the axillary field. Spectral surface readings often display contained emissive variations aligned with the clavicle or scapular border, contrasting with diffuse patterns of muscular activation.

These signatures reveal how subtle skeletal misalignment projects into external biosignals, aiding the recognition of articular dysfunction in a region often clinically confounded by overlapping soft tissue findings.

Step 2,3,4: ROI Classification and Interpretive Questions

Hyperemission suggests tissue reactivity or acute skeletal injury such as fractures or costal joint separation.

- Is there localized tenderness, swelling, or warmth?
- Are symptoms worsened by movement or palpation?

Hypoemission indicates chronic degeneration or hypoperfusion in skeletal tissues.

- Are symptoms persistent with dull pain or stiffness?
- Is there a history of trauma or repetitive stress?

Step 5: Confirmatory Evaluations

Test	Purpose & Justification	Relevance to Emissive Pattern
X-ray	Detects fractures, dislocations, and degenerative changes.	Supports interpretive understanding of skeletal signal behavior.
MRI	Visualizes soft tissue involvement and bone marrow edema.	Correlates with activation and structural adaptation.

Bone scan	Assesses bone metabolism and detects occult lesions.	Confirms active skeletal field dynamics or remodeling processes.
Physical exam	Evaluates tenderness, mobility, and neurological signs.	Complements imaging and emissive findings.

Step 6: Care Strategies and Intervention Pathways

Naturopathic Approach

Support bone health with calcium, magnesium, vitamin D, and collagen peptides (Kruger & Kruger, 2019). Use anti-inflammatory herbs such as *Boswellia serrata* for joint inflammation. Physical therapy focusing on posture and mobility enhances recovery. Acupuncture and bioresonance provide pain relief and inflammation control.

Standard Medical Approaches

Treatment includes analgesics, anti-inflammatory medication, and rehabilitation. Surgical intervention may be necessary in severe cases.

Specialty / Practitioner Care Strategies Table

Specialty Group	Practitioners Included	Hyperemissive Strategies	Hypoemissive Strategies
Biochemistry	Nutritionists, Orthomolecular, Herbalists, Naturopaths	Bone-supportive nutrients, anti-inflammatory herbs	Nutritional support for bone repair
Rehabilitation	Physiotherapists, Osteopaths / Chiropractors, Massage Therapists	Manual therapy, posture correction, pain management	Ergonomic training, spinal mobilization
Energetics	Acupuncturists (TCM), Bioenergetic Therapists	Acupuncture, PEMF, energy healing	Energy balancing and stimulation
Psychological	GNM practitioners, Psychotherapists, Vibrational therapists, Family constellation facilitators	Psychotherapy, bioresonance, stress management	Emotional balancing and coping strategies

Educational Pearls & Considerations.

- Early diagnosis and treatment prevent chronic skeletal dysfunction.
- Nutritional support is essential for bone healing.
- Manual therapies combined with rehabilitation optimize outcomes.
- Monitor for complications requiring specialist referral.

GROUP 3 - ZONE 14 – LEFT AXILLARY

Category 4: *Nervous*

Step 1: Functional Anatomy and Interpretive Importance

The left axillary region is supplied by the brachial plexus, which provides sensory and motor innervation to the upper limb through multiple peripheral branches (Standring, 2016).

Compression or traction injuries within the axilla can result in neuropathic pain, sensory disturbance, and motor weakness, often complicating diagnosis. Ferrante (2004) documented that brachial plexopathies frequently arise from trauma, postsurgical scarring, or radiation therapy, producing complex patterns of dysfunction.

Such neural compromise alters vascular and muscular regulation within the shoulder girdle, creating emissive variations visible on the body surface.

Biospectral asymmetries in the axillary field often appear as focal signals tracing the clavicular border or scapular margin, contrasting with the diffuse emissions of muscular strain.

These patterns externalize the impact of brachial plexus injury, providing a valuable noninvasive marker for identifying neurogenic contributions to axillary and shoulder dysfunction.

Step 2,3,4: ROI Classification and Interpretive Questions

Hyperemission indicates nerve irritation or neurogenic reactivity.

- Are there burning, tingling, or sharp pains in the region?
- Is there localized hypersensitivity or swelling?

Hypoemission suggests nerve hypoperfusion, compression, or denervation with decreased autonomic activity.

- Are numbness, weakness, or muscle atrophy present?
- Do symptoms worsen with movement or specific positions?

Step 5: Confirmatory Evaluations

Test	Purpose & Justification	Relevance to Emissive Pattern
Nerve conduction studies (NCS), Electromyography (EMG)	Assess nerve and muscle function (Janis et al., 2010).	Correlates with hypoemissive neurofunctional disruption.
Quantitative sensory testing (QST)	Measures sensory nerve thresholds.	Supports interpretation of neurofunctional patterns.
MRI	Detects nerve root compression or structural abnormalities.	Identifies origin of neural signal disturbance.
Blood tests (glucose, vitamin B12)	Evaluates metabolic causes of neuropathy.	Supports interpretive understanding of systemic neuroregulatory involvement.

Step 6: Care Strategies and Intervention Pathways

Naturopathic Approach

Support nerve repair with B-complex vitamins, alpha-lipoic acid, and Acetyl-L-carnitine (Papanas & Ziegler, 2014). Use *Hypericum perforatum* for neuropathic pain relief (Kasper et al., 2010). Neural mobilization and bioresonance therapies promote recovery. Mind-body approaches modulate neurovascular and autonomic function.

Standard Medical Approaches

Pharmacologic treatments include anticonvulsants, antidepressants, and analgesics. Surgical decompression may be required. Managing metabolic contributors like diabetes is critical.

Specialty / Practitioner Care Strategies Table

Specialty Group	Practitioners Included	Hyperemissive Strategies	Hypoemissive Strategies
Biochemistry	Nutritionists, Orthomolecular, Herbalists, Naturopaths	Neurotrophic vitamins, alpha-lipoic acid, anti-inflammatory botanicals	Circulatory stimulants, metabolic support, neuroprotective nutrients
Rehabilitation	Physiotherapists, Massage Therapists, Osteopaths / Chiropractors	Neural mobilization, myofascial release, gentle massage	Neural gliding exercises, ergonomic guidance, neurorehabilitation
Energetics	Acupuncturists (TCM), Bioenergetic Therapists	Acupuncture, moxibustion, PEMF	Warming acupuncture, frequency therapy, energy healing
Psychological	GNM practitioners, Psychotherapists, Vibrational therapists, Family constellation facilitators	Psychotherapy, bioresonance, mindfulness	Psychosomatic conflict resolution, vibrational medicine

Educational Pearls & Considerations.

- Early recognition of nerve injury prevents chronic deficits.
- Nutritional and energetic therapies support nerve regeneration.
- Monitor for metabolic causes of neuropathy.
- Avoid aggressive therapy during acute inflammatory phases.
- Tailor rehabilitation to patient tolerance.

GROUP 3 - ZONE 14 – LEFT AXILLARY

Category 5: *Lymphatic*

Step 1: Functional Anatomy and Interpretive Importance

The left axilla functions as a major lymphatic basin, collecting drainage from the ipsilateral upper limb, chest wall, and breast before directing it toward central venous return (Standring, 2016).

This region is central to both immune surveillance and systemic fluid balance. Petrek and Heelan (1998) emphasized that axillary lymph node dissection is the leading cause of chronic upper-limb lymphedema, imposing long-term immune and mechanical burden.

When this basin is compromised, adjacent tissues adapt with altered vascular tone and fascial compliance, producing changes that extend outward to the emissive surface.

These external expressions often appear as confined emissive fields at the axillary dome or clavicular border, reflecting the geometry of disrupted flow.

By providing a visible correlate of axillary dysfunction, emissive analysis strengthens the clinician's ability to detect immune drainage compromise in its earlier stages, even before overt swelling becomes manifest.

Step 2,3,4: ROI Classification and Interpretive Questions

Hyperemission reflects acute lymphatic reactivity, microbial activity, or lymphatic congestion presenting with swelling and spectral intensification.

- Is there redness, tenderness, or rapid swelling?
- Has the patient experienced recent trauma or infection?

Hypoemission indicates chronic lymphatic stasis with fibrosis and impaired lymph flow causing decreased biosignal.

- Is swelling persistent and firm?
- Are recurrent infections or delayed wound healing present?

Step 5: Confirmatory Evaluations

Test	Purpose & Justification	Relevance to Emissive Pattern
Lymphoscintigraphy	Assesses lymphatic flow and identifies obstructions.	Confirms lymphatic retention or reduced perfusion.
Doppler ultrasound	Rules out venous insufficiency contributing to swelling.	Differentiates vascular from lymphatic causes.

Blood tests (CBC, inflammatory markers)	Detects infection or systemic inflammation.	Supports hyperemissive tissue activation states.
Physical exam (Stemmer's sign, limb measurements)	Identifies clinical signs of lymphedema.	Correlates with biospectral findings.

Step 6: Care Strategies and Intervention Pathways

Naturopathic Approach

Use herbal lymphagogues such as *Hedera helix* and *Vitis vinifera* to stimulate lymphatic drainage (Godoy et al., 2012). Manual lymphatic drainage by trained therapists promotes fluid movement. Compression therapy supports lymph return and requires proper fitting. Nutritional antioxidants and anti-inflammatory nutrients support tissue repair. Hydrotherapy with alternating warm and cold applications enhances lymphatic circulation.

Standard Medical Approaches

Standard care includes manual lymphatic drainage, compression garments, physical therapy, and infection management. Surgery is reserved for refractory cases.

Specialty / Practitioner Care Strategies Table

Specialty Group	Practitioners Included	Hyperemissive Strategies	Hypoemissive Strategies
Biochemistry	Nutritionists, Orthomolecular, Herbalists, Naturopaths	Herbal lymphagogues, antioxidants, anti-inflammatory nutrients	Circulatory support, nutritional tissue repair support
Rehabilitation	Physiotherapists, Massage Therapists, Osteopaths / Chiropractors	Manual lymphatic drainage, gentle massage, postural retraining	Compression therapy, graded exercise, ergonomic guidance
Energetics	Acupuncturists (TCM), Bioenergetic Therapists	Acupuncture, herbal formulas, PEMF	Warming acupuncture, energy balancing
Psychological	GNM practitioners, Psychotherapists, Vibrational therapists, Family constellation facilitators	Mind-body therapies supporting immune function and healing	Psychosomatic conflict resolution, emotional balancing

Educational Pearls & Considerations.

- Early intervention prevents progression to chronic lymphedema.
- Manual lymphatic drainage should be performed by certified therapists.
- Compression therapy requires proper fitting and monitoring.
- Nutritional support enhances lymphatic function and tissue repair.
- Prompt infection control is essential.

GROUP 3 - ZONE 14 – LEFT AXILLARY

Category 6: *Organ-Related (GNM)*

Step 1: Functional Anatomy and Interpretive Importance

The left axillary region is bounded by the pectoralis major, latissimus dorsi, and thoracic wall, containing lymph nodes, neurovascular bundles, and connective tissues that communicate directly with the upper thorax (Standring, 2016).

Within GNM, this region is linked to biological conflicts affecting the heart and lungs, where resolution is seen as hyperemissive intensification and active conflict as hypoemissive suppression. Hamer (2012) described how these visceral programs are projected outward, producing emissive signatures in adjacent fields.

On surface assessment, such expressions may appear as confined signals along the axillary dome or extending into the anterior thoracic margin. Lutgendorf and Costanzo (2003) highlighted the bidirectional relationship between psychosocial stress and immune–cardiopulmonary regulation, reinforcing the plausibility of these observations.

Thus, emissive mapping of the left axilla provides a visible correlate of heart–lung adaptation, extending interpretation beyond purely musculoskeletal or lymphatic explanations.

Step 2,3,4: ROI Classification and Interpretive Questions

Hyperemission indicates reactive or healing phases with increased metabolic activity.

- Are there symptoms like localized pain, chest discomfort, or respiratory issues?
- Is infection or inflammation present?

Hypoemission corresponds to conflict-active phases with tissue loss or functional suppression.

- Are symptoms chronic with fatigue or decreased organ function?
- Is psychological stress or unresolved conflict evident?

Step 5: Confirmatory Evaluations

Test	Purpose & Justification	Relevance to Emissive Pattern
Chest imaging (X-ray, CT, MRI)	Visualizes thoracic organ morphology and pathology.	Correlates with emissive anomalies indicating organ involvement.
Cardiac and pulmonary function tests	Assess heart and lung function.	Supports interpretive understanding of organ field dysregulation.
Inflammatory markers, CBC	Detect systemic inflammation or infection.	Supports hyperemissive resolution phases.
Psychological assessment	Evaluates biological conflicts and psychosomatic factors.	Complements GNM interpretive approach.

Step 6: Care Strategies and Intervention Pathways

Naturopathic Approach

Use cardioprotective and anti-inflammatory botanicals such as *Crataegus monogyna* and *Curcuma longa* (Tattelman, 2001). Support respiratory health with expectorants and antioxidants. Stress management and psychotherapy assist conflict resolution. Nutritional antioxidants aid tissue repair.

Standard Medical Approaches

Medical management guided by imaging and functional tests. Pharmacologic therapies target cardiac and pulmonary conditions. Lifestyle modification and rehabilitation support recovery.

Specialty / Practitioner Care Strategies Table

Specialty Group	Practitioners Included	Hyperemissive Strategies	Hypoemissive Strategies
Biochemistry	Nutritionists, Orthomolecular, Herbalists, Naturopaths	Cardioprotective herbs, antioxidants, anti-inflammatories	Nutritional support for organ function and repair
Rehabilitation	Physiotherapists, Massage Therapists, Osteopaths / Chiropractors	Respiratory therapy, circulation enhancement	Gentle mobilization and relaxation techniques
Energetics	Acupuncturists (TCM), Bioenergetic Therapists	Acupuncture for cardiac and pulmonary support	Energy balancing and harmonization
Psychological	GNM practitioners, Psychotherapists, Vibrational therapists, Family constellation facilitators	Psychotherapy, bioresonance, conflict resolution	Emotional balancing and stress management

Educational Pearls & Considerations.

- Consider psychosomatic influences per GNM in thoracic organ pathology.
- Integrate physical and psychological therapies for best outcomes.
- Regular monitoring of cardiac and pulmonary function is essential.
- Multidisciplinary approach enhances patient care.

GROUP 3 - ZONE 14 – LEFT AXILLARY

Category 7: *Acupuncture / Meridian*

Step 1: Functional Anatomy and Interpretive Importance

The left axillary region includes neurovascular bundles, lymph nodes, and fascia bridging the thoracic wall with the upper limb (Standring, 2016). TCM associates this zone with the Heart (HT), Pericardium (PC), and Lung (LU) meridians.

Deadman et al. (2007) noted the therapeutic use of LU1 and PC1 in regulating respiratory and emotional balance via the axillary entry points. Maciocia (2015) emphasized how disruptions in LU and HT channels contribute to fatigue, chest pain, or dyspnea. Clinically, tension or fullness in the axilla may accompany cardiovascular or pulmonary imbalance.

On biosignal assessment, surface emissive variations appear as localized hyper- or hypoemission along axillary arcs, reflecting the trajectory of LU, HT, and PC channels. These externalized signals reinforce the view that axillary biospectral asymmetries can represent both thoracic meridian dysfunction and systemic energy disturbance.

Step 2,3,4: ROI Classification and Interpretive Questions

Hyperemission suggests Qi stagnation or energetic reactivity along the meridians.

- Are there localized pain, tightness, or discomfort?
- Are symptoms aggravated by emotional stress or physical exertion?

Hypoemission indicates Qi deficiency or chronic stagnation with poor circulation and cold sensations.

- Does the patient report fatigue, coldness, or palpitations?
- Are symptoms persistent or worsening?

Step 5: Confirmatory Evaluations

Test	Purpose & Justification	Relevance to Emissive Pattern
Pulse diagnosis and tongue examination	TCM methods assessing meridian Qi and Blood status (Flaws, 2000).	Helps differentiate hyper- and hypoemissive patterns.
Biospectral imaging	Visualizes thermal asymmetries along meridian pathways.	Correlates with Qi imbalances in the axillary region.
Patient symptom questionnaire	Assesses chest discomfort, palpitations, and emotional state.	Assists clinical differentiation of meridian signal disruption.

Step 6: Care Strategies and Intervention Pathways

Naturopathic Approach

Acupuncture points such as HT7, PC6, and LU1 regulate Qi flow and relieve stagnation (Lao et al., 2004). Moxibustion warms hypoemissive meridian areas. Herbal formulas like *Tian Wang Bu Xin Dan* and *Bao Yuan Tang* support thoracic meridians (Bensky et al., 2004). Lifestyle and stress management complement treatment.

Standard Medical Approaches

Acupuncture is used adjunctively for pain relief and improved thoracic function.

Specialty / Practitioner Care Strategies Table

Specialty Group	Practitioners Included	Hyperemissive Strategies	Hypoemissive Strategies
Biochemistry	Nutritionists, Orthomolecular, Herbalists, Naturopaths	Cardiovascular and respiratory herbs, antioxidants	Qi tonics and nutritional support
Rehabilitation	Physiotherapists, Massage Therapists, Osteopaths / Chiropractors	Thoracic mobilization, myofascial release	Gentle mobilization, warming massage
Energetics	Acupuncturists (TCM), Bioenergetic Therapists	Acupuncture, moxibustion, PEMF	Warming acupuncture, energy balancing
Psychological	GNM practitioners, Psychotherapists, Vibrational therapists, Family constellation facilitators	Psychotherapy, bioresonance, energy clearing	Psychosomatic conflict resolution, emotional balancing

Educational Pearls & Considerations.

- Accurate acupuncture point selection enhances effectiveness.
- Moxibustion should be used cautiously in heat-sensitive patients.
- Herbal prescriptions require qualified supervision.
- Combine acupuncture with rehabilitative therapies for best outcomes.

GROUP 3 - ZONE 14 – LEFT AXILLARY

Category 8: *Energetic*

Step 1: Functional Anatomy and Interpretive Importance

The left axillary region incorporatees lymph nodes, neurovascular bundles, and musculature that link the thoracic wall to the upper limb (Standring, 2016). Energetically, it acts as a transitional node, mediating between central thoracic coherence and peripheral regulation.

Hammerschlag et al. (2015) reviewed evidence linking biofield therapies with autonomic modulation, a concept that parallels emissive signals observed in this region.

Clinically, patients may experience diffuse axillary heaviness, immune strain, or shoulder instability. Spectral surface readings commonly display hypoemissive hollows indicating stagnation of systemic flow, interspersed with hyperemissive arcs reflecting immune activation or reparative effort.

These emissive dynamics extend across fascial and lymphatic pathways, underscoring their interpretive value beyond localized pathology. The left axillary region therefore provides visible evidence of how systemic regulation and immune resilience are expressed through surface energy signatures, linking thoracic, lymphatic, and upper limb coherence.

Step 2,3,4: ROI Classification and Interpretive Questions

Hyperemission indicates localized energetic congestion or field reactivity.

- Does the patient experience heat, tension, or discomfort in the axillary area?
- Are stress or emotional factors present?

Hypoemission suggests energetic deficiency or stagnation.

- Does the patient report fatigue, coldness, or low vitality?
- Are symptoms chronic or resistant to standard treatments?

Step 5: Confirmatory Evaluations

Test	Purpose & Justification	Relevance to Emissive Pattern
Bioresonance testing	Measures energy frequencies and tissue imbalances.	Correlates with emissive energetic anomalies.
Electrodermal screening (EDS)	Assesses skin conductance linked to energetic pathways.	Supports interpretive understanding of energetic imbalance.
Patient emotional and symptom history	Provides context for energetic dysfunction and stress factors.	Assists biospectral differentiation.

Step 6: Care Strategies and Intervention Pathways

Naturopathic Approach

Utilize bioresonance, pulsed electromagnetic fields (PEMF), and adaptogens to restore energetic balance and promote healing (Matsumoto et al., 2010). Nutritional antioxidants and adaptogens enhance systemic resilience. Mindfulness and stress reduction techniques complement energetic therapies.

Standard Medical Approaches

Energetic treatments act as adjuncts to conventional and rehabilitative care, optimizing patient outcomes.

Specialty / Practitioner Care Strategies Table

Specialty Group	Practitioners Included	Hyperemissive Strategies	Hypoemissive Strategies
Biochemistry	Nutritionists, Orthomolecular, Herbalists, Naturopaths	Adaptogens, antioxidants, herbal energetics	Nutritional support for energy deficiency
Rehabilitation	Physiotherapists, Massage Therapists, Osteopaths / Chiropractors	Energy-based manual therapies, PEMF, therapeutic touch	Gentle stimulation, mobilization
Energetics	Acupuncturists (TCM), Bioenergetic Therapists	Bioresonance, PEMF, acupuncture	Warming acupuncture, energy balancing
Psychological	GNM practitioners, Psychotherapists, Vibrational therapists, Family constellation facilitators	Psychotherapy, bioresonance, mindfulness	Emotional balancing, vibrational medicine

Educational Pearls & Considerations.

- Energetic therapies complement but do not replace standard medical treatments.
- Patient response and practitioner skill influence effectiveness.
- Regular reassessment and adaptation optimize outcomes.
- Holistic approach addressing psychological and physical factors is essential.

GROUP 3 - ZONE 14 – LEFT AXILLARY

Category 9: *Metabolic / Endocrine*

Step 1: Functional Anatomy and Interpretive Importance

The left axillary region contains lymph nodes, neurovascular structures, and fascial supports connecting thorax and upper limb (Standring, 2016). Endocrine and metabolic systems strongly influence this area, particularly through immune–metabolic interactions.

Brent (2012) highlighted thyroid hormones as modulators of vascular tone and immune function, processes that converge in the axillary field. Clinically, patients may describe immune fatigue, left-sided thoracic heaviness, or recurrent strain.

Biospectral imaging reveals hypoemissive hollows consistent with suppressed metabolic or thyroid drive, contrasted with focal hyperemissive arcs representing immune or reparative intensification.

These emissive signals extend beyond local structures, emphasizing systemic interpretation. The left axillary field thus integrates metabolic–endocrine and immune regulation, making it a key biospectral marker of systemic resilience.

Step 2,3,4: ROI Classification and Interpretive Questions

Hyperemission indicates localized reactivity, metabolic overactivity, or microbial activity.

- Is there warmth, redness, or swelling in the region?
- Is systemic metabolic control optimal?

Hypoemission suggests hypoperfusion, neuropathy, or impaired perfusion due to metabolic/endocrine dysfunction.

- Are cold sensations, numbness, or delayed healing present?
- Are systemic symptoms like fatigue or temperature intolerance reported?

Step 5: Confirmatory Evaluations

Test	Purpose & Justification	Relevance to Emissive Pattern
HbA1c, fasting glucose	Assesses glycemic control in diabetes.	Correlates with hypoemissive neurofunctional or perfusion-restricted areas.
Thyroid function tests (TSH, Free T4)	Evaluates thyroid dysfunction affecting metabolism and circulation.	Associated with altered emissive regulation.
Lipid profile	Assesses cardiovascular risk impacting tissue perfusion.	Supports metabolic vascular adaptation.
Inflammatory markers (CRP, ESR)	Detects systemic inflammation influencing tissue health.	Correlates with hyperemissive tissue activation states.

Step 6: Care Strategies and Intervention Pathways

Naturopathic Approach

Support metabolic balance through low glycemic diets, antioxidants, and adaptogens (Alberti et al., 2006). Use herbs like *Panax ginseng* and *Gymnema sylvestre* to support endocrine function. Supplement chromium, magnesium, and alpha-lipoic acid to aid glucose metabolism and neuroprotection. Encourage regular aerobic exercise to improve circulation.

Standard Medical Approaches

Medical management includes pharmacologic and lifestyle interventions for metabolic control. Thyroid hormone replacement and lipid management reduce complications.

Specialty / Practitioner Care Strategies Table

Specialty Group	Practitioners Included	Hyperemissive Strategies	Hypoemissive Strategies
Biochemistry	Nutritionists, Orthomolecular, Herbalists, Naturopaths	Antioxidants, adaptogens, insulin sensitizers, micronutrients	Metabolic support, neuroprotective nutrients, dietary management
Rehabilitation	Physiotherapists, Massage Therapists, Osteopaths / Chiropractors	Exercise therapy, circulation enhancement	Neuromuscular re-education, aerobic conditioning
Energetics	Acupuncturists (TCM), Bioenergetic Therapists	Acupuncture supporting metabolic function	Energy balancing, PEMF
Psychological	GNM practitioners, Psychotherapists, Vibrational therapists, Family constellation facilitators	Mind-body therapies supporting metabolic regulation	Stress reduction, emotional balancing

Educational Pearls & Considerations.

- Monitor metabolic parameters regularly to prevent complications.
- Dietary and lifestyle changes enhance clinical management.
- Adaptogens support but do not replace standard therapies.
- Educate patients on skin care to prevent ulcerations.

GROUP 3

ZONE 15 – RIGHT AXILLARY

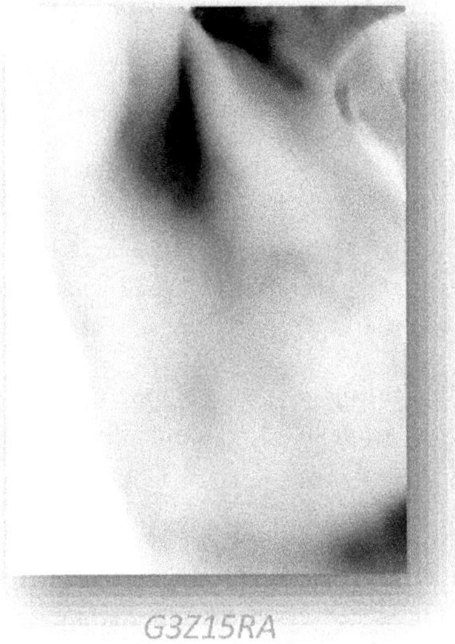

G3Z15RA

The right axillary region mirrors the density of its left counterpart, containing lymphatic nodes, neurovascular bundles, and muscular attachments that create a complex field for emissive observation. It houses the axillary vein and artery, branches of the brachial plexus, and a concentration of lymph nodes draining the right upper limb, thoracic wall, and portions of the breast (Standring, 2016).

Emissive asymmetries here are particularly important for recognizing lymphatic burden and vascular compromise. Axillary lymphadenopathy is common in systemic immune responses, reported in up to 38% of patients following infection or immunologic activation (Cohen et al., 2014), making this region a sentinel of immune adaptation. In women, the right axillary nodes are equally relevant for breast surveillance, with irregularities potentially indicating vascular or lymphatic change before structural detection.

From a neurovascular perspective, this zone is implicated in thoracic outlet syndromes, with compression affecting venous and neural pathways; prevalence of symptomatic neurovascular compression is estimated at 3–8%, often with subclinical circulatory irregularities (Illig et al., 2010).

Musculoskeletal tension in the pectoralis minor, latissimus dorsi, or serratus anterior can also generate persistent hyperactivity or suppression. A further interpretive dimension is systemic: the right axilla may correspond to hepatic or right-sided lymphatic burden, reflecting drainage patterns shaped by central circulation.

Biospectrally, subtle emissive asymmetry here thus serves as a peripheral marker of visceral regulation, particularly in hepatic metabolic stress or right-dominant lymphatic load. For integrative interpretation, the right axilla unites muscular, vascular, lymphatic, and systemic influences, making it a pivotal region for early recognition of immune and metabolic adaptation.

Zone 15 – Right Axillary: Emission-Relevant Structures

Category	Relevant Structures	Emission Relevance
1. Vascular / Circulatory	- Axillary artery and vein - Branches of the subclavian vessels	Hyperemission indicates vascular retention or tissue activation; Hypoemission suggests perfusion decline or impaired blood flow due to compression or spasm.
2. Muscular / Myofascial	- Pectoralis minor and major (proximal insertions) - Serratus anterior - Subscapularis	Hyperemission corresponds to muscle overuse or fascial activation; Hypoemission may indicate muscle atrophy or fascial tension limiting function.
3. Skeletal / Articular	- Clavicle (medial third) - Scapula (coracoid process) - Ribs (first and second)	Hyperemission suggests periosteal field reactivity or joint signal excitation; Hypoemission reflects degenerative or perfusion-restricted bony changes.
4. Nervous System / Spine	- Brachial plexus trunks and cords - Sympathetic cervical and thoracic ganglia	Hyperemission may indicate nerve field irritation or thoracic outlet compression; Hypoemission suggests nerve compression or autonomic dysfunction.
5. Lymphatic / Immune	- Axillary lymph nodes (central, lateral, posterior groups) - Superficial lymphatic vessels	Hyperemissive zones suggest lymphatic signal activation or immune field response; Hypoemission may reflect lymphatic stasis or fibrosis.
6. Organs / GNM (German New Medicine)	- Lymphatic drainage pathways from upper limb and thorax	Hyperemission may represent active immune field stress; Hypoemission correlates with healing or impaired drainage.
7. Acupuncture / Meridians	- Large Intestine Meridian - Lung Meridian - Heart Meridian (axillary branch points)	Hyperemission indicates Qi stagnation or excess; Hypoemission suggests Qi deficiency or dampness affecting respiratory and immune function.
8. Energetic / Frequency	- Reflex energetic zones associated with immune and neurovascular regulation	Hyperemission linked to bioenergetic activation or emotional stress; Hypoemission indicates regulatory depletion or autonomic imbalance.
9. Metabolic / Endocrine	- Reflex zones impacting systemic immune and metabolic activities	Hypoemissive patterns indicate metabolic downregulation or adrenal underperformance; Hyperemission correlates with tissue activation or increased metabolic demand.

GROUP 3 - ZONE 15 – RIGHT AXILLARY

Category 1: *Vascular / Circulatory*

Step 1: Functional Anatomy and Interpretive Importance

The right axillary region mirrors the left, with the axillary artery divided into three parts by the pectoralis minor and giving rise to branches that supply the shoulder girdle, thoracic wall, and proximal upper limb. Venous return through the axillary vein parallels this distribution, continuing as the subclavian vein (Standring, 2016).

Clinical reports describe the axillary vessels as crucial landmarks in both vascular and oncological surgery, particularly for maintaining perfusion during dissection (Clough et al., 2010).

On spectral surface reading, emissive asymmetries in this region frequently align with the axillary arterial and venous courses. These patterns may signal transient venous overload, regulatory adjustments of arterial tone, or adaptive circulatory stress from upper-limb movement. As a transitional hub between thoracic and limb circulation, the axilla often yields meaningful emissive markers for vascular assessment.

Step 2,3,4: ROI Classification and Interpretive Questions

Hyperemission suggests vascular reactivity, venous congestion, or patterns suggestive of thrombotic involvement.

- Are there signs of redness, swelling, or tenderness?
- Are systemic symptoms like fever or malaise present?

Hypoemission indicates hypoperfusion or compromised blood flow.

- Is coldness, pallor, or delayed wound healing observed?
- Is there a history of vascular or lymphatic disease?

Step 5: Confirmatory Evaluations

Test	Purpose & Justification	Relevance to Emissive Pattern
Doppler ultrasound	Assesses arterial and venous flow in axillary vessels.	Correlates hyperemissive tissue activation and hypoemissive perfusion decline..
CT or MRI angiography	Visualizes vessel patency and detects occlusions or thrombosis.	Confirms vascular flow restriction or signal intensification.
Blood tests (CBC, CRP, coagulation profile)	Detect infection, inflammation, or coagulation disorders.	Supports hyperemissive retention or circulatory impedance states.
Physical exam	Inspects and palpates for vascular compromise signs.	Complements biospectral findings.

Step 6: Care Strategies and Intervention Pathways

Naturopathic Approach

Botanical venotonics such as *Aesculus hippocastanum* and *Ruscus aculeatus* improve microcirculation and reduce edema (Chrubasik et al., 2011). Anti-inflammatory diets rich in antioxidants and omega-3 fatty acids support vascular health (Calder, 2017). Contrast hydrotherapy stimulates circulation (Sutkowy et al., 2019). Vitamins C, E, and bioflavonoids enhance endothelial function. Limb elevation and gentle massage promote venous return.

Standard Medical Approaches

Imaging guides anticoagulation, anti-inflammatory medication, or surgical intervention as necessary. Management of systemic contributors like coagulopathies is essential.

Specialty / Practitioner Care Strategies Table

Specialty Group	Practitioners Included	Hyperemissive Strategies	Hypoemissive Strategies
Biochemistry	Nutritionists, Orthomolecular, Herbalists, Naturopaths	Botanical venotonics, antioxidants, anti-inflammatory diet	Circulatory stimulants, endothelial support nutrients
Rehabilitation	Physiotherapists, Massage Therapists, Osteopaths / Chiropractors	Gentle massage, lymphatic drainage, postural correction	Graded exercise, circulatory enhancement
Energetics	Acupuncturists (TCM), Bioenergetic Therapists	Acupuncture, moxibustion, herbal formulas	Warming acupuncture, energy balancing
Psychological	GNM practitioners, Psychotherapists, Vibrational therapists, Family constellation facilitators	Psychotherapy, bioresonance, mindfulness	Stress reduction, emotional balancing

Educational Pearls & Considerations.

- Early diagnosis of thrombophlebitis or vascular inflammation is critical.
- Botanical venotonics, diet, and hydrotherapy effectively support vascular health.
- Nitric oxide boosters and omega-3 fatty acids improve endothelial function and perfusion.
- Compression therapy contraindicated in severe arterial insufficiency.
- Early mobilization and limb elevation help prevent chronic complications.

GROUP 3 - ZONE 15 – RIGHT AXILLARY

Category 2: *Muscular*

Step 1: Functional Anatomy and Interpretive Importance

The right axillary region mirrors the structural composition of the left, with pectoralis major and minor, subscapularis, latissimus dorsi, and serratus anterior forming its muscular framework.

These muscles, supplied by axillary and thoracodorsal branches, ensure coordinated arm elevation, internal rotation, and scapular stability (Standring, 2016). Clinical investigations have linked pectoralis minor tightness and altered scapular kinematics to the development of shoulder impingement and chronic pain syndromes (Borstad & Ludewig, 2006).

Biospectral examination of this region often identifies emissive variations across the anterior axillary fold or posterior scapular margin, reflecting asymmetry in shoulder stabilization. Such findings reveal early compensations in neuromuscular recruitment, positioning the axilla as a sensitive biosignal region for detecting dysfunction in upper limb integration.

Step 2,3,4: ROI Classification and Interpretive Questions

Hyperemission indicates acute muscle strain, muscular reactivity, or active trigger points.

- Has the patient experienced trauma, repetitive use, or overexertion?
- Is there localized tenderness, swelling, or muscle tightness?

Hypoemission suggests chronic hypoperfusion, fibrosis, or neurogenic muscle atrophy.

- Are symptoms such as weakness, stiffness, or limited mobility present?
- Is muscle wasting or altered sensation observed?

Step 5: Confirmatory Evaluations

Test	Purpose & Justification	Relevance to Emissive Pattern
Creatine kinase (CK), LDH	Detects muscle injury or inflammation (Simons et al., 1999).	Elevated in hyperemissive tissue activation states.
MRI	Visualizes muscle edema, inflammation, or fibrosis.	Supports hyper- or hypoemissive findings.
Electromyography (EMG)	Assesses muscle and nerve function.	Correlates with hypoemissive neurofunctional causes.
Blood tests (CBC, inflammatory markers)	Detects systemic inflammation or infection.	Supports hyperemissive regulatory field conditions.

Step 6: Care Strategies and Intervention Pathways

Naturopathic Approach

Utilize anti-inflammatory botanicals such as *Curcuma longa* and *Boswellia serrata* to reduce muscle inflammation (Hewlings & Kalman, 2017). Magnesium supplementation supports muscle relaxation. Hydrotherapy with alternating warm and cold applications improves circulation (Sutkowy et al., 2019). Progressive stretching and strengthening promote recovery. Adequate protein and antioxidants support tissue repair.

Standard Medical Approaches

Rest, NSAIDs, and physical therapy are standard treatments for muscle injuries (Simons et al., 1999). Neurological evaluation is advised if weakness or sensory changes occur.

Specialty / Practitioner Care Strategies Table

Specialty Group	Practitioners Included	Hyperemissive Strategies	Hypoemissive Strategies
Biochemistry	Nutritionists, Orthomolecular, Herbalists, Naturopaths	Anti-inflammatory botanicals, magnesium, antioxidants, protein	Circulatory support, neurotrophic nutrients, protein support
Rehabilitation	Physiotherapists, Massage Therapists, Osteopaths / Chiropractors	Myofascial release, trigger point therapy, gentle massage	Graded aerobic exercise, neurorehabilitation, ergonomic guidance
Energetics	Acupuncturists (TCM), Bioenergetic Therapists	Acupuncture, moxibustion, PEMF	Warming acupuncture, frequency therapy
Psychological	GNM practitioners, Psychotherapists, Vibrational therapists, Family constellation facilitators	Psychotherapy, bioresonance, mindfulness	Psychosomatic conflict resolution, emotional balancing

Educational Pearls & Considerations.

- Early identification and treatment of myofascial trigger points improves prognosis.
- Magnesium supports muscle relaxation and reduces spasms.
- Hydrotherapy protocols should align with inflammation phases.
- Neurological assessment is necessary for weakness or sensory deficits.
- Gradual rehabilitation prevents chronic dysfunction.

GROUP 3 - ZONE 15 – RIGHT AXILLARY

Category 3: *Skeletal*

Step 1: Functional Anatomy and Interpretive Importance

The skeletal configuration of the right axilla mirrors the contralateral clavicle, scapula, and rib complex, establishing a framework that supports shoulder stability and thoracic-limb integration (Standring, 2016).

These osseous structures protect neurovascular pathways while enabling a broad range of arm movements. Trauma, dislocation, or degenerative processes at the scapuloclavicular or costosternal articulations often manifest clinically as localized pain or restricted motion. Miller et al. (2014) highlight the diagnostic difficulty of differentiating skeletal irritation from soft tissue pathology in this area.

Yet these osseous changes leave a clear regulatory signature, where spectral surface readings often display biospectral asymmetries concentrated along clavicular or scapular margins. The contained nature of these emissive fields reflects their skeletal origin, offering visual contrast to the wider signals of muscular strain.

This integration enhances diagnostic precision by projecting hidden skeletal dysfunctions into visible biosignals, providing a more complete assessment of axillary articular stress.

Step 2,3,4: ROI Classification and Interpretive Questions

Hyperemission indicates acute tissue reactivity or injury such as fractures or costal joint separation.

- Is there localized tenderness, swelling, or warmth?
- Are symptoms exacerbated by movement or palpation?

Hypoemission suggests chronic degeneration or hypoperfusion in skeletal tissues.

- Are there persistent dull pain or stiffness?
- Is there a history of trauma or repetitive strain?

Step 5: Confirmatory Evaluations

Test	Purpose & Justification	Relevance to Emissive Pattern
X-ray	Detects fractures, dislocations, and degenerative changes.	Confirms acute or chronic skeletal signal alterations..
MRI	Visualizes soft tissue involvement and bone marrow edema.	Correlates with activation and structural adaptation.

Bone scan	Assesses bone metabolism and identifies occult lesions.	Confirms active skeletal field dynamics or remodeling processes.
Physical exam	Evaluates tenderness, mobility, and neurological signs.	Supports imaging and biospectral findings.

Step 6: Care Strategies and Intervention Pathways

Naturopathic Approach

Provide bone-supportive nutrients such as calcium, magnesium, vitamin D, and collagen peptides (Kruger & Kruger, 2019). Use anti-inflammatory herbs like *Boswellia serrata* to reduce joint inflammation. Physical therapy focusing on posture and mobility aids recovery. Acupuncture and bioresonance support pain relief and inflammation modulation.

Standard Medical Approaches

Standard treatments include analgesics, anti-inflammatory medications, and rehabilitation. Surgical intervention may be indicated in severe cases.

Specialty / Practitioner Care Strategies Table

Specialty Group	Practitioners Included	Hyperemissive Strategies	Hypoemissive Strategies
Biochemistry	Nutritionists, Orthomolecular, Herbalists, Naturopaths	Bone-supportive nutrients, anti-inflammatory herbs	Nutritional support for bone repair
Rehabilitation	Physiotherapists, Osteopaths / Chiropractors, Massage Therapists	Manual therapy, posture correction, pain management	Ergonomic training, spinal mobilization
Energetics	Acupuncturists (TCM), Bioenergetic Therapists	Acupuncture, PEMF, energy healing	Energy balancing and stimulation
Psychological	GNM practitioners, Psychotherapists, Vibrational therapists, Family constellation facilitators	Psychotherapy, bioresonance, stress management	Emotional balancing and coping strategies

Educational Pearls & Considerations.

- Early intervention prevents chronic skeletal dysfunction.
- Nutritional support is vital for bone healing.
- Combining manual therapies with rehabilitation optimizes outcomes.
- Monitor for complications necessitating specialist referral.

GROUP 3 - ZONE 15 – RIGHT AXILLARY

Category 4: *Nervous*

Step 1: Functional Anatomy and Interpretive Importance

The right axillary region shares the same brachial plexus innervation, supplying motor and sensory function to the upper limb (Standring, 2016). Lesions of the plexus may result from trauma, inflammatory neuropathy, or entrapment, producing weakness, pain, and sensory changes.

Wilbourn (1999) emphasized that brachial plexopathies often present with patchy deficits that challenge localization. These neural disturbances also alter autonomic balance, reshaping regional emissive behavior.

On the surface, biospectral asymmetries appear as confined signals following the clavicular contour or extending toward the scapular margin, whose sharply bounded geometry reflects the neural distribution.

Such surface markers provide a window into plexus dysfunction, helping distinguish neurogenic origins of axillary pain from muscular or vascular conditions.

Step 2,3,4: ROI Classification and Interpretive Questions

Hyperemission indicates nerve irritation or neurogenic reactivity.

- Are there symptoms such as burning, tingling, or sharp pains?
- Is localized swelling or hypersensitivity present?

Hypoemission suggests nerve hypoperfusion, compression, or denervation with decreased autonomic activity.

- Are numbness, weakness, or muscle atrophy reported?
- Do symptoms worsen with posture or movement?

Step 5: Confirmatory Evaluations

Test	Purpose & Justification	Relevance to Emissive Pattern
Nerve conduction studies (NCS), Electromyography (EMG)	Assess nerve and muscle function (Janis et al., 2010).	Correlates with hypoemissive neurofunctional disruption.
Quantitative sensory testing (QST)	Measures sensory nerve thresholds.	Supports interpretation of neurofunctional patterns.
MRI	Detects nerve root compression or structural abnormalities.	Identifies origin of neural signal disturbance.
Blood tests (glucose, vitamin B12)	Evaluates metabolic causes of neuropathy.	Supports interpretive understanding of systemic neuroregulatory involvement.

Step 6: Care Strategies and Intervention Pathways

Naturopathic Approach

Support nerve regeneration with B-complex vitamins, alpha-lipoic acid, and Acetyl-L-carnitine (Papanas & Ziegler, 2014). Use *Hypericum perforatum* for neuropathic pain relief (Kasper et al., 2010). Neural mobilization and bioresonance therapies aid recovery. Mind-body therapies modulate neurovascular and autonomic function.

Standard Medical Approaches

Pharmacologic treatments include anticonvulsants, antidepressants, and analgesics. Surgical decompression may be necessary. Managing metabolic contributors such as diabetes is essential.

Specialty / Practitioner Care Strategies Table

Specialty Group	Practitioners Included	Hyperemissive Strategies	Hypoemissive Strategies
Biochemistry	Nutritionists, Orthomolecular, Herbalists, Naturopaths	Neurotrophic vitamins, alpha-lipoic acid, anti-inflammatory botanicals	Circulatory stimulants, metabolic support, neuroprotective nutrients
Rehabilitation	Physiotherapists, Massage Therapists, Osteopaths / Chiropractors	Neural mobilization, myofascial release, gentle massage	Neural gliding exercises, ergonomic guidance, neurorehabilitation
Energetics	Acupuncturists (TCM), Bioenergetic Therapists	Acupuncture, moxibustion, PEMF	Warming acupuncture, frequency therapy, energy healing
Psychological	GNM practitioners, Psychotherapists, Vibrational therapists, Family constellation facilitators	Psychotherapy, bioresonance, mindfulness	Psychosomatic conflict resolution, vibrational medicine

Educational Pearls & Considerations.

- Early diagnosis prevents chronic nerve damage.
- Nutritional and energetic therapies support nerve repair.
- Monitor metabolic contributors such as diabetes.
- Avoid aggressive therapy during acute inflammation.
- Tailor neural mobilization to patient tolerance.

GROUP 3 - ZONE 15 – RIGHT AXILLARY

Category 5: *Lymphatic*

Step 1: Functional Anatomy and Interpretive Importance

The right axilla mirrors the functional role of the left, serving as a primary hub for lymphatic return from the arm, chest wall, and breast (Standring, 2016). Effective clearance in this region safeguards systemic immune integrity.

Paskett et al. (2007) observed that axillary lymphedema following oncologic therapy often persists for years, with profound quality-of-life impact. Functional impairment alters neurovascular coordination and fascial dynamics, producing regulatory imprints that are projected outward.

On emissive mapping, clinicians may observe focal fields extending along the clavicle or scapular edge, whose sharply defined geometry reflects lymphatic flow lines. These signals provide an external indicator of axillary lymphatic stress, enabling more precise interpretation of shoulder girdle dysfunction when immune burden is a hidden driver.

Their recognition is vital for distinguishing neural or vascular contributors from lymphatic origins of upper thoracic imbalance.

Step 2,3,4: ROI Classification and Interpretive Questions

Hyperemission reflects acute lymphatic reactivity, microbial activity, or lymphatic congestion characterized by swelling and spectral intensification.

- Is there redness, tenderness, or rapid swelling?
- Has the patient had recent trauma or infection?

Hypoemission indicates chronic lymphatic stasis with fibrosis and impaired drainage causing reduced biosignal.

- Is swelling persistent and firm?
- Are recurrent infections or delayed wound healing present?

Step 5: Confirmatory Evaluations

Test	Purpose & Justification	Relevance to Emissive Pattern
Lymphoscintigraphy	Assesses lymphatic flow and identifies obstructions.	Confirms lymphatic retention or reduced perfusion.
Doppler ultrasound	Rules out venous insufficiency contributing to swelling.	Differentiates vascular from lymphatic causes.

Blood tests (CBC, inflammatory markers)	Detects infection or systemic inflammation.	Supports hyperemissive tissue activation states.
Physical exam (Stemmer's sign, limb measurements)	Identifies clinical signs of lymphedema.	Correlates with biospectral findings.

Step 6: Care Strategies and Intervention Pathways

Naturopathic Approach

Use herbal lymphagogues such as *Hedera helix* and *Vitis vinifera* to stimulate lymphatic drainage (Godoy et al., 2012). Manual lymphatic drainage by trained therapists promotes fluid movement. Compression therapy supports lymph return and requires proper fitting. Nutritional antioxidants and anti-inflammatory nutrients aid tissue repair. Hydrotherapy with alternating warm and cold applications enhances lymphatic circulation.

Standard Medical Approaches

Standard treatment includes manual lymphatic drainage, compression garments, physical therapy, and infection management. Surgery is reserved for refractory cases.

Specialty / Practitioner Care Strategies Table

Specialty Group	Practitioners Included	Hyperemissive Strategies	Hypoemissive Strategies
Biochemistry	Nutritionists, Orthomolecular, Herbalists, Naturopaths	Herbal lymphagogues, antioxidants, anti-inflammatory nutrients	Circulatory support, nutritional tissue repair support
Rehabilitation	Physiotherapists, Massage Therapists, Osteopaths / Chiropractors	Manual lymphatic drainage, gentle massage, postural retraining	Compression therapy, graded exercise, ergonomic guidance
Energetics	Acupuncturists (TCM), Bioenergetic Therapists	Acupuncture, herbal formulas, PEMF	Warming acupuncture, energy balancing
Psychological	GNM practitioners, Psychotherapists, Vibrational therapists, Family constellation facilitators	Mind-body therapies supporting immune function and healing	Psychosomatic conflict resolution, emotional balancing

Educational Pearls & Considerations.

- Early intervention prevents chronic lymphedema progression.
- Manual lymphatic drainage requires certified practitioners.
- Compression therapy must be properly fitted and regularly monitored.
- Nutritional support enhances lymphatic function and tissue repair.
- Prompt infection control is vital.

GROUP 3 - ZONE 15 – RIGHT AXILLARY

Category 6: *Organ-Related (GNM)*

Step 1: Functional Anatomy and Interpretive Importance

The right axillary space, similarly defined by surrounding thoracic musculature, overlies structures that connect with hepatic and biliary systems as well as the ascending colon (Standring, 2016).

In GNM, conflicts tied to survival, territoriality, or digestion are associated with liver and gallbladder programs, which externalize through right-sided axillary fields. Hamer (2012) noted that conflict-active phases result in biosignal withdrawal (hypoemission), while reparative phases manifest as hyperemission due to cellular and immune activity.

These emissive responses may present along the clavicular border or posterior axillary fold, with sharp outlines reflecting organ-related projection. Black (2002) discussed the growing evidence for psychoneuroimmunology as a framework linking stress to hepatic and gastrointestinal function, supporting the external observation of such programs.

This interpretation situates the right axilla as a surface field where visceral adaptation becomes visible, complementing structural and lymphatic assessment.

Step 2,3,4: ROI Classification and Interpretive Questions

Hyperemission indicates reactive or healing phases with increased metabolic activity.

- Are there symptoms such as chest pain, respiratory difficulties, or palpitations?
- Is infection or inflammation present?

Hypoemission corresponds to conflict-active phases with tissue loss or functional suppression.

- Are chronic symptoms like fatigue or reduced organ function noted?
- Is unresolved psychological conflict or stress evident?

Step 5: Confirmatory Evaluations

Test	Purpose & Justification	Relevance to Emissive Pattern
Chest imaging (X-ray, CT, MRI)	Visualizes thoracic organ structure and pathology.	Correlates with emissive anomalies.
Cardiac and pulmonary function tests	Assess function of heart and lungs.	Supports interpretive understanding of organ field dysregulation.
Inflammatory markers, CBC	Detect systemic inflammation or infection.	Supports hyperemissive resolution phases.
Psychological assessment	Evaluates psychosomatic conflicts and stress factors.	Complements GNM interpretation.

Step 6: Care Strategies and Intervention Pathways

Naturopathic Approach

Utilize cardioprotective and anti-inflammatory herbs such as *Crataegus monogyna* and *Curcuma longa* (Tattelman, 2001). Support respiratory health with expectorants and antioxidants. Employ stress management and psychotherapy to aid conflict resolution. Nutritional antioxidants assist tissue repair.

Standard Medical Approaches

Management is guided by imaging and functional tests. Pharmacologic therapy targets cardiac and pulmonary conditions. Lifestyle and rehabilitative interventions support recovery.

Specialty / Practitioner Care Strategies Table

Specialty Group	Practitioners Included	Hyperemissive Strategies	Hypoemissive Strategies
Biochemistry	Nutritionists, Orthomolecular, Herbalists, Naturopaths	Cardioprotective herbs, antioxidants, anti-inflammatories	Nutritional support for organ repair and function
Rehabilitation	Physiotherapists, Massage Therapists, Osteopaths / Chiropractors	Respiratory therapy, circulation enhancement	Gentle mobilization, relaxation techniques
Energetics	Acupuncturists (TCM), Bioenergetic Therapists	Acupuncture for cardiac and pulmonary support	Energy balancing and harmonization
Psychological	GNM practitioners, Psychotherapists, Vibrational therapists, Family constellation facilitators	Psychotherapy, bioresonance, conflict resolution	Emotional balancing and stress management

Educational Pearls & Considerations.

- Recognize psychosomatic influences on thoracic organ pathology per GNM.
- Integrate physical and psychological therapies for optimal outcomes.
- Monitor cardiac and pulmonary function regularly.
- Multidisciplinary care improves patient prognosis.

GROUP 3 - ZONE 15 – RIGHT AXILLARY

Category 7: *Acupuncture / Meridian*

Step 1: Functional Anatomy and Interpretive Importance

The right axillary space mirrors the anatomy of the left, with neurovascular bundles and lymphatic structures integrated into fascial planes (Standring, 2016). It corresponds in meridian mapping to the Heart (HT), Pericardium (PC), and Lung (LU) channels, which converge into the axillary region before traversing the upper limb.

Flaws (2000) emphasized their role in harmonizing circulation, respiration, and emotional expression. Cheng (1987) described the LU meridian's importance for regulating Qi flow through the thoracic wall and upper extremities.

Clinically, disruptions are reported as chest tightness, shortness of breath, or axillary tension. On biosignal imaging, surface emissive asymmetries are often localized along the anterior axillary fold, correlating with HT–PC–LU pathways.

These patterns reveal how emotional, cardiovascular, and respiratory imbalance may be projected externally into the axilla, aligning with both classical meridian mapping and biospectral observation.

Step 2,3,4: ROI Classification and Interpretive Questions

Hyperemission indicates Qi stagnation or energetic congestion along the meridians.

- Are there localized pain, tightness, or discomfort?
- Are symptoms aggravated by emotional stress or physical exertion?

Hypoemission suggests Qi deficiency or chronic stagnation, leading to poor circulation and biosignal suppression.

- Does the patient report fatigue, coldness, or palpitations?
- Are symptoms persistent or worsening?

Step 5: Confirmatory Evaluations

Test	Purpose & Justification	Relevance to Emissive Pattern
Pulse diagnosis and tongue examination	Traditional TCM methods assessing meridian Qi and Blood status (Flaws, 2000).	Helps differentiate hyper- and hypoemissive patterns.
Biospectral imaging	Visualizes thermal asymmetries along meridian pathways.	Correlates with Qi imbalances in the axillary region.
Patient symptom questionnaire	Assesses chest discomfort, palpitations, and emotional state.	Assists clinical differentiation of meridian signal disruption.

Step 6: Care Strategies and Intervention Pathways

Naturopathic Approach

Acupuncture points such as HT7, PC6, and LU1 regulate Qi flow and relieve stagnation (Lao et al., 2004). Moxibustion warms hypoemissive meridian areas. Herbal formulas like *Tian Wang Bu Xin Dan* and *Bao Yuan Tang* support thoracic meridians (Bensky et al., 2004). Stress reduction and lifestyle modifications complement treatment.

Standard Medical Approaches

Acupuncture serves as adjunctive therapy for chest discomfort and thoracic function improvement.

Specialty / Practitioner Care Strategies Table

Specialty Group	Practitioners Included	Hyperemissive Strategies	Hypoemissive Strategies
Biochemistry	Nutritionists, Orthomolecular, Herbalists, Naturopaths	Cardiovascular and respiratory herbs, antioxidants	Qi tonics and nutritional support
Rehabilitation	Physiotherapists, Massage Therapists, Osteopaths / Chiropractors	Thoracic mobilization, myofascial release	Gentle mobilization, warming massage
Energetics	Acupuncturists (TCM), Bioenergetic Therapists	Acupuncture, moxibustion, PEMF	Warming acupuncture, energy balancing
Psychological	GNM practitioners, Psychotherapists, Vibrational therapists, Family constellation facilitators	Psychotherapy, bioresonance, energy clearing	Psychosomatic conflict resolution, emotional balancing

Educational Pearls & Considerations.

- Precise acupuncture point selection is critical for treatment efficacy.
- Moxibustion should be applied cautiously in heat-sensitive individuals.
- Herbal prescriptions require qualified practitioner oversight.
- Integration with rehabilitative therapies improves outcomes.

GROUP 3 - ZONE 15 – RIGHT AXILLARY

Category 8: *Energetic*

Step 1: Functional Anatomy and Interpretive Importance

The right axilla shares structural features with the left, containing lymphatic nodes, neurovascular elements, and muscular supports of the shoulder girdle (Standring, 2016). Energetically, it reflects systemic processing related to circulation, detoxification, and autonomic balance.

Baldwin et al. (2017) demonstrated that energy therapies influence heart rate variability, reinforcing the association between axillary fields and systemic autonomic control. Patients may present with recurrent shoulder tightness, vague thoracic discomfort, or immune susceptibility.

Biospectral imaging highlights diffuse hypoemissive shadows aligned with stagnated energy processing, while narrow hyperemissive bands often signify reparative signaling or immune regulation.

These emissive variations integrate both local and systemic processes, revealing how peripheral zones serve as mirrors of central physiologic adaptation. The right axillary field thus offers interpretive access to systemic detoxification and autonomic coherence, visible as surface biosignals prior to overt dysfunction.

Step 2,3,4: ROI Classification and Interpretive Questions

Hyperemission suggests localized energetic congestion or biosignal overload.

- Does the patient report sensations of heat, tension, or discomfort in the axilla?
- Are stress or emotional factors prominent?

Hypoemission indicates energetic deficiency or signal stagnation.

- Does the patient experience fatigue, coldness, or low vitality?
- Are symptoms chronic or refractory to standard treatment?

Step 5: Confirmatory Evaluations

Test	Purpose & Justification	Relevance to Emissive Pattern
Bioresonance testing	Measures tissue energy frequencies and imbalances.	Correlates with emissive energetic anomalies..
Electrodermal screening (EDS)	Assesses skin conductance linked to energy pathways.	Supports interpretive understanding of energetic imbalance.
Patient emotional and symptom history	Provides context for energetic dysfunction and stress factors.	Assists in biospectral interpretation.

Step 6: Care Strategies and Intervention Pathways

Naturopathic Approach

Employ bioresonance, pulsed electromagnetic fields (PEMF), and adaptogenic botanicals to restore energetic balance and promote healing (Matsumoto et al., 2010). Nutritional antioxidants and adaptogens enhance systemic resilience. Mindfulness and stress reduction complement energetic therapies.

Standard Medical Approaches

Energetic therapies act as adjuncts to conventional and rehabilitative care to optimize patient outcomes.

Specialty / Practitioner Care Strategies Table

Specialty Group	Practitioners Included	Hyperemissive Strategies	Hypoemissive Strategies
Biochemistry	Nutritionists, Orthomolecular, Herbalists, Naturopaths	Adaptogens, antioxidants, herbal energetics	Nutritional support for energy deficiency
Rehabilitation	Physiotherapists, Massage Therapists, Osteopaths / Chiropractors	Energy-based manual therapies, PEMF, therapeutic touch	Gentle stimulation, mobilization
Energetics	Acupuncturists (TCM), Bioenergetic Therapists	Bioresonance, PEMF, acupuncture	Warming acupuncture, energy balancing
Psychological	GNM practitioners, Psychotherapists, Vibrational therapists, Family constellation facilitators	Psychotherapy, bioresonance, mindfulness	Emotional balancing, vibrational medicine

Educational Pearls & Considerations.

- Energetic therapies complement but do not replace standard medical treatments.
- Practitioner skill and patient receptivity affect outcomes.
- Regular reassessment optimizes therapeutic efficacy.
- Address psychological and physical factors holistically.

GROUP 3 - ZONE 15 – RIGHT AXILLARY

Category 9: *Metabolic / Endocrine*

Step 1: Functional Anatomy and Interpretive Importance

The right axillary region mirrors the left anatomically but is often influenced by hepatic–metabolic pathways due to its association with right thoracic drainage (Standring, 2016).

Endocrine and metabolic dysfunction, especially diabetes and metabolic syndrome, frequently manifest here through circulatory or immune irregularities. Vinik et al. (2003) noted that peripheral neuropathy and vascular compromise in metabolic disease extend to regional nodes and fascial lines.

Patients may present with right-sided thoracic discomfort, shoulder tension, or systemic fatigue. Spectral surface readings demonstrate hypoemissive depressions consistent with impaired perfusion or glycoregulatory decline, alongside hyperemissive foci reflecting compensatory or immune-driven activation.

These emissive variations often trace along fascial continuities, reinforcing their systemic rather than local significance. Clinically, the right axillary field reveals how metabolic stress projects into peripheral zones, making it an important biospectral marker of systemic load.

Step 2,3,4: ROI Classification and Interpretive Questions

Hyperemission suggests metabolic overactivity, localized biosignal reactivity, or underlying systemic stress.

- Is there warmth, redness, or swelling?
- Is metabolic control adequate?

Hypoemission indicates perfusion deficits, neuropathic signal suppression, or autonomic downregulation related to endocrine imbalance.

- Are cold sensations, numbness, or delayed healing present?
- Are systemic symptoms like fatigue or temperature intolerance reported?

Step 5: Confirmatory Evaluations

Test	Purpose & Justification	Relevance to Emissive Pattern
HbA1c, fasting glucose	Measures glycemic control in diabetes.	Correlates with hypoemissive neurofunctional or perfusion-restricted areas.
Thyroid function tests (TSH, Free T4)	Evaluates thyroid disorders affecting metabolism and circulation.	Associated with altered emissive regulation.

Lipid profile	Assesses cardiovascular risk influencing tissue perfusion.	Supports metabolic vascular adaptation.
Inflammatory markers (CRP, ESR)	Detects systemic inflammation impacting tissue health.	Correlates with hyperemissive tissue activation states.

Step 6: Care Strategies and Intervention Pathways

Naturopathic Approach

Promote metabolic health through low glycemic diets, antioxidants, and adaptogens (Alberti et al., 2006). Herbs such as *Panax ginseng* and *Gymnema sylvestre* support endocrine function. Supplement chromium, magnesium, and alpha-lipoic acid to improve glucose metabolism and neuroprotection. Encourage regular aerobic exercise for vascular health.

Standard Medical Approaches

Medical management includes pharmacologic therapy and lifestyle modification for metabolic control. Thyroid hormone replacement and lipid management reduce complications.

Specialty / Practitioner Care Strategies Table

Specialty Group	Practitioners Included	Hyperemissive Strategies	Hypoemissive Strategies
Biochemistry	Nutritionists, Orthomolecular, Herbalists, Naturopaths	Antioxidants, adaptogens, insulin sensitizers, micronutrients	Metabolic support, neuroprotective nutrients, dietary management
Rehabilitation	Physiotherapists, Massage Therapists, Osteopaths / Chiropractors	Exercise therapy, circulation enhancement	Neuromuscular re-education, aerobic conditioning
Energetics	Acupuncturists (TCM), Bioenergetic Therapists	Acupuncture supporting metabolic function	Energy balancing, PEMF
Psychological	GNM practitioners, Psychotherapists, Vibrational therapists, Family constellation facilitators	Mind-body therapies supporting metabolic regulation	Stress reduction, emotional balancing

Educational Pearls & Considerations.

- Regular metabolic monitoring prevents complications.
- Lifestyle and dietary changes support clinical treatment.
- Adaptogens complement but do not replace standard care.
- Patient education on skin and wound care is essential.

GROUP 3

ZONE 16 – UPPER BACK

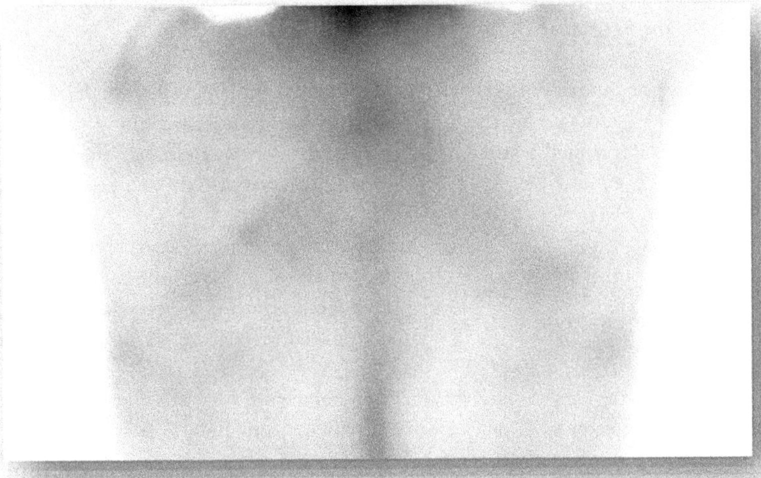

G3Z16UB

The upper back, comprising the dorsal thoracic musculature, scapular attachments, and vertebral segments of the thoracic spine, is one of the body's most diagnostically versatile surfaces. It includes the trapezius, rhomboids, latissimus dorsi, and spinal extensors, together with the thoracic vertebrae and associated neurovascular structures (Standring, 2016).

Functionally, this zone sustains postural stabilization and upper limb mechanics, making it vulnerable to strain and overuse. Chronic upper back pain affects up to 20% of adults, often linked to muscular imbalance and sedentary behavior (Hoy et al., 2014).

Biospectrally, the region often shows hyperemissive activity from lactic acid accumulation in overworked musculature, especially in repetitive arm elevation or sustained tension. Athletes and manual laborers frequently demonstrate lateralized asymmetries from compensatory overactivation of scapular stabilizers (Kibler & Sciascia, 2010).

Respiratory mechanics add another dimension: asymmetries may reflect altered rib excursion or postural restriction influencing pulmonary function. Neurofunctionally, sympathetic chain ganglia adjacent to thoracic vertebrae heighten the emissive sensitivity of this region, allowing autonomic dysregulation to surface (Baron et al., 2013). Psychosomatic influences are also evident, as chronic stress increases trapezius and upper thoracic activation, correlating with emissive asymmetries (Lundberg, 1999).

Systemically, the upper back may mirror visceral dysfunction through compensatory postural adaptations linked to abdominal or pelvic imbalance. Its diagnostic strength lies in multidimensionality: simultaneously reflecting musculoskeletal load, autonomic balance, emotional stress, and postural integration, making it one of the most clinically revealing zones for biospectral interpretation.

Zone 16 – Upper Back: Emission-Relevant Structures

Category	Relevant Structures	Emission Relevance
1. Vascular / Circulatory	- Posterior intercostal arteries and veins - Dorsal scapular vessels - Paraspinal venous plexus	Hyperemission suggests vascular retention, tissue activation, or increased blood flow; Hypoemission may indicate perfusion decline, vascular spasm, or sympathetic vasoconstriction.
2. Muscular / Myofascial	- Trapezius - Rhomboids - Levator scapulae - Erector spinae (thoracic portion)	Hyperemission often corresponds to muscle spasm, fascial strain, or overuse; Hypoemission may be seen with disuse, chronic myofascial restriction, or fascial adhesions.
3. Skeletal / Articular	- Thoracic vertebrae (T1-T12) - Scapula - Costovertebral joints	Hyperemission may be linked to vertebral signal activity or joint field excitation; Hypoemission can indicate chronic degenerative changes or decreased bone perfusion.
4. Nervous System / Spine	- Dorsal rami of thoracic spinal nerves - Sympathetic chain (thoracic portion)	Hyperemission may indicate nerve field irritation or segmental activation; Hypoemission suggests chronic nerve compression or autonomic dysfunction affecting dorsal spinal innervation.
5. Lymphatic / Immune	- Thoracic lymphatic vessels - Axillary and posterior cervical lymph nodes	Hyperemission often reflects immune-related signal response or lymphatic field activation; Hypoemission may indicate lymphatic congestion or fibrosis in drainage pathways.
6. Organs / GNM (German New Medicine)	- Upper thoracic viscera reflex zones (lungs, heart)	Elevated emissive expression may represent active visceral conflict or terrain-level activation; Hypoemission corresponds to healing phases or functional suppression via somatovisceral reflex.
7. Acupuncture / Meridians	- Bladder Meridian (thoracic segment) - Governing Vessel (Du Mai)	Hyperemission suggests Qi stagnation or excess; low-emission areas may indicate Qi deficiency or blood stasis affecting thoracic autonomic and musculoskeletal function.
8. Energetic / Frequency	- Energetic reflex zones related to respiratory and postural regulation	Hyperemission may be linked to sympathetic signal dominance or emotional stress; Hypoemission may indicate regulatory depletion or impaired autonomic balance.
9. Metabolic / Endocrine	- Reflex zones for pulmonary metabolism and systemic autonomic influence	Hypoemissive patterns suggest metabolic downregulation or adrenal underperformance; Hyperemission may indicate tissue activation or regulatory stress in upper back tissues.

GROUP 3 - ZONE 16 – UPPER BACK

Category 1: *Vascular / Circulatory*

Step 1: Functional Anatomy and Interpretive Importance

The upper back is vascularized by the dorsal scapular artery, the transverse cervical artery, and branches of the subscapular and intercostal systems. These vessels perfuse the trapezius, rhomboids, levator scapulae, and paraspinal musculature, together with overlying cutaneous territories.

Venous return occurs through the dorsal scapular and transverse cervical veins, which drain into the subclavian and axillary systems (Standring, 2016). Anatomical and imaging studies have highlighted the role of the dorsal scapular artery in supplying the scapular region, particularly in reconstructive surgery (Kim et al., 2010).

On spectral surface reading, emissive asymmetries often follow the paraspinal or scapular axes, reflecting postural strain, venous retention, or adaptive shifts in regional arterial tone. Because this zone supports continuous load-bearing in posture and movement, emissive patterns here provide important orientation to dorsal circulatory physiology.

Step 2,3,4: ROI Classification and Interpretive Questions

Hyperemission indicates vascular reactivity, venous overload, or signal retention in the region.

- Is there localized redness, swelling, or tenderness?
- Is there a systemic inflammatory response?

Hypoemission suggests reduced perfusion, vascular insufficiency, or autonomic underactivation.

- Are there cold sensations, pallor, or delayed healing?
- Is there a history of vascular disease or risk factors?

Step 5: Confirmatory Evaluations

Test	Purpose & Justification	Relevance to Emissive Pattern
Doppler ultrasound	Evaluates arterial and venous flow in upper back vessels.	Correlates hyperemissive tissue activation and hypoemissive perfusion decline.
CT or MRI angiography	Visualizes vessel patency and occlusions.	Confirms vascular flow restriction or signal intensification.
Blood tests (CBC, CRP, coagulation profile)	Detects systemic inflammation or coagulation abnormalities.	Supports hyperemissive retention or circulatory impedance states.
Physical exam	Assesses for signs of vascular compromise.	Complements biospectral findings.

Step 6: Care Strategies and Intervention Pathways

Naturopathic Approach

Use botanical venotonics such as *Aesculus hippocastanum* and *Ruscus aculeatus* to improve microcirculation and reduce edema (Chrubasik et al., 2011). Implement anti-inflammatory diet rich in antioxidants and omega-3 fatty acids (Calder, 2017). Employ contrast hydrotherapy to stimulate circulation (Sutkowy et al., 2019). Supplement vitamins C, E, and bioflavonoids for endothelial support. Encourage posture correction and gentle massage to aid venous return.

Standard Medical Approaches

Imaging guides anticoagulant therapy, anti-inflammatory medication, or surgery when indicated. Manage systemic contributors such as coagulation disorders.

Specialty / Practitioner Care Strategies Table

Specialty Group	Practitioners Included	Hyperemissive Strategies	Hypoemissive Strategies
Biochemistry	Nutritionists, Orthomolecular, Herbalists, Naturopaths	Botanical venotonics, antioxidants, anti-inflammatory diet	Circulatory stimulants, endothelial support nutrients
Rehabilitation	Physiotherapists, Massage Therapists, Osteopaths / Chiropractors	Gentle massage, lymphatic drainage, postural correction	Graded exercise, circulatory enhancement
Energetics	Acupuncturists (TCM), Bioenergetic Therapists	Acupuncture, moxibustion, herbal formulas	Warming acupuncture, energy balancing
Psychological	GNM practitioners, Psychotherapists, Vibrational therapists, Family constellation facilitators	Psychotherapy, bioresonance, mindfulness	Stress reduction, emotional balancing

Educational Pearls & Considerations.

- Early identification of vascular inflammation prevents complications.
- Botanical venotonics and diet effectively support vascular health.
- Nitric oxide boosters and omega-3 fatty acids enhance endothelial function.
- Compression therapy contraindications must be respected.
- Posture and mobilization aid venous return.

GROUP 3 - ZONE 16 – UPPER BACK

Category 2: *Muscular*

Step 1: Functional Anatomy and Interpretive Importance

The upper back musculature consists of the trapezius, rhomboids, levator scapulae, and the upper fibers of the erector spinae, all of which are responsible for scapular movement, cervical stabilization, and thoracic posture.

These muscles receive innervation primarily from the dorsal scapular, spinal accessory, and cervical nerves, coordinating shoulder mechanics with spinal alignment (Standring, 2016).

Clinical reviews note that trapezius myalgia and rhomboid strain are frequent in individuals exposed to prolonged desk work or repetitive lifting, often producing tension-related pain and reduced scapular control (Szeto et al., 2005).

Spectral evaluation of this region commonly identifies band-like emissive asymmetries tracking the trapezial lines or paraspinal zones, where hypertonicity and fatigue alter fascial tone. Such signals often accompany postural syndromes, demonstrating the functional link between static load, muscle endurance, and the biospectral surface profile of the upper back.

Step 2,3,4: ROI Classification and Interpretive Questions

Hyperemission indicates myofascial strain, neuromuscular activation, or active trigger point activity.

- Is there localized tenderness, swelling, or muscle tightness?
- Has the patient experienced trauma or repetitive strain?

Hypoemission suggests chronic fascial rigidity, reduced perfusion, or neurogenic muscle suppression.

- Are symptoms such as weakness, stiffness, or reduced mobility present?
- Is muscle wasting or sensory change noted?

Step 5: Confirmatory Evaluations

Test	Purpose & Justification	Relevance to Emissive Pattern
Creatine kinase (CK), LDH	Detects muscle injury or inflammation (Simons et al., 1999).	Elevated in hyperemissive tissue activation states.
MRI	Visualizes muscle edema, inflammation, or fibrosis.	Correlates with biospectral findings.
Electromyography (EMG)	Assesses muscle and nerve function.	Supports neurofunctional causes of Hypoemission.
Blood tests (CBC, inflammatory markers)	Detects systemic inflammation or infection.	Supports muscular field activation patterns.

Step 6: Care Strategies and Intervention Pathways

Naturopathic Approach

Anti-inflammatory herbs such as *Curcuma longa* and *Boswellia serrata* reduce muscle inflammation (Hewlings & Kalman, 2017). Magnesium supports muscle relaxation. Hydrotherapy with alternating warm and cold applications improves circulation (Sutkowy et al., 2019). Progressive stretching and strengthening promote recovery. Adequate protein and antioxidants support tissue repair.

Standard Medical Approaches

Rest, NSAIDs, and physical therapy are standard treatments for muscle injury (Simons et al., 1999). Neurological evaluation is recommended if weakness or sensory changes occur.

Specialty / Practitioner Care Strategies Table

Specialty Group	Practitioners Included	Hyperemissive Strategies	Hypoemissive Strategies
Biochemistry	Nutritionists, Orthomolecular, Herbalists, Naturopaths	Anti-inflammatory botanicals, magnesium, antioxidants, protein	Circulatory support, neurotrophic nutrients, protein support
Rehabilitation	Physiotherapists, Massage Therapists, Osteopaths / Chiropractors	Myofascial release, trigger point therapy, gentle massage	Graded aerobic exercise, neurorehabilitation, ergonomic guidance
Energetics	Acupuncturists (TCM), Bioenergetic Therapists	Acupuncture, moxibustion, PEMF	Warming acupuncture, frequency therapy
Psychological	GNM practitioners, Psychotherapists, Vibrational therapists, Family constellation facilitators	Psychotherapy, bioresonance, mindfulness	Psychosomatic conflict resolution, emotional balancing

Educational Pearls & Considerations.

- Early treatment of trigger points improves outcomes.
- Magnesium assists in muscle relaxation and spasm reduction.
- Hydrotherapy should be tailored to inflammation stage.
- Neurological assessment is important for persistent weakness.
- Gradual rehabilitation prevents chronic dysfunction.

GROUP 3 - ZONE 16 – UPPER BACK

Category 3: *Skeletal*

Step 1: Functional Anatomy and Interpretive Importance

The upper back includes the thoracic vertebrae, scapulae, and posterior rib articulations, forming a stabilizing scaffold for trunk posture and spinal protection (Standring, 2016). These skeletal elements transmit forces between the cervical and lumbar regions and serve as pivotal anchors for respiratory and scapular musculature.

Structural compromise, whether through vertebral degeneration, costovertebral restriction, or scapulothoracic dysfunction, can generate persistent discomfort and altered mechanics. Miller et al. (2014) emphasize that thoracic vertebral and costal changes are underappreciated contributors to chronic dorsal pain.

Such skeletal influences extend into regulatory dynamics, producing biospectral asymmetries across the thoracic surface.

Spectral surface readings often reveal linear or segmental emissive variations aligned with vertebral columns, distinct from the broader fields of paraspinal muscles.

These patterns externalize the hidden skeletal load of the thoracic spine, illustrating the integration of vertebral stress, articular function, and surface biosignals in a region central to postural stability.

Step 2,3,4: ROI Classification and Interpretive Questions

Hyperemission indicates active structural overload, acute skeletal injury, or signal amplification due to biomechanical stress.

- Is there localized swelling, tenderness, or warmth?
- Are symptoms worsened by movement or palpation?

Hypoemission suggests chronic degenerative remodeling, signal depletion, or neuro-osseous compromise.

- Are symptoms persistent with stiffness or dull pain?
- Is there a history of trauma or repetitive strain?

Step 5: Confirmatory Evaluations

Test	Purpose & Justification	Relevance to Emissive Pattern
X-ray	Detects fractures, dislocations, and degenerative changes.	Confirms acute or chronic skeletal signal alterations.
MRI	Visualizes soft tissue and bone marrow edema.	Correlates with activation or structural adaptation.

Bone scan	Assesses bone metabolism and detects occult lesions.	Confirms active skeletal field dynamics.
Physical exam	Evaluates tenderness, mobility, and neurological signs.	Complements imaging and biospectral findings.

Step 6: Care Strategies and Intervention Pathways

Naturopathic Approach

Support bone health with calcium, magnesium, vitamin D, and collagen peptides (Kruger & Kruger, 2019). Use anti-inflammatory herbs such as *Boswellia serrata* to reduce inflammation. Physical therapy focusing on posture and spinal mobility aids recovery. Acupuncture and bioresonance may help relieve pain and modulate inflammation.

Standard Medical Approaches

Treatment involves analgesics, anti-inflammatory drugs, and rehabilitation. Surgery may be required in severe cases.

Specialty / Practitioner Care Strategies Table

Specialty Group	Practitioners Included	Hyperemissive Strategies	Hypoemissive Strategies
Biochemistry	Nutritionists, Orthomolecular, Herbalists, Naturopaths	Bone-supportive nutrients, anti-inflammatory herbs	Nutritional support for bone repair
Rehabilitation	Physiotherapists, Osteopaths / Chiropractors, Massage Therapists	Manual therapy, posture correction, pain management	Ergonomic training, spinal mobilization
Energetics	Acupuncturists (TCM), Bioenergetic Therapists	Acupuncture, PEMF, energy healing	Energy balancing and stimulation
Psychological	GNM practitioners, Psychotherapists, Vibrational therapists, Family constellation facilitators	Psychotherapy, bioresonance, stress management	Emotional balancing and coping strategies

Educational Pearls & Considerations.

- Early diagnosis prevents chronic skeletal dysfunction.
- Nutritional support is crucial for bone healing.
- Combine manual therapies with rehabilitation for best results.
- Monitor for complications that require specialist care.

GROUP 3 - ZONE 16 – UPPER BACK

Category 4: *Nervous*

Step 1: Functional Anatomy and Interpretive Importance

The upper back receives innervation from the dorsal rami of thoracic spinal nerves, which supply paraspinal musculature and cutaneous tissues (Standring, 2016). These small nerves are prone to irritation from vertebral dysfunction, joint restriction, or chronic postural strain.

Dreyfuss et al. (1994) highlighted that thoracic zygapophyseal joint pain is commonly mediated by dorsal rami irritation, contributing to persistent dorsal pain. Neural dysfunction in this region influences both muscular recruitment and sympathetic regulation, projecting its effects outward as emissive patterns.

Biospectral asymmetries in the upper back typically align with vertebral segments or paraspinal fields, exhibiting a geometry distinct from broader myofascial emissions. Such externalized signals provide a noninvasive representation of dorsal rami stress, enhancing the interpretation of upper back dysfunction in clinical assessment.

Step 2,3,4: ROI Classification and Interpretive Questions

Hyperemission suggests localized neurogenic signal amplification or irritative biospectral activity.

- Are there burning, tingling, or sharp pain symptoms?
- Is there localized hypersensitivity or swelling?

Hypoemission indicates signal suppression, such as nerve ischemia, compression, or segmental denervation, with reduced autonomic tone.

- Are numbness, weakness, or muscle atrophy present?
- Do symptoms worsen with posture or certain movements?

Step 5: Confirmatory Evaluations

Test	Purpose & Justification	Relevance to Emissive Pattern
Nerve conduction studies (NCS), Electromyography (EMG)	Evaluate nerve and muscle function (Janis et al., 2010).	Correlates with hypoemissive neurofunctional disruption.
Quantitative sensory testing (QST)	Measures sensory thresholds.	Supports interpretation of neurofunctional patterns.
MRI	Identifies nerve root compression or structural abnormalities.	Detects origins of neural signal disturbance.
Blood tests (glucose, vitamin B12)	Evaluates metabolic causes of neuropathy.	Supports interpretive understanding of systemic neuroregulatory involvement.

Step 6: Care Strategies and Intervention Pathways

Naturopathic Approach

Support nerve regeneration with B-complex vitamins, alpha-lipoic acid, and Acetyl-L-carnitine (Papanas & Ziegler, 2014). Use *Hypericum perforatum* for neuropathic pain relief (Kasper et al., 2010). Neural mobilization and bioresonance therapies facilitate recovery. Mind-body interventions modulate neurovascular and autonomic functions.

Standard Medical Approaches

Pharmacologic treatments include anticonvulsants, antidepressants, and analgesics. Surgical decompression may be indicated. Addressing metabolic contributors like diabetes is essential.

Specialty / Practitioner Care Strategies Table

Specialty Group	Practitioners Included	Hyperemissive Strategies	Hypoemissive Strategies
Biochemistry	Nutritionists, Orthomolecular, Herbalists, Naturopaths	Neurotrophic vitamins, alpha-lipoic acid, anti-inflammatory botanicals	Circulatory stimulants, metabolic support, neuroprotective nutrients
Rehabilitation	Physiotherapists, Massage Therapists, Osteopaths / Chiropractors	Neural mobilization, myofascial release, gentle massage	Neural gliding exercises, ergonomic guidance, neurorehabilitation
Energetics	Acupuncturists (TCM), Bioenergetic Therapists	Acupuncture, moxibustion, PEMF	Warming acupuncture, frequency therapy, energy healing
Psychological	GNM practitioners, Psychotherapists, Vibrational therapists, Family constellation facilitators	Psychotherapy, bioresonance, mindfulness	Psychosomatic conflict resolution, vibrational medicine

Educational Pearls & Considerations.

- Early recognition prevents chronic nerve damage.
- Nutritional and energetic therapies support nerve repair.
- Monitor metabolic causes such as diabetes.
- Avoid aggressive therapy during acute inflammation.
- Tailor neural mobilization to patient tolerance.

GROUP 3 - ZONE 16 – UPPER BACK

Category 5: *Lymphatic*

Step 1: Functional Anatomy and Interpretive Importance

The upper back lymphatics converge laterally toward axillary nodes and centrally into the thoracic duct, forming a network that supports clearance of interstitial fluid and immune elements from the dorsal thorax (Standring, 2016).

This system is critical for balancing dorsal load and systemic immune transport. Szuba et al. (2002) highlighted that dorsal truncal lymphedema often arises as a late consequence of breast cancer therapy, with subtle changes preceding obvious edema.

Functional compromise alters paraspinal compliance and modifies autonomic regulation, producing effects that extend to the surface. These appear as vertical or paramedian emissive fields following thoracic vertebrae, distinguishable from diffuse muscular activation.

Such externally visible markers allow clinicians to identify dorsal lymphatic strain, improving early recognition of immune dysfunction in the posterior thorax and guiding more targeted management strategies.

Step 2,3,4: ROI Classification and Interpretive Questions

Hyperemission suggests acute lymphatic signal congestion with possible energetic overload or immune activation.

- Is there redness, tenderness, or rapid swelling?
- Any recent infections or trauma?

Hypoemission indicates chronic lymphatic stagnation with reduced flow and fibrotic signal depletion.

- Is swelling persistent and firm?
- Are recurrent infections or delayed healing present?

Step 5: Confirmatory Evaluations

Test	Purpose & Justification	Relevance to Emissive Pattern
Lymphoscintigraphy	Evaluates lymphatic flow and obstruction sites.	Confirms lymphatic retention or reduced perfusion.
Doppler ultrasound	Excludes venous insufficiency contributing to edema.	Differentiates vascular from lymphatic causes.

Blood tests (CBC, inflammatory markers)	Detects infection or systemic inflammation.	Supports hyperemissive tissue activation states.
Physical exam (Stemmer's sign, limb measurements)	Identifies clinical signs of lymphedema.	Correlates with biospectral findings.

Step 6: Care Strategies and Intervention Pathways

Naturopathic Approach

Use herbal lymphagogues like *Hedera helix* and *Vitis vinifera* to stimulate lymphatic drainage (Godoy et al., 2012). Manual lymphatic drainage by certified therapists promotes fluid mobilization. Compression therapy supports lymph return and requires appropriate fitting. Nutritional antioxidants and anti-inflammatory nutrients support tissue repair. Hydrotherapy with alternating warm and cold applications enhances lymphatic circulation.

Standard Medical Approaches

Standard management includes manual lymphatic drainage, compression garments, physical therapy, and infection control. Surgical options are reserved for refractory cases.

Specialty / Practitioner Care Strategies Table

Specialty Group	Practitioners Included	Hyperemissive Strategies	Hypoemissive Strategies
Biochemistry	Nutritionists, Orthomolecular, Herbalists, Naturopaths	Herbal lymphagogues, antioxidants, anti-inflammatory nutrients	Circulatory support, nutritional tissue repair support
Rehabilitation	Physiotherapists, Massage Therapists, Osteopaths / Chiropractors	Manual lymphatic drainage, gentle massage, postural retraining	Compression therapy, graded exercise, ergonomic guidance
Energetics	Acupuncturists (TCM), Bioenergetic Therapists	Acupuncture, herbal formulas, PEMF	Warming acupuncture, energy balancing
Psychological	GNM practitioners, Psychotherapists, Vibrational therapists, Family constellation facilitators	Mind-body therapies supporting immune function and healing	Psychosomatic conflict resolution, emotional balancing

Educational Pearls & Considerations.

- Early intervention prevents progression to chronic lymphedema.
- Manual lymphatic drainage should be performed by trained therapists.
- Compression therapy requires proper fitting and ongoing monitoring.
- Nutritional support enhances lymphatic function and tissue healing.
- Prompt infection control is critical.

GROUP 3 - ZONE 16 – UPPER BACK

Category 6: *Organ-Related (GNM)*

Step 1: **Functional Anatomy and Interpretive Importance**

The upper back overlies thoracic structures including the lungs and paraspinal elements of the thoracic spine, integrating musculoskeletal support with respiratory mechanics (Standring, 2016).

In GNM, conflicts involving breathing capacity or relational themes may engage pulmonary tissues, projecting their adaptive phases into dorsal emissive fields. Hamer (2012) explained that hypoemission corresponds to conflict-active states, while hyperemission reflects reparative phases.

These emissive variations often align vertically with thoracic vertebral segments, differentiating them from diffuse paraspinal muscular activity. Cohen et al. (2007) demonstrated that psychological stress significantly increases susceptibility to respiratory illness, providing contemporary evidence that links conflict-related stress with pulmonary adaptation.

Such findings reinforce the interpretation of dorsal emissive fields as reflections of organ-related programs, enabling clinicians to distinguish psychosomatic contributions from mechanical or vascular causes in the upper back.

Step 2,3,4: **ROI Classification and Interpretive Questions**

Hyperemission signals biospectral intensification consistent with healing processes or metabolic overactivation.

- Is there chest discomfort, respiratory symptoms, or signs of infection?
- Is systemic inflammatory response evident?

Hypoemission corresponds to conflict-active phases with suppressed biosignal output linked to unresolved psycho-organic processes.

- Is chronic fatigue, reduced thoracic function, or a psychological stressor reported?
- Does the patient exhibit a long-term emotional conflict impacting thoracic structures?

Step 5: **Confirmatory Evaluations**

Test	Purpose & Justification	Relevance to Emissive Pattern
Chest imaging (X-ray, CT, MRI)	Visualizes thoracic organ structure and pathology.	Correlates with emissive anomalies indicating organ involvement.
Cardiac and pulmonary function tests	Assess heart and lung function.	Supports interpretive understanding of organ field dysregulation.

Inflammatory markers, CBC	Detect systemic inflammation or infection.	Supports hyperemissive resolution phases.
Psychological assessment	Evaluates biological conflicts and psychosomatic factors.	Complements GNM interpretive approach.

Step 6: Care Strategies and Intervention Pathways

Naturopathic Approach

Employ cardioprotective and anti-inflammatory botanicals such as *Crataegus monogyna* and *Curcuma longa* (Tattelman, 2001). Support respiratory health with expectorants and antioxidants. Stress management and psychotherapy facilitate conflict resolution. Nutritional antioxidants assist tissue repair.

Standard Medical Approaches

Management guided by imaging and functional testing. Pharmacologic therapy addresses cardiac and pulmonary conditions. Lifestyle and rehabilitative measures support recovery.

Specialty / Practitioner Care Strategies Table

Specialty Group	Practitioners Included	Hyperemissive Strategies	Hypoemissive Strategies
Biochemistry	Nutritionists, Orthomolecular, Herbalists, Naturopaths	Cardioprotective herbs, antioxidants, anti-inflammatories	Nutritional support for organ repair
Rehabilitation	Physiotherapists, Massage Therapists, Osteopaths / Chiropractors	Respiratory therapy, circulation enhancement	Gentle mobilization, relaxation techniques
Energetics	Acupuncturists (TCM), Bioenergetic Therapists	Acupuncture for cardiac and pulmonary support	Energy balancing and harmonization
Psychological	GNM practitioners, Psychotherapists, Vibrational therapists, Family constellation facilitators	Psychotherapy, bioresonance, conflict resolution	Emotional balancing and stress management

Educational Pearls & Considerations.

- Psychosomatic factors play a key role in thoracic organ pathology per GNM.
- Multidisciplinary approach integrating physical and psychological therapies optimizes care.
- Regular monitoring of cardiac and pulmonary function is essential.
- Early intervention improves outcomes.

GROUP 3 - ZONE 16 – UPPER BACK

Category 7: *Acupuncture / Meridian*

Step 1: Functional Anatomy and Interpretive Importance

The upper back comprises the thoracic vertebrae, scapulae, paraspinal musculature, and posterior rib cage, stabilizing respiration and posture (Standring, 2016). In TCM, this region is traversed by the Bladder (BL) and Small Intestine (SI) meridians, both of which parallel the vertebral column.

Deadman et al. (2007) highlighted the therapeutic use of BL13 (Feishu) and SI11 for respiratory, spinal, and immune regulation. Maciocia (2015) emphasized the BL channel's influence on autonomic balance and resistance to illness. Clinically, disruptions manifest as stiffness, scapular pain, or respiratory vulnerability.

In emissive mapping, biosignal variations appear as bilateral vertical bands along the thoracic spine, aligning with BL–SI trajectories rather than diffuse muscular activation.

These fields illustrate how posterior meridian function becomes visible through biospectral signatures, enabling clinicians to interpret dorsal emissive asymmetries as reflections of Qi stagnation or deficiency in thoracic channels.

Step 2,3,4: ROI Classification and Interpretive Questions

Hyperemission suggests localized Qi congestion or active meridian disturbance.

- Is there localized pain, tension, or tightness?
- Are symptoms exacerbated by stress or physical activity?

Hypoemission suggests Qi deficiency or chronic stagnation with poor circulation and cold sensations.

- Does the patient report fatigue, coldness, or chronic pain?
- Are symptoms persistent despite conventional treatments?

Step 5: Confirmatory Evaluations

Test	Purpose & Justification	Relevance to Emissive Pattern
Pulse diagnosis and tongue examination	Traditional TCM methods assessing Qi and Blood flow (Flaws, 2000).	Helps differentiate hyper- and hypoemissive patterns.
Biospectral imaging	Visualizes thermal asymmetries along meridian pathways.	Correlates with Qi imbalances in the upper back region.
Patient symptom questionnaire	Assesses musculoskeletal discomfort and emotional factors.	Assists clinical differentiation of meridian signal disruption.

Step 6: Care Strategies and Intervention Pathways

Naturopathic Approach

Acupuncture points such as BL13, BL15, and SI11 regulate Qi flow and relieve stagnation (Lao et al., 2004). Moxibustion warms hypoemissive meridian areas. Herbal formulas supporting meridian function are indicated (Bensky et al., 2004). Stress management and lifestyle modifications complement treatment.

Standard Medical Approaches

Acupuncture is utilized adjunctively for pain management and autonomic regulation.

Specialty / Practitioner Care Strategies Table

Specialty Group	Practitioners Included	Hyperemissive Strategies	Hypoemissive Strategies
Biochemistry	Nutritionists, Orthomolecular, Herbalists, Naturopaths	Anti-inflammatory and circulation-supporting herbs	Qi tonics and nutritional support
Rehabilitation	Physiotherapists, Massage Therapists, Osteopaths / Chiropractors	Myofascial release, thoracic mobilization	Gentle mobilization, warming massage
Energetics	Acupuncturists (TCM), Bioenergetic Therapists	Acupuncture, moxibustion, PEMF	Warming acupuncture, energy balancing
Psychological	GNM practitioners, Psychotherapists, Vibrational therapists, Family constellation facilitators	Psychotherapy, bioresonance, energy clearing	Psychosomatic conflict resolution, emotional balancing

Educational Pearls & Considerations.

- Correct point selection and technique optimize acupuncture outcomes.
- Moxibustion should be used cautiously in heat-sensitive patients.
- Herbal treatments require qualified supervision.
- Combining acupuncture with rehabilitation enhances results.

GROUP 3 - ZONE 16 – UPPER BACK

Category 8: *Energetic*

Step 1: Functional Anatomy and Interpretive Importance

The upper back is defined by the thoracic vertebrae, paraspinal muscles, scapular stabilizers, and overlying fascia that support posture and respiration (Standring, 2016). Energetically, this region functions as a stabilizing field, regulating coherence between autonomic activity, musculoskeletal coordination, and systemic resilience.

Becker and Selden (1985) emphasized the role of bioelectric signaling in maintaining structural and regulatory stability, a principle directly relevant here.

Patients often report chronic tension, restricted mobility, or diffuse discomfort resistant to conventional intervention. Spectral surface readings reveal broad hypoemissive depressions consistent with systemic depletion, alternating with hyperemissive arcs aligned with adaptive repair or compensatory activation.

These emissive features trace along spinal and fascial continuities, illustrating how the upper back functions as both an anatomical support and an energetic anchor. Clinically, it serves as a window into systemic resilience, autonomic load, and emotional adaptation, offering biospectral insight into otherwise elusive dysfunctions.

Step 2,3,4: ROI Classification and Interpretive Questions

Hyperemission suggests localized energetic congestion or signal overload.

- Does the patient report heat, tension, or discomfort in the upper back?
- Are emotional or stress factors contributing?

Hypoemission indicates energetic depletion or stagnation.

- Are fatigue, coldness, or low vitality present?
- Are symptoms chronic or refractory?

Step 5: Confirmatory Evaluations

Test	Purpose & Justification	Relevance to Emissive Pattern
Bioresonance testing	Measures tissue energy frequencies and imbalances.	Correlates with emissive energetic anomalies.
Electrodermal screening (EDS)	Assesses skin conductance linked to energetic pathways.	Supports interpretive understanding of energetic imbalance.
Patient emotional and symptom history	Provides context for energetic dysfunction and stress factors.	Assists biospectral differentiation.

Step 6: Care Strategies and Intervention Pathways

Naturopathic Approach

Use bioresonance, pulsed electromagnetic fields (PEMF), and adaptogenic herbs to restore energetic balance and promote healing (Matsumoto et al., 2010). Nutritional antioxidants and adaptogens improve systemic resilience. Mindfulness and stress reduction techniques complement energetic therapies.

Standard Medical Approaches

Energetic therapies serve as adjuncts to conventional and rehabilitative care, enhancing overall patient outcomes.

Specialty / Practitioner Care Strategies Table

Specialty Group	Practitioners Included	Hyperemissive Strategies	Hypoemissive Strategies
Biochemistry	Nutritionists, Orthomolecular, Herbalists, Naturopaths	Adaptogens, antioxidants, herbal energetics	Nutritional support for energy deficiency
Rehabilitation	Physiotherapists, Massage Therapists, Osteopaths / Chiropractors	Energy-based manual therapies, PEMF, therapeutic touch	Gentle stimulation, mobilization
Energetics	Acupuncturists (TCM), Bioenergetic Therapists	Bioresonance, PEMF, acupuncture	Warming acupuncture, energy balancing
Psychological	GNM practitioners, Psychotherapists, Vibrational therapists, Family constellation facilitators	Psychotherapy, bioresonance, mindfulness	Emotional balancing, vibrational medicine

Educational Pearls & Considerations.

- Energetic therapies complement but do not replace standard medical care.
- Practitioner skill and patient receptivity influence effectiveness.
- Regular reassessment enhances therapeutic success.
- Address psychological and physical aspects holistically.

GROUP 3 - ZONE 16 – UPPER BACK

Category 9: *Metabolic / Endocrine*

Step 1: Functional Anatomy and Interpretive Importance

The upper back includes the thoracic spine, scapular stabilizers, and overlying fascial tracts crucial for posture and autonomic stability (Standring, 2016). Endocrine and metabolic conditions, including diabetes, thyroid imbalance, and adrenal dysregulation, frequently manifest here through muscular fatigue and vascular irregularities.

Chrousos (2009) emphasized the role of the hypothalamic–pituitary–adrenal axis in systemic stress adaptation, a concept that aligns with emissive findings in this field. Patients often report chronic tension, fatigue, or pain resistant to localized interventions.

Spectral surface readings highlight diffuse hypoemissive depressions associated with systemic depletion, alongside hyperemissive arcs reflecting adaptive or compensatory activation. These emissive signatures extend across spinal and fascial planes, situating the upper back as both a mechanical and metabolic anchor.

Clinically, this zone provides biospectral insight into systemic resilience and stress–endocrine adaptation.

Step 2,3,4: ROI Classification and Interpretive Questions

Hyperemission eflects localized tissue reactivity, metabolic overactivity, or systemic challenge.

- Is there warmth, redness, or swelling?
- Is systemic metabolic control adequate?

Hypoemission indicates perfusion deficits, neuropathy, or circulatory impairment related to metabolic or endocrine dysfunction.

- Are cold sensations, numbness, or delayed healing present?
- Are systemic symptoms like fatigue or temperature intolerance reported?

Step 5: Confirmatory Evaluations

Test	Purpose & Justification	Relevance to Emissive Pattern
HbA1c, fasting glucose	Measures glycemic control in diabetes.	Correlates with hypoemissive neurofunctional or perfusion-restricted areas.
Thyroid function tests (TSH, Free T4)	Evaluates thyroid disorders affecting metabolism and circulation.	Associated with altered emissive regulation.

Lipid profile	Assesses cardiovascular risk influencing tissue perfusion.	Supports metabolic vascular adaptation.
Inflammatory markers (CRP, ESR)	Detects systemic inflammation impacting tissue health.	Correlates with hyperemissive tissue activation states.

Step 6: Care Strategies and Intervention Pathways

Naturopathic Approach

Support metabolic health through low glycemic diets, antioxidants, and adaptogens (Alberti et al., 2006). Herbs such as *Panax ginseng* and *Gymnema sylvestre* support endocrine function. Supplement chromium, magnesium, and alpha-lipoic acid to improve glucose metabolism and neuroprotection. Encourage regular aerobic exercise for vascular health.

Standard Medical Approaches

Medical management includes pharmacologic therapy and lifestyle modification for metabolic control. Thyroid hormone replacement and lipid management reduce complications.

Specialty / Practitioner Care Strategies Table

Specialty Group	Practitioners Included	Hyperemissive Strategies	Hypoemissive Strategies
Biochemistry	Nutritionists, Orthomolecular, Herbalists, Naturopaths	Antioxidants, adaptogens, insulin sensitizers, micronutrients	Metabolic support, neuroprotective nutrients, dietary management
Rehabilitation	Physiotherapists, Massage Therapists, Osteopaths / Chiropractors	Exercise therapy, circulation enhancement	Neuromuscular re-education, aerobic conditioning
Energetics	Acupuncturists (TCM), Bioenergetic Therapists	Acupuncture supporting metabolic function	Energy balancing, PEMF
Psychological	GNM practitioners, Psychotherapists, Vibrational therapists, Family constellation facilitators	Mind-body therapies supporting metabolic regulation	Stress reduction, emotional balancing

Educational Pearls & Considerations.

- Regular monitoring of metabolic parameters prevents complications.
- Lifestyle and dietary changes enhance clinical outcomes.
- Adaptogens support but do not replace standard treatments.
- Patient education on skin and wound care is essential.

GROUP 4

NECK AND FACE

The neck and face zones present a biospectrally rich and clinically complex anatomical region where vascular, neurological, lymphatic, and musculoskeletal structures converge, offering high interpretive yield. These areas are uniquely responsive to subtle changes in autonomic tone, inflammatory processes, and microcirculatory behavior, often revealing both systemic regulation and localized dysfunction.

Emissive patterns in the cervical region provide critical insights into vascular perfusion, nerve root stress, and fascial tension, allowing early identification of conditions such as lymphatic stasis, autonomic dysregulation, or neurovascular strain. In the facial zone, with its dense sensory-motor innervation and intricate vascular architecture, biospectral imaging can visualize neurogenic activation, vasomotor imbalance, and superficial muscular tension, often before clinical symptoms are reported.

Also, emissive responses in the neck and face frequently mirror emotional and autonomic shifts, reinforcing the diagnostic interface between psychosomatic dynamics and physiological regulation. This group's patterns significantly aid in distinguishing functional disturbances from structural changes, supporting refined interpretation and personalized care in regions that often elude precise characterization by conventional imaging tools.

Zones 17 to 19: Neck and Face Regions

The neck and face regions represent an anatomically and functionally complex area where vascular, neurological, lymphatic, and musculoskeletal systems intricately converge, producing a rich spectrum of emissive signals.

These zones involve vital structures including the cervical spine, carotid and vertebral vessels, jugular and facial veins, cranial nerve pathways, particularly trigeminal branches, and an extensive lymphatic network.

Given their high metabolic demand and dense innervation, the neck and face areas exhibit dynamic emissive patterns that reflect both localized imbalances and systemic autonomic regulation.

Emissive interpretation of the neck often reveals patterns associated with vascular load, muscular tension, lymphatic burden, and autonomic imbalance. Cervical emissive asymmetries may correspond to nerve root stress, cervical musculature strain, or circulatory restriction, sometimes preceding overt symptoms.

The neck's unique role as a conduit between the brain and body makes its emissive profile particularly sensitive to subtle alterations in sympathetic tone and regulatory dynamics. Ring and

Ammer (2012) emphasize that early recognition of such variations through infrared imaging can enhance interpretive clarity in relation to cervical regulatory changes.

Facial emissive mapping highlights neurogenic activation, vascular dysregulation, and myofascial imbalance, which may present in association with trigeminal stress, temporomandibular strain, or vascular-type headaches. The superficial vascularity and innervation of the face render it highly responsive to both emotional and systemic physiological influences, making emissive patterns in this area a sensitive marker of neurovascular and psychosomatic interaction.

Lahiri et al. (2012) note how emissive assessment of facial zones provides valuable adjunctive information for identifying regulatory disturbances involving vascular or autonomic systems.

The neck and face are also key regions where emotional and autonomic nervous system responses can be visualized emissively, linking psychophysiological states with somatic presentation.

Myers (2014) highlights the importance of fascial continuity and muscular chains in shaping emissive patterns, reinforcing the need for integrative interpretation in these zones. Additionally, Reitz (2024) points to the modulation of these emissive dynamics by metabolic and energetic influences, reinforcing the functional complexity inherent to this anatomical group.

This group includes three primary zones:

17. Frontal Neck and Supraclavicular
18. Cervical Spine and Nuchal Zone
19. Facial Area (Frontal and Lateral)

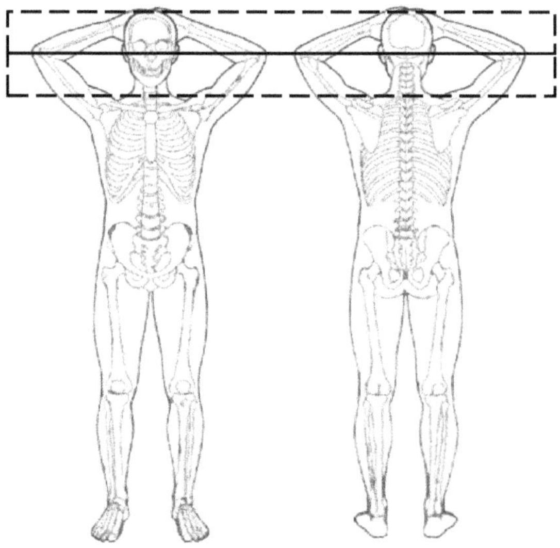

Each zone contributes specific diagnostic relevance within neurovascular, musculoskeletal, and lymphatic systems. Together, they provide a functional mapping of the interface between cranial and systemic regulation. Early emissive deviations in these regions assist in identifying regulatory disturbances and support clinical interpretation of autonomic, circulatory, and postural imbalances.

GROUP 4

ZONE 17 – FRONTAL NECK AND SUPRACLAVICULAR EGION

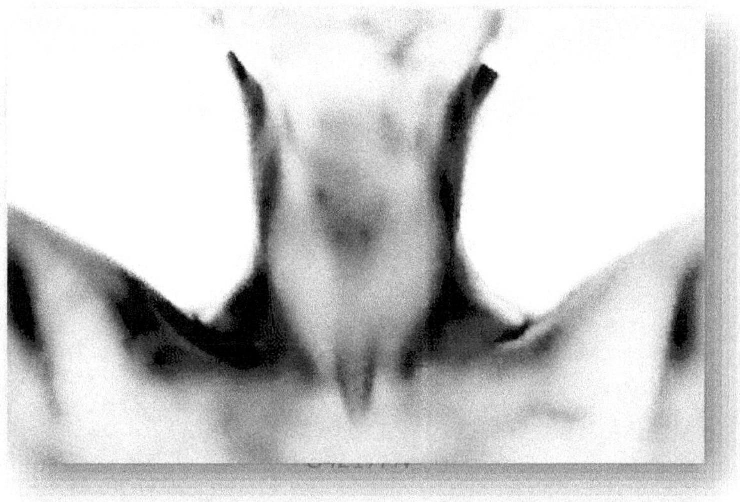

The frontal neck and supraclavicular region is among the body's most clinically sensitive surfaces, combining neurovascular, lymphatic, and endocrine structures within minimal soft tissue. It includes the anterior cervical musculature, carotid arteries and jugular veins, the thyroid gland, and the supraclavicular lymphatic chain (Standring, 2016). Because of this convergence, emissive asymmetries are rarely incidental.

The carotid arteries supply 80% of cerebral blood flow, and even minor regulatory alterations may produce detectable irregularities (Spence, 2006). The thyroid, one of the most metabolically active organs, shows perfusion changes in early dysfunction that affects 5–10% of the global population, often before clinical manifestation (Vanderpump, 2011).

The supraclavicular nodes drain both thoracic and abdominal territories; their enlargement, particularly Virchow's node, is a classic sign of systemic burden (Suárez et al., 2002). Biospectrally, even slight asymmetry may indicate immune or visceral adaptation. Autonomic density further heightens interpretive value, with the cervical plexus and vagus nerve contributing to neurovascular modulation (Benarroch, 2006).

Clinically, hyperactivity in the supraclavicular fossae may signal lymphatic congestion, respiratory demand, or early endocrine strain, while hypoactivity may reflect vascular suppression or reduced neural engagement. Thus, this zone provides an early, non-invasive perspective on vascular, immune, and endocrine states of major systemic significance.

Zone 17 – Frontal Neck and Supraclavicular: Emission-Relevant Structures.

Category	Relevant Structures	Emission Relevance
1. Vascular / Circulatory	- Carotid arteries - Jugular veins - Superficial cervical vessels	Hyperemission may indicate vascular activation, congestion, or vasodilation; Hypoemission suggests vasospasm or reduced perfusion in cervical vessels.
2. Muscular / Myofascial	- Sternocleidomastoid - Platysma - Suprahyoid and infrahyoid muscles	Hyperemission often reflects muscle tension, inflammation, or fascial strain; Hypoemission may indicate disuse or fascial restriction.
3. Skeletal / Articular	- Cervical vertebrae anterior aspects - Clavicles - First ribs	Hyperemission may reflect periosteal inflammation or joint irritation; Hypoemission may be due to chronic structural adaptation or reduced perfusion.
4. Nervous System / Spine	- Cervical spinal nerves (C1-C4) - Sympathetic chain ganglia	Hyperemissive zones indicate nerve irritation or radiculopathy; Hypoemission may correspond to compressive or autonomic patterns.
5. Lymphatic / Immune	- Supraclavicular lymph nodes - Superficial cervical lymphatics	Hyperemission often corresponds with lymphatic activity or immune engagement; Hypoemission may reveal stagnation or altered drainage capacity.
6. Organs / GNM (German New Medicine)	- Thyroid gland - Parathyroid glands - Larynx and pharynx	Hyperemissive patterns may reflect functional activation of organ-related zones; Hypoemission corresponds to regulatory downshift or resolution phase.
7. Acupuncture / Meridians	- Lung Meridian (cervical and supraclavicular) - Large Intestine Meridian	Hyperemission suggests Qi stagnation or excess; Hypoemission reflects Qi deficiency or dampness affecting cervical and respiratory meridians.
8. Energetic / Frequency	- Energetic reflex zones for autonomic and emotional regulation	Hyperemission may reflect sympathetic arousal or regulatory stress; Hypoemission indicates depletion or lowered autonomic tone.
9. Metabolic / Endocrine	- Thyroid reflex zones - Adrenal influence on cervical musculature	Hypoemission suggests reduced metabolic drive; Hyperemission may indicate increased metabolic demand or regulatory activation.

GROUP 4 - ZONE 17 – FRONTAL NECK AND SUPRACLAVICULAR

Category 1: *Vascular / Circulatory*

Step 1: Functional Anatomy and Interpretive Importance

The anterior neck and supraclavicular region receive arterial inflow from branches of the external carotid system, including the superior thyroid, lingual, and facial arteries, together with contributions from the subclavian system.

Venous return occurs through tributaries of the internal and external jugular veins, which drain the cervical musculature, thyroid, and fascial layers (Standring, 2016). Vascular research has emphasized the jugular system as a major pathway for cranio-cervical venous outflow, with functional importance in circulatory adaptation (Valdueza et al., 2000).

Spectral surface readings of this zone often reveal band-like emissive asymmetries along the vertical carotid–jugular axis. Such findings may indicate venous congestion, circulatory overload, or localized arterial reactivity.

Because of the region's integration of vascular, endocrine, and lymphatic structures, this area frequently displays emissive patterns of systemic significance.

Step 2,3,4: ROI Classification and Interpretive Questions

Hyperemission suggests tissue reactivity, venous congestion, or superficial vasodilation.

- Is there localized redness, swelling, or tenderness?
- Are systemic signs of inflammation present?

Hypoemission indicates compromised perfusion due to arterial compromise or chronic vascular insufficiency.

- Is coldness, pallor, or delayed tissue healing reported?
- Is there a history of vascular disease or systemic risk factors?

Step 5: Confirmatory Evaluations

Test	Purpose & Justification	Relevance to Emissive Pattern
Doppler ultrasound	Evaluates carotid and jugular vessel patency and flow dynamics.	Confirms vessel pathology corresponding to emissive changes.
CT or MRI angiography	Visualizes vascular structures and detects obstructions.	Confirms vessel pathology corresponding to emissive changes.
Blood tests (CBC, CRP, coagulation profile)	Detects systemic inflammation, infection, or coagulation abnormalities.	Supports biospectral or thrombotic states.
Physical exam	Assesses for vascular compromise signs such as swelling or bruit.	Complements biospectral findings.

Step 6: Care Strategies and Intervention Pathways

Naturopathic Approach

Botanical venotonics like *Aesculus hippocastanum* and *Ruscus aculeatus* improve microcirculation and reduce edema (Chrubasik et al., 2011). An anti-inflammatory diet rich in antioxidants and omega-3 fatty acids supports vascular health (Calder, 2017). Contrast hydrotherapy enhances circulation (Sutkowy et al., 2019). Supplementation with vitamins C, E, and bioflavonoids supports endothelial function. Gentle massage and postural correction aid venous return.

Standard Medical Approaches

Management includes imaging-guided anticoagulation, anti-inflammatory treatment, or surgical intervention when necessary. Address systemic risk factors such as hypertension or coagulopathies.

Specialty / Practitioner Care Strategies Table

Specialty Group	Practitioners Included	Hyperemissive Strategies	Hypoemissive Strategies
Biochemistry	Nutritionists, Orthomolecular, Herbalists, Naturopaths	Botanical venotonics, antioxidants, anti-inflammatory diet	Circulatory stimulants, endothelial support nutrients
Rehabilitation	Physiotherapists, Massage Therapists, Osteopaths / Chiropractors	Gentle massage, lymphatic drainage, postural correction	Graded exercise, circulatory enhancement
Energetics	Acupuncturists (TCM), Bioenergetic Therapists	Acupuncture, moxibustion, herbal formulas	Warming acupuncture, energy balancing
Psychological	GNM practitioners, Psychotherapists, Vibrational therapists, Family constellation facilitators	Psychotherapy, bioresonance, mindfulness	Stress reduction, emotional balancing

Educational Pearls & Considerations.

- Early detection of vascular inflammation or obstruction prevents complications.
- Botanical venotonics and anti-inflammatory nutrition support vascular integrity.
- Nitric oxide boosters and omega-3 fatty acids enhance endothelial function and perfusion.
- Compression therapy is contraindicated in significant arterial insufficiency.
- Gentle mobilization and posture correction aid venous return.

GROUP 4 - ZONE 17 – FRONTAL NECK AND SUPRACLAVICULAR

Category 2: *Muscular*

Step 1: Functional Anatomy and Interpretive Importance

The anterior neck and supraclavicular zone are supported by the sternocleidomastoid, scalenes, platysma, and superior trapezius fibers, muscles that facilitate head rotation, cervical stability, and accessory breathing.

These muscles are innervated by the spinal accessory and cervical plexus nerves, integrating cervical posture with thoracic mechanics (Standring, 2016). Clinical observations confirm that overactivation of the sternocleidomastoid and scalene groups contributes to tension headaches, cervical dysfunction, and compromised respiratory patterns (Fernández-de-las-Peñas et al., 2005).

Biospectral surface mapping of this region often reveals emissive asymmetries along the sternocleidomastoid trajectory or supraclavicular fossae, where muscular strain and fascial stress modify emissive output.

These findings frequently correspond to patient-reported tension or dysregulated breathing mechanics, marking the anterior neck as an important indicator of both musculoskeletal and autonomic adaptation.

Step 2,3,4: ROI Classification and Interpretive Questions

Hyperemission indicates active muscle strain, fascial tension, or localized signal retention.

- Has the patient experienced trauma, repetitive motion, or poor posture?
- Are symptoms such as tenderness, swelling, or tightness present?

Hypoemission suggests chronic perfusion deficit, fibrotic adaptation, or neurogenic atrophy.

- Are symptoms such as stiffness, weakness, or restricted mobility present?
- Is there muscle wasting or altered sensation?

Step 5: Confirmatory Evaluations

Test	Purpose & Justification	Relevance to Emissive Pattern
Creatine kinase (CK), LDH	Detects muscle injury or inflammation (Simons et al., 1999).	Elevated in hyperemissive activation states.
MRI	Visualizes muscle edema, inflammation, or fibrosis.	Correlates with emissive findings.

Electromyography (EMG)	Assesses muscle and nerve function.	Supports neurogenic causes of Hypoemission.
Blood tests (CBC, inflammatory markers)	Detects systemic inflammation or infection.	Supports biospectral muscle conditions.

Step 6: Care Strategies and Intervention Pathways

Naturopathic Approach

Use anti-inflammatory botanicals such as *Curcuma longa* and *Boswellia serrata* to reduce muscle inflammation (Hewlings & Kalman, 2017). Magnesium supports muscle relaxation and reduces spasms. Hydrotherapy with alternating warm and cold applications improves circulation (Sutkowy et al., 2019). Progressive stretching and strengthening promote recovery. Adequate protein and antioxidants support tissue repair.

Standard Medical Approaches

Rest, NSAIDs, and physical therapy are standard treatments for muscle injury (Simons et al., 1999). Neurological evaluation is recommended if weakness or sensory changes occur.

Specialty / Practitioner Care Strategies Table

Specialty Group	Practitioners Included	Hyperemissive Strategies	Hypoemissive Strategies
Biochemistry	Nutritionists, Orthomolecular, Herbalists, Naturopaths	Anti-inflammatory botanicals, magnesium, antioxidants, protein	Circulatory support, neurotrophic nutrients, protein support
Rehabilitation	Physiotherapists, Massage Therapists, Osteopaths / Chiropractors	Myofascial release, trigger point therapy, gentle massage	Graded aerobic exercise, neurorehabilitation, ergonomic guidance
Energetics	Acupuncturists (TCM), Bioenergetic Therapists	Acupuncture, moxibustion, PEMF	Warming acupuncture, frequency therapy
Psychological	GNM practitioners, Psychotherapists, Vibrational therapists, Family constellation facilitators	Psychotherapy, bioresonance, mindfulness	Psychosomatic conflict resolution, emotional balancing

Educational Pearls & Considerations.

- Early treatment of trigger points improves outcomes.
- Magnesium assists muscle relaxation and reduces spasms.
- Hydrotherapy protocols should be aligned with inflammation stages.
- Neurological assessment is important for persistent weakness.
- Gradual rehabilitation prevents chronic dysfunction.

GROUP 4 ZONE 17 – FRONTAL NECK AND SUPRACLAVICULAR

Category 3: *Skeletal*

Step 1: Functional Anatomy and Interpretive Importance

The frontal neck and supraclavicular region incorporates the clavicle, upper ribs, and lower cervical vertebrae, structures that form a transitional skeletal platform between thorax and head (Standring, 2016).

These bones stabilize the shoulder girdle and protect vascular and neural conduits traversing the thoracic outlet. Mechanical stress, degenerative remodeling, or postural compression at the clavicle or first rib often produces discomfort radiating into adjacent compartments.

Clinical research has highlighted the contribution of subtle costoclavicular alterations to thoracic outlet syndromes, with patients frequently presenting nonspecific upper limb symptoms (Illig et al., 2010). Such skeletal dysfunctions modify regional load transmission and fascial tension, and their emissive imprint can be discerned through spectral surface readings.

Biospectral asymmetries in this region frequently align along clavicular contours or supraclavicular depressions, revealing how bone and joint adaptations externalize into visible surface signals. These emissive patterns provide valuable context for distinguishing skeletal load issues from vascular or soft tissue influences in a complex anatomical crossroad.

Step 2,3,4: ROI Classification and Interpretive Questions

Hyperemission flects acute structural stress, mechanical overload, or periosteal reactivity.

- Is there localized swelling, tenderness, or warmth?
- Are symptoms exacerbated by movement or palpation?

Hypoemission suggests chronic degeneration, reduced perfusion, or neurogenic involvement.

- Are symptoms persistent with stiffness, dull pain, or reduced mobility?
- Is there a history of trauma or repetitive strain?

Step 5: Confirmatory Evaluations

Test	Purpose & Justification	Relevance to Emissive Pattern
X-ray	Detects fractures, dislocations, and degenerative changes.	Confirms skeletal pathology correlating with emissive patterns.
MRI	Visualizes soft tissues, bone marrow edema, and nerve involvement.	Supports interpretive recognition of reactive or degenerative patterns.
Bone scan	Assesses bone metabolism and detects occult lesions.	Identifies active skeletal remodeling or activation.

Physical exam	Evaluates tenderness, range of motion, and neurological signs.	Complements imaging and emissive findings.

Step 6: Care Strategies and Intervention Pathways

Naturopathic Approach

Support bone health with calcium, magnesium, vitamin D, and collagen peptides (Kruger & Kruger, 2019). Anti-inflammatory herbs like *Boswellia serrata* reduce joint inflammation. Physical therapy focused on posture and mobility aids recovery. Acupuncture and bioresonance may assist pain relief and modulate inflammation.

Standard Medical Approaches

Treatment includes analgesics, anti-inflammatory medications, and rehabilitation. Surgical intervention may be needed in severe cases.

Specialty / Practitioner Care Strategies Table

Specialty Group	Practitioners Included	Hyperemissive Strategies	Hypoemissive Strategies
Biochemistry	Nutritionists, Orthomolecular, Herbalists, Naturopaths	Bone-supportive nutrients, anti-inflammatory herbs	Nutritional support for bone repair
Rehabilitation	Physiotherapists, Osteopaths / Chiropractors, Massage Therapists	Manual therapy, posture correction, pain management	Ergonomic training, spinal mobilization
Energetics	Acupuncturists (TCM), Bioenergetic Therapists	Acupuncture, PEMF, energy healing	Energy balancing and stimulation
Psychological	GNM practitioners, Psychotherapists, Vibrational therapists, Family constellation facilitators	Psychotherapy, bioresonance, stress management	Emotional balancing and coping strategies

Educational Pearls & Considerations.

- Early diagnosis prevents chronic skeletal dysfunction.
- Nutritional support is essential for bone healing.
- Combining manual therapies with rehabilitation optimizes outcomes.
- Monitor for complications requiring specialist referral.

GROUP 4 - ZONE 17 – FRONTAL NECK AND SUPRACLAVICULAR

Category 4: *Nervous*

Step 1: Functional Anatomy and Interpretive Importance

The frontal neck and supraclavicular region is innervated by the cervical plexus (C1–C4) and branches of the brachial plexus, supplying sensory input to the anterior neck and motor control to muscles stabilizing the shoulder and upper thorax (Standring, 2016). These pathways are vulnerable to thoracic outlet compression, producing pain, paresthesia, and motor fatigue. Illig et al. (2010) note that thoracic outlet syndromes often involve both sensory and autonomic components, with neurovascular compromise influencing distal performance.

Such disturbances alter perfusion and fascial recruitment, projecting externally as surface biosignals. In emissive analysis, biospectral asymmetries commonly appear along the clavicular contour or supraclavicular fossa, reflecting nerve course and autonomic modulation. These patterns provide a noninvasive marker of neural compression at this junction, supporting differentiation from muscular or vascular causes of supraclavicular discomfort.

Step 2,3,4: ROI Classification and Interpretive Questions

Hyperemission indicates nerve irritation or neurogenic signaling consistent with heightened activity in affected neural pathways.

- Are there burning, tingling, or shooting pain symptoms?
- Is there localized swelling or hypersensitivity?

Hypoemission suggests signal interruption due to ischemia, mechanical compression, or denervation, resulting in reduced autonomic outflow and neuromuscular support.

- Are numbness, weakness, or muscle wasting present?
- Do symptoms worsen with certain postures or movements?

Step 5: Confirmatory Evaluations

Test	Purpose & Justification	Relevance to Emissive Pattern
Nerve conduction studies (NCS), Electromyography (EMG)	Evaluate nerve and muscle function (Janis et al., 2010).	Correlate with hypoemissive neurofunctional dysfunction.
Quantitative sensory testing (QST)	Measures sensory nerve thresholds.	Supports interpretive recognition of neuropathic patterns."
MRI	Identifies nerve root compression or structural abnormalities.	Detects causes of neurological symptoms.
Blood tests (glucose, vitamin B12)	Evaluates metabolic contributors to neuropathy.	Supports interpretive understanding of systemic neuroregulation.

Step 6: Care Strategies and Intervention Pathways

Naturopathic Approach

Use neurotrophic vitamins (B-complex), alpha-lipoic acid, and Acetyl-L-carnitine to support nerve regeneration (Papanas & Ziegler, 2014). *Hypericum perforatum* may alleviate neuropathic pain (Kasper et al., 2010). Neural mobilization and bioresonance therapies facilitate recovery. Mind-body therapies regulate autonomic function.

Standard Medical Approaches

Pharmacologic treatments include anticonvulsants, antidepressants, and analgesics. Surgical decompression is considered for severe compression. Managing metabolic causes such as diabetes is essential.

Specialty / Practitioner Care Strategies Table

Specialty Group	Practitioners Included	Hyperemissive Strategies	Hypoemissive Strategies
Biochemistry	Nutritionists, Orthomolecular, Herbalists, Naturopaths	Neurotrophic vitamins, alpha-lipoic acid, anti-inflammatory botanicals	Circulatory stimulants, metabolic support, neuroprotective nutrients
Rehabilitation	Physiotherapists, Massage Therapists, Osteopaths / Chiropractors	Neural mobilization, myofascial release, gentle massage	Neural gliding exercises, ergonomic guidance, neurorehabilitation
Energetics	Acupuncturists (TCM), Bioenergetic Therapists	Acupuncture, moxibustion, PEMF	Warming acupuncture, frequency therapy, energy healing
Psychological	GNM practitioners, Psychotherapists, Vibrational therapists, Family constellation facilitators	Psychotherapy, bioresonance, mindfulness	Psychosomatic conflict resolution, vibrational medicine

Educational Pearls & Considerations.

- Early diagnosis prevents chronic nerve damage.
- Nutritional and energetic therapies support nerve repair.
- Monitor metabolic contributors such as diabetes.
- Avoid aggressive therapy during acute inflammation.
- Tailor neural mobilization to patient tolerance.

GROUP 4 - ZONE 17 – FRONTAL NECK AND SUPRACLAVICULAR

Category 5: *Lymphatic*

Step 1: Functional Anatomy and Interpretive Importance

The The frontal neck and supraclavicular region contains superficial and deep lymphatic vessels that drain from the head, neck, and upper thorax toward supraclavicular and deep cervical nodes (Standring, 2016).

These nodal stations are among the most significant for filtering immune cells and monitoring systemic circulation from both thoracic and abdominal territories. McLaughlin et al. (2008) documented that lymphatic disruption in this region, often following surgical or oncologic procedures, leads to persistent stasis and tissue tension. Altered transport modifies fascial mobility and vascular signaling, changes that extend to surface emissive expression.

On clinical imaging, emissive irregularities may appear as confined fields across the supraclavicular fossa or extending along the clavicle, their geometry reflecting lymphatic pathways rather than muscular activation.

These signals provide a visible indication of cervical lymphatic congestion, assisting clinicians in distinguishing immune-related drainage disturbances from neuromuscular or vascular contributors to supraclavicular discomfort.

Step 2,3,4: ROI Classification and Interpretive Questions

Hyperemission indicates acute lymphatic overload, localized infection, or signal congestion presenting with swelling and warmth.

- Is there redness, tenderness, or rapid swelling?
- Has the patient had recent infections, trauma, or malignancy?

Hypoemission suggests chronic lymphatic stagnation with tissue remodeling and reduced biosignal flow leading to reduced tissue perfusion.

- Is swelling persistent, firm, or non-pitting?
- Are recurrent infections or delayed healing present?

Step 5: Confirmatory Evaluations

Test	Purpose & Justification	Relevance to Emissive Pattern
Lymphoscintigraphy	Assesses lymphatic flow and identifies obstructions.	Confirms lymphatic congestion or flow restriction.
Doppler ultrasound	Differentiates venous insufficiency from lymphatic causes.	Clarifies fluid retention etiology.

Blood tests (CBC, inflammatory markers)	Detects systemic infection or inflammation.	Supports hyperemissive activation states.
Physical exam (Stemmer's sign, limb measurements)	Identifies clinical signs of lymphedema.	Correlates with emissive findings.

Step 6: Care Strategies and Intervention Pathways

Naturopathic Approach

Use herbal lymphagogues such as *Hedera helix* and *Vitis vinifera* to stimulate lymphatic drainage (Godoy et al., 2012). Certified manual lymphatic drainage therapy promotes fluid movement. Properly fitted compression garments aid lymph return. Nutritional antioxidants and anti-inflammatory nutrients support tissue repair. Hydrotherapy with alternating warm and cold enhances circulation.

Standard Medical Approaches

Treatment includes manual lymphatic drainage, compression therapy, physical rehabilitation, and infection management. Surgical interventions reserved for refractory cases.

Specialty / Practitioner Care Strategies Table

Specialty Group	Practitioners Included	Hyperemissive Strategies	Hypoemissive Strategies
Biochemistry	Nutritionists, Orthomolecular, Herbalists, Naturopaths	Herbal lymphagogues, antioxidants, anti-inflammatory nutrients	Circulatory support, nutritional tissue repair support
Rehabilitation	Physiotherapists, Massage Therapists, Osteopaths / Chiropractors	Manual lymphatic drainage, gentle massage, postural retraining	Compression therapy, graded exercise, ergonomic guidance
Energetics	Acupuncturists (TCM), Bioenergetic Therapists	Acupuncture, herbal formulas, PEMF	Warming acupuncture, energy balancing
Psychological	GNM practitioners, Psychotherapists, Vibrational therapists, Family constellation facilitators	Mind-body therapies supporting immune function and healing	Psychosomatic conflict resolution, emotional balancing

Educational Pearls & Considerations.

- Early intervention prevents chronic lymphedema progression.
- Manual lymphatic drainage requires trained professionals.
- Compression therapy must be properly fitted and monitored.
- Nutritional support enhances lymphatic and tissue health.
- Infection control is critical.

GROUP 4 - ZONE 17 – FRONTAL NECK AND SUPRACLAVICULAR

Category 6: *Organ-Related (GNM)*

Step 1: Functional Anatomy and Interpretive Importance

The frontal neck and supraclavicular area contain the thyroid and parathyroid glands, as well as major vascular and lymphatic conduits of the cervical region (Standring, 2016). In German New Medicine (GNM), biological conflicts tied to communication, fear of attack, or existential threat may manifest through thyroid-related organ programs.

Hamer (2012) explained that active conflicts often suppress emissive activity (hypoemission), whereas reparative phases are marked by hyperemissive fields reflecting cellular recovery.

These externalized biosignal variations may be observed along the lower cervical and supraclavicular zones, distinct from vascular or muscular signals. Heim et al. (2000) demonstrated how early-life stress and trauma can alter hypothalamic–pituitary–thyroid regulation, aligning with the psychosomatic links described in GNM.

This integration strengthens the interpretation of surface emission patterns as visible correlates of endocrine stress responses, providing insight into psychobiological influences on thyroid function.

Step 2,3,4: ROI Classification and Interpretive Questions

Hyperemission indicates active healing or energetic activation with increased metabolic signaling.

- Are there symptoms such as neck discomfort, swelling, or endocrine dysfunction?
- Is systemic inflammation present?

Hypoemission corresponds to conflict-active phases with functional suppression or signal reduction.

- Are there chronic symptoms such as fatigue, hormonal imbalance, or unresolved psychological stress?
- Are there signs of ongoing low energy, poor regulation, or emotional conflict?

Step 5: Confirmatory Evaluations

Test	Purpose & Justification	Relevance to Emissive Pattern
Thyroid function tests (TSH, Free T4, Free T3)	Evaluate thyroid hormonal status and dysfunction.	Correlates with biospectral changes in thyroid-related conditions.

Ultrasound of thyroid and neck	Visualizes gland morphology, nodules, or inflammation.	Supports correlation with biosignal findings.
Inflammatory markers, CBC	Detect systemic or local inflammation.	Supports hyperemissive activation phases.
Psychological assessment	Identifies psychosomatic conflicts relevant to GNM diagnosis.	Complements interpretation of emissive patterns.

Step 6: Care Strategies and Intervention Pathways

Naturopathic Approach

Use thyroid-supportive nutrients such as iodine, selenium, and zinc. Anti-inflammatory botanicals like *Withania somnifera* (Ashwagandha) may support endocrine balance (Singh et al., 2011). Stress management and psychotherapy assist in resolving psychosomatic conflicts. Nutritional antioxidants support tissue repair.

Standard Medical Approaches

Thyroid hormone replacement and anti-inflammatory treatments are tailored to specific diagnoses. Regular monitoring and imaging guide management.

Specialty / Practitioner Care Strategies Table

Specialty Group	Practitioners Included	Hyperemissive Strategies	Hypoemissive Strategies
Biochemistry	Nutritionists, Orthomolecular, Herbalists, Naturopaths	Endocrine support nutrients, antioxidants, anti-inflammatory herbs	Nutritional support for hormone synthesis and balance
Rehabilitation	Physiotherapists, Massage Therapists, Osteopaths / Chiropractors	Gentle neck mobilization, myofascial release	Postural correction, relaxation techniques
Energetics	Acupuncturists (TCM), Bioenergetic Therapists	Acupuncture for endocrine regulation	Energy balancing and harmonization
Psychological	GNM practitioners, Psychotherapists, Vibrational therapists, Family constellation facilitators	Psychotherapy, bioresonance, conflict resolution	Emotional balancing, stress reduction

Educational Pearls & Considerations.

- Monitor thyroid function regularly in patients with thermal abnormalities in this zone.
- Integrate physical and psychological therapies for comprehensive care.
- Nutritional support is critical for endocrine health.
- Early recognition of psychosomatic factors improves outcomes.

GROUP 4 - ZONE 17 – FRONTAL NECK AND SUPRACLAVICULAR

Category 7: *Acupuncture / Meridian*

Step 1: Functional Anatomy and Interpretive Importance

The frontal neck and supraclavicular region contain the thyroid gland, cervical fascia, and major vascular conduits, with musculature including sternocleidomastoid and scalene groups (Standring, 2016).

In acupuncture mapping, this area corresponds to the Kidney (KI), Lung (LU), and Stomach (ST) meridians, which intersect at the base of the neck and influence systemic circulation and respiratory control. Flaws (2000) highlighted the role of LU1 and ST9 in regulating breathing and fluid dynamics.

Deadman et al. (2007) emphasized that Kidney channel points in the supraclavicular region stabilize endocrine and metabolic regulation, linking surface palpation with systemic effects. Clinically, disruptions in these channels may be associated with throat tension, swallowing difficulty, or fatigue.

On emissive imaging, biosignal changes are often observed as vertical or oblique fields across the supraclavicular fossa, sharply defined in comparison to vascular or muscular activity.

These fields provide external evidence of Qi stagnation, deficiency, or hyperactivity in upper thoracic meridians, reinforcing the integration of TCM channel mapping with biospectral observation.

Step 2,3,4: ROI Classification and Interpretive Questions

Hyperemission indicates Qi stagnation or excessive signal expression along meridian trajectories.

- Are there localized tightness, pain, or discomfort?
- Are symptoms exacerbated by emotional stress or physical exertion?

Hypoemission suggests Qi deficiency or chronic stagnation contributing to reduced circulatory dynamics and diminished signal expression.

- Does the patient report fatigue, coldness, or chronic discomfort?
- Are symptoms persistent or worsening?

Step 5: Confirmatory Evaluations

Test	Purpose & Justification	Relevance to Emissive Pattern
Pulse diagnosis and tongue examination	Traditional TCM diagnostic tools assessing Qi and Blood status (Flaws, 2000).	Helps differentiate between hyper- and hypoemissive patterns.
Biospectral imaging	Visualizes thermal asymmetries along meridian courses.	Correlates with Qi stagnation in the neck region.
Symptom questionnaire	Assesses chest discomfort, breathing difficulties, and emotional state.	Supports differentiation of meridian patterns.

Step 6: Care Strategies and Intervention Pathways

Naturopathic Approach

Acupuncture points such as KI27, LU1, and ST9 regulate Qi flow and relieve stagnation (Lao et al., 2004). Moxibustion is used to warm hypoemissive meridians. Herbal formulas like *Liu Wei Di Huang Wan* support kidney and lung function (Bensky et al., 2004). Lifestyle and stress management complement these therapies.

Standard Medical Approaches

Acupuncture serves as an adjunct to conventional care for symptom relief and improved autonomic regulation.

Specialty / Practitioner Care Strategies Table

Specialty Group	Practitioners Included	Hyperemissive Strategies	Hypoemissive Strategies
Biochemistry	Nutritionists, Orthomolecular, Herbalists, Naturopaths	Respiratory and kidney-supportive herbs, antioxidants	Qi tonics and nutritional support
Rehabilitation	Physiotherapists, Massage Therapists, Osteopaths / Chiropractors	Thoracic mobilization, myofascial release	Gentle mobilization, warming massage
Energetics	Acupuncturists (TCM), Bioenergetic Therapists	Acupuncture, moxibustion, PEMF	Warming acupuncture, energy balancing
Psychological	GNM practitioners, Psychotherapists, Vibrational therapists, Family constellation facilitators	Psychotherapy, bioresonance, energy clearing	Psychosomatic conflict resolution, emotional balancing

Educational Pearls & Considerations.

- Accurate acupuncture point selection is vital for therapeutic success.
- Moxibustion should be used cautiously, particularly in heat-sensitive individuals.
- Herbal treatments require practitioner supervision.
- Integration with rehabilitative therapies enhances outcomes.

GROUP 4 - ZONE 17 – FRONTAL NECK AND SUPRACLAVICULAR

Category 8: *Energetic*

Step 1: Functional Anatomy and Interpretive Importance

The frontal neck and supraclavicular region contain the thyroid gland, vascular conduits, cervical fascia, and neural branches linking thorax and head (Standring, 2016). Energetically, this surface functions as a field of systemic communication, integrating endocrine regulation, vocal expression, and autonomic stability. Motoyama (1977) demonstrated electrophysiological correlations between supraclavicular energy flow and meridian pathways, supporting its clinical interpretation.

Patients often report vocal fatigue, thyroid strain, or diffuse neck tension. Spectral readings reveal hypoemissive depressions linked to suppressed output and hyperemissive arcs reflecting reparative or expressive intensification. These dynamics extend along fascial and vascular lines, projecting systemic regulation beyond localized anatomy. Clinically, the region operates as a biospectral node of metabolic, communicative, and autonomic integration, with surface signatures that can precede systemic imbalance or adaptation.

Step 2,3,4: ROI Classification and Interpretive Questions

Hyperemission suggests localized energetic congestion or excessive signal expression.

- Does the patient experience sensations of heat, tension, or discomfort?
- Are stress or emotional factors prominent?

Hypoemission indicates energetic signal depletion or prolonged stagnation.

- Are symptoms such as fatigue, coldness, or low vitality reported?
- Are symptoms chronic or resistant to treatment?

Step 5: Confirmatory Evaluations

Test	Purpose & Justification	Relevance to Emissive Pattern
Bioresonance testing	Measures tissue energy frequencies and imbalances.	Correlates with biosignal energetic variations.
Electrodermal screening (EDS)	Assesses skin conductance linked to energy pathways.	Supports interpretive recognition of energetic pattern expressions.
Patient emotional and symptom history	Provides context for energetic dysfunction and stress factors.	Assists differential interpretation.

Step 6: Care Strategies and Intervention Pathways

Naturopathic Approach

Utilize bioresonance, pulsed electromagnetic fields (PEMF), and adaptogenic botanicals to restore energetic balance and promote healing (Matsumoto et al., 2010). Nutritional antioxidants and adaptogens enhance systemic resilience. Mindfulness and stress reduction techniques support energetic therapies.

Standard Medical Approaches

Energetic therapies complement conventional and rehabilitative care, enhancing overall patient outcomes.

Specialty / Practitioner Care Strategies Table

Specialty Group	Practitioners Included	Hyperemissive Strategies	Hypoemissive Strategies
Biochemistry	Nutritionists, Orthomolecular, Herbalists, Naturopaths	Adaptogens, antioxidants, herbal energetics	Nutritional support for energy deficiency
Rehabilitation	Physiotherapists, Massage Therapists, Osteopaths / Chiropractors	Energy-based manual therapies, PEMF, therapeutic touch	Gentle stimulation, mobilization
Energetics	Acupuncturists (TCM), Bioenergetic Therapists	Bioresonance, PEMF, acupuncture	Warming acupuncture, energy balancing
Psychological	GNM practitioners, Psychotherapists, Vibrational therapists, Family constellation facilitators	Psychotherapy, bioresonance, mindfulness	Emotional balancing, vibrational medicine

Educational Pearls & Considerations.

- Energetic therapies support but do not replace standard medical care.
- Practitioner skill and patient receptivity influence effectiveness.
- Ongoing reassessment improves therapeutic success.
- Holistic addressing of psychological and physical factors is essential.

GROUP 4 - ZONE 17 – FRONTAL NECK AND SUPRACLAVICULAR

Category 9: *Metabolic / Endocrine*

Step 1: Functional Anatomy and Interpretive Importance

The frontal neck and supraclavicular region contain the thyroid and parathyroid glands, vascular conduits, and fascial networks that regulate systemic metabolism and calcium balance (Standring, 2016).

Dysfunctions such as thyroid disease or parathyroid imbalance manifest here with systemic consequences on energy regulation and vascular tone. Brent (2012) detailed how thyroid dysfunction alters basal metabolic rate, thermogenesis, and muscular tone, providing context for observed biospectral changes.

Clinically, patients may present with vocal strain, fatigue, or systemic dysregulation. Spectral surface readings reveal hypoemissive depressions consistent with thyroid suppression and hyperemissive fields associated with reparative or overactive states.

These emissive variations frequently extend beyond glandular borders, mapping endocrine balance onto visible surface patterns. Clinically, this field offers direct biospectral insight into thyroid and parathyroid regulation as central components of metabolic health.

Step 2,3,4: ROI Classification and Interpretive Questions

Hyperemission uggests signal intensification associated with increased metabolic demand or regulatory activation.

- Is there warmth, swelling, or tenderness?
- Are systemic symptoms such as heat intolerance or palpitations present?

Hypoemission indicates reduced metabolic expression, vascular insufficiency, or regulatory suppression potentially linked to endocrine imbalance.

- Are cold intolerance, fatigue, or tissue hypoxia reported?
- Is there a history of thyroid or parathyroid disease?

Step 5: Confirmatory Evaluations

Test	Purpose & Justification	Relevance to Emissive Pattern
Thyroid function tests (TSH, Free T4, Free T3)	Assess thyroid hormone levels and function.	Correlates with biospectral changes in thyroid function.
Calcium and parathyroid hormone (PTH) levels	Evaluate parathyroid function and calcium metabolism.	Supports interpretive recognition of parathyroid-related patterns.

Ultrasound of thyroid and parathyroid glands	Detects nodules, inflammation, or structural abnormalities.	Correlates with localized emissive variations.
Inflammatory markers, CBC	Detects systemic or local inflammation.	Supports hyperemissive activation states.

Step 6: Care Strategies and Intervention Pathways

Naturopathic Approach

Support thyroid and parathyroid function with selenium, iodine, zinc, and antioxidants (Rajput et al., 2013). Use anti-inflammatory botanicals such as *Withania somnifera* to modulate endocrine balance (Singh et al., 2011). Stress management and psychotherapy assist in resolving psychosomatic contributors. Nutritional antioxidants promote tissue repair.

Standard Medical Approaches

Pharmacological therapy includes hormone replacement or suppression depending on diagnosis. Regular imaging and lab monitoring guide management.

Specialty / Practitioner Care Strategies Table

Specialty Group	Practitioners Included	Hyperemissive Strategies	Hypoemissive Strategies
Biochemistry	Nutritionists, Orthomolecular, Herbalists, Naturopaths	Endocrine support nutrients, antioxidants, anti-inflammatory herbs	Nutritional support for hormone synthesis and balance
Rehabilitation	Physiotherapists, Massage Therapists, Osteopaths / Chiropractors	Gentle neck mobilization, myofascial release	Postural correction, relaxation techniques
Energetics	Acupuncturists (TCM), Bioenergetic Therapists	Acupuncture for endocrine regulation	Energy balancing and harmonization
Psychological	GNM practitioners, Psychotherapists, Vibrational therapists, Family constellation facilitators	Psychotherapy, bioresonance, conflict resolution	Emotional balancing, stress reduction

Educational Pearls & Considerations.

- Regular thyroid and parathyroid monitoring is essential in this zone.
- Nutritional and botanical support aids endocrine health.
- Psychosomatic factors may influence symptomatology.
- Early intervention improves prognosis.

GROUP 4

ZONE 18 – CERVICAL SPINE AND NUCHAL REGION

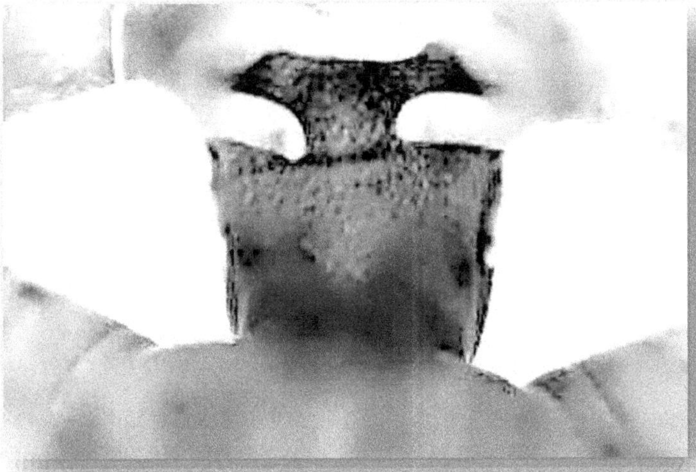

G4Z18CS

The cervical spine and nuchal region forms a biomechanical and neurofunctional hub where musculoskeletal, vascular, and autonomic influences converge. It includes the cervical vertebrae, posterior musculature such as splenius capitis and semispinalis, and associated structures including the vertebral arteries and cervical sympathetic chain (Standring, 2016).

This zone is highly sensitive to muscular strain and neural compression, often manifesting as emissive asymmetries. Neck pain affects nearly 30% of adults annually, with recurrence in up to 50% of cases (Fejer et al., 2006). Hyperactivity here frequently reflects acute muscular tension or sympathetic overactivity, while hypoactivity may correspond to denervation, reduced perfusion, or fascial rigidity.

The vertebral arteries, supplying up to 20% of cerebral circulation, demonstrate flow alterations in vertebrobasilar insufficiency that can produce early surface-detectable microcirculatory changes (Caplan, 2000).

Chronic postural strain, particularly from screen use, has been linked with cervical myofascial overload and persistent nuchal asymmetries (Hoy et al., 2014). Neurogenic mechanisms also contribute: radiculopathy or neuropathic irritation often generate surface changes before imaging reveals compression (Baron et al., 2013).

Emotional stress adds another dimension, as trapezius and cervical extensors increase activity under mental load, a response reflected emissively (Lundberg, 1999). Clinically, this makes the cervical spine and nuchal zone a critical surface for early recognition of biomechanical overload, neurovascular compromise, and autonomic strain, bridging localized and systemic interpretation.

.

Zone 18 – Cervical Spine and Nuchal Region: Emission-Relevant Structures

Category	Relevant Structures	Emission Relevance
1. Vascular / Circulatory	- Vertebral arteries - Posterior cervical arteries and veins	Hyperemission may indicate vascular activation or congestion; Hypoemission can reflect arterial spasm or sympathetic vasoconstriction.
2. Muscular / Myofascial	- Trapezius - Splenius capitis - Semispinalis capitis and cervicis	Hyperemission corresponds to muscle spasm, tissue activation, or overuse; Hypoemission may indicate disuse, fibrosis, or chronic myofascial restriction.
3. Skeletal / Articular	- Cervical vertebrae (C1-C7) - Occipital bone	Local Hyperemission may reflect arthritic activity or tissue reactivity; Hypoemission may indicate degenerative changes or reduced blood flow.
4. Nervous System / Spine	- Cervical spinal nerves (C1-C8) - Sympathetic cervical chain ganglia	Hyperemission suggests nerve irritation or radicular activation; Hypoemission corresponds to chronic nerve compression or autonomic suppression.
5. Lymphatic / Immune	- Deep cervical lymph nodes - Superficial cervical lymphatics	Hyperemission reflects immune node activation; Hypoemission may indicate lymphatic congestion or fibrosis.
6. Organs / GNM (German New Medicine)	- Spinal cord segments related to cervical spine reflexes	Biosignal variations may correspond to visceral-somatic reflex activity related to organ response patterns or conflict phases.
7. Acupuncture / Meridians	- Bladder Meridian (cervical region) - Governing Vessel (Du Mai)	Hyperemission indicates Qi stagnation or excess; hypoemissive regions reflect deficiency or blood stasis affecting cervical spinal and autonomic regulation.
8. Energetic / Frequency	- Energetic reflex centers related to cervical autonomic and neuromuscular regulation	Hyperemission may be linked to sympathetic overactivity or excitatory load; Hypoemission suggests energetic depletion or autonomic downregulation.
9. Metabolic / Endocrine	- Reflex zones for thyroid and adrenal influence	Hypoemission suggests hormonal underexpression; Hyperemission may indicate tissue activation or hypermetabolic behavior in cervical tissues.

GROUP 4 - ZONE 18 – CERVICAL SPINE AND NUCHAL ZONE

Category 1: *Vascular / Circulatory*

Step 1: Functional Anatomy and Interpretive Importance

The posterior cervical region is supplied by the vertebral arteries, which ascend through the transverse foramina of the cervical vertebrae, together with contributions from the occipital artery and deep cervical branches. V

enous return occurs through the vertebral venous plexus and tributaries of the internal and external jugular systems (Standring, 2016). Neuroangiographic studies have detailed the vertebral and occipital systems extensively, underlining their importance in cervical and cranio-cervical perfusion (Lasjaunias & Berenstein, 2001).

On spectral surface reading, emissive asymmetries are frequently observed along the vertebrobasilar and occipital tracks. These may reflect circulatory strain from postural demand, venous stasis in the posterior cervical plexus, or adaptive vascular changes linked to spinal mechanics.

This zone therefore provides an essential window into the vascular dynamics of cervical and nuchal regulation.

Step 2,3,4: ROI Classification and Interpretive Questions

Hyperemission indicates signal intensification associated with venous stasis or superficial vascular expansion.

- Is there localized swelling, redness, or tenderness?
- Are systemic inflammatory symptoms present?

Hypoemission suggests vascular insufficiency or reduced circulatory adaptation.

- Is coldness, pallor, or delayed tissue healing reported?
- Is there a history of vascular disease or systemic risk factors?

Step 5: Confirmatory Evaluations

Test	Purpose & Justification	Relevance to Emissive Pattern
Doppler ultrasound	Assesses vertebral and cervical artery patency and flow.	Correlates with hyperemissive vascular activation or hypoemissive perfusion reduction.
CT or MRI angiography	Visualizes vascular structures and identifies occlusions.	Confirms vascular involvement related to biosignal findings.

Blood tests (CBC, CRP, coagulation profile)	Detects systemic inflammation or coagulation abnormalities.	Supports congestive or occlusive processes.
Physical exam	Evaluates vascular compromise signs such as swelling or bruit.	Complements emissive observations.

Step 6: Care Strategies and Intervention Pathways

Naturopathic Approach

Botanical venotonics like *Aesculus hippocastanum* and *Ruscus aculeatus* enhance microcirculation and reduce edema (Chrubasik et al., 2011). An anti-inflammatory diet rich in antioxidants and omega-3 fatty acids supports vascular health (Calder, 2017). Contrast hydrotherapy stimulates circulation (Sutkowy et al., 2019). Supplementation with vitamins C, E, and bioflavonoids supports endothelial function. Gentle massage and postural correction promote venous return.

Standard Medical Approaches

Management may include anticoagulation, anti-inflammatory medications, or surgical intervention guided by imaging. Address systemic risk factors such as hypertension and coagulopathies.

Specialty / Practitioner Care Strategies Table

Specialty Group	Practitioners Included	Hyperemissive Strategies	Hypoemissive Strategies
Biochemistry	Nutritionists, Orthomolecular, Herbalists, Naturopaths	Botanical venotonics, antioxidants, anti-inflammatory diet	Circulatory stimulants, endothelial support nutrients
Rehabilitation	Physiotherapists, Massage Therapists, Osteopaths / Chiropractors	Gentle massage, lymphatic drainage, postural correction	Graded exercise, circulatory enhancement
Energetics	Acupuncturists (TCM), Bioenergetic Therapists	Acupuncture, moxibustion, herbal formulas	Warming acupuncture, energy balancing
Psychological	GNM practitioners, Psychotherapists, Vibrational therapists, Family constellation facilitators	Psychotherapy, bioresonance, mindfulness	Stress reduction, emotional balancing

Educational Pearls & Considerations.

- Early identification of vascular issues prevents complications.
- Botanical venotonics and anti-inflammatory nutrition support vascular integrity.
- Nitric oxide boosters and omega-3 fatty acids enhance endothelial health and perfusion.
- Avoid compression therapy if significant arterial insufficiency exists.
- Posture and mobilization support venous return.

GROUP 4 - ZONE 18 – CERVICAL SPINE AND NUCHAL ZONE

Category 2: *Muscular*

Step 1: Functional Anatomy and Interpretive Importance

The posterior cervical region includes the trapezius, splenius capitis, semispinalis, and the deep suboccipital group, innervated by dorsal rami and the spinal accessory nerve. These muscles provide extension, rotation, and fine control of the head and cervical spine, functioning in close synergy with ligamentous and fascial structures (Standring, 2016).

Research demonstrates that inhibition or maladaptation of the deep cervical extensors contributes significantly to chronic neck pain and impaired sensorimotor control (Falla et al., 2004).

Emissive changes in this zone often appear as focal biospectral asymmetries across the nuchal ridge or suboccipital area, reflecting strain, fatigue, or adaptive overuse of stabilizers.

Because the cervical musculature is closely tied to proprioception and balance, spectral deviations here are especially valuable for understanding the interplay between neuromuscular integrity and postural regulation.

Step 2,3,4: ROI Classification and Interpretive Questions

Hyperemission indicates signal intensification associated with muscle strain or myofascial irritative foci.

- Has the patient experienced trauma, poor posture, or repetitive strain?
- Are symptoms of tenderness, swelling, or stiffness present?

Hypoemission suggests chronic vascular insufficiency, fascial densification, or neurogenic regulation loss.

- Are there symptoms of weakness, stiffness, or decreased range of motion?
- Is muscle wasting or neurological deficit evident?

Step 5: Confirmatory Evaluations

Test	Purpose & Justification	Relevance to Emissive Pattern
Creatine kinase (CK), LDH	Detects muscle injury or inflammation (Simons et al., 1999).	Elevated in hyperemissive activation states.
MRI	Visualizes muscle edema, inflammation, or fibrosis.	Correlates with biosignal findings.
Electromyography (EMG)	Assesses muscle and nerve function.	Supports neuromuscular contributors to Hypoemission.
Blood tests (CBC, inflammatory markers)	Detects systemic inflammation or infection.	Supports myofascial response patterns.

Step 6: Care Strategies and Intervention Pathways

Naturopathic Approach

Anti-inflammatory herbs such as *Curcuma longa* and *Boswellia serrata* reduce muscle inflammation (Hewlings & Kalman, 2017). Magnesium supports muscle relaxation and reduces spasms. Hydrotherapy with alternating warm and cold applications improves circulation (Sutkowy et al., 2019). Progressive stretching and strengthening promote recovery. Adequate protein and antioxidants support tissue repair.

Standard Medical Approaches

Rest, NSAIDs, and physical therapy remain standard treatment for muscle injury and myofascial pain (Simons et al., 1999). Neurological evaluation is advised if weakness or sensory changes persist.

Specialty / Practitioner Care Strategies Table

Specialty Group	Practitioners Included	Hyperemissive Strategies	Hypoemissive Strategies
Biochemistry	Nutritionists, Orthomolecular, Herbalists, Naturopaths	Anti-inflammatory botanicals, magnesium, antioxidants, protein	Circulatory support, neurotrophic nutrients, protein support
Rehabilitation	Physiotherapists, Massage Therapists, Osteopaths / Chiropractors	Myofascial release, trigger point therapy, gentle massage	Graded aerobic exercise, neurorehabilitation, ergonomic guidance
Energetics	Acupuncturists (TCM), Bioenergetic Therapists	Acupuncture, moxibustion, PEMF	Warming acupuncture, frequency therapy
Psychological	GNM practitioners, Psychotherapists, Vibrational therapists, Family constellation facilitators	Psychotherapy, bioresonance, mindfulness	Psychosomatic conflict resolution, emotional balancing

Educational Pearls & Considerations.

- Early treatment of myofascial trigger points improves recovery.
- Magnesium supplementation aids in muscle relaxation.
- Hydrotherapy protocols must be aligned with inflammation phase.
- Neurological evaluation is necessary for persistent weakness.
- Gradual rehabilitation prevents chronic dysfunction.

GROUP 4 - ZONE 18 – CERVICAL SPINE AND NUCHAL ZONE

Category 3: *Skeletal*

Step 1: Functional Anatomy and Interpretive Importance

The cervical spine comprises seven vertebrae (C1–C7), interconnected by facet joints and stabilized by ligaments, forming the most mobile segment of the vertebral column (Standring, 2016). This region balances structural support with flexibility, protecting the spinal cord while allowing wide ranges of head and neck movement.

Skeletal disturbances such as vertebral misalignment, degenerative remodeling, or facet joint restriction are common clinical findings and can lead to mechanical pain or mobility loss. Bogduk and Mercer (2000) highlighted the importance of cervical facet joints as frequent generators of chronic neck pain.

These skeletal dysfunctions influence vascular and periarticular regulation, and their signatures emerge as biospectral asymmetries on spectral surface readings. Emissive variations often appear as linear fields following vertebral alignment or as focal intensifications at upper cervical levels, patterns distinct from diffuse muscular signals.

By mapping these emissive expressions, clinicians can visualize how skeletal imbalance of the cervical spine projects into external regulatory biosignals, supporting early recognition of articular dysfunction.

Step 2,3,4: ROI Classification and Interpretive Questions

Hyperemission indicates signal intensification associated with recent tissue stress, structural overload, or articular sensitization.

- Is there localized swelling, tenderness, or warmth?
- Are symptoms exacerbated by movement or palpation?

Hypoemission suggests chronic structural adaptation, vascular insufficiency, or neuromuscular regulation loss.

- Are symptoms persistent with stiffness, dull pain, or reduced mobility?
- Is there a history of trauma or chronic strain?

Step 5: Confirmatory Evaluations

Test	Purpose & Justification	Relevance to Emissive Pattern
X-ray	Detects fractures, subluxations, and degenerative changes.	Confirms skeletal findings correlating with biosignal findings.

MRI	Visualizes soft tissue, disc pathology, and nerve root involvement.	Supports interpretive recognition of reactive or structural patterns.
Bone scan	Assesses bone metabolism and detects occult lesions.	Identifies active bone remodeling or tissue activation.
Physical exam	Evaluates tenderness, range of motion, and neurological status.	Complements imaging and emissive findings.

Step 6: Care Strategies and Intervention Pathways

Naturopathic Approach

Support bone and joint health with calcium, magnesium, vitamin D, and collagen peptides (Kruger & Kruger, 2019). Use anti-inflammatory herbs such as *Boswellia serrata* to reduce joint inflammation. Employ manual therapies focusing on spinal alignment and posture correction. Acupuncture and bioresonance may alleviate pain and modulate inflammation.

Standard Medical Approaches

Management includes analgesics, anti-inflammatory drugs, physical therapy, and in some cases, surgical intervention.

Specialty / Practitioner Care Strategies Table

Specialty Group	Practitioners Included	Hyperemissive Strategies	Hypoemissive Strategies
Biochemistry	Nutritionists, Orthomolecular, Herbalists, Naturopaths	Bone-supportive nutrients, anti-inflammatory herbs	Nutritional support for repair and regeneration
Rehabilitation	Physiotherapists, Osteopaths / Chiropractors, Massage Therapists	Manual therapy, posture correction, pain management	Ergonomic training, spinal mobilization
Energetics	Acupuncturists (TCM), Bioenergetic Therapists	Acupuncture, PEMF, energy healing	Energy balancing and stimulation
Psychological	GNM practitioners, Psychotherapists, Vibrational therapists, Family constellation facilitators	Psychotherapy, bioresonance, stress management	Emotional balancing and coping strategies

Educational Pearls & Considerations.

- Early detection of degenerative changes improves prognosis.
- Nutritional support is key to bone and joint repair.
- Combine manual therapies with rehabilitation for optimal outcomes.
- Monitor for neurological signs requiring specialist referral.

GROUP 4 - ZONE 18 – CERVICAL SPINE AND NUCHAL ZONE

Category 4: *Nervous*

Step 1: Functional Anatomy and Interpretive Importance

The cervical spine and nuchal region are innervated by cervical spinal nerves (C1–C8), whose dorsal rami supply paraspinal musculature while ventral branches contribute to cervical plexus formation (Standring, 2016).

This dual role supports both mobility and stability, while protecting the spinal cord. Neural irritation here may arise from degenerative changes, disc pathology, or facet joint dysfunction. Bogduk and Govind (2009) highlighted the cervical facet joints as common generators of neck pain mediated by nerve irritation.

Such disturbances affect local conduction and autonomic control, with downstream impact on vascular and fascial regulation.

On the surface, these regulatory shifts appear as biospectral asymmetries aligned with cervical vertebral levels or focal signals at the upper cervical spine. Their precise geometry reflects the neural topography, offering an externalized view of cervical nerve stress that aids differentiation from purely muscular or postural contributors to nuchal dysfunction.

Step 2,3,4: ROI Classification and Interpretive Questions

Hyperemission indicates neural signal amplification associated with irritative phenomena or neurogenic regulatory activation.

- Are symptoms such as burning, tingling, or shooting pain present?
- Is there localized swelling or hypersensitivity?

Hypoemission suggests neurovascular suppression, compressive interference, or reduced autonomic modulation.

- Are numbness, weakness, or muscle wasting noted?
- Do symptoms worsen with posture or movement?

Step 5: Confirmatory Evaluations

Test	Purpose & Justification	Relevance to Emissive Pattern
Nerve conduction studies (NCS), Electromyography (EMG)	Assess nerve and muscle function (Janis et al., 2010).	Correlate with hypoemissive neurogenic suppression.
Quantitative sensory testing (QST)	Measures sensory thresholds.	Supports interpretation of neuropathic patterns.

MRI	Identifies nerve root compression or structural abnormalities.	Detects contributors to neurological expression.
Blood tests (glucose, vitamin B12)	Evaluate metabolic causes of neuropathy.	Supports interpretive understanding of systemic neural behavior..

Step 6: Care Strategies and Intervention Pathways

Naturopathic Approach

Support nerve regeneration with B-complex vitamins, alpha-lipoic acid, and Acetyl-L-carnitine (Papanas & Ziegler, 2014). Use *Hypericum perforatum* for neuropathic pain relief (Kasper et al., 2010). Neural mobilization and bioresonance therapies facilitate recovery. Mind-body techniques support autonomic balance.

Standard Medical Approaches

Pharmacologic treatments include anticonvulsants, antidepressants, and analgesics. Surgical decompression may be necessary for severe nerve compression. Manage metabolic contributors such as diabetes.

Specialty / Practitioner Care Strategies Table

Specialty Group	Practitioners Included	Hyperemissive Strategies	Hypoemissive Strategies
Biochemistry	Nutritionists, Orthomolecular, Herbalists, Naturopaths	Neurotrophic vitamins, alpha-lipoic acid, anti-inflammatory botanicals	Circulatory stimulants, metabolic support, neuroprotective nutrients
Rehabilitation	Physiotherapists, Massage Therapists, Osteopaths / Chiropractors	Neural mobilization, myofascial release, gentle massage	Neural gliding exercises, ergonomic guidance, neurorehabilitation
Energetics	Acupuncturists (TCM), Bioenergetic Therapists	Acupuncture, moxibustion, PEMF	Warming acupuncture, frequency therapy, energy healing
Psychological	GNM practitioners, Psychotherapists, Vibrational therapists, Family constellation facilitators	Psychotherapy, bioresonance, mindfulness	Psychosomatic conflict resolution, vibrational medicine

Educational Pearls & Considerations.

- Early recognition prevents permanent nerve damage.
- Nutritional and energetic therapies support nerve repair.
- Monitor metabolic causes such as diabetes.
- Avoid aggressive therapy during acute inflammation.
- Tailor neural mobilization to patient tolerance.

GROUP 4 - ZONE 18 – CERVICAL SPINE AND NUCHAL ZONE

Category 5: *Lymphatic*

Step 1: Functional Anatomy and Interpretive Importance

The cervical and nuchal region contains both superficial collectors and deeper lymphatics that channel fluid toward cervical and jugular nodes, forming an essential link between cranial and thoracic drainage systems (Standring, 2016). Effective clearance here supports tissue equilibrium in the upper spine and posterior scalp.

Piller and Thelander (1998) described how cervical lymphatic failure, often post-radiation, contributes to chronic tissue stiffness and reduced mobility. These disturbances affect both immune regulation and neurovascular dynamics, creating changes visible at the surface.

On emissive assessment, one may observe vertical or localized fields overlying the upper cervical vertebrae or nuchal ridge, distinguished from diffuse muscular emissions by their bounded geometry.

Such externally observable signatures indicate compromised lymphatic flow, offering a noninvasive method for identifying hidden immune burden in the cervical spine and refining evaluation of chronic nuchal dysfunction.

Step 2,3,4: ROI Classification and Interpretive Questions

Hyperemission indicates lymphatic signal retention associated with immune field activation or acute fluid stagnation.

- Is there redness, tenderness, or rapid swelling?
- Has the patient had recent infections or trauma?

Hypoemission suggests chronic lymphodynamic restriction with tissue densification and reduced interstitial flow, potentially leading to diminished biosignal expression.

- Is swelling persistent, firm, or non-pitting?
- Are recurrent infections or delayed healing noted?

Step 5: Confirmatory Evaluations

Test	Purpose & Justification	Relevance to Emissive Pattern
Lymphoscintigraphy	Evaluates lymphatic flow and obstruction sites.	Confirms lymphatic congestion or hypoperfusion.
Doppler ultrasound	Differentiates venous insufficiency from lymphatic causes.	Helps identify fluid retention patterns.

Blood tests (CBC, inflammatory markers)	Detects systemic infection or inflammation.	Supports hyperemissive activation states.
Physical exam (Stemmer's sign, limb measurements)	Identifies clinical signs of lymphedema.	Correlates with biosignal findings.

Step 6: Care Strategies and Intervention Pathways

Naturopathic Approach

Use herbal lymphagogues such as *Hedera helix* and *Vitis vinifera* to promote lymphatic drainage (Godoy et al., 2012). Certified manual lymphatic drainage aids fluid mobilization. Compression therapy supports lymph return, requiring proper fitting and monitoring. Nutritional antioxidants and anti-inflammatory nutrients promote tissue repair. Hydrotherapy with alternating warm and cold enhances lymphatic circulation.

Standard Medical Approaches

Treatment involves manual lymphatic drainage, compression garments, physical rehabilitation, and infection control. Surgery is reserved for refractory cases.

Specialty / Practitioner Care Strategies Table

Specialty Group	Practitioners Included	Hyperemissive Strategies	Hypoemissive Strategies
Biochemistry	Nutritionists, Orthomolecular, Herbalists, Naturopaths	Herbal lymphagogues, antioxidants, anti-inflammatory nutrients	Circulatory support, nutritional tissue repair support
Rehabilitation	Physiotherapists, Massage Therapists, Osteopaths / Chiropractors	Manual lymphatic drainage, gentle massage, postural retraining	Compression therapy, graded exercise, ergonomic guidance
Energetics	Acupuncturists (TCM), Bioenergetic Therapists	Acupuncture, herbal formulas, PEMF	Warming acupuncture, energy balancing
Psychological	GNM practitioners, Psychotherapists, Vibrational therapists, Family constellation facilitators	Mind-body therapies supporting immune function and healing	Psychosomatic conflict resolution, emotional balancing

Educational Pearls & Considerations.

- Early treatment prevents chronic lymphedema.
- Manual lymphatic drainage should be performed by trained therapists.
- Compression therapy requires careful fitting and monitoring.
- Nutritional support enhances lymphatic and tissue health.
- Prompt infection control is vital.

GROUP 4 - ZONE 18 – CERVICAL SPINE AND NUCHAL ZONE

Category 6: *Organ-Related (GNM)*

Step 1: Functional Anatomy and Interpretive Importance

The cervical spine and nuchal region include the vertebrae, facet joints, and deep ligamentous structures that support the craniovertebral junction (Standring, 2016). While primarily musculoskeletal, GNM associates this area with systemic regulation, where conflicts tied to intellectual burden or coordination of control may reflect in organ-related adaptation.

Hamer (2012) described that conflict-active states lead to hypoemissive suppression, while reparative activity generates hyperemissive intensification.

These emissive patterns often appear as linear fields aligned with the cervical vertebrae, distinguishing them from diffuse muscular contraction. McEwen (1998) introduced the concept of allostatic load, showing how chronic psychosocial stress accumulates in neuroendocrine systems, providing a biological framework for cervical surface patterns linked to systemic conflict.

Such findings support the interpretation of nuchal emissive fields as markers of psychobiological stress regulation visible through spectral surface assessment.

Step 2,3,4: ROI Classification and Interpretive Questions

Hyperemission suggests regulatory reactivation or biosignal intensification consistent with healing-phase expression.

- Is there muscle tightness, discomfort, or signs of systemic recovery?
- Are psychosocial stressors present?

Hypoemission indicates an active psychobiological conflict associated with tissue signal suppression or regulatory inhibition.

- Are symptoms of chronic tension, fatigue, or unresolved stress noted?
- Is there a history of emotional or psychosomatic conditions?

Step 5: Confirmatory Evaluations

Test	Purpose & Justification	Relevance to Emissive Pattern
Psychological evaluation	Identifies psychosomatic conflicts and emotional stressors.	Supports GNM-related interpretation of biosignal imaging.
Musculoskeletal exam	Assesses muscle tension, range of motion, and neurological status.	Correlates physical findings with emissive asymmetries.
Inflammatory markers (CRP, ESR)	Evaluates systemic inflammatory state.	Differentiates tissue responses from conflict-phase expressions.

Step 6: Care Strategies and Intervention Pathways

Naturopathic Approach

Integrate stress reduction techniques such as mindfulness, meditation, and family constellation therapy. Herbal adaptogens like *Rhodiola rosea* support resilience (Panossian & Wikman, 2010). Bioenergetic therapies including bioresonance facilitate energetic harmonization.

Standard Medical Approaches

Psychotherapy and psychosomatic medicine approaches are essential. Supportive care may include physical therapy and pharmacologic symptom management as needed.

Specialty / Practitioner Care Strategies Table

Specialty Group	Practitioners Included	Hyperemissive Strategies	Hypoemissive Strategies
Biochemistry	Nutritionists, Orthomolecular, Herbalists, Naturopaths	Adaptogens, antioxidants, stress-supportive herbs	Nutritional support for stress modulation
Rehabilitation	Physiotherapists, Massage Therapists, Osteopaths / Chiropractors	Relaxation techniques, myofascial release	Postural correction, gentle mobilization
Energetics	Acupuncturists (TCM), Bioenergetic Therapists	Bioresonance, PEMF, energy balancing	Energetic harmonization, frequency therapy
Psychological	GNM practitioners, Psychotherapists, Vibrational therapists, Family constellation facilitators	Psychotherapy, bioresonance, family constellation therapy	Emotional balancing and conflict resolution

Educational Pearls & Considerations.

- Psychosomatic factors significantly influence symptoms in this zone.
- Multimodal therapy addressing mind-body connections yields best results.
- Early psychological support reduces chronicity.
- Careful monitoring of physical and emotional progress is essential.

GROUP 4 - ZONE 18 – CERVICAL SPINE AND NUCHAL ZONE

Category 7: *Acupuncture / Meridian*

Step 1: Functional Anatomy and Interpretive Importance

The cervical spine and nuchal zone incorporate vertebral elements (C1–C7), ligamentous structures, and musculature such as trapezius and semispinalis capitis, all vital for craniovertebral stability (Standring, 2016).

In TCM, this zone corresponds to the Bladder (BL), Gallbladder (GB), and Small Intestine (SI) meridians, which course longitudinally along the posterior neck. Deadman et al. (2007) noted that BL10 and GB20 are critical points for alleviating tension, regulating autonomic balance, and influencing cranial function.

Langevin and Yandow (2002) suggested that meridian pathways often align with connective tissue planes, supporting their anatomical plausibility.

Clinically, blockages along these channels manifest as neck stiffness, headaches, or visual disturbances. On biosignal imaging, emissive fields appear as linear or nodal variations tracking posterior cervical lines, distinct from diffuse muscular contractions.

Such findings illustrate how nuchal emissive asymmetries can represent stagnation or excess in BL–GB–SI pathways, aligning traditional channel theory with modern biospectral assessment.

Step 2,3,4: ROI Classification and Interpretive Questions

Hyperemission indicates Qi stagnation or excessive signal expression along meridian trajectories.

- Is there localized pain, muscle tightness, or tension?
- Are symptoms worsened by stress or physical exertion?

Hypoemission suggests Qi deficiency or chronic stagnation resulting in reduced signal circulation and diminished surface expression.

- Does the patient report fatigue, coldness, or chronic neck discomfort?
- Are symptoms persistent despite previous treatments?

Step 5: Confirmatory Evaluations

Test	Purpose & Justification	Relevance to Emissive Pattern
Pulse diagnosis and tongue examination	Traditional TCM diagnostics assessing Qi and Blood flow (Flaws, 2000).	Helps differentiate hyper- and hypoemissive patterns.

Biospectral imaging	Visualizes thermal asymmetries along meridian courses.	Correlates with energetic signal variations in cervical region.
Symptom questionnaire	Assesses musculoskeletal and emotional symptoms.	Supports interpretation of meridian pattern expressions.

Step 6: Care Strategies and Intervention Pathways

Naturopathic Approach

Acupuncture points such as BL10, GB20, and SI15 are targeted to relieve neck tension and restore Qi flow (Lao et al., 2004). Moxibustion warms hypoemissive areas. Herbal formulas supporting the Bladder and Gallbladder meridians assist recovery (Bensky et al., 2004). Lifestyle and stress management complement these therapies.

Standard Medical Approaches

Acupuncture is used adjunctively for pain relief and autonomic regulation.

Specialty / Practitioner Care Strategies Table

Specialty Group	Practitioners Included	Hyperemissive Strategies	Hypoemissive Strategies
Biochemistry	Nutritionists, Orthomolecular, Herbalists, Naturopaths	Anti-inflammatory and circulation-supportive herbs	Qi tonics and nutritional support
Rehabilitation	Physiotherapists, Massage Therapists, Osteopaths / Chiropractors	Myofascial release, cervical mobilization	Gentle mobilization, warming massage
Energetics	Acupuncturists (TCM), Bioenergetic Therapists	Acupuncture, moxibustion, PEMF	Warming acupuncture, energy balancing
Psychological	GNM practitioners, Psychotherapists, Vibrational therapists, Family constellation facilitators	Psychotherapy, bioresonance, energy clearing	Psychosomatic conflict resolution, emotional balancing

Educational Pearls & Considerations.

- Accurate point selection is crucial for efficacy.
- Moxibustion should be used cautiously in heat-sensitive patients.
- Herbal treatment should be supervised by qualified practitioners.
- Combining acupuncture with physical therapy enhances outcomes.

GROUP 4 - ZONE 18 – CERVICAL SPINE AND NUCHAL ZONE

Category 8: *Energetic*

Step 1: Functional Anatomy and Interpretive Importance

The cervical spine and nuchal area include vertebrae, ligamentous supports, paraspinal musculature, and neurovascular pathways essential for stability and communication (Standring, 2016).

Energetically, this region serves as a bridge linking cranial regulation with systemic balance, often mirroring stress adaptation. Oschman (2016) described connective tissue as a living matrix for energy conduction, a model that aligns with emissive changes observed in this zone. Patients frequently report headaches, restricted cervical mobility, or stress-related tension.

Biospectral readings highlight hypoemissive depressions aligned with suppressed energy flow, alternating with hyperemissive streaks reflecting compensatory activation. These emissive fields follow fascial and neural distributions more than isolated muscles, underscoring the integrative role of this region.

Clinically, the cervical spine and nuchal field offer biospectral evidence of systemic stress processing, where surface emissive variations reflect the balance between resilience and strain.

Step 2,3,4: ROI Classification and Interpretive Questions

Hyperemission indicates localized energetic congestion or excessive signal expression.

- Does the patient feel heat, tension, or discomfort in the neck region?
- Are stress or emotional factors significant?

Hypoemission suggests energetic depletion or persistent stagnation.

- Are fatigue, coldness, or low vitality reported?
- Are symptoms chronic or resistant to treatment?

Step 5: Confirmatory Evaluations

Test	Purpose & Justification	Relevance to Emissive Pattern
Bioresonance testing	Measures tissue energy frequencies and imbalances.	Correlates with energetic signal variations observed through biosignal imaging.
Electrodermal screening (EDS)	Assesses skin conductance linked to energetic pathways.	Supports interpretive understanding of energetic pattern behavior.
Patient emotional and symptom history	Provides context for energetic dysfunction and stress factors.	Aids in differential interpretation.

Step 6: **Care Strategies and Intervention Pathways**

Naturopathic Approach

Employ bioresonance, pulsed electromagnetic fields (PEMF), and adaptogenic herbs to restore energetic balance and promote healing (Matsumoto et al., 2010). Nutritional antioxidants and adaptogens enhance systemic resilience. Mindfulness and stress reduction techniques complement energetic therapies.

Standard Medical Approaches

Energetic therapies serve as adjuncts to conventional care, enhancing overall patient outcomes.

Specialty / Practitioner Care Strategies Table

Specialty Group	Practitioners Included	Hyperemissive Strategies	Hypoemissive Strategies
Biochemistry	Nutritionists, Orthomolecular, Herbalists, Naturopaths	Adaptogens, antioxidants, herbal energetics	Nutritional support for energy deficiency
Rehabilitation	Physiotherapists, Massage Therapists, Osteopaths / Chiropractors	Energy-based manual therapies, PEMF, therapeutic touch	Gentle stimulation, mobilization
Energetics	Acupuncturists (TCM), Bioenergetic Therapists	Bioresonance, PEMF, acupuncture	Warming acupuncture, energy balancing
Psychological	GNM practitioners, Psychotherapists, Vibrational therapists, Family constellation facilitators	Psychotherapy, bioresonance, mindfulness	Emotional balancing, vibrational medicine

Educational Pearls & Considerations.

- Energetic therapies complement but do not replace standard medical treatment.
- Practitioner skill and patient receptivity influence outcomes.
- Regular reassessment improves therapeutic success.
- Holistic care addressing mind and body is essential.

GROUP 4 - ZONE 18 – CERVICAL SPINE AND NUCHAL ZONE

Category 9: *Metabolic / Endocrine*

Step 1: Functional Anatomy and Interpretive Importance

The cervical spine and nuchal zone support neural pathways and vascular channels while reflecting systemic metabolic regulation (Standring, 2016). Endocrine imbalance, particularly adrenal and thyroid dysfunction, often alters muscle tone, vascular supply, and repair capacity in this region.

DeFronzo & Ferrannini (1991) noted that metabolic dysfunction extends beyond peripheral tissues into spinal physiology, influencing systemic stability. Patients frequently present with tension headaches, fatigue, or cervical stiffness linked to systemic dysregulation.

Spectral surface readings highlight broad hypoemissive depressions reflecting metabolic depletion, contrasted with hyperemissive streaks signaling compensatory repair or endocrine overactivation.

These emissive fields trace fascial and neural planes, reinforcing their systemic basis. Clinically, the cervical spine and nuchal field serve as a biospectral indicator of metabolic endurance and systemic regulatory adaptation.

Step 2,3,4: ROI Classification and Interpretive Questions

Hyperemission indicates signal intensification associated with increased metabolic activity or regulatory excitation.

- Is there warmth, swelling, or tenderness?
- Are systemic symptoms like heat intolerance or palpitations present?

Hypoemission suggests metabolic downregulation, vascular insufficiency, or reduced perfusion dynamics possibly related to endocrine imbalance.

- Are cold intolerance, fatigue, or tissue hypoxia reported?
- Is there a history of thyroid or parathyroid disease?

Step 5: Confirmatory Evaluations

Test	Purpose & Justification	Relevance to Emissive Pattern
Thyroid function tests (TSH, Free T4, Free T3)	Assess thyroid hormone levels and function.	Correlates with biospectral changes in thyroid function.
Calcium and parathyroid hormone (PTH) levels	Evaluate parathyroid function and calcium metabolism.	Supports interpretive understanding of parathyroid regulatory variations.

Ultrasound of thyroid and parathyroid glands	Detects nodules, inflammation, or structural abnormalities.	Correlates with localized emissive signal deviations.
Inflammatory markers, CBC	Detects systemic or local inflammation.	Supports hyperemissive activation states.

Step 6: Care Strategies and Intervention Pathways

Naturopathic Approach

Support endocrine function with selenium, iodine, zinc, and antioxidants (Rajput et al., 2013). Use adaptogenic herbs like *Withania somnifera* to modulate hormonal balance (Singh et al., 2011). Stress management and psychotherapy assist psychosomatic aspects. Nutritional antioxidants support tissue repair.

Standard Medical Approaches

Medical management includes hormone replacement or suppression therapy guided by diagnostics. Regular imaging and lab tests monitor disease progression.

Specialty / Practitioner Care Strategies Table

Specialty Group	Practitioners Included	Hyperemissive Strategies	Hypoemissive Strategies
Biochemistry	Nutritionists, Orthomolecular, Herbalists, Naturopaths	Endocrine support nutrients, antioxidants, anti-inflammatory herbs	Nutritional support for hormone synthesis and balance
Rehabilitation	Physiotherapists, Massage Therapists, Osteopaths / Chiropractors	Gentle neck mobilization, myofascial release	Postural correction, relaxation techniques
Energetics	Acupuncturists (TCM), Bioenergetic Therapists	Acupuncture for endocrine regulation	Energy balancing and harmonization
Psychological	GNM practitioners, Psychotherapists, Vibrational therapists, Family constellation facilitators	Psychotherapy, bioresonance, conflict resolution	Emotional balancing, stress reduction

Educational Pearls & Considerations.

- Regular monitoring of thyroid and parathyroid function is essential.
- Nutritional and botanical support benefits endocrine health.
- Psychosomatic factors can influence symptoms and outcomes.
- Early detection and intervention improve prognosis.

GROUP 4

ZONE 19 – FACIAL AREA (FRONTAL AND LATERAL)

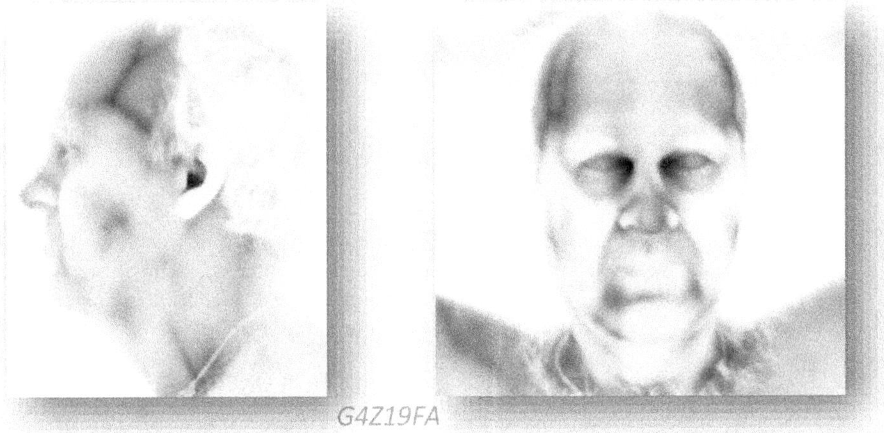

The facial area, containing the forehead, periorbital region, cheeks, jawline, and mandibular zones, is among the most richly vascularized and innervated surfaces of the body. It includes branches of the trigeminal and facial nerves, the superficial temporal and facial arteries, and an extensive lymphatic network (Standring, 2016).

This dense integration makes the face highly responsive to neurogenic and vascular influences, explaining its diagnostic sensitivity in biospectral interpretation. Because the skin is thin and vessels lie close to the surface, emissive asymmetries here strongly reflect systemic and local states.

Neurogenic disorders such as trigeminal neuralgia or temporomandibular dysfunction often create focal irregularities before overt pain, consistent with evidence that trigeminal activation alters microvascular flow even in preclinical states (Borsook et al., 2012). Vascular dynamics are equally prominent: the face is one of the earliest sites to reveal microangiogenesis, central to tumor biology and chronic remodeling (Hanahan & Weinberg, 2011), with angiogenic signatures in perioral or submandibular zones sometimes preceding tumor formation.

The temporomandibular joint and dental arcades also influence emissive patterns, with bruxism, necrotic teeth, or occlusal asymmetry frequently producing mandibular field irregularities. Temporomandibular disorders affect up to 12% of the population, and such changes often provide early functional cues (Scrivani et al., 2008).

Metabolic and endocrine influences are also visible: diabetes and thyroid dysfunction alter facial microcirculation, supported by findings of reduced vasodilatory response in these conditions (Tooke, 1996). Emotional stress modulates blood flow and tone through autonomic shifts, producing emissive variations that parallel sympathetic activity (Kreibig, 2010). Lymphatic drainage via submandibular and preauricular nodes adds another interpretive layer, with congestion often signaling immune or toxic burden.

Zone 19 – Facial Area (Frontal and Lateral): Emission-Relevant Structures

Category	Relevant Structures	Emission Relevance
1. Vascular / Circulatory	- Superficial temporal artery and vein - Facial artery and vein - Angular artery	Hyperemission may indicate vascular dilation, neurogenic activation, or congestion; Hypoemission suggests vasospasm or reduced peripheral perfusion.
2. Muscular / Myofascial	- Masseter - Temporalis - Orbicularis oculi and oris - Buccinator	Hyperemission often reflects muscle spasm, tension, or tissue reactivity; Hypoemission may signal disuse or chronic fascial restrictions impacting facial expression and mobility.
3. Skeletal / Articular	- Temporomandibular joint (TMJ) - Zygomatic arch - Mandibular ramus	Hyperemission may reflect joint reactivity or trauma; Hypoemission may indicate chronic structural adaptation or hypoperfusion.
4. Nervous System / Spine	- Trigeminal nerve branches (V1, V2, V3) - Facial nerve (VII)	Hyperemissive zones may indicate neuralgia, neuropathic signal activity, or autonomic dysregulation; Hypoemission may reflect nerve compression or neurogenic suppression.
5. Lymphatic / Immune	- Parotid and submandibular lymph nodes - Facial lymphatic vessels	Hyperemission suggests immune node activation; Hypoemission may correspond to lymphatic stasis or immune suppression.
6. Organs / GNM (German New Medicine)	- Salivary glands - Nasal mucosa and sinuses	Biosignal variations may reflect active visceral response patterns or conflict in these glands or mucosal tissues.
7. Acupuncture / Meridians	- Large Intestine Meridian - Stomach Meridian - Gallbladder Meridian	Hyperemissive expression indicates Qi stagnation or excess; hypoemissive regions reflect Qi deficiency or dampness impacting neurovascular and digestive meridians in the facial region.
8. Energetic / Frequency	- Energetic reflex zones linked to cranial autonomic regulation	Hyperemission may reflect sympathetic hyperactivity or emotional excitation; Hypoemission may indicate energetic depletion or autonomic regulatory decline.
9. Metabolic / Endocrine	- Reflex zones for thyroid and adrenal influence	Hypoemission suggests hormonal underexpression; Hyperemission may indicate tissue activation or hypermetabolic states affecting facial tissues.

GROUP 4 - ZONE 19 – FACIAL AREA (FRONTAL AND LATERAL)

Category 1: *Vascular / Circulatory*

Step 1: Functional Anatomy and Interpretive Importance

The superficial face is perfused primarily by branches of the external carotid artery, including the facial, angular, and superficial temporal arteries. Venous return follows the facial, angular, and retromandibular veins, with important connections to the ophthalmic system, creating a rich venous network between superficial and deep territories (Standring, 2016).

Anatomical mapping of facial vasculature has emphasized the angular and facial systems as key landmarks in both reconstructive and aesthetic surgery (Behrens et al., 2011).

Spectral surface readings of the face often show emissive asymmetries around the perioral, nasolabial, and temporal zones. These may correspond to venous congestion, circulatory reactivity, or adaptive modulation in areas of high muscular and expressive activity.

Because the face is among the most vascularized regions of the body, its emissive profile offers a detailed view of localized and systemic circulatory adaptation.

Step 2,3,4: ROI Classification and Interpretive Questions

Hyperemission suggests localized signal intensification associated with vascular expansion, immune field activation, or superficial regulatory overload.

- Are there signs of erythema, swelling, or tenderness?
- Is there a history of skin infections, trauma, or vascular conditions?

Hypoemission indicates vascular insufficiency, vasoregulatory restriction, or chronic perfusion deficit.

- Are cold sensations, pallor, or delayed healing reported?
- Is there a history of Raynaud's phenomenon, migraines, or vascular disorders?

Step 5: Confirmatory Evaluations

Test	Purpose & Justification	Relevance to Emissive Pattern
Doppler ultrasound	Assesses arterial and venous blood flow in facial vessels.	Correlates with hyperemissive vascular activation or hypoemissive perfusion reduction..
Skin biopsy or swab	Identifies infection or inflammation source if needed.	Supports interpretive confirmation of hyperemissive patterns.

Blood tests (CBC, inflammatory markers)	Detect systemic inflammation or infection.	Supports activation-related signal behavior.
Physical exam	Assesses for vascular abnormalities, skin changes, or swelling.	Complements biosignal findings.

Step 6: Care Strategies and Intervention Pathways

Naturopathic Approach

Use anti-inflammatory botanicals such as *Calendula officinalis* and antioxidants like vitamin C to support vascular health and skin repair (Rafieian-Kopaei et al., 2017). Promote circulation with gentle massage and hydrotherapy. Nutritional support includes omega-3 fatty acids to improve endothelial function.

Standard Medical Approaches

Treat underlying vascular or infectious conditions. Use topical or systemic medications as indicated. Refer to dermatology or vascular specialists as needed.

Specialty / Practitioner Care Strategies Table

Specialty Group	Practitioners Included	Hyperemissive Strategies	Hypoemissive Strategies
Biochemistry	Nutritionists, Orthomolecular, Herbalists, Naturopaths	Anti-inflammatory herbs, antioxidants, vascular support	Circulatory stimulants, endothelial support nutrients
Rehabilitation	Physiotherapists, Massage Therapists	Gentle facial massage, lymphatic drainage	Thermal protection, circulation enhancement
Energetics	Acupuncturists (TCM), Bioenergetic Therapists	Acupuncture, moxibustion, PEMF	Warming acupuncture, energy balancing
Psychological	GNM practitioners, Psychotherapists, Vibrational therapists, Family constellation facilitators	Psychotherapy, bioresonance, mindfulness	Emotional balancing, stress reduction

Educational Pearls & Considerations.

- Facial vascular conditions may indicate systemic disease.
- Early intervention prevents complications such as skin ulceration.
- Gentle techniques avoid aggravating sensitive facial tissues.
- Nutritional and botanical therapies support tissue repair.

GROUP 4 - ZONE 19 – FACIAL AREA (FRONTAL AND LATERAL)

Category 2: *Muscular*

Step 1: Functional Anatomy and Interpretive Importance

The facial musculature is composed of the frontalis, orbicularis oculi, zygomaticus major and minor, orbicularis oris, and masseter, among others, all innervated by branches of the facial nerve.

These muscles regulate facial expression, mastication, and speech, with their intricate fascial interconnections ensuring fluid communication across the face (Standring, 2016). Studies in orofacial pain confirm that hyperactivity of the masseter and temporalis is strongly associated with temporomandibular dysfunction and bruxism, conditions that alter bite mechanics and muscular balance (Manfredini et al., 2011).

Spectral evaluation of this zone frequently reveals emissive asymmetries along the masseteric or periorbital regions, where muscular overactivation or imbalance modifies the biosignal.

Such findings provide insight into stress-related motor activity, integrating facial expression, chewing function, and regulatory adaptation into a coherent biospectral profile.

Step 2,3,4: ROI Classification and Interpretive Questions

Hyperemission indicates myofascial signal intensification associated with muscular contraction patterns, focal tension, or irritative foci.

- Is there localized tenderness, stiffness, or spasms?
- Is there history of trauma, overuse, or stress-related clenching?

Hypoemission suggests chronic perfusion limitation, fascial densification, or neuromuscular regulation loss.

- Are there symptoms of weakness, atrophy, or reduced facial mobility?
- Is there evidence of neuropathic involvement?

Step 5: Confirmatory Evaluations

Test	Purpose & Justification	Relevance to Emissive Pattern
Creatine kinase (CK), LDH	Detects muscle injury or inflammation (Simons et al., 1999).	Elevated in hyperemissive myofascial activation.
Electromyography (EMG)	Assesses facial muscle and nerve function.	Supports neural contributors to Hypoemission.
MRI	Visualizes muscle edema or atrophy.	Correlates with biosignal findings.
Physical exam	Evaluates muscle tone, strength, and trigger points.	Complements emissive observations.

Step 6: Care Strategies and Intervention Pathways

Naturopathic Approach

Use anti-inflammatory botanicals like *Curcuma longa* and magnesium supplementation for muscle relaxation (Hewlings & Kalman, 2017). Gentle facial massage and trigger point therapy improve circulation and relieve tension. Stress management and relaxation techniques reduce muscle spasm.

Standard Medical Approaches

Physical therapy, muscle relaxants, and nerve blocks may be indicated. Neurological evaluation is necessary for persistent weakness or neuropathy.

Specialty / Practitioner Care Strategies Table

Specialty Group	Practitioners Included	Hyperemissive Strategies	Hypoemissive Strategies
Biochemistry	Nutritionists, Orthomolecular, Herbalists, Naturopaths	Anti-inflammatory herbs, magnesium, antioxidants	Neurotrophic nutrients, circulatory support
Rehabilitation	Physiotherapists, Massage Therapists	Myofascial release, facial massage	Neuromuscular re-education, ergonomic guidance
Energetics	Acupuncturists (TCM), Bioenergetic Therapists	Acupuncture, moxibustion, PEMF	Energy balancing, warming acupuncture
Psychological	GNM practitioners, Psychotherapists, Vibrational therapists, Family constellation facilitators	Psychotherapy, bioresonance, mindfulness	Emotional balancing, conflict resolution

Educational Pearls & Considerations.

- Early intervention improves muscle function and prevents chronic pain.
- Magnesium is effective for reducing muscle spasms.
- Facial muscles are sensitive; gentle techniques are essential.
- Neurological causes must be ruled out in refractory cases.

GROUP 4 - ZONE 19 – FACIAL AREA (FRONTAL AND LATERAL)

Category 3: *Skeletal*

Step 1: Functional Anatomy and Interpretive Importance

The skeletal framework of the face includes the frontal bone, zygomatic arches, maxilla, mandible, and nasal bones, each providing structural support for facial muscles and protection for sensory organs (Standring, 2016).

These osseous structures articulate at mobile sites such as the temporomandibular joints, where mechanical stress or misalignment can generate pain and secondary muscular imbalance. Clinical studies recognize temporomandibular joint dysfunction and maxillofacial skeletal asymmetry as significant contributors to chronic orofacial pain and altered biomechanics (Okeson, 2013).

Such skeletal alterations reshape vascular and neuromuscular regulation, leaving emissive imprints that become perceptible on spectral surface readings.

Biospectral asymmetries in the facial zone often present as localized intensifications around the mandible, zygomatic arch, or temporomandibular region, distinct from diffuse cutaneous emissions.

These patterns externalize the subtle interplay of bone alignment, joint function, and adjacent soft tissue regulation, offering clinicians a noninvasive method of detecting skeletal imbalance in one of the most functionally expressive regions of the body.

Step 2,3,4: ROI Classification and Interpretive Questions

Hyperemission indicates signal intensification associated with structural overload, osseous disruption, or articular sensitization.

- Is there localized swelling, redness, or tenderness?
- Are symptoms aggravated by movement or palpation?

Hypoemission suggests chronic structural adaptation, reduced circulatory support, or neuromuscular regulation loss.

- Are symptoms persistent with stiffness, dull pain, or restricted movement?
- Is there a history of trauma or chronic strain?

Step 5: Confirmatory Evaluations

Test	Purpose & Justification	Relevance to Emissive Pattern
X-ray, CT scan	Detect fractures, joint pathology, or bone abnormalities.	Confirms skeletal causes correlating with biosignal findings.

MRI	Visualizes soft tissues, TMJ components, and bone marrow edema.	Supports interpretive recognition of reactive or structural patterns.
Physical exam	Assesses tenderness, range of motion, and joint function.	Complements imaging and emissive analysis.

Step 6: Care Strategies and Intervention Pathways

Naturopathic Approach

Support bone health with calcium, magnesium, vitamin D, and collagen peptides (Kruger & Kruger, 2019). Use anti-inflammatory herbs like *Boswellia serrata* to reduce joint inflammation. Manual therapies focused on TMJ mobilization and posture improve function. Acupuncture and bioenergetic therapies aid in pain relief.

Standard Medical Approaches

Management includes analgesics, anti-inflammatories, physical therapy, and surgical consultation when necessary.

Specialty / Practitioner Care Strategies Table

Specialty Group	Practitioners Included	Hyperemissive Strategies	Hypoemissive Strategies
Biochemistry	Nutritionists, Orthomolecular, Herbalists, Naturopaths	Bone-supportive nutrients, anti-inflammatory herbs	Nutritional support for repair and regeneration
Rehabilitation	Physiotherapists, Osteopaths / Chiropractors, Massage Therapists	Manual therapy, TMJ mobilization, pain management	Ergonomic training, joint mobilization
Energetics	Acupuncturists (TCM), Bioenergetic Therapists	Acupuncture, PEMF, energy healing	Energy balancing and stimulation
Psychological	GNM practitioners, Psychotherapists, Vibrational therapists, Family constellation facilitators	Psychotherapy, bioresonance, stress management	Emotional balancing and coping strategies

Educational Pearls & Considerations.

- Early detection of TMJ and facial skeletal issues prevents chronic pain.
- Nutritional support aids tissue repair.
- Manual and energetic therapies complement conventional treatments.
- Monitor for complications requiring specialist referral.

GROUP 4 - ZONE 19 – FACIAL AREA (FRONTAL AND LATERAL)

Category 4: *Nervous*

Step 1: Functional Anatomy and Interpretive Importance

The face is innervated by cranial nerves, principally the trigeminal nerve (CN V) for sensory distribution and the facial nerve (CN VII) for motor control of expression (Standring, 2016). These pathways are crucial for both protective sensation and social communication.

Dysfunction may occur through compression, trauma, or idiopathic processes, resulting in pain, numbness, or motor asymmetry. Zakrzewska (2013) reported that trigeminal neuropathies are a leading cause of chronic facial pain, often associated with autonomic disturbances in the affected dermatome.

Such neural alterations influence vascular and muscular regulation, leaving emissive imprints externally visible as biospectral asymmetries across the mandible, zygomatic arch, or perioral region.

These signals differ from diffuse cutaneous fields by their sharply defined distribution, reflecting the precision of neural topography. By translating cranial nerve dysfunction into surface emissive patterns, clinicians gain a noninvasive tool for evaluating neurogenic contributions to facial imbalance and discomfort.

Step 2,3,4: ROI Classification and Interpretive Questions

Hyperemission suggests neural signal amplification associated with irritative responses or neurogenic regulatory activation.

- Are there symptoms such as burning, tingling, or facial pain?
- Is there localized swelling or hypersensitivity?

Hypoemission indicates neurovascular suppression, compressive interference, or reduced neural output leading to diminished autonomic modulation.

- Are numbness, weakness, or facial muscle atrophy present?
- Do symptoms worsen with movement or certain postures?

Step 5: Confirmatory Evaluations

Test	Purpose & Justification	Relevance to Emissive Pattern
Nerve conduction studies (NCS), Electromyography (EMG)	Assess facial nerve and muscle function (Janis et al., 2010).	Correlates with hypoemissive neurogenic suppression.
Quantitative sensory testing (QST)	Measures sensory nerve function.	Supports interpretation of neuropathic patterns.

MRI	Detects nerve compression or structural abnormalities.	Identifies contributors to neurological expression.
Blood tests (glucose, vitamin B12)	Evaluate metabolic causes of neuropathy.	Supports interpretive understanding of systemic neural behavior.

Step 6: Care Strategies and Intervention Pathways

Naturopathic Approach

Administer neurotrophic vitamins (B-complex), alpha-lipoic acid, and Acetyl-L-carnitine to promote nerve regeneration (Papanas & Ziegler, 2014). *Hypericum perforatum* may relieve neuropathic pain (Kasper et al., 2010). Neural mobilization and bioresonance therapies support recovery. Mindfulness and stress reduction aid autonomic regulation.

Standard Medical Approaches

Use anticonvulsants, antidepressants, analgesics, and consider surgical decompression for severe nerve entrapment. Manage metabolic contributors like diabetes.

Specialty / Practitioner Care Strategies Table

Specialty Group	Practitioners Included	Hyperemissive Strategies	Hypoemissive Strategies
Biochemistry	Nutritionists, Orthomolecular, Herbalists, Naturopaths	Neurotrophic vitamins, alpha-lipoic acid, anti-inflammatory botanicals	Circulatory support, metabolic and neuroprotective nutrients
Rehabilitation	Physiotherapists, Massage Therapists, Osteopaths / Chiropractors	Neural mobilization, myofascial release, gentle massage	Neural gliding exercises, ergonomic guidance, neurorehabilitation
Energetics	Acupuncturists (TCM), Bioenergetic Therapists	Acupuncture, moxibustion, PEMF	Warming acupuncture, frequency therapy, energy healing
Psychological	GNM practitioners, Psychotherapists, Vibrational therapists, Family constellation facilitators	Psychotherapy, bioresonance, mindfulness	Psychosomatic conflict resolution, vibrational medicine

Educational Pearls & Considerations.

- Early treatment prevents permanent nerve damage.
- Nutritional and energetic therapies support nerve repair.
- Monitor metabolic factors such as diabetes.
- Avoid aggressive interventions during acute inflammation.
- Tailor neural mobilization to patient tolerance.

GROUP 4 - ZONE 19 – FACIAL AREA (FRONTAL AND LATERAL)

Category 5: *Lymphatic*

Step 1: Functional Anatomy and Interpretive Importance

The facial lymphatic network consists of superficial and deep vessels draining into submandibular, submental, and parotid nodes, with final convergence toward deep cervical stations (Standring, 2016).

This system regulates clearance of interstitial fluid and supports immune surveillance of highly vascularized tissues. Ridner et al. (2012) noted that facial and head-and-neck lymphedema frequently follow oncologic interventions, with even mild dysfunction contributing to discomfort and functional impairment.

Altered drainage in the facial network influences tissue compliance, cutaneous signaling, and vascular reactivity, leaving distinct traces on the surface. Emissive fields in this region often appear as localized variations along the mandibular contour, perioral region, or zygomatic arch, their sharply defined distribution contrasting with diffuse cutaneous signals.

These external expressions provide clinicians with a visible indicator of facial lymphatic strain, enhancing recognition of immune congestion and clarifying its contribution to orofacial imbalance.

Step 2,3,4: ROI Classification and Interpretive Questions

Hyperemission indicates lymphatic signal retention associated with immune field activation, acute fluid stagnation, or superficial regulatory overload.

- Are redness, tenderness, or rapid swelling present?
- Is there a recent history of infection, trauma, or surgery?

Hypoemission suggests chronic lymphodynamic restriction with tissue densification and reduced interstitial flow.

- Is swelling persistent, firm, or non-pitting?
- Are recurrent infections or delayed healing reported?

Step 5: Confirmatory Evaluations

Test	Purpose & Justification	Relevance to Emissive Pattern
Lymphoscintigraphy	Evaluates lymphatic drainage and obstruction.	Confirms lymphatic congestion or hypoperfusion.

Doppler ultrasound	Differentiates venous insufficiency from lymphatic causes.	Helps determine fluid retention origin.
Blood tests (CBC, inflammatory markers)	Detects systemic infection or inflammation.	Supports hyperemissive activation states.
Physical exam (Stemmer's sign, measurements)	Identifies clinical signs of lymphedema.	Correlates with biosignal findings.

Step 6: Care Strategies and Intervention Pathways

Naturopathic Approach

Herbal lymphagogues such as *Hedera helix* and *Vitis vinifera* stimulate lymphatic flow (Godoy et al., 2012). Certified manual lymphatic drainage promotes fluid movement. Compression garments aid lymph return but require correct fitting. Nutritional antioxidants and anti-inflammatory nutrients support tissue repair. Hydrotherapy with alternating warm and cold applications enhances circulation.

Standard Medical Approaches

Treatment includes manual lymphatic drainage, compression therapy, physical rehabilitation, and infection management. Surgery is reserved for refractory cases.

Specialty / Practitioner Care Strategies Table

Specialty Group	Practitioners Included	Hyperemissive Strategies	Hypoemissive Strategies
Biochemistry	Nutritionists, Orthomolecular, Herbalists, Naturopaths	Herbal lymphagogues, antioxidants, anti-inflammatory nutrients	Circulatory support, nutritional tissue repair support
Rehabilitation	Physiotherapists, Massage Therapists, Osteopaths / Chiropractors	Manual lymphatic drainage, gentle massage, postural retraining	Compression therapy, graded exercise, ergonomic guidance
Energetics	Acupuncturists (TCM), Bioenergetic Therapists	Acupuncture, herbal formulas, PEMF	Warming acupuncture, energy balancing
Psychological	GNM practitioners, Psychotherapists, Vibrational therapists, Family constellation facilitators	Mind-body therapies supporting immune function and healing	Psychosomatic conflict resolution, emotional balancing

Educational Pearls & Considerations.

- Early intervention prevents progression of lymphedema.
- Manual lymphatic drainage must be performed by trained therapists.
- Compression garments need to be properly fitted and monitored.
- Nutritional support aids lymphatic and tissue health.
- Prompt infection control is critical.

GROUP 4 - ZONE 19 – FACIAL AREA (FRONTAL AND LATERAL)

Category 6: *Organ-Related (GNM)*

Step 1: Functional Anatomy and Interpretive Importance

The facial region includes the frontal bone, maxilla, mandible, and sensory systems, integrated with superficial vasculature and lymphatic drainage (Standring, 2016).

Though primarily musculoskeletal and integumentary, GNM highlights that unresolved conflicts tied to identity, self-image, or communication may manifest through organ-related programs reflected in the face. Hamer (2012) described that active phases suppress surface biosignals, producing hypoemission, while reparative phases amplify emissive intensity.

These variations may localize around the mandibular and perioral fields, sometimes mirroring psychosomatic conflict themes. Lane et al. (2009) emphasized the role of emotional awareness and regulation in shaping autonomic and physiological expression, supporting the idea that facial biospectral changes can embody unresolved psychobiological conflicts.

Through this lens, the face becomes a unique surface field where organ-related programs project visible correlates of psychosomatic regulation, accessible to emissive interpretation.

Step 2,3,4: ROI Classification and Interpretive Questions

Hyperemission reflects healing-phase expression or regulatory signal intensification.

- Are there signs of tissue repair, redness, or swelling?
- Are emotional or psychological stressors present?

Hypoemission indicates an active psychobiological conflict associated with tissue signal suppression or functional regulation loss.

- Are symptoms of chronic tension, fatigue, or unresolved psychosomatic issues evident?
- Is there a history of emotional stress or trauma?

Step 5: Confirmatory Evaluations

Test	Purpose & Justification	Relevance to Emissive Pattern
Psychological assessment	Identifies psychosomatic conflicts and emotional stressors.	Supports GNM-based interpretation of biosignal findings.
Physical exam	Assesses muscle tension, inflammation, and neurological status.	Correlates with emissive asymmetries.
Inflammatory markers (CRP, ESR)	Differentiates inflammatory from psychosomatic patterns.	Helps refine interpretive recognition.

Step 6: Care Strategies and Intervention Pathways

Naturopathic Approach

Implement stress reduction techniques including mindfulness, meditation, and family constellation therapy. Use adaptogenic herbs like *Rhodiola rosea* to support resilience (Panossian & Wikman, 2010). Employ bioenergetic therapies such as bioresonance for energetic harmonization.

Standard Medical Approaches

Psychotherapy and psychosomatic medicine approaches are fundamental. Physical rehabilitation and pharmacologic symptom management may support recovery.

Specialty / Practitioner Care Strategies Table

Specialty Group	Practitioners Included	Hyperemissive Strategies	Hypoemissive Strategies
Biochemistry	Nutritionists, Orthomolecular, Herbalists, Naturopaths	Adaptogens, antioxidants, stress-supportive botanicals	Nutritional support for emotional balance
Rehabilitation	Physiotherapists, Massage Therapists, Osteopaths / Chiropractors	Relaxation therapies, myofascial release	Postural correction, gentle mobilization
Energetics	Acupuncturists (TCM), Bioenergetic Therapists	Bioresonance, PEMF, energy balancing	Energetic harmonization, frequency therapy
Psychological	GNM practitioners, Psychotherapists, Vibrational therapists, Family constellation facilitators	Psychotherapy, bioresonance, family constellation therapy	Emotional balancing and conflict resolution

Educational Pearls & Considerations.

- Psychosomatic factors are significant contributors to symptoms in the facial area.
- Multimodal mind-body therapies enhance treatment outcomes.
- Early psychological support reduces symptom chronicity.
- Close monitoring of emotional and physical progress is essential.

GROUP 4 - ZONE 19 – FACIAL AREA (FRONTAL AND LATERAL)

Category 7: *Acupuncture / Meridian*

Step 1: Functional Anatomy and Interpretive Importance

The facial region comprises the frontal bone, zygomatic arch, mandible, and associated musculature, with dense innervation and vascular supply supporting sensory and expressive functions (Standring, 2016).

Acupuncture meridian theory associates this zone with the Stomach (ST), Large Intestine (LI), and Governing Vessel (GV) channels. Flaws (2000) described their influence on digestion, sinus regulation, and systemic Qi flow. Deadman et al. (2007) emphasized the therapeutic significance of ST4, LI20, and GV26 for facial paralysis, sinus congestion, and resuscitation, highlighting both local and systemic impact.

Kaptchuk (2000) linked these facial meridians to the integration of identity and expression in TCM, showing how energetic balance extends beyond physiology.

Clinically, imbalance is expressed as tension, numbness, or sensitivity in facial fields. On biosignal imaging, emissive asymmetries often trace the course of ST and LI channels across the cheeks, jawline, and nasal bridge, providing external markers of Qi disturbance projected into the face.

Step 2,3,4: ROI Classification and Interpretive Questions

Hyperemission suggests Qi stagnation or excessive signal expression along meridian trajectories.

- Are localized pain, tension, or redness present?
- Are symptoms aggravated by emotional stress or environmental factors?

Hypoemission indicates Qi deficiency or prolonged stagnation resulting in diminished surface responsiveness and reduced signal circulation.

- Does the patient report fatigue, cold sensations, or persistent discomfort?
- Are symptoms unresponsive to prior therapies?

Step 5: Confirmatory Evaluations

Test	Purpose & Justification	Relevance to Emissive Pattern
Pulse diagnosis and tongue examination	TCM methods to evaluate Qi and Blood status (Flaws, 2000).	Helps differentiate emissive patterns.

Biospectral imaging	Visualizes thermal asymmetries along meridian pathways.	Correlates with meridian signal variations.
Symptom questionnaire	Assesses facial discomfort and systemic symptoms.	Supports meridian-based interpretation.

Step 6: Care Strategies and Intervention Pathways

Naturopathic Approach

Acupuncture points such as ST4, LI20, and GV26 regulate facial Qi flow and alleviate tension (Lao et al., 2004). Moxibustion warms hypoemissive areas. Herbal formulas like *Xiao Feng San* support meridian balance (Bensky et al., 2004). Stress management and lifestyle modifications complement therapy.

Standard Medical Approaches

Acupuncture serves as adjunctive treatment for symptom relief and autonomic regulation.

Specialty / Practitioner Care Strategies Table

Specialty Group	Practitioners Included	Hyperemissive Strategies	Hypoemissive Strategies
Biochemistry	Nutritionists, Orthomolecular, Herbalists, Naturopaths	Anti-inflammatory herbs, circulation-supportive botanicals	Qi tonics and nutritional support
Rehabilitation	Physiotherapists, Massage Therapists, Osteopaths / Chiropractors	Facial mobilization, myofascial release	Gentle warming massage
Energetics	Acupuncturists (TCM), Bioenergetic Therapists	Acupuncture, moxibustion, PEMF	Warming acupuncture, energy balancing
Psychological	GNM practitioners, Psychotherapists, Vibrational therapists, Family constellation facilitators	Psychotherapy, bioresonance, energy clearing	Emotional balancing, psychosomatic conflict resolution

Educational Pearls & Considerations.

- Precise acupuncture point selection improves outcomes.
- Moxibustion should be applied carefully in heat-sensitive patients.
- Herbal prescriptions require practitioner expertise.
- Combining acupuncture with rehabilitative therapies enhances results.

GROUP 4 - ZONE 19 – FACIAL AREA (FRONTAL AND LATERAL)

Category 8: *Energetic*

Step 1: Functional Anatomy and Interpretive Importance

The facial region includes expressive musculature, sensory organs, craniofacial structures, and fascial planes interconnecting with the cervical spine (Standring, 2016). Energetically, the face acts as a communicative and regulatory surface, reflecting systemic adaptation, emotional signaling, and psychosomatic dynamics.

Van Wijk (2014) documented that ultraweak photon emissions fluctuate with physiologic states, offering a biophysical rationale for observed emissive changes in this zone. Patients often describe asymmetry, unexplained fatigue, or chronic tension in facial muscles.

Spectral surface readings reveal localized hyperemissive foci around expressive muscles such as orbicularis oris or frontalis, indicative of reparative activity or heightened emotional output.

Diffuse hypoemissive shadows may also emerge, consistent with suppressed regulation or systemic exhaustion. These emissive signals align with fascial and neurovascular continuities rather than isolated structures, reinforcing the role of the face as an energetic interface.

Clinically, interpretation of facial emissive signatures allows insight into the integration of systemic vitality, emotional adaptation, and psychosomatic coherence, situating this zone as a visible nexus of inner regulation and outward expression.

Step 2,3,4: ROI Classification and Interpretive Questions

Hyperemission indicates localized energetic congestion or excessive signal expression.

- Does the patient report sensations of heat, tension, or discomfort in the face?
- Are emotional or stress-related factors evident?

Hypoemission suggests energetic depletion or prolonged stagnation.

- Are symptoms of fatigue, coldness, or low vitality present?
- Are symptoms persistent or resistant to conventional treatments?

Step 5: Confirmatory Evaluations

Test	Purpose & Justification	Relevance to Emissive Pattern
Bioresonance testing	Measures tissue energy imbalances and frequencies.	Correlates with biosignal energetic variations.

Electrodermal screening (EDS)	Assesses skin conductance linked to energetic pathways.	Supports interpretive understanding of energetic pattern behavior.
Patient emotional and symptom history	Assesses psychological stress and energetic dysfunction.	Aids differential interpretation.

Step 6: Care Strategies and Intervention Pathways

Naturopathic Approach

Use bioresonance, pulsed electromagnetic fields (PEMF), and adaptogenic herbs to restore energetic balance (Matsumoto et al., 2010). Nutritional antioxidants and adaptogens support systemic resilience. Mindfulness and stress-reduction techniques complement energetic therapies.

Standard Medical Approaches

Energetic therapies serve as adjuncts to standard care, enhancing overall patient recovery.

Specialty / Practitioner Care Strategies Table

Specialty Group	Practitioners Included	Hyperemissive Strategies	Hypoemissive Strategies
Biochemistry	Nutritionists, Orthomolecular, Herbalists, Naturopaths	Adaptogens, antioxidants, herbal energetics	Nutritional support for energetic deficiency
Rehabilitation	Physiotherapists, Massage Therapists, Osteopaths / Chiropractors	Energy-based manual therapies, PEMF, therapeutic touch	Gentle stimulation, mobilization
Energetics	Acupuncturists (TCM), Bioenergetic Therapists	Bioresonance, PEMF, acupuncture	Warming acupuncture, energy balancing
Psychological	GNM practitioners, Psychotherapists, Vibrational therapists, Family constellation facilitators	Psychotherapy, bioresonance, mindfulness	Emotional balancing, vibrational medicine

Educational Pearls & Considerations.

- Energetic therapies complement but do not replace conventional treatments.
- Practitioner expertise and patient receptivity affect effectiveness.
- Ongoing reassessment optimizes therapy.
- Holistic mind-body care is essential.

GROUP 4 - ZONE 19 – FACIAL AREA (FRONTAL AND LATERAL)

Category 9: *Metabolic / Endocrine*

Step 1: Functional Anatomy and Interpretive Importance

The facial area incorporatees muscles of expression, sensory fields, and superficial glands influenced by systemic metabolic regulation (Standring, 2016). Endocrine conditions, including thyroid imbalance, adrenal dysregulation, and glycoregulatory disturbance, often project visibly into this region.

Larsen et al. (2016) emphasized the role of endocrine hormones in cutaneous physiology and vascular control, providing a framework for interpreting emissive findings here.

Patients may present with asymmetry, skin changes, or chronic fatigue expressed through facial tension. Spectral surface readings highlight localized hyperemissive foci around expressive musculature, consistent with endocrine-driven activation, while diffuse hypoemissive shadows reflect systemic suppression or depletion.

These emissive signatures follow fascial and vascular vectors more than isolated muscles, situating the face as both a communicative surface and a biospectral indicator of systemic metabolic balance. Clinically, the facial region provides one of the most visible maps of endocrine and metabolic health.

Step 2,3,4: ROI Classification and Interpretive Questions

Hyperemission reflects signal intensification associated with regulatory excitation, immune field activation, or elevated metabolic demand.

- Are there symptoms like warmth, redness, or tenderness?
- Are systemic symptoms such as heat intolerance or hormonal imbalance present?

Hypoemission indicates metabolic downregulation, vascular insufficiency, or tissue underactivation related to endocrine dysregulation.

- Are cold intolerance, fatigue, or skin changes reported?
- Is there known thyroid, adrenal, or metabolic disease?

Step 5: Confirmatory Evaluations

Test	Purpose & Justification	Relevance to Emissive Pattern
Thyroid function tests (TSH, Free T4, Free T3)	Assesses thyroid hormone status.	Correlates with emissive variations in facial tissues.
Blood glucose and HbA1c	Evaluates glycemic control and diabetes status.	Supports interpretive recognition of metabolic patterns linked to neural suppression or tissue repair delay.

Adrenal hormone panel	Assesses cortisol and related hormones.	Identifies emotional-endocrine regulatory shifts.
Inflammatory markers, CBC	Detects systemic or local inflammation.	Supports hyperemissive activation dynamics.

Step 6: Care Strategies and Intervention Pathways

Naturopathic Approach

Support endocrine and metabolic balance with antioxidants, chromium, magnesium, and adaptogens like *Withania somnifera* (Singh et al., 2011). Address glycemic control with diet and supplements. Stress management and psychotherapy support hormonal regulation.

Standard Medical Approaches

Medical management includes hormone replacement, diabetes control, and treatment of underlying metabolic conditions. Monitoring and imaging guide therapy.

Specialty / Practitioner Care Strategies Table

Specialty Group	Practitioners Included	Hyperemissive Strategies	Hypoemissive Strategies
Biochemistry	Nutritionists, Orthomolecular, Herbalists, Naturopaths	Antioxidants, adaptogens, metabolic support nutrients	Nutritional support for endocrine balance
Rehabilitation	Physiotherapists, Massage Therapists, Osteopaths / Chiropractors	Relaxation and circulation-enhancing therapies	Postural correction and gentle mobilization
Energetics	Acupuncturists (TCM), Bioenergetic Therapists	Acupuncture for metabolic and endocrine regulation	Energy balancing and harmonization
Psychological	GNM practitioners, Psychotherapists, Vibrational therapists, Family constellation facilitators	Psychotherapy, bioresonance, stress reduction	Emotional balancing and hormonal support

Educational Pearls & Considerations.

- Monitor metabolic and endocrine parameters regularly.
- Nutritional and botanical support optimize hormonal health.
- Psychosomatic factors influence metabolic function.
- Early intervention improves prognosis.

CHAPTER

4

CASE STUDIES IN BIOSPECTRAL MEDICINE

INTEGRATIVE CLINICAL APPLICATION OF THE R-CIIM METHOD ACROSS ALL ZONES

The clinical application of Biospectral Medicine demands both precision and perspective. While the six-step interpretive methodology offers a structured pathway for identifying dysfunction within specific emission zones, its true strength lies in its ability to integrate localized findings within the totality of the patient's biosignal field.

Each of the following case studies serves as a practical and instructional model, demonstrating how the Biospectral system guides diagnosis and therapy across a wide range of clinical conditions. Every case is written using the same methodological steps, allowing readers to follow the logic from symptom to zone, from emission pattern to interpretive category, and from testing to individualized therapeutic action.

Importantly, although each case study centres on a primary anatomical zone aligned with the patient's main clinical complaint, all 19 zones are consistently examined during patient evaluations. This full-body assessment is central to the philosophy of Biospectral Medicine, which views human dysfunction not as isolated to single locations but as emerging from interconnected biofunctional fields.

While one emission zone may carry the primary signal, it is common to observe compensatory, referred, or downstream biosignal changes in secondary zones. These may reflect regulatory strain, autonomic imbalance, or unresolved metabolic terrain stress. Such patterns often help identify the true origin of the problem, which is frequently missed in conventional, complaint-focused evaluations.

In fact, one of the foundational principles of natural and integrative medicine is that a localized symptom may only represent the terminal expression of a broader systemic dysfunction. As such, biosignal mapping through infrared emission provides localized interpretive understanding and a functional cartography of systemic dysregulation.

Practitioners trained in naturopathy, orthomolecular therapy, or terrain-based approaches already recognize this dynamic: gastrointestinal dysfunction may manifest in skin zones; emotional repression may alter jaw and facial emissions; vascular stagnation may originate from musculoskeletal or postural imbalance.

This integrative view aligns with emerging models in systems biology and regulatory medicine, which emphasize that complex health disturbances arise not from isolated events but from interlinked dysfunctions across structural, metabolic, and energetic systems (Biron et al., 2020).

Likewise, research in developmental and theoretical biology confirms that biofunctional unity, the coordinated regulation of distant systems through feedback networks, is central to all healing processes (Rosslenbroich, 2007). Biospectral interpretation captures these signals at the site of the complaint and throughout the interconnected terrain.

From a technical standpoint, this whole-body evaluation is also justified by studies on infrared interpretation methodology, which emphasize the need for anatomical precision and multisite analysis to differentiate local pathology from systemic expressions (Ring & Ammer, 2012; Lahiri et al., 2012).

Therefore, even when the analysis is directed toward a single zone, practitioners are encouraged to maintain a wide-field interpretive logic, comparing symmetrical and adjacent emissions to understand the directionality and depth of biosignal propagation.

In summary, the case studies presented in this Atlas reflect a true clinical workflow. Each begins with a defined complaint and zone but ultimately moves through an integrative evaluation of bodywide biosignals, respecting the dynamic, multifactorial nature of human dysfunction. This structure offers a bridge between pattern recognition and interpretive precision, between subjective complaint and objective evidence.

For practitioners and researchers alike, it demonstrates why Biospectral Medicine must evolve into the next interpretive language, one capable of decoding health at the speed and complexity of the body itself.

CASE STUDY

1

Zone 1: Frontal Lower Legs

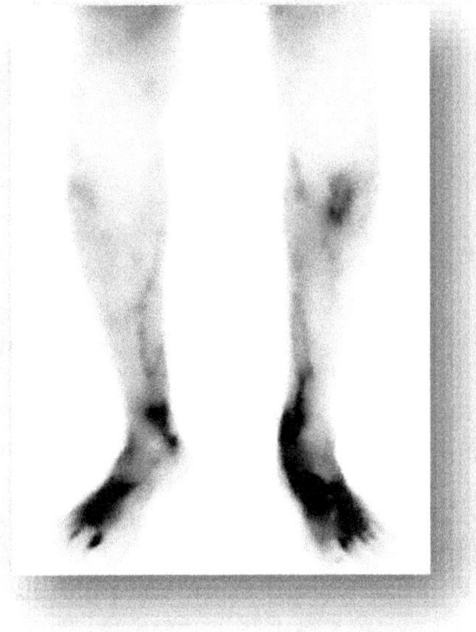

Interpretive Category: Vascular / Circulatory
Clinical Condition: Venous Insufficiency
Patient Profile: Female, 58 years old
Date of Birth: 2 February 1967

Step 1 – Zone Relevance: Anatomical and Biospectral Context

The patient reported a long-standing complaint of heaviness and visible swelling in the lower legs, particularly worsening at the end of the day after long hours of standing at her job. This type of symptomatology immediately pointed to Zone 1 – Frontal Lower Legs as a relevant anatomical region to evaluate.

This zone covers the anterior aspect of the tibial region and the perimalleolar area, a physiologically dependent region strongly influenced by superficial venous drainage, microcirculatory integrity, and the muscle pump mechanism of the tibialis anterior. It is also one of the key zones in upright circulation, prone to gravity-induced pooling of venous blood and lymphatic fluid.

In Biospectral Medicine, this region often expresses early signs of stasis, superficial venous incompetence, and dermal congestion, which makes it essential to investigate thoroughly when symptoms of postural swelling or fatigue are present.

Step 2 – ROI Classification (Emission Pattern)

During the image review, we observed an irregular pattern of biospectral emissions in the anterior tibial zone bilaterally, with greater intensity on the left side. The emission zones were characterized by blotchy, patchy elevation along the paths commonly occupied by the great saphenous vein and its tributaries.

These findings were classified as hyperemissive according to our system, indicating regions with elevated spectral output typically associated with increased superficial flow, stagnation, or low-grade reactivity. The asymmetry and focal distribution of these emissions fit the clinical hypothesis of superficial venous congestion rather than diffuse systemic reactivity or deeper vascular impairment.

Step 3 – Interpretive Category Determination

Given the anatomical features and the nature of the emissions observed, the most consistent classification was Category 1 – Vascular / Circulatory. The location, distribution, and symmetry of the biospectral elevation aligned with superficial venous pathways, particularly the great saphenous vein, which commonly shows overload in patients with gravitational pooling and reduced valve competence.

Other categories such as muscular or lymphatic were considered but excluded due to the absence of structural overload or dermal lymphatic emission spread. The overall biosignal supported the interpretation of venous stasis rather than arterial insufficiency or lymphedema, which would have presented with different emission profiles, such as hyporeactivity or plateaued dermatomal zones.

> **BIOSPECTRAL INTERPRETATION RULE**
>
> *In vascular cases, emissions appear as irregular, patchy, or blotchy zones that follow known venous trajectories rather than muscular or dermatomal structures. In the frontal lower legs, these signals commonly mirror the course of the great saphenous vein and its tributaries, especially in gravity-dependent regions. When asymmetrical, dense, and surface-bound, such patterns reflect superficial venous congestion or early valvular insufficiency. Unlike arterial insufficiency, which may present with hyporeactive zones, or lymphatic stagnation, which tends to appear nodular and lateral, venous biosignals in this zone cluster along linear drainage pathways and intensify after prolonged standing.*

Step 4 – Differential Interpretive Confirmation Through Patient History

In conversation, the patient confirmed that her legs often felt tired and heavy by late afternoon, particularly after prolonged periods of standing. She described visible swelling in the ankle area and occasional itching and warmth in the lower legs, which were more intense on the left side.

When asked about colder extremities, numbness, or cramping while walking, symptoms often associated with arterial insufficiency, she denied any such experiences. She reported that her legs did not feel cold to the touch and she had no pain while walking, only after extended periods of standing still. She also had no history of skin discoloration on the toes or delayed wound healing.

These answers helped reinforce the hypothesis of venous congestion while effectively excluding arterial disease and neurological deficits, both of which would have led us to different interpretive categories. Her verbal confirmation, when contextualized with the biospectral pattern, guided the case toward a confident vascular diagnosis.

Step 5 – Confirmatory Clinical Tests

To validate the interpretive hypothesis, we referred the patient for vascular imaging and functional tests. Doppler ultrasound of the lower limbs confirmed bilateral venous insufficiency with delayed valve closure times, especially in the left great saphenous pathway. Ankle-Brachial Index (ABI) was 1.1 on both sides, ruling out arterial compromise. Capillary refill tests were normal, indicating preserved microcirculatory dynamics, while inflammatory markers (CRP and ESR) were mildly elevated, consistent with chronic low-grade vascular inflammation.

These findings confirmed the biospectral observation and demonstrated that the CBI findings had accurately identified the functional disturbance, narrowing the interpretive process and avoiding unnecessary testing.

Step 6 – Therapeutic Suggestions and Clinical Outcome

The integrative therapeutic strategy was built around improving venous return, reducing microinflammation, and supporting vascular tone. We recommended botanical venotonics, including *Aesculus hippocastanum* and *Centella asiatica*, along with daily hydrotherapy using contrast foot baths to stimulate calf pump activity and fluid mobilization.

The patient also adopted a high-flavonoid diet, rich in citrus bioflavonoids and polyphenols, and began taking vitamin C and omega-3 supplements to support capillary stability and reduce endothelial stress. She was instructed to elevate her legs at regular intervals throughout the day and was fitted for graduated compression stockings to support passive venous return.

Psychophysiological insights during the consultation suggested a pattern of "feeling unsupported" and "overburdened," which were gently addressed through emotional counselling and mindfulness practices, helping her reconnect circulation with a sense of flow and internal rhythm.

Therapeutic Outcome

At her six-week follow-up, the patient reported a clear reduction in swelling and heaviness, particularly after work. She described being able to "stand longer without that pressure building up" and had resumed light evening walks, which had previously been too uncomfortable. From her own words: *"Before, I would come home and collapse with swollen feet. Now I still feel tired, but I don't feel broken anymore."*

This case demonstrated how Biospectral Medicine, applied correctly, provided both accurate interpretive orientation and effective therapeutic guidance using an integrative logic that respects physiology and the lived experience of the patient.

CASE STUDY

2

Zone 2: Dorsal Lower Legs

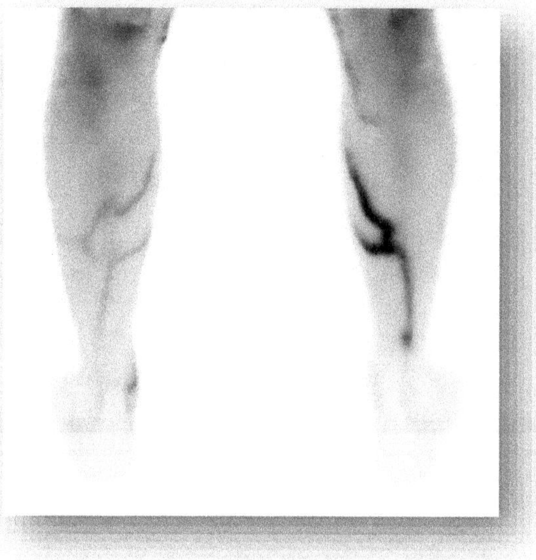

Interpretive Category: Muscular / Myofascial
Clinical Condition: Post-Exertional Muscular Pain
Patient Profile: Male, 45 years old
Date of Birth: 14 August 1979

Step 1 – Zone Relevance: Anatomical and Biospectral Context

The patient presented with a recurring complaint of muscular tightness and aching in the posterior legs, particularly aggravated after hiking or long walks. This led us directly to examine Zone 2 – Dorsal Lower Legs, which includes the gastrocnemius, soleus, and Achilles tendon structures, as well as the deep myofascial compartments and their vascular and neural interfaces.

This zone is structurally dependent on coordinated calf muscle contraction to support upright locomotion and venous return.

In Biospectral Medicine, this area frequently emits compensatory biosignals in response to myofascial overload, impaired metabolic recovery, or postural fatigue. Given the patient's complaint and activity pattern, this zone became the primary emission area for investigation.

Step 2 – ROI Classification (Emission Pattern)

The spectral scan of Zone 2 showed symmetrical but pronounced emission elevation along the medial and lateral gastrocnemius bulk, more prominent on the left side. The pattern revealed dense, columnar hyperemissive zones that followed the muscular striations and terminated near the Achilles insertion.

These biospectral markers were classified as hyperemissive, suggesting ongoing myofascial activation or metabolic congestion, rather than acute reactivity or neuropathy.

The bilateral symmetry and reproducibility of the emission further aligned with functional muscular overuse rather than structural trauma.

Step 3 – Interpretive Category Determination

The pattern observed clearly aligned with Category 2 – Muscular / Myofascial. The emission followed muscular contours rather than neurovascular trajectories or dermatomal lines, ruling out a neuropathic or circulatory category. The absence of hyporeactive zones also excluded fascial adhesion or deep compartment stagnation.

Based on the emission distribution, history of exertional onset, and absence of systemic reactive features, we classified the case as a muscular terrain imbalance with probable delayed metabolic clearance and mild microtrauma accumulation.

Step 4 – Differential Interpretive Confirmation Through Patient History

The patient confirmed that symptoms would begin 12 to 24 hours after moderate physical activity, such as hiking or climbing stairs, and resolved gradually over several days. He denied sharp or electric-like pain, which could indicate nerve involvement, and noted that pain was dull, tight, and sometimes accompanied by morning stiffness. He had no history of swelling, varicosities, or skin colour changes.

There were no signs of impaired mobility or trauma. He also denied any heat or redness in the area, which excluded deeper reactivity or vascular events. These patient responses reinforced the muscular interpretation and excluded circulatory, skeletal, or neurological involvement.

> **BIOSPECTRAL INTERPRETATION RULE**
>
> *In Biospectral Medicine, emissions that appear linear or vertical on the legs are not automatically vascular; their classification depends on pattern logic. Vascular biosignals tend to show irregular branching, pooling, or diffuse patchiness, reflecting stagnation or overload in the superficial vein network. In contrast, muscular/myofascial emissions are typically dense, columnar, and symmetrical, aligning with the shape and function of major muscle groups. When an emission follows the contours of the gastrocnemius or soleus, terminates near a tendon insertion, and shows reproducibility with exertional history, it indicates myofascial activation or metabolic stress, not venous congestion, even if visually similar at first glance.*

Step 5 – Confirmatory Clinical Tests

To support the diagnosis, the patient underwent a musculoskeletal ultrasound which showed mild thickening and reactive changes in the left gastrocnemius without any tear or fascial disruption. Creatine kinase levels were mildly elevated post-exertion, confirming ongoing muscular microtrauma. Range of motion and resistance testing of the ankle and knee showed reduced dorsiflexion and increased muscle tone in the posterior chain.

A myofascial flexibility scan using manual palpation confirmed taut bands and trigger point reactivity bilaterally. These findings matched the biospectral emissions and validated the muscular/myofascial origin of the discomfort.

Step 6 – Therapeutic Suggestions and Clinical Outcome

The therapeutic strategy aimed to reduce myofascial tension, enhance post-exercise recovery, and improve muscular resilience. The patient began magnesium bisglycinate supplementation to support muscular relaxation and reduce excitability. Arnica montana and Ruta graveolens were used in low potency for soft tissue recovery.

Deep tissue massage was introduced once weekly, focusing on myofascial release of the posterior compartments. Hydrotherapy using warm water immersion followed by cold rinses was prescribed post-activity to promote clearance of metabolites.

He was also instructed to perform eccentric calf exercises and daily stretches, particularly targeting the Achilles and posterior chain. Emotional assessment suggested a "need for movement and escape," which was integrated through nature-based exercise with structured rest periods, reducing overexertion as a coping mechanism.

Therapeutic Outcome

At his six-week follow-up, the patient reported a significant reduction in post-exertional soreness and improved flexibility. He had resumed weekly hiking without experiencing the previous muscle heaviness and tightness. "Before, I would feel like my calves were turning into bricks the day after a walk," he said. "Now, it feels like they've finally learned to recover."

This case demonstrated the muscular interpretive value of Zone 2 in Biospectral Medicine, and how a targeted integrative plan can restore musculoskeletal balance by reading the functional language of biospectral emission.

CASE STUDY

3

Zone 3: Internal Left Leg

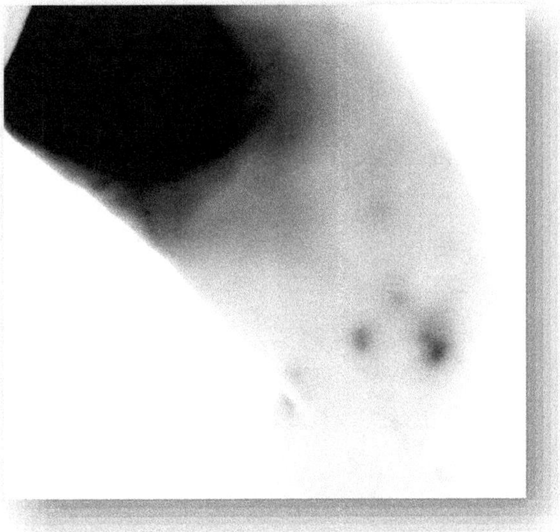

Interpretive Category: Skeletal / Articular
Clinical Condition: Medial Knee Pain Due to Degenerative Articular Stress
Patient Profile: Female, 50 years old
Date of Birth: 7 November 1974

Step 1 – Zone Relevance: Anatomical and Biospectral Context

The patient presented with persistent discomfort and stiffness along the medial side of the left knee, especially during weight-bearing activities such as climbing stairs or rising from a seated position. This presentation directed our focus to Zone 3 – Internal Left Leg, which anatomically incorporates the medial femoral condyle, medial tibial plateau, and pes anserinus insertion, all of which are common sites of early articular stress.

In Biospectral Medicine, this zone often emits skeletal biosignals in response to joint surface overload, periarticular irritation, or enthesopathic reactions. Given the localized medial pain and mechanical pattern of onset, Zone 3 was considered a skeletal emission site of high interpretive value.

Step 2 – ROI Classification (Emission Pattern)

The spectral image revealed a focal, intense hyperemissive zone directly over the left medial knee joint, without spread to the surrounding thigh or lower leg. The emission was sharply demarcated and confined to the region of the medial femoral-tibial interface. No dermatomal, fascial, or vascular branching was present, which reinforced its articular nature.

The right knee showed a neutral spectral field with no signs of compensatory loading. This emission was classified as a localized skeletal biosignal, suggesting increased metabolic activity or irritation at the joint level, most likely related to early degenerative or mechanical articular processes.

Step 3 – Interpretive Category Determination

The biospectral features, focal hyperemission, joint-level localization, and absence of systemic or soft tissue involvement, were characteristic of Category 3 – Skeletal / Articular. The image did not align with muscular activation, vascular congestion, or neurogenic distribution.

The structural nature of the complaint and the emission's confinement to the knee joint supported the interpretation of mechanical overload or early osteoarticular degeneration.

This category was further reinforced by the emission's stability over repeated scans, indicating a chronic structural pattern rather than a transient reactive or neural event.

BIOSPECTRAL INTERPRETATION RULE

Skeletal and articular biosignals present as localized, joint-centered emissions that are sharply defined and confined to periarticular zones. These emissions do not follow muscular, vascular, or dermatomal pathways but instead concentrate over bony landmarks, joint lines, or enthesis regions. They often reflect mechanical stress, early degenerative changes, or subclinical articular overload. The spectral pattern is typically focal, stable, and reproducible across postures, indicating structural imbalance rather than dynamic tissue response. In Biospectral Medicine, these emissions help identify biomechanical dysfunction before radiological findings emerge, supporting early intervention in load-bearing joints.

Step 4 – Differential Interpretive Confirmation Through Patient History

Upon further exploration, the patient described the knee pain as deep, dull, and pressure-like, intensified during movement and relieved by rest. She denied sensations of burning, tingling, or shooting pain, which excluded neuropathic involvement.

There was no visible swelling, redness, or temperature change in the area, and no morning stiffness exceeding 15 minutes, ruling out systemic reactive arthritis.

She recalled a long history of mild valgus alignment and prior episodes of patellofemoral discomfort. She reported no trauma, but described her daily habits as sedentary with frequent knee flexion. This confirmed a mechanical and degenerative etiology, consistent with the spectral findings.

Step 5 – Confirmatory Clinical Tests

A standing X-ray of the left knee demonstrated mild medial joint space narrowing and early signs of subchondral sclerosis, consistent with incipient medial compartment osteoarthritis. There was no evidence of fracture, effusion, or severe deformity.

Orthopedic testing revealed pain on medial compression and valgus stress, without joint instability. Manual palpation confirmed localized tenderness over the pes anserinus insertion and medial collateral ligament.

Gait analysis showed mild compensation on left foot strike, further validating the articular load imbalance. These findings matched the biospectral emission and confirmed a skeletal-articular origin for the patient's complaint.

Step 6 – Therapeutic Suggestions and Clinical Outcome

The therapeutic strategy aimed to reduce joint stress, support cartilage metabolism, and correct postural load imbalance. The patient began Boswellia serrata and Curcuma longa supplementation to modulate articular catabolism and low-grade inflammation. Hyaluronic acid-rich collagen peptides were introduced to support cartilage hydration. Daily corrective exercises were prescribed to improve medial quadriceps activation and reduce valgus strain.

Infrared compresses were applied locally to promote periarticular microcirculation. She adopted a wedge insole to slightly offload the medial knee compartment. Emotional inquiry revealed a pattern of overcommitment without grounding, and grounding techniques were introduced to reinforce pelvic-knee alignment.

Therapeutic Outcome

After eight weeks, the patient reported marked improvement in joint fluidity and reduced discomfort when climbing stairs. She no longer needed to support herself when rising from a chair. In her words: "It feels like my knee is moving again, instead of grinding."

This case illustrates the precision of Biospectral Medicine in identifying focal skeletal emissions linked to mechanical overload, allowing for early intervention before structural deterioration becomes radiologically advanced.

CASE STUDY

4

Zone 4: Internal Right Leg

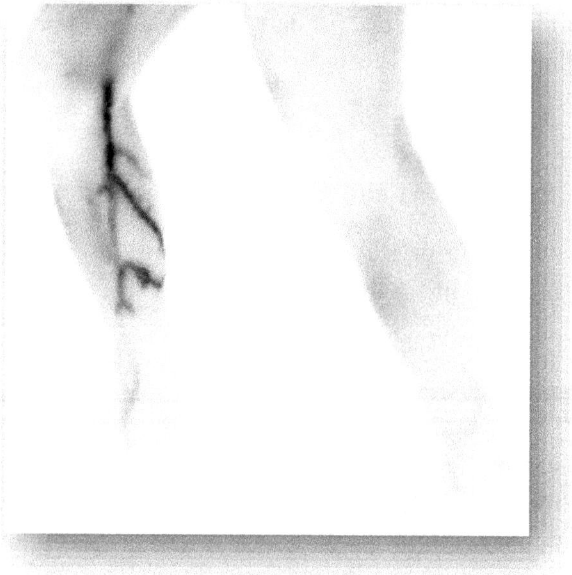

Interpretive Category: Vascular / Circulatory
Clinical Condition: Medial Venous Congestion with Postural Overload
Patient Profile: Male, 34 years old
Date of Birth: 11 March 1991

Step 1 – Zone Relevance: Anatomical and Biospectral Context

The patient presented with heaviness, intermittent aching, and mild swelling along the inner right leg, particularly after prolonged standing or intense leg workouts.

These symptoms pointed toward Zone 4 – Internal Right Leg, which anatomically includes the great saphenous vein, its perforating tributaries, and the deep medial venous plexus. This region is also biomechanically influenced by pelvic tilt, knee valgus, and postural venous return dynamics.

In Biospectral Medicine, this zone frequently emits vascular biosignals under conditions of valvular insufficiency, venous pooling, or orthostatic congestion. Given the symptom timing, location, and mechanical context, this zone became the primary area of biospectral investigation.

Step 2 – ROI Classification (Emission Pattern)

The spectral scan revealed a distinct, branching hyperemissive pattern following the medial course of the right thigh and knee, extending from the upper adductor region to the lower leg. The emission mirrored the trajectory of the great saphenous vein, with visible bifurcations and perforating branches.

The left leg showed no comparable emission, reinforcing the lateralized vascular hypothesis. The biospectral pattern was not linear or muscular but rather diffuse, lobulated, and venous in morphology, consistent with regional circulatory overload.

Step 3 – Interpretive Category Determination

The emission characteristics, vascular trajectory, medial distribution, branching architecture, and unilateral expression, clearly aligned with Category 1 – Vascular / Circulatory. There was no striated muscular emission, dermatomal alignment, or skeletal joint localization.

The pattern was incompatible with neural or articular origin. The presence of tributary-like branching further excluded soft tissue strain and pointed toward superficial venous stress, possibly due to valvular fatigue or orthostatic pooling in the saphenous system.

> **BIOSPECTRAL INTERPRETATION RULE**
>
> *Vascular biosignals are identified by their branching, irregular, or lobulated emission patterns that follow known venous or circulatory pathways rather than structural anatomy. These emissions often appear as asymmetric pooling, linear streaks with tributary spread, or diffuse congestion in areas of venous drainage. Unlike muscular emissions, which are dense and aligned with striated tissue, vascular signals reflect dynamic flow disturbances such as valvular fatigue, orthostatic stasis, or regional circulatory overload. Their morphology often mimics the course of superficial veins and is most pronounced in gravitational zones, making vascular mapping a key tool for assessing hemodynamic stress and return inefficiency.*

Step 4 – Differential Interpretive Confirmation Through Patient History

The patient confirmed that the symptoms worsened after standing long hours at work or intense gym sessions focused on lower body strength.

He described the sensation as a "pressure build-up" rather than pain, with occasional mild swelling and throbbing localized to the inner thigh and knee. He denied redness, heat, or skin discoloration, and had no history of trauma, surgery, or neurological symptoms.

Compression garments provided partial relief, and the discomfort typically subsided after leg elevation. These responses ruled out musculoskeletal strain and supported a venous congestion pattern related to posture and circulatory return inefficiency.

Step 5 – Confirmatory Clinical Tests

A venous Doppler ultrasound of the right leg revealed mild valvular incompetence in the proximal great saphenous vein with reflux under Valsalva maneuver. There was no evidence of thrombosis, phlebitis, or deep vein involvement. Orthopedic and neurological exams were unremarkable.

Postural analysis revealed anterior pelvic tilt and medial knee collapse during stance, increasing venous pressure along the inner limb. Manual palpation revealed mild tenderness over the adductor canal and femoral triangle, consistent with venous stasis. These findings correlated directly with the spectral emission map, confirming the vascular evaluation interpretation.

Step 6 – Therapeutic Suggestions and Clinical Outcome

The therapeutic plan focused on improving venous return, reducing regional pooling, and correcting postural contributors. The patient began Ruscus aculeatus and Aesculus hippocastanum to improve venous tone and capillary resistance. Bioflavonoid-rich citrus extract was added to support endothelial function. He was advised to wear graduated compression stockings during prolonged standing, and to implement ankle-pump exercises throughout the day.

Pelvic realignment work included gluteal activation and internal hip rotator stretching to reduce medial knee collapse. Cold leg rinses and inversion exercises were introduced to mechanically stimulate venous drainage. Emotionally, a theme of "inability to move forward without resistance" was explored and addressed with journaling and symbolic movement therapy.

Therapeutic Outcome

After five weeks, the patient reported substantial relief of heaviness and swelling, especially at the end of workdays. He resumed gym training with corrected biomechanics and described the leg as feeling "lighter, more reactive, and less trapped." The follow-up biospectral scan showed reduced emission intensity along the saphenous trajectory, confirming clinical and circulatory improvement.

This case demonstrates how Zone 4 can effectively reveal subclinical venous dysfunction before structural complications arise, enabling early vascular intervention through integrative, non-invasive care.

CASE STUDY

5

Zone 5: External Left Leg

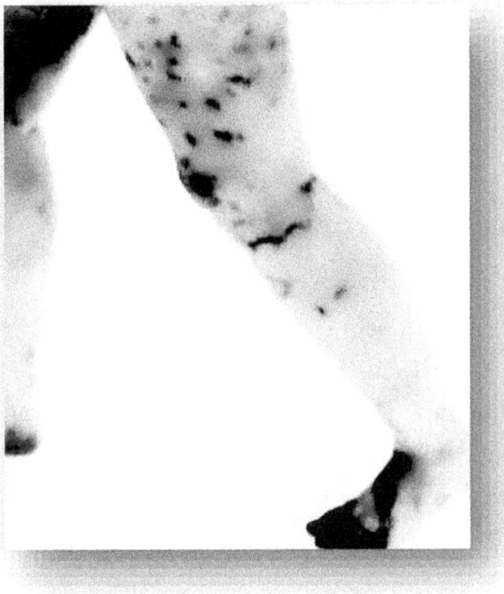

Interpretive Category: Lymphatic / Immune
Clinical Condition: Lateral Dermal Congestion with Regional Lymphatic Reactivity
Patient Profile: Male, 41 years old
Date of Birth: 25 May 1984

Step 1 – Zone Relevance: Anatomical and Biospectral Context

The patient reported a chronic sensation of discomfort, heaviness, and "dermal irritation" along the lateral aspect of his left leg, extending from the outer thigh to the calf. These symptoms, particularly their vague, migratory nature and surface-level distribution, directed our focus to Zone 5 – External Left Leg, which includes the iliotibial region, lateral thigh fascia, popliteal drainage pathways, and superficial lymphatic territories.

In Biospectral Medicine, this zone frequently emits irregular, blotchy hyperemission patterns when there is lymphatic congestion, immune terrain stress, or toxic tissue burden. The absence of mechanical or vascular indicators and the diffuse nature of symptoms pointed to this zone as a likely site of lymphatic emission expression.

Step 2 – ROI Classification (Emission Pattern)

The spectral analysis revealed multiple irregular, nodular hyperemissive patches scattered across the lateral left thigh and calf, with no continuity along muscular striations or vascular lines.

The emission appeared patchy and diffuse, with uneven clustering suggestive of immune dermal signalling and lymphatic stagnation rather than linear or mechanical overload. Especially, there was no similar pattern on the contralateral leg, emphasizing regional immune terrain imbalance.

This emission was classified as a lymphatic-dominant biosignal, indicative of interstitial immune activation or compromised drainage efficiency within the superficial lymphatic network.

Step 3 – Interpretive Category Determination

The pattern morphology, distribution, and lack of alignment with structural anatomy were consistent with Category 5 – Lymphatic / Immune. The emission did not follow any muscular, nervous, or vascular architecture. It was multifocal, surface-bound, and non-linear, excluding meridian-based or fascial explanations.

Given the absence of systemic symptoms, the pattern likely reflected localized immune burden, perhaps from environmental toxin exposure, post-infectious tissue retention, or dysregulated tissue detoxification. The biospectral expression was typical of a low-grade, chronic immune stress terrain, not an acute reactive response.

BIOSPECTRAL INTERPRETATION RULE

Lymphatic and immune biosignals appear as diffuse, blotchy, or clustered hyperemissions that lack anatomical alignment. Unlike muscular or vascular patterns, they do not follow striated, linear, or branching trajectories. Instead, they localize in regions of dermal congestion or nodal stagnation, often reflecting tissue detoxification burden, immune terrain reactivity, or impaired lymphatic flow. These emissions are typically asymmetric and surface-oriented, serving as early visual markers of systemic or regional immune stress.

Step 4 – Differential Interpretive Confirmation Through Patient History

In detailed history-taking, the patient noted that symptoms had persisted for over a year, waxing and waning with no clear musculoskeletal trigger. He described a "crawling under the skin" sensation, particularly after travel, heat exposure, or eating processed foods.

He denied joint pain, muscle fatigue, or neuropathic symptoms. Notably, he had a past history of recurrent upper respiratory infections and food sensitivities, and reported persistent post-exertional fatigue.

He also experienced mild facial puffiness in the morning and described himself as "sluggish to detox." There was no trauma, medication use, or dermatological diagnosis. These findings reinforced the hypothesis of lymphatic immune congestion, consistent with the biospectral scan.

Step 5 – Confirmatory Clinical Tests

Capillary phase contrast microscopy revealed evidence of proteinaceous debris, immune cell aggregation, and early signs of rouleaux, consistent with low-grade immune activation and hemorheological stress.

Manual lymphatic palpation showed reduced mobility of lateral superficial nodes in the inguinal chain and signs of tissue stiffness in the iliotibial region. A live blood analysis revealed activated neutrophils, oxidative stress markers, and reduced membrane flexibility.

Bioresonance testing pointed toward chemical burden and immune terrain dysregulation. Together, these findings confirmed that the emission pattern observed in Zone 5 reflected a lymphatic and immune response pattern, not a structural or energetic imbalance.

Step 6 – Therapeutic Suggestions and Clinical Outcome

Therapy focused on stimulating lymphatic flow, modulating immune reactivity, and supporting tissue detoxification. The patient began a lymphotropic protocol including Galium aparine, Echinacea purpurea, and Calendula officinalis, supported by dry brushing and rebound stimulation to enhance drainage. Contrast hydrotherapy and manual lymphatic drainage sessions were introduced weekly.

To reduce immune reactivity, dietary adjustments removed histamine-rich foods and supported gut–immune regulation with L-glutamine and lactobacillus strains. Emotional processing revealed a long-standing sense of "being overloaded and under-supported," which was addressed using reflective journaling and guided body awareness techniques to release internalized tension.

Therapeutic Outcome

At his six-week follow-up, the patient reported a significant reduction in tissue discomfort and an overall sense of "lightness" in the leg and body. He noted improved tolerance to temperature changes and less morning facial puffiness. In his words: "It's like my system is no longer clogged. I feel like something is finally moving again." A follow-up biospectral scan confirmed reduction in nodular emission clusters, supporting clinical resolution.

This case illustrates how Zone 5 can manifest immune terrain overload long before systemic reactivity becomes evident, allowing for precise early intervention through spectral lymphatic mapping.

CASE STUDY

6

Zone 6: External Right Leg

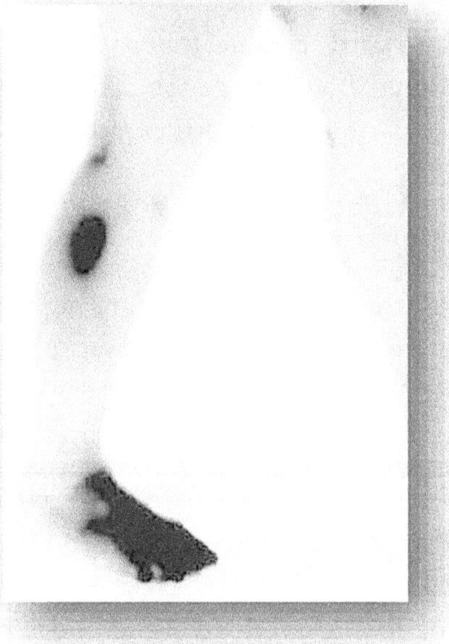

NOTE: *In this case, the image shows a focal hyperemissive area on the external right leg, with no anatomical alignment, no venous branching, and no muscular striation. It does not follow the shape, spread, or bruising behaviour of a physical injury or trauma. Bruised tissue typically shows irregular, mottled, or peripheral emission changes, often with a gradient or surrounding compensatory cold zone. In contrast, this emission is geometrically precise, stable, and confined to the energetic field, indicating a frequency-based amplification or congestion, not reactivity or trauma.*

Interpretive Category: Energetic / Frequency
Clinical Condition: Lateral Energy Blockade with Localized Field Hypoactivity
Patient Profile: Female, 45 years old
Date of Birth: 8 October 1979

Step 1 – Zone Relevance: Anatomical and Biospectral Context

The patient reported an unusual sensation of "emptiness" or "energy collapse" along the outer right leg, particularly around the calf and ankle, without associated pain or fatigue. She described it as a sense of energetic disconnection, especially after emotionally stressful days or prolonged computer work.

These non-anatomical, field-based descriptions directed our attention to Zone 6 – External Right Leg, which includes the lateral thigh, IT band, fibular territory, and energetic field interfaces aligned with the external meridian grid.

In Biospectral Medicine, this zone is often used to detect lateral frequency disruptions related to emotional dissociation, field collapse, or interference in electromagnetic coherence. The patient's lateralized, non-structural complaints pointed toward this zone as a candidate for energetic biosignal evaluation.

Step 2 – ROI Classification (Emission Pattern)

The spectral imaging revealed discrete, sharply defined hyporeactive zones over the lateral right calf and ankle, appearing as dark circular depressions in the biospectral field. These focal hypoemissions were clearly not aligned with vascular or muscular anatomy, nor did they reflect reactive or structural overload. The surrounding tissue showed normal signal intensity, emphasizing the localized energetic collapse.

The morphology of the pattern, circular, sharply bordered, and asymmetric, is characteristic of energetic field deactivation, not consistent with lymphatic, neural, or articular profiles. This image was classified as a frequency-related biosignal disturbance, suggestive of energetic stagnation, suppression, or dissociation.

Step 3 – Interpretive Category Determination

Given the non-anatomical location, distinct focal cold zones, and absence of mechanical or physiological correlations, this case was classified under Category 8 – Energetic / Frequency.

The emissions did not follow dermatomes, meridians, vasculature, or muscular striations. Instead, they presented as spatially stable hypoactive zones, which in Biospectral interpretation often indicate field suppression, blocked biophysical resonance, or chronic energetic depletion.

BIOSPECTRAL INTERPRETATION RULE

Energetic biosignals are characterized by discrete, sharply localized hyperemissions or hypoemissions that do not follow anatomical, vascular, or musculoskeletal pathways. These patterns often appear in symbolic or geometrically unusual forms, such as focal spots, rings, or mirrored zones, and are typically unresponsive to mechanical testing. They reflect disturbances in biofield coherence, resonance imbalance, or energy accumulation, rather than tissue damage or structural dysfunction.

The clarity and reproducibility of the hypoemission ruled out artifact or imaging inconsistency and supported a true energetic signature.

Step 4 – Differential Interpretive Confirmation Through Patient History

In dialogue, the patient confirmed that her main complaint was not pain but a persistent feeling of "loss of sensation or energy integrity" on the outer right leg. She described feeling like her body "didn't extend into that area anymore."

The sensation was most prominent in moments of emotional stress, mental exhaustion, or after social conflict. She denied any weakness, numbness, swelling, or discomfort during movement.

There were no signs of varicosities, trauma, or prior surgeries. These details reinforced the non-structural, non-reactive nature of the issue and supported the hypothesis of energetic field disruption, possibly involving localized coherence loss in subtle energy systems.

Step 5 – Confirmatory Clinical Tests

Conventional imaging and orthopedic exams were unremarkable. However, bioresonance assessment revealed coherence loss in the right lower field with low amplitude wave readings in the lateral limb segment. HRV analysis showed elevated sympathetic tone with poor coherence under stress testing.

A bioterrain scan identified frequency dropout zones over the lateral calf, matching the biospectral hypoemission. Manual energetic field palpation noted a "cold spot" on the lateral gastrocnemius corresponding precisely to the image. Together, these findings validated the energetic interpretation and ruled out musculoskeletal, vascular, or neurological origins.

Step 6 – Therapeutic Suggestions and Clinical Outcome

The therapeutic strategy focused on restoring energetic coherence, reintegrating dissociated field zones, and supporting the body's self-regulation mechanisms. Care plan began with low-frequency PEMF (Pulsed Electromagnetic Field) sessions targeting the lateral right leg, combined with bioresonance harmonization protocols.

The patient used a daily practice of grounding techniques, walking barefoot, and focused visualization, imagining light re-entering the hypoactive zones. She received a blend of flower essences aimed at reconnection and integration (including Clematis and Olive), and applied essential oils of rosemary and juniper over the emission sites to stimulate subtle field circulation.

Emotional inquiry revealed themes of personal boundary loss and energetic withdrawal under pressure, which were integrated through breath-led journaling and creative somatic movement.

Therapeutic Outcome

At her seven-week follow-up, the patient reported a clear shift in perception and physical awareness. "It's like that side of my body came back online," she said. She described improved sensory awareness in the right leg and reduced emotional detachment under stress. A follow-up biospectral scan revealed normalization of the previous hypoemissive zones, with symmetrical field balance restored across both legs.

This case illustrates the power of Biospectral Medicine to detect and resolve non-physical energetic disruptions, offering precise mapping of frequency-based imbalances and integrative strategies for full-spectrum recovery.

CASE STUDY

7

Zone 7: Frontal Upper Legs

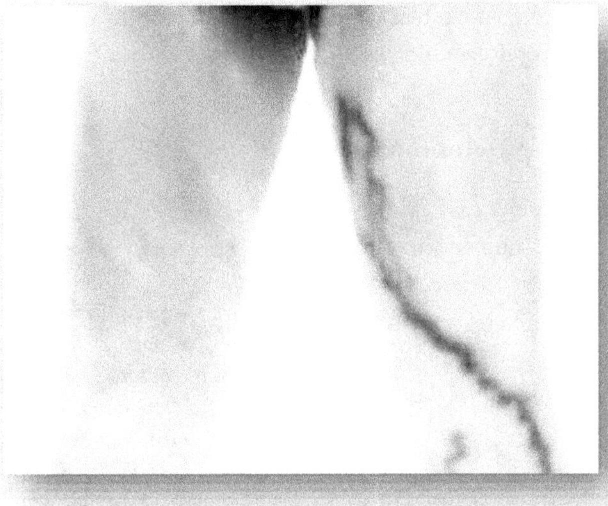

Interpretive Category: Vascular / Circulatory
Clinical Condition: Unilateral Saphenous Overload with Early Valvular Insufficiency
Patient Profile: Female, 50 years old
Date of Birth: 27 June 1975

Step 1 – Zone Relevance: Anatomical and Biospectral Context

The patient reported localized heaviness and pressure along the inner right thigh, particularly after prolonged standing or during late afternoon hours. She described the sensation as "deep fatigue" with occasional itching, without overt swelling.

These symptoms directed our assessment to Zone 7 – Frontal Upper Legs, a region containing the great saphenous vein, inguinal lymphatic collectors, and key superficial venous routes of the lower limb.

In Biospectral Medicine, this zone often expresses superficial venous stress when valvular tone, gravitational drainage, or postural venous return is compromised. Due to the anatomical concentration of superficial veins along the medial thigh, this area becomes a sensitive biospectral site for detecting early venous overload before visible varicosities emerge.

Step 2 – ROI Classification (Emission Pattern)

The spectral image showed a well-defined, branching hyperemissive pattern along the right medial thigh, following the exact trajectory of the great saphenous vein. The emission extended from the inguinal region to the medial knee, with lobulated tributary patterns, and no signal on the contralateral side.

The emission was linear yet irregular, with signs of venous turbulence or pooling, a hallmark of venous reflux or valvular fatigue. There was no striated muscular activation, no dermatomal shape, and no pattern suggestive of fascial or energetic emission. The sharp contrast between legs further confirmed a unilateral vascular event.

Step 3 – Interpretive Category Determination

Given the morphology, trajectory, and unilateral localization of the emission, the most accurate classification was Category 1 – Vascular / Circulatory. The image precisely reflected a superficial venous pathway, with emission density and shape characteristic of saphenous system overload.

There were no signs of muscular compensation or energetic field collapse, and the lymphatic distribution would have appeared nodular or dermal rather than linear and vascular.

The emission profile clearly indicated superficial venous congestion, likely due to valvular insufficiency or gravitational pooling in the absence of mechanical or systemic disease.

BIOSPECTRAL INTERPRETATION RULE

When a biospectral emission follows the precise anatomical path of a known superficial vein, such as the great saphenous, and presents as a branching, lobulated, or linear hyperemissive pattern, the signal reflects superficial venous overload or valvular fatigue. These vascular biosignals are typically unilateral, anatomically consistent, and lack muscular striation or dermatomal logic. In contrast to diffuse edema or metabolic stagnation, this type of emission is sharply defined, pathway-bound, and often intensifies with gravitational stress, making it a clear marker of superficial circulatory strain.

Step 4 – Differential Interpretive Confirmation Through Patient History

During consultation, the patient described a history of right-sided leg heaviness and skin sensitivity along the inner thigh, particularly after long work shifts standing. She denied numbness, cramping, or cold feet, ruling out neuropathic and arterial causes.

She reported a mild visible vein in the groin area that had become more prominent over the past year. There was no trauma, orthopedic limitation, or muscle soreness.

Her symptoms worsened in warm weather and improved with elevation. These descriptions reinforced the hypothesis of superficial venous dilation, especially in the great saphenous territory, and excluded muscular, lymphatic, or neural contributions.

Step 5 – Confirmatory Clinical Tests

A Doppler ultrasound confirmed mild reflux in the right great saphenous vein, with preserved deep venous competence. Venous diameter was slightly enlarged compared to the contralateral limb. An Ankle-Brachial Index was 1.1 bilaterally, ruling out arterial disease. No thrombotic signs or deep vein involvement were observed.

Capillary refill and postural drainage tests revealed sluggish superficial flow on the right side. Bioimpedance analysis detected slight extracellular fluid retention in the right thigh.

These findings confirmed the biospectral hypothesis: early-stage superficial venous insufficiency with no systemic or deep vascular compromise.

Step 6 – Therapeutic Suggestions and Clinical Outcome

The therapeutic strategy focused on restoring venous tone, improving postural drainage, and reducing superficial reflux. The patient was prescribed Aesculus hippocastanum and Centella asiatica in venotonic phytotherapeutic form, with added rutin and hesperidin for endothelial support. Daily elevation breaks and quadriceps-pump activation exercises were introduced to assist in superficial drainage.

Gentle fascial release of the medial thigh and hip flexor area supported decompression of the saphenous path. She began wearing graduated compression shorts during standing hours. On the emotional level, a theme of "bearing pressure without movement" was explored, and somatic therapy encouraged reconnection with right-leg vitality through guided movement and symbolic visualization of flow.

Therapeutic Outcome

At her six-week follow-up, the patient reported a significant reduction in heaviness and skin irritation, with visible flattening of the groin vein. "It no longer feels like my leg is filling up," she said. She resumed moderate walks and daily standing without discomfort. Follow-up imaging showed decreased emission intensity and improved symmetry between legs.

This case demonstrated how Zone 7, when read with vascular logic, offers early detection of superficial circulatory overload, allowing timely, non-invasive correction before degenerative or cosmetic complications emerge.

CASE STUDY

8

Zone 8: Dorsal Upper Legs

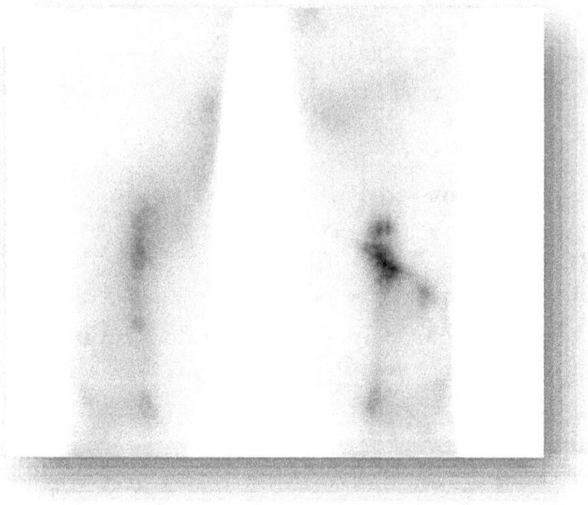

Interpretive Category: Acupuncture / Meridians
Clinical Condition: Bilateral Meridian Overload Along Bladder Channel
Patient Profile: Male, 38 years old
Date of Birth: 11 November 1986

Step 1 – Zone Relevance: Anatomical and Biospectral Context

The patient presented with a sensation of persistent tension and postural fatigue centered in the posterior thighs, often described as "tightness along the back of the legs into the hips," especially after extended periods of standing, driving, or emotional stress. This directed our evaluation to Zone 8 – Dorsal Upper Legs, which anatomically includes the hamstrings, ischial tuberosity region, and gluteal-pelvic interface.

In Biospectral Medicine, this zone is also a major energetic field associated with the Bladder meridian, a vertically aligned acupuncture channel responsible for regulating postural tone, fear response, and energetic grounding. Given the bilateral nature and the emotional context described by the patient, this zone became the primary region of meridian-based field investigation.

Step 2 – ROI Classification (Emission Pattern)

Biospectral imaging revealed symmetrical, vertically aligned hyperemissive fields extending from the gluteal folds through the posterior thighs and into the popliteal region on both legs. The emissions followed the precise trajectory of the Bladder meridian, particularly the segment from BL36 (Chengfu) through BL40 (Weizhong) toward the upper calf.

The emission morphology was non-vascular, non-muscular, and non-dermatomal, with no signs of mechanical strain or reactive hotspots.

The pattern was sharply defined, field-coherent, and resonant with meridian activation, suggesting Qi excess, emotional overload, or unresolved energetic tension held along the Water element channel.

Step 3 – Interpretive Category Determination

Given the bilateral symmetry, energetic alignment, and anatomical irrelevance of the emission, the case was classified under Category 7 – Acupuncture / Meridians. The emission did not correspond to muscle strain, vascular drainage, or structural dysfunction. Instead, it followed a known acupuncture meridian line with precise consistency, ruling out structural categories such as myofascial, skeletal, or nervous system.

The emission's clarity, symmetry, and reproducibility strongly indicated a functional field activation of the Bladder meridian, often linked to emotional containment, fear-pattern holding, and postural energetic rigidity in traditional Chinese energetic interpretation.

BIOSPECTRAL INTERPRETATION RULE

In Biospectral Medicine, when hyperemissive patterns align with known meridian pathways, yet show no correspondence to muscles, nerves, or vessels, they are interpreted as field-level activations of the acupuncture system. These emissions are typically geometrically stable, energetically coherent, and reflect disruptions in the subtle regulatory networks rather than structural dysfunction. In Zone 8 – Dorsal Upper Legs, the Bladder meridian is particularly prone to such expression. The image presented shows symmetrical, vertically aligned hyperemissions following the Bladder channel from BL36 through the popliteal space, consistent with Qi overload, postural energetic stress, or emotional holding within the Water element. This pattern reveals meridian-specific reactivity, not pathological reactivity, making it a clear example of acupuncture-field activation visible through spectral imaging.

Step 4 – Differential Interpretive Confirmation Through Patient History

The patient described a persistent feeling of "tension held behind me", exacerbated during emotionally charged conversations or long static postures. He reported no pain, numbness, or weakness, but noted that the area felt "heavy and reactive", particularly during high-stress periods.

He practiced yoga and reported that deep forward folds would sometimes trigger an emotional release, especially when stretching the posterior chain.

There was no history of trauma, sciatica, or vascular compromise. He also reported frequent feelings of withdrawal, difficulty expressing fear, and a sense of emotional pressure without outlet. These experiences aligned closely with a diagnosis of Qi stagnation along the Bladder meridian, especially linked to unresolved emotional retention in the Water element terrain.

Step 5 – Confirmatory Clinical Tests

A pulse-tongue diagnosis by an acupuncturist revealed tight wiry pulses in the Bladder channel, particularly on the left side, with slight tongue scalloping, indicating internalized stress and Qi tension. Manual palpation along the posterior thigh confirmed tenderness at BL36, BL37, and BL40, consistent with energetic nodal overload.

A biofield scan using resonance-based field imaging showed dense energetic accumulation in the posterior leg fields, matching the spectral hyperemissions.

No abnormalities were found in orthopedic or neurological testing. These findings confirmed the meridian-based energetic congestion and validated the image as an evaluation field expression.

Step 6 – Therapeutic Suggestions and Clinical Outcome

The therapeutic strategy protocol centered on discharging meridian overload, restoring energetic flow, and liberating somato-emotional stagnation. Acupuncture sessions focused on BL36, BL40, BL57, and distal Bladder points (e.g. BL60), supported by moxibustion and cupping on the posterior thigh to stimulate movement of retained Qi. Jin Shin Jyutsu techniques and breath-led hamstring lengthening exercises were integrated daily.

The patient began using Schisandra chinensis and Eleutherococcus senticosus to support adaptive balance in the Water element. Emotional therapy explored the theme of contained fear and chronic internalization, guiding the patient to visualize energetic release through the legs and connection to grounding.

Therapeutic Outcome

At his six-week follow-up, the patient reported increased leg flexibility, reduced emotional rigidity, and a feeling of “being able to let go from the back of my body.” He described a newfound sense of energetic grounding and the ability to navigate difficult conversations without somatic recoil. “It feels like my legs aren't carrying fear anymore,” he said.

A follow-up spectral scan showed reduced emission intensity and more diffused posterior leg fields, indicating meridian rebalancing.

This case confirmed how Biospectral Medicine can visually map acupuncture meridian activation, revealing deeply held energetic patterns and offering precise tools for therapeutic liberation.

CASE STUDY

9

Zone 9: Frontal Abdomen

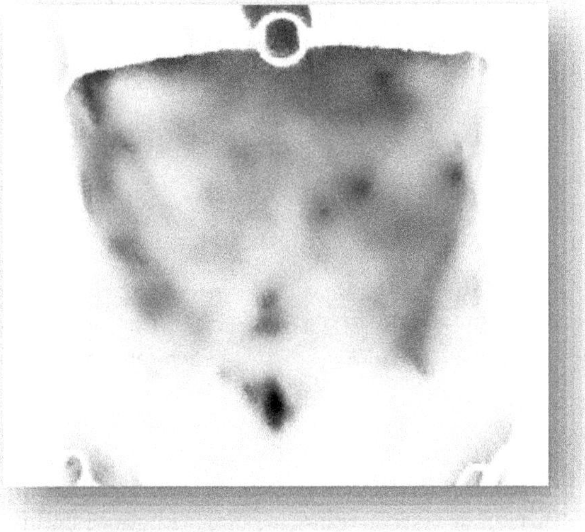

Interpretive Category: Organs / GNM
Clinical Condition: Digestive Terrain Dysregulation with Emotional-Indigestive Conflict
Patient Profile: Female, 41 years old
Date of Birth: 7 May 1984

Step 1 – Zone Relevance: Anatomical and Biospectral Context

The patient presented with long-standing complaints of postprandial discomfort, bloating, and unpredictable bowel movements. These symptoms were described as worse under emotional stress, often accompanied by a sensation of "knots" in the stomach and a vague pressure behind the navel.

This constellation of complaints directed our attention to Zone 9 – Frontal Abdomen, involving the epigastric, periumbilical, and hypogastric regions.

In Biospectral Medicine, this zone is a key interpretive field for assessing visceral regulation, including the stomach, intestines, pancreas, and gut–brain axis. The area also overlaps with somatic expressions of identity conflict, emotional assimilation, and digestive boundary processing, as explored through the lens of German New Medicine (GNM) and integrative terrain theory.

Step 2 – ROI Classification (Emission Pattern)

The biospectral scan revealed centralized, sharply defined hyperemissive zones with dense black emission fields in the epigastric, periumbilical, and hypogastric quadrants, particularly surrounding the navel and suprapubic region.

The emission was non-linear, non-vascular, and did not follow muscular or fascial structures. The pattern showed a static, localized saturation, suggesting organ-level field overload rather than mechanical, circulatory, or reactive stress.

The surrounding abdominal tissue remained neutral, highlighting the emission's specificity and reinforcing its classification as an organ-regulatory signal. The profile strongly indicated functional digestive distress, consistent with visceral stagnation and emotional digestive terrain reactivity.

Step 3 – Interpretive Category Determination

The emission pattern and clinical narrative aligned clearly with Category 6 – Organs / GNM. The central location, depth of signal saturation, and emotional triggers pointed to gastric and intestinal field dysregulation, particularly within the anterior stomach–pancreas–small intestine zones. No evidence of muscular strain, lymphatic pooling, or vascular overload was present.

The emission profile matched the biospectral characteristics of organ-specific energetic tension, a hallmark of unresolved digestive conflict themes, such as nourishment, assimilation, or boundary collapse.

> **BIOSPECTRAL INTERPRETATION RULE**
>
> Organ-related biosignals in Biospectral Medicine typically appear as centralized, irregular hyperemissions in the epigastric, periumbilical, or hypogastric zones, unrelated to vascular, muscular, or dermatomal anatomy. These patterns reflect functional organ field dysregulation and often correspond to emotional-biological conflicts, as described in German New Medicine. In this image, the sharp, focal emissions around the umbilicus and lower abdomen represent digestive field overload and unresolved visceral tension, interpreted as functional distress within the enteric system, linked to emotional themes of assimilation, nourishment, and identity processing.

This categorization was supported by image morphology and by the GNM interpretive model, which views the abdomen as a territory for biologically encoded responses to stress around safety, identity, and absorption, both physical and emotional.

Step 4 – Differential Interpretive Confirmation Through Patient History

During the consultation, the patient described a lifelong pattern of digestive irregularity, particularly worsening in periods of emotional stress, relationship conflict, or professional tension. She reported a deep sense of being unable to digest what life throws at her, and often experienced a post-meal sensation of "tightness or blockage behind the belly button."

She ate a clean, whole-food diet but noted that even healthy meals sometimes led to bloating or fatigue. She denied reflux, gallbladder pain, or rectal symptoms. She had never been diagnosed with IBS but had explored elimination diets without lasting resolution. Her emotional narrative included early family mealtimes marked by control, anxiety, and self-suppression.

These insights aligned precisely with a GNM-oriented organ field conflict, confirming the functional and terrain-based nature of her complaint.

Step 5 – Confirmatory Clinical Tests

Functional testing confirmed the presence of non-structural, organ-level dysfunction. Stool analysis showed low pancreatic elastase, mild dysbiosis, and elevated fermentation markers.

Serum zonulin was elevated, indicating early intestinal permeability, and organic acids revealed incomplete carbohydrate metabolism with low short-chain fatty acid production. Micronutrient markers suggested subclinical B-vitamin depletion and oxidative stress.

Abdominal ultrasound showed no lesions, and routine labs were normal. These results validated the biospectral signature as an accurate representation of functional digestive dysregulation, not pathological damage, reinforcing the case's placement within Organ / GNM terrain mapping.

Step 6 – Therapeutic Suggestions and Clinical Outcome

Therapeutic strategy focused on restoring organ field resilience, improving digestive vitality, and releasing emotional compression associated with the abdominal region. A tailored protocol included plant-based digestive enzymes, slippery elm, and bitter extracts before meals to stimulate organ flow. Probiotic support was provided using soil-based strains alongside fermented vegetables.

Emotional terrain therapy involved abdominal breathing practices, somatic journaling, and use of Bach flowers (particularly *Centaury*, *Agrimony*, and *Walnut*) to support emotional digestion and self-boundary integration. She engaged in daily abdominal self-contact, reconnecting sensory awareness with safety and presence during meals.

A four-week dietary rotation excluded gluten and dairy while emphasizing warm, cooked, enzyme-rich foods with fennel, ginger, and turmeric infusions.

Therapeutic Outcome

At the eight-week follow-up, the patient reported marked improvement in digestion, less bloating, and regular, complete bowel movements. She described post-meal sensations as "peaceful" for the first time in years.

Emotionally, she felt more centered and resilient, noting, "I can finally process what I'm feeling, food and emotions, without freezing."

Follow-up biospectral imaging showed reduced emission intensity and restored abdominal symmetry. This case illustrates how Biospectral Medicine can detect organ-specific terrain imbalances, integrate GNM-based emotional logic, and guide non-invasive strategies for digestive regulation.

CASE STUDY

10

Zone 10: Lateral Right Abdomen

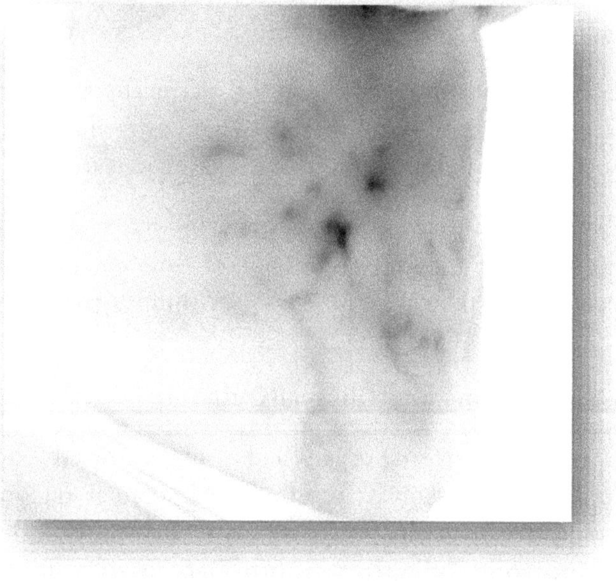

Interpretive Category: Organs / GNM
Clinical Condition: Hepatic Terrain Overload with Emotional Retention Pattern
Patient Profile: Male, 50 years old
Date of Birth: 3 November 1974

Step 1 – Zone Relevance: Anatomical and Biospectral Context

The patient reported persistent fatigue, mood fluctuations, and discomfort localized to the right upper abdominal quadrant, particularly after consuming fatty or processed foods. These symptoms pointed directly to Zone 10 – Lateral Right Abdomen, which anatomically overlays the liver, gallbladder, and hepatic flexure of the colon.

In Biospectral Medicine, this zone is one of the most organ-specific spectral regions, often expressing signs of hepatobiliary congestion, detoxification strain, or terrain stagnation.

The field is also deeply reactive to emotional conflicts involving pressure, control, or injustice, particularly in individuals who suppress frustration. Spectral changes in this zone provide early visualization of functional hepatic burden before structural disease arises.

Step 2 – ROI Classification (Emission Pattern)

The biospectral image revealed a rounded, sharply localized hyperemissive zone on the right lateral rib margin, directly overlying the hepatic projection field. The emission was unilateral, dense, and morphologically distinct from vascular or muscular patterns. No dermatomal or fascial involvement was present.

The signal tone suggested organ-field metabolic saturation, not reactivity or hypoperfusion. The shape and location of the emission precisely matched known hepatic field stress zones, consistent with subclinical detoxification overload or emotional-liver field compression.

Step 3 – Interpretive Category Determination

Given the anatomical precision, emission character, and patient complaint, the case was classified under Category 6 – Organs / GNM. The absence of striated muscle activation, dermatomal spread, or lymphatic pooling ruled out other categories. The hepatic field became the primary focus, and the biospectral signature confirmed an internalized hepatic burden.

In GNM mapping, this area often corresponds to themes of territorial frustration, injustice, or silent anger, which was later echoed in the patient's emotional narrative. The convergence of spectral, anatomical, and emotional indicators confirmed this category with high specificity.

BIOSPECTRAL INTERPRETATION RULE

When a unilateral, well-defined hyperemission appears over the right lateral upper abdomen, particularly along the hepatic projection zone, and shows no correlation with muscular or vascular anatomy, it reflects organ-specific biosignal activation. In Biospectral Medicine, this pattern indicates functional liver strain or detoxification overload, especially when segmental, rounded, and field-stable. Such emissions are often linked to emotional conflicts associated with the liver terrain in German New Medicine, including injustice, suppressed frustration, or unprocessed anger. The clarity and localization of the signal confirm the liver as the primary emission source and differentiate it from diffuse metabolic or structural pathologies.

Step 4 – Differential Interpretive Confirmation Through Patient History

The patient confirmed that for the past two years, he had experienced post-meal sluggishness, mild nausea, and frequent irritability, especially after high-fat meals or under emotional strain. He denied epigastric burning, reflux, or left-sided symptoms.

When specifically questioned, he admitted to a longstanding pattern of internalized anger, often directed at slow decision-making in his corporate environment. "I always swallow my frustration," he said. He also noted tension under his right ribs when lying on his side and a dislike of pressure in that area.

There was no history of liver disease, medication burden, or alcohol overuse. These statements strongly supported a hepatobiliary terrain dysfunction, rooted in both biochemical strain and emotional suppression.

Step 5 – Confirmatory Clinical Tests

A hepatic terrain panel showed mildly elevated GGT and borderline ALT, with normal bilirubin and CRP. Organic acid testing revealed sluggish bile metabolism markers and reduced phase II detox indicators.

Liver ultrasound showed grade I hepatic steatosis without ductal dilation or structural lesions. Hair mineral analysis showed a zinc–copper imbalance, often associated with impaired detoxification and emotional rigidity.

These findings confirmed a functional liver overload, validating the biospectral signature and emotional hypothesis, and distinguishing it from reactive or structural liver disease.

Step 6 – Therapeutic Suggestions and Clinical Outcome

Therapy was designed to support hepatobiliary clearance, reduce terrain stagnation, and address emotional compression. The patient began Silybum marianum, Bupleurum falcatum, and Schisandra chinensis to enhance Phase I/II detoxification. Dietary adjustments emphasized bitter greens, artichoke, and cruciferous vegetables, along with lemon water and apple cider vinegar to support bile flow.

Emotional therapy focused on recognizing and expressing repressed frustration, supported by Bach flowers (Holly and Willow) and right-side-directed breathing exercises to release stored tension. He practiced a daily diaphragmatic breathing protocol and began PEMF sessions targeting the hepatic field.

Therapeutic Outcome

After seven weeks, the patient reported lighter digestion, fewer episodes of post-meal fogginess, and improved mood regulation. "It's like there's more flow inside me, less internal pressure," he said. Follow-up testing showed normalized liver enzymes and improved bile acid metabolism markers. The follow-up biospectral scan revealed significantly reduced emission density over Zone 10, indicating hepatic field recovery.

This case demonstrates how Biospectral Medicine, grounded in the organ–emotion interface, can detect early functional liver stress and guide integrative strategies for restoring both metabolic vitality and emotional resilience.

CASE STUDY

11

Zone 11 – Lateral Left Abdomen

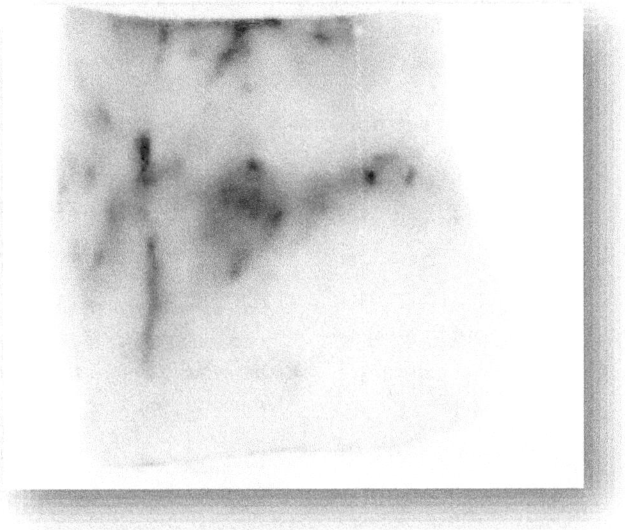

Interpretive Category: Metabolic / Endocrine
Clinical Condition: Functional colonic terrain overload with metabolic retention
Patient Profile: Female, 49 years old
Date of Birth: 3 February 1976

Step 1 – Zone Relevance: Anatomical and Biospectral Context

Zone 11 incorporates the lateral left abdominal quadrant, overlying the descending colon, a critical segment for the compaction, retention, and final preparation of stool. Biospectrally, this region is highly responsive to microbiome imbalance, mucosal burden, and terrain-level endocrine-metabolic retention, particularly when detoxification pathways or hormonal rhythms are disrupted.

In Biospectral Medicine, this zone is often activated in cases of digestive stasis, slow colonic transit, or terrain suppression resulting from emotional inhibition, particularly involving themes of control and "holding in."

Step 2 – ROI Classification (Emission Pattern)

The spectral scan revealed a diffuse, irregular hyperemissive pattern covering the left lower lateral abdomen. The emission was non-axial, non-vascular, and lacked dermatomal logic. Its presentation was terrain-like, consistent with subclinical metabolic retention along the colonic route.

There was no muscular striation or lymphatic spread, and the pattern was sharply confined to the descending colon field. The tone and texture of the emission suggested mucosal metabolic saturation, not reactive or obstructive pathology. This profile aligned with chronic colonic stagnation and functional terrain burden.

Step 3 – Interpretive Category Determination

The emission behavior, anatomical location, and spectral signature clearly aligned with Category 9 – Metabolic / Endocrine. The pattern did not conform to any musculoskeletal or vascular zone logic and was inconsistent with lymphatic or energetic systems. Its diffuse but clearly zoned appearance supports an interpretation of terrain-level metabolic dysfunction, rather than focal organ disease.

In Biospectral Medicine, this type of emission frequently corresponds to retention terrain, especially in patients exhibiting hormonal imbalance, colonic dysbiosis, and subclinical stagnation across elimination systems. The emission's shape, density, and position confirmed its metabolic classification.

BIOSPECTRAL INTERPRETATION RULE

When hyperemissive terrain patterns appear along the lateral abdominal wall without vascular, muscular, or dermatomal alignment, and especially when centered over the descending colon, they suggest metabolic or mucosal burden rather than structural pathology. These emissions tend to be irregular, non-linear, and dispersed, often reflecting stagnation in the colon-liver axis, terrain acidification, or emotional retention conflicts. In Biospectral Medicine, such field-type patterns on the lateral abdomen align with metabolic-endocrine terrain imbalance, particularly when supported by gastrointestinal symptoms or bioresonance findings.

Step 4 – Differential Interpretive Confirmation Through Patient History

The patient described longstanding postprandial bloating, worsened by bread, cheese, and sweets. She reported emotional heaviness, particularly around unprocessed grief and familial tension.

Although she followed a relatively clean diet, she experienced unpredictable digestion, occasional alternating constipation and soft stools, and a chronic sense of internal pressure in the lower abdomen.

She denied rectal bleeding, fever, or weight loss, and had no family history of colorectal disease. Emotional exploration revealed a pattern of emotional holding, perfectionism, and boundary rigidity, psychosocial traits frequently reflected in descending colon terrain reactivity and metabolic compression.

Step 5 – Confirmatory Clinical Tests and Interpretive Integration

Live blood analysis demonstrated rouleaux formation, microbial imbalance, and protein fermentation markers, consistent with fermentative dysbiosis. Stool ecology revealed elevated methane-producing flora and low levels of short-chain fatty acid output, pointing to mucosal terrain depletion. A hair mineral test showed zinc–copper inversion, often linked to endocrine fatigue and poor detoxification.

No structural abnormalities were observed on abdominal ultrasound. These findings confirmed a pattern of metabolic terrain stagnation with corresponding spectral organ field activation on the left abdomen. The test results supported the biospectral impression of a non-reactive yet metabolically burdened colon segment.

Step 6 – Therapeutic Suggestions and Clinical Outcome

The patient began a terrain regulation protocol focused on restoring colon motility, endocrine tone, and mucosal resilience. Her program included L-glutamine, zinc carnosine, and curcuma longa for mucosal repair, along with bitter tonics and prebiotic-fiber rotation.

A probiotic blend targeting methane-dominant dysbiosis was introduced. She followed a warming, anti-inflammatory diet, emphasizing root vegetables, fermented foods, and gentle liver support.

Emotionally, she engaged in somatic journaling and symbolic decluttering, reflecting the GNM-oriented theme of letting go. Flower essences (*Walnut* and *Honeysuckle*) were used to support emotional transition. Light movement, abdominal breathing, and rhythmic outdoor walking helped restore metabolic parasympathetic tone.

Therapeutic Outcome

By her eight-week follow-up, the patient reported regular bowel movements, reduced bloating, and a distinct lightness in the lower abdomen. She noted spontaneous emotional release and described the experience as "feeling lighter both physically and emotionally."

A repeat spectral scan showed clear reduction in hyperemission across Zone 11, with rebalancing of the terrain signal. The resolution of both symptoms and field expression confirmed a successful terrain-based intervention using biosignal-guided therapy aligned with metabolic and emotional rhythms.

CASE STUDY

12

Zone 12 – Lumbar Region

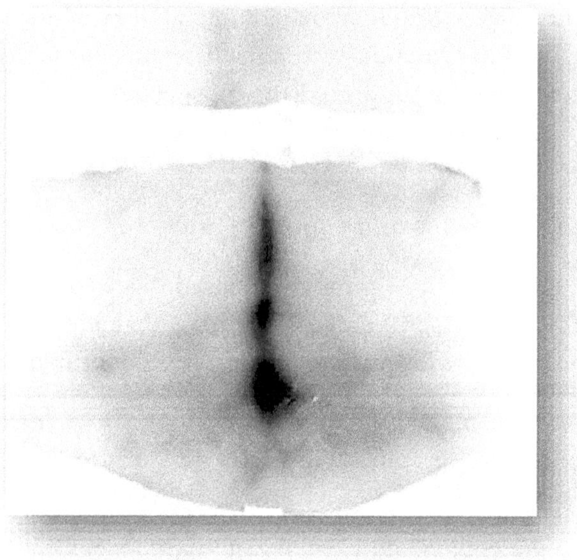

Interpretive Category: Skeletal / Articular
Clinical Condition: Chronic lumbosacral overload with axial compression
Patient Profile: Male, 47 years old
Date of Birth: 25 November 1977

Step 1 – Zone Relevance: Anatomical and Biospectral Context

The patient presented with a long-standing complaint of axial lumbar discomfort, marked by stiffness, postural fatigue, and pain after prolonged standing. This led to the selection of Zone 12 – Lumbar Region, which contains the vertebral column from L2 to S2 and its articulations with the sacroiliac junctions.

Biospectrally, this region reflects skeletal stress, facet joint overload, and vertebrogenic compensation. Because this axial region serves as the central postural fulcrum of the body, emission changes here are strongly correlated with load-bearing imbalance, segmental fixation, or chronic structural strain.

In the context of this case, the emission field aligned anatomically with vertebral and articular structures rather than muscle planes or nerve tracts.

Step 2 – ROI Classification (Emission Pattern)

The CBI scan demonstrated a vertically aligned, symmetrical hyperemissive column running along the midline of the lower back. The emission was dense and sharply demarcated, centered from L3 through the sacral base, without significant lateral spread. There was no evidence of dermatomal radiation, muscular banding, or vascular tributary involvement.

The signal was classified as hyperemissive, consistent with persistent articular stress and deep vertebral activation. The geometric alignment, tone, and spatial coherence of the emission supported a primary mechanical category, rather than reactive or neural.

Step 3 – Interpretive Category Determination

Given the emission's anatomical precision, geometric linearity, and lack of neurovascular patterning, the case was classified as Category 3 – Skeletal / Articular. The hyperemissive ROI followed the vertebral midline without deviation, ruling out muscular compensation or energetic field effects. Importantly, the emission terminated at the sacral base, consistent with SI joint overload and lumbosacral transition stress.

There was no indication of discogenic or myofascial contribution based on the absence of paraspinal spill or peripheral banding. These elements confirmed the diagnosis as a segmental articular compensation along the axial skeleton.

Step 4 – Differential Interpretive Confirmation Through Patient History

The patient reported a five-year history of low back stiffness and dull pain that worsened with prolonged standing or walking on hard surfaces. He denied sharp pain, numbness, or leg symptoms, helping to exclude nerve root involvement. He also described a sensation of internal compression and a recurring "locked" feeling in the lower back.

He had no prior diagnosis of herniation but recalled years of poor posture and pelvic asymmetry due to prior athletic overuse. His professional role required long hours standing, which correlated with mechanical axial fatigue. The absence of reactive flares, systemic symptoms, or sciatica reinforced the articular category.

BIOSPECTRAL INTERPRETATION RULE

When a symmetrical, vertically aligned hyperemissive column appears along the lumbar midline, without lateral radiation or muscular diffusion, the pattern is best interpreted as skeletal-articular activation. In Biospectral Medicine, these emissions reflect chronic axial loading, vertebral facet stress, or sacroiliac compensation, particularly when centered over L4–S1. The emission's geometric regularity, central anchoring, and absence of dermatomal or vascular features distinguish it from muscular overuse or neuropathic signaling. This pattern indicates mechanical overload or fixation within the axial skeleton and is especially relevant in postural fatigue, facet joint hypertrophy, or vertebrogenic stiffness syndromes.

Step 5 – Confirmatory Clinical Tests

Orthopedic testing revealed limited lumbar extension and localized pain on facet loading at L4–L5. The Stork test indicated mild instability at the sacroiliac joint, while palpation showed segmental stiffness across the lower lumbar spine. Neurological screening, including straight leg raise and reflexes, was unremarkable.

Postural evaluation showed anterior pelvic tilt and slight leg-length discrepancy. Imaging revealed moderate facet joint hypertrophy at L5–S1 without disc herniation. Spectrovascular Response Test (SVRT) revealed delayed thermal recovery over the lumbosacral zone, supporting chronic mechanical stress and vertebral compensatory behavior. These findings confirmed the articular-skeletal origin of the biospectral emission.

Step 6 – Therapeutic Suggestions and Clinical Outcome

A targeted structural support protocol was developed to reduce segmental compression and enhance vertebral articulation. The approach included axial decompression maneuvers, sacroiliac joint balancing techniques, and the use of Boswellia serrata and collagen type II for articular support.

Daily posture correction routines and core activation exercises were prescribed to stabilize the lumbar spine and correct pelvic tilt.

Emotional mapping revealed themes of "rigidity under pressure" and long-term structural holding. Therapeutic support included flower essences (*Oak* and *Rock Water*) and guided movement therapy to reestablish lumbopelvic fluidity.

Therapeutic Outcome

By week seven, the patient reported a marked decrease in morning stiffness and improved ease during weight-bearing tasks. He described a "feeling of vertical space" returning to his lower back and greater ease in transitions from standing to sitting.

A follow-up biospectral scan showed clear reduction in the midline hyperemission and restored field balance across the lumbosacral arc. The therapeutic response confirmed both the interpretive accuracy and biomechanical relevance of Zone 12 as a window into axial skeletal overload, enabling targeted non-invasive correction guided by biospectral insight.

CASE STUDY

13

Zone 13 – Chest and Sternum

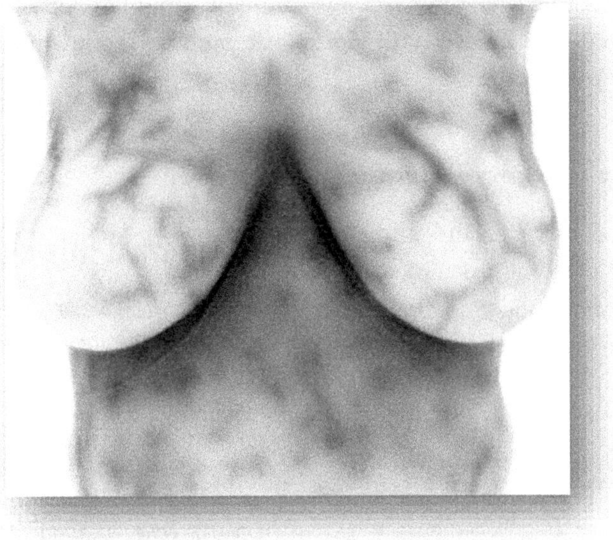

Interpretive

Category: Metabolic / Endocrine
Clinical Condition: Cyclical breast tension, emotional instability, and fatigue worsening before menstruation
Patient Profile: Female, 38 years old
Date of Birth: 22 May 1987

Step 1 – Zone Relevance: Anatomical and Biospectral Context

The patient reported recurring premenstrual symptoms, including breast congestion, mood instability, and progressive fatigue during the second half of her cycle. These complaints directed clinical attention to Zone 13 – Chest and Sternum, a region frequently impacted in hormonal dysregulation, particularly involving estrogen–progesterone imbalances.

In Biospectral Medicine, the anterior thoracic fascia and parasternal tissues are recognized as sensitive zones for systemic endocrine signaling, especially in women presenting with cyclical vascular and emotional symptoms.

The anterior chest, due to its integration with lymphatic drainage, cardiac-autonomic fields, and mammary endocrine receptors, often reflects metabolic or detoxification impairments that do not localize to glandular structures but manifest peripherally through biosignal patterns.

Step 2 – ROI Classification (Emission Pattern)

The biospectral image showed a bilaterally diffuse, branching hyperemissive field extending across the upper and medial breast regions and converging over the sternum. The emission lacked dermatomal or muscular patterning and followed a vascular distribution, consistent with capillary dilation under systemic influence. The pattern was symmetrical but more pronounced on the left parasternal line.

There were no signs of reactive foci, neuromuscular segmentation, or nodular concentration. This spectral field presented as a low-grade, hormonally modulated vascular biosignal, consistent with systemic estrogenic influence and inefficient metabolic clearance pathways rather than structural or reactive pathology.

Step 3 – Interpretive Category Determination

Based on the spectral findings and clinical correspondence, the pattern was classified under Category 9 – Metabolic / Endocrine. The diffuse emission field, vascular mapping, and cyclical timing supported an interpretation of functional estrogen dominance, often linked to hepatic clearance inefficiencies, gut-liver axis imbalance, and altered steroid metabolism.

The absence of spectral features suggestive of lymphatic stagnation, immune reactivity, or neuromuscular tension further excluded other categories. The biosignal expression in Zone 13 was interpreted as a peripheral indicator of endocrine retention and biochemical overload, with systemic hormonal signatures visualized through the anterior thoracic fascia and microvasculature.

BIOSPECTRAL INTERPRETATION RULE

When a diffuse, vascular-patterned hyperemissive field appears bilaterally across the upper thoracic region, especially over the medial breast quadrants and parasternal line, without myofascial segmentation or inflammatory foci, the pattern is best interpreted as metabolic–endocrine signaling. In Biospectral Medicine, this emission reflects hormonal terrain overload, most commonly associated with estrogenic retention, impaired hepatic clearance, or altered steroid metabolism. The branching vascular geometry, cyclical reproducibility, and thoracic localization distinguish it from lymphatic congestion or autonomic activation. This pattern indicates systemic hormonal influence on peripheral vasculature, particularly in the context of endocrine–hepatic–intestinal axis dysfunction, and is frequently observed in cases of estrogen dominance, premenstrual terrain dysregulation, or detoxification fatigue.

Step 4 – Differential Interpretive Confirmation Through Patient History

The patient described symptoms that intensified in the luteal phase, including breast heaviness, fluid retention, irritability, and fatigue. She reported a long history of oral contraceptive use and irregular bowel function, particularly during PMS. She had no history of mastitis, breast nodules, or dermatological conditions in the region.

Cardiopulmonary symptoms were absent. The symptoms did not appear in response to exertion, mechanical posture, or seasonal shifts, ruling out myofascial, respiratory, or immune origins.

The cyclicity, hormonal history, and digestive profile reinforced the hypothesis of estrogen recirculation, likely linked to reduced hepatic conjugation and microbiota imbalance, confirming a metabolic–endocrine source for the spectral findings.

Step 5 – Confirmatory Clinical Tests

Salivary hormone analysis showed an elevated estradiol-to-progesterone ratio in the second half of the cycle. Urinary organic acid testing revealed markers of reduced methylation and phase II liver detoxification strain. A dried urine hormone profile (DUTCH) confirmed the dominance of the 16-OH estrone metabolic pathway, associated with increased estrogenic activity and poor clearance.

Functional stool testing revealed reduced B-glucuronidase clearance capacity, reinforcing enterohepatic recirculation of estrogens. Spectrovascular Response Testing revealed a delayed recovery curve in Zone 13, consistent with metabolic retention. No structural imaging was required. These findings collectively confirmed a functional metabolic overload with peripheral biospectral signature in the thoracic hormonal field.

Step 6 – Therapeutic Suggestions and Clinical Outcome

The therapeutic strategy protocol was focused on supporting estrogen detoxification, restoring hepatic conjugation, and improving hormonal terrain resilience. Nutritional interventions included a fiber-rich, cruciferous vegetable-based diet, with targeted use of indole-3-carbinol, calcium-D-glucarate, and flaxseed lignans to support estrogen modulation.

A methylation support formula (B6, B12, folate, betaine) was introduced, along with liver support using Silybum marianum and Taraxacum officinale.

Castor oil packs were applied over the liver five times per week. Emotional support focused on Pulsatilla and flower essences addressing hormonal sensitivity and emotional release. Breathing exercises and thoracic fascia opening were prescribed to encourage spectral flow. A bioresonance protocol was used to modulate estrogen receptor resonance and terrain frequency.

Therapeutic Outcome

At her seven-week review, the patient reported a clear reduction in premenstrual symptoms, with breast congestion becoming minimal and emotional stability greatly improved. Energy levels were more consistent, and she noted a “sense of flow” in her chest that had not been present before. Repeat spectral imaging showed a significant decrease in emission density across Zone 13, with resolution of the branching vascular pattern.

Follow-up hormone testing showed a shift toward the protective 2-OH estrogen pathway, and improved methylation capacity. The case demonstrated how metabolic and endocrine dysfunctions can be precisely localized and monitored using spectral zone-based logic, with non-invasive therapies producing measurable terrain resolution.

CASE STUDY

14

Zone 14 – Left Axillary

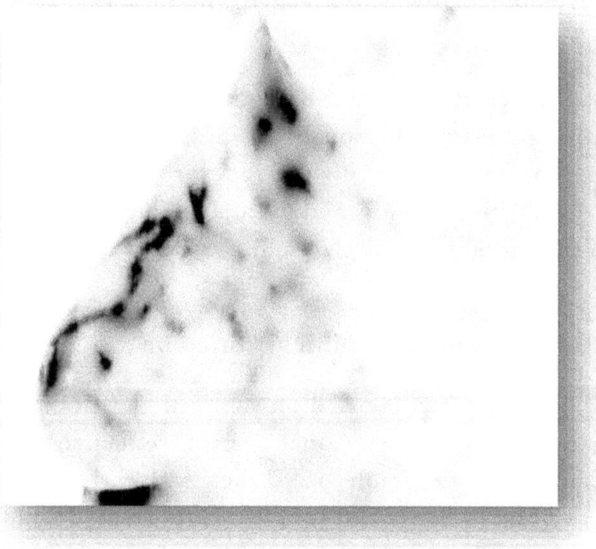

Interpretive Category: Lymphatic / Immune
Clinical Condition: Post-Infectious Terrain Retention with Localized Lymphatic **Stagnation**
Patient Profile: Female, 45 years old
Date of Birth: 7 April 1980

Step 1 – Zone Relevance: Anatomical and Biospectral Context

The patient reported a lingering sense of fullness and intermittent discomfort beneath the left axilla, persisting for several weeks following recovery from a respiratory infection. Although systemic symptoms had resolved, she described a vague "blocked" sensation that was more evident during arm movement or emotional stress.

This led us to evaluate Zone 14 – Left Axillary, a key lymphatic field responsible for drainage from the lateral thoracic wall, breast tissue, and upper extremity.

In Biospectral Medicine, this zone is a primary receptor of immune terrain residue, especially post-infectious or reactive states. It frequently registers biospectral changes even when no clinical reactivity is visible, due to stagnation of lymphatic fluid, fascial resistance, or incomplete terrain clearance.

Based on the history and anatomical specificity of the symptom, Zone 14 was prioritized for spectral investigation.

Step 2 – ROI Classification (Emission Pattern)

The biospectral image revealed a localized, terrain-like hyperemissive field beneath the left axilla, forming a cluster of non-linear, rounded emission zones. The signal extended slightly into the upper medial arm and lateral thoracic wall but did not cross dermatomal, vascular, or muscular boundaries.

The emission had a blunted and static appearance, lacking directional flow or segmentation. This geometry is consistent with lymphatic terrain retention, not active reactivity, not vascular dilation, and not neural projection.

No corresponding signal was observed on the right side, confirming unilateral dysfunction. The spectral tone was low to moderate in intensity and remained topographically anchored to the lymphatic drainage basin.

Step 3 – Interpretive Category Determination

Based on the emission pattern, clinical context, and zone anatomy, the signal was classified under Category 5 – Lymphatic / Immune. The lack of radiation, vascular trace, or neuromuscular involvement ruled out adjacent interpretive categories.

The unilateral nature and terrain-like tone of the emission suggested residual immune load following infection, a pattern frequently observed in Biospectral Medicine after the immune system has resolved acute reactivity but terrain drainage remains incomplete.

There was no suggestion of autoimmune reactivation, nor any features consistent with endocrine or metabolic biosignatures. The case fit the classical profile of low-grade immune stagnation in the axillary nodal field.

BIOSPECTRAL INTERPRETATION RULE

When a blunted, non-linear hyperemissive field appears unilaterally beneath the axillary fold, without vascular branching or muscular segmentation, the pattern is best interpreted as lymphatic–immune terrain retention. In Biospectral Medicine, this emission reflects post-infectious or post-inflammatory stagnation, often due to unresolved nodal clearance or fascial impedance. The absence of dermatomal radiation, bilateral symmetry, or dynamic vascular tone distinguishes it from endocrine, neural, or circulatory patterns. This configuration typically indicates low-grade immune load or residual microbial terrain in the superficial axillary system.

Step 4 – Differential Interpretive Confirmation Through Patient History

The patient had experienced a strong respiratory infection two months prior, requiring antibiotics. Though acute symptoms resolved, she began noticing localized fullness beneath the left arm, particularly during exertion or long periods of standing.

There was no redness, swelling, or pain, but she described the area as "congested" or "unresolved." She denied fever, fatigue, joint stiffness, or systemic flare-ups. She reported that the sensation worsened before menstruation and improved slightly after sweating or sauna use.

These details, combined with the localized biospectral findings, ruled out vascular, neural, and muscular causes. The cyclical aggravation suggested mild hormonal influence on terrain drainage, but the primary source was interpreted as post-infectious lymphatic retention.

Step 5 – Confirmatory Clinical Tests

Palpation of the axillary fold showed mild tenderness and limited fascial glide, without nodal hardness or acute reactivity. Lymphatic ultrasound revealed slight swelling of superficial nodes, consistent with past immune activation but no structural change.

Laboratory markers were normal, excluding systemic reactivity. Bioresonance indicated low-level microbial patterns with terrain retention, and Spectrovascular Response Testing in Zone 14 showed delayed post-cooling recovery, typical of lymphatic biospectral congestion.

Findings confirmed an unresolved lymphatic terrain burden following infection.

Step 6 – Therapeutic Suggestions and Clinical Outcome

Therapy focused on clearing local terrain stagnation, enhancing lymphatic flow, and completing immune recovery. A lymphatic herbal blend with Galium aparine, Calendula officinalis, and Echinacea angustifolia supported drainage and modulation.

Castor oil packs were applied to the left axilla and thorax three times weekly, combined with dry brushing, contrast hydrotherapy, thoracic breathing, and light rebounding to stimulate lymphatic dynamics.

From a terrain standpoint, Carcinosinum was used to address residual post-infectious biosignatures and internal tension, while emotional review explored suppressed resentment through journaling and somatic release.

Therapeutic Outcome

After four weeks of care, the patient reported that the sensation of axillary fullness had completely resolved. She described feeling "lighter and more mobile," particularly in the left side of her upper body. She resumed physical activity with ease and noted that her breathing felt "more open" after morning stretching.

Repeat biospectral imaging demonstrated complete resolution of emission in Zone 14, with no compensatory activation in adjacent territories. Spectrovascular Response Testing showed normalized recovery. In her own words: "It's like I moved something that had been stuck there for months. I feel clearer."

This case exemplifies how subtle, unresolved lymphatic dysfunctions can be identified early through spectral imaging and resolved using non-invasive, terrain-oriented interventions in Biospectral Medicine.

CASE STUDY

15

Zone 15 – Right Axillary

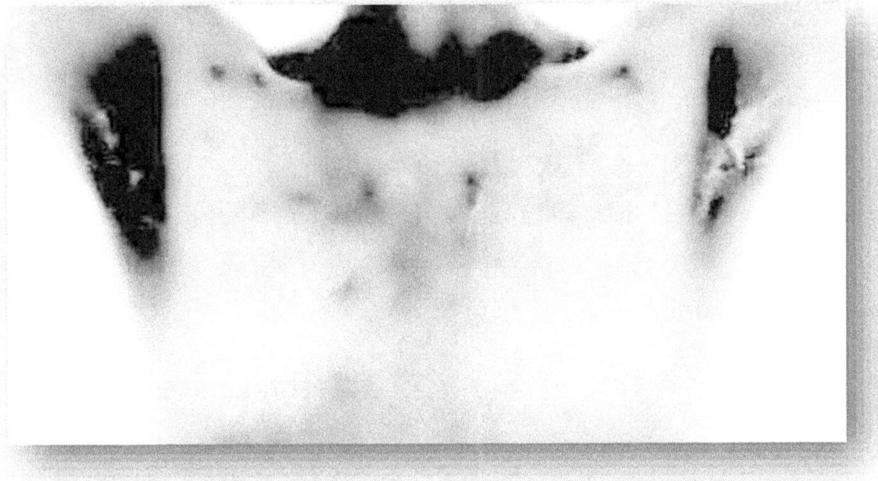

The emission seen in this image is not consistent with lymphatic or immune patterns, as it lacks nodal clustering, drainage geometry, or terrain-like stagnation. It also does not reflect dermal or inflammatory processes, which typically present with focal, peaked emissions and defined borders. Instead, the diffuse, radiant, non-structural signal extending beyond anatomical boundaries is characteristic of energetic–frequency imbalance. This image illustrates a non-local biospectral disturbance, likely linked to biofield disruption or environmental frequency overload, and is best classified under Category 8 – Energetic / Frequency.

Interpretive Category: Energetic / Frequency
Clinical Condition: Localized Axillary Emission with Biofield Disruption
Patient Profile: Male, 52 years old
Date of Birth: 3 March 1973

Step 1 – Zone Relevance: Anatomical and Biospectral Context

The patient presented with a sensation of internal agitation on the right side of the chest, a vague fullness in the axillary region, and a recurrent sense of energetic "imbalance" or "pull" without physical pain. These complaints, while difficult to localize using conventional anatomical frameworks, pointed toward Zone 15 – Right Axillary, a region that in Biospectral Medicine acts as a subtle receptor for field-based interference and vibrational terrain imbalance.

While anatomically the axillary zone contains lymphatic structures, neurovascular bundles, and connective tissue, in energetic evaluations it is also sensitive to biofield distortions arising from electromagnetic exposure, unresolved vibrational conflict, or polarity imbalances within the chest's energetic architecture. The unusual nature of the patient's symptoms and their lateralized presence led to targeted biospectral evaluation of this zone.

Step 2 – ROI Classification (Emission Pattern)

Biospectral imaging revealed a diffuse, radiant hyperemissive field concentrated in the right axillary basin, extending medially toward the anterior thoracic wall. The emission was asymmetrical, with no corresponding signal on the left side, and lacked vascular, lymphatic, or muscular patterning. Its geometry was soft-edged, planar, and field-like, without nodal localization or structural contour.

The emission extended into regions that are not anatomically connected through tissue continuity, suggesting a non-structural origin. There were no signs of focal reactivity, dermatomal radiation, or muscular segmentation. The signal's diffuse nature and spectral tone pointed toward energetic field disruption rather than anatomical dysfunction.

Step 3 – Interpretive Category Determination

Given the absence of vascular, lymphatic, reactive, or mechanical features, the emission was classified under Category 8 – Energetic / Frequency.

The biosignal behavior, its diffuse geometry, non-local spread, and disconnection from structural anatomy, aligned with known spectral patterns of biofield interference, often seen in individuals exposed to electromagnetic fields, geopathic stress, or unresolved terrain-based energetic stressors.

The lateralization and non-reactivity of the emission excluded nervous system or autonomic categories. In Biospectral Medicine, such patterns reflect vibrational incoherence, where spectral data reveals energetic blockage, resonance overload, or field compression affecting a specific zone without physical correlates.

> **BIOSPECTRAL INTERPRETATION RULE**
>
> *When a diffuse, asymmetrical emission appears without anatomical boundaries, segmentation, or vascular structure, the pattern is classified as energetic–frequency, reflecting vibrational incoherence, biofield disruption, or environmental frequency overload. In this image, the right axillary signal presents as a radiant, unstructured field extending beyond zone borders, lacking nodal, muscular, or dermatomal anchors, and is best interpreted as a localized spectral distortion within Category 8 – Energetic / Frequency.*

Step 4 – Differential Interpretive Confirmation Through Patient History

The patient reported no pain, swelling, or trauma in the axillary or thoracic regions. Instead, he described a persistent sense of "charge" or "static" under the right arm, often intensified when near certain electronic devices or during prolonged screen exposure. He denied respiratory, lymphatic, or cardiovascular symptoms.

He noted difficulty sleeping on the right side and described episodes of inexplicable agitation or restlessness, especially in crowded environments or after long hours indoors.

He had a history of high sensitivity to noise, fluorescent lights, and certain wireless devices. There were no infectious triggers or immune burdens in recent history. These responses, along with the emission profile, supported a diagnosis of localized energetic terrain distortion rather than structural or immune dysfunction.

Step 5 – Confirmatory Clinical Tests

No structural abnormalities were found on ultrasound or palpation. Laboratory markers were within normal range, including CRP, white blood cells, and liver enzymes. Lymphatic testing was negative for retention or nodal strain.

Biofield resonance testing revealed a pattern of electromagnetic hypersensitivity and incoherent frequency imprinting, particularly in the right thoracic and axillary meridians. Auricular terrain mapping showed energetic congestion in zones correlating with right lung polarity and upper thoracic field tension.

Spectrovascular Response Testing demonstrated anomalous spectral persistence post-cooling, with non-linear decay curves, a finding commonly associated with frequency-based field disturbances rather than metabolic or vascular stagnation. These findings validated the classification as an energetic/frequency terrain imbalance.

Step 6 – Therapeutic Suggestions and Clinical Outcome

Care plan centered on realigning the biofield, clearing environmental frequency overload, and stabilizing energetic terrain flow. The patient was instructed to reduce exposure to high-frequency EMFs, install grounding mechanisms near sleep and work areas, and use protective shielding fabrics during high-exposure periods. A vibrational protocol was initiated, including homeopathic resonance drops matched to terrain distortion patterns, as well as regular pulsed light and bioresonance sessions to restore spectral coherence.

He began a morning routine involving barefoot grounding, coherence breathing, and polarity balancing exercises. The remedy Phosphorus was prescribed to address energetic permeability and upper field dysregulation. A terrain-specific frequency imprint was customized and delivered weekly to recalibrate spectral flow.

Therapeutic Outcome

After six weeks, the patient reported a marked reduction in the sensation of static or charge under the right arm. He noted that he could sleep on his right side without discomfort and felt more resilient in urban environments. His subjective clarity and emotional balance improved, and he described a sense of "reconnection" with his chest and upper body.

Repeat biospectral imaging showed complete resolution of the axillary emission, with reestablished symmetry across both axillary fields. The case illustrates the role of Biospectral Medicine in detecting and correcting non-structural, frequency-based disruptions, offering clear therapeutic pathways for individuals with invisible but measurable energetic terrain imbalances.

CASE STUDY

16

Zone 16 – Upper Back

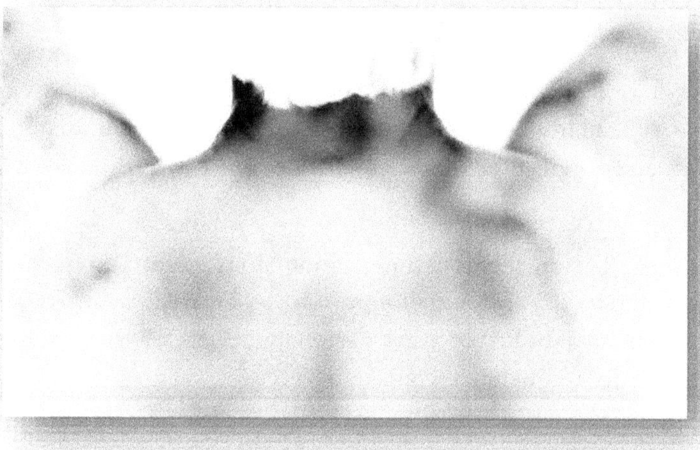

The descending emission from the cervical base to the scapular region is not vascular, as it lacks branching or tubular structure, nor is it neural, since it does not follow dermatomal or unilateral nerve paths. Instead, its diffuse, symmetrical, and terrain-like geometry is characteristic of metabolic–endocrine biosignals, often reflecting adrenal strain, thyroid dysregulation, or systemic biochemical overload expressed through the cervicothoracic fascia.

Interpretive Category: Metabolic / Endocrine
Clinical Condition: Chronic fatigue, cognitive slowdown, and upper thoracic tension
Patient Profile: Female, 41 years old
Date of Birth: 2 December 1983

Step 1 – Zone Relevance: Anatomical and Biospectral Context

The patient reported persistent fatigue, difficulty concentrating, and a sensation of upper back tension that worsened in the afternoon. These symptoms had no clear musculoskeletal trigger and were resistant to posture correction, massage, or physical activity. This profile directed attention to Zone 16 – Upper Back, covering the paravertebral and scapular regions from T1 to T5.

In Biospectral Medicine, this zone acts as a peripheral receptor for metabolic load, often reflecting dysfunctions of the thyroid axis, adrenal regulation, or hepatic detoxification pathways. The upper back fascia and connective matrix serve as conduits for systemic biochemical strain, especially in cases of hormonal imbalance, terrain exhaustion, or subclinical endocrine dysregulation.

Step 2 – ROI Classification (Emission Pattern)

The biospectral image revealed a broad, symmetrical hyperemissive field across the upper thoracic region, with a descending spectral line originating at the cervical-thoracic junction, passing through the trapezius, and extending toward the scapular margins. The emission showed no dermatomal or myofascial segmentation and lacked vascular branching.

The tone was diffuse and terrain-like, without focal peaks or reactive hyperemissions. The geometry suggested systemic rather than localized pathology. The descending line, while linear, was non-vascular and non-neural, fitting the known presentation of neuroendocrine overflow or biochemical retention expressed through the upper thoracic fascia.

Step 3 – Interpretive Category Determination

Based on its symmetrical distribution, non-structural geometry, and association with cognitive and fatigue symptoms, the emission was classified under Category 9 – Metabolic / Endocrine. There were no signs of myofascial strain, nerve compression, or reactive reaction.

The absence of vascular or dermatomal architecture confirmed that the spectral signature was not circulatory or neurological. Instead, the bilateral terrain expression aligned with chronic metabolic overload, likely involving HPA axis fatigue, thyroid underregulation, or detoxification strain. This spectral pattern is frequently seen in individuals with burnout syndromes, adrenal flattening, or mid-phase endocrine dysfunction.

Step 4 – Differential Interpretive Confirmation Through Patient History

The patient described constant low energy, poor mental focus, and increasing difficulty recovering after stress or exertion. She denied physical pain in the upper back, but noted a sensation of "weight" or internal tightness in that area. Symptoms worsened with mental effort or poor sleep. She had a history of irregular cycles, poor tolerance to fasting, and caffeine overuse.

There was no history of reactive conditions, trauma, or musculoskeletal injury. Her lifestyle included long screen hours and disrupted circadian rhythms. These findings excluded postural or structural causes and instead suggested a functional metabolic collapse with probable adrenal and thyroid involvement.

BIOSPECTRAL INTERPRETATION RULE

When a diffuse, symmetrical hyperemissive field appears across the upper thoracic region, often descending from the cervicothoracic junction without muscular or dermatomal segmentation, the pattern is best interpreted as metabolic–endocrine in origin. In Biospectral Medicine, this emission reflects systemic biochemical burden, adrenal flattening, or thyroid signaling imbalance expressed through the upper back fascia. Its bilateral terrain-like geometry and absence of structural anchors distinguish it from myofascial, neural, or reactive categories.

Step 5 – Confirmatory Clinical Tests

Salivary cortisol revealed flattened diurnal rhythm with low morning and high evening levels, indicating adrenal dysregulation. Serum TSH was borderline elevated with suboptimal free T3, consistent with compensated hypothyroidism. Organic acid testing revealed impaired phase II detoxification markers and mild mitochondrial stress.

Blood glucose was within normal range, but the patient showed signs of reactive hypoglycemia under fasting. Thermographic Spectrovascular Response Testing confirmed delayed cooling recovery in Zone 16, suggesting spectral stagnation linked to metabolic congestion. These findings confirmed the presence of systemic metabolic and endocrine terrain imbalance, correlating directly with the spectral emission pattern.

Step 6 – Therapeutic Suggestions and Clinical Outcome

Care plan aimed to support adrenal recovery, thyroid regulation, and metabolic terrain clearance. Nutritional support focused on protein-rich breakfasts, stabilizing blood sugar, and adding iodine-rich foods and selenium to improve thyroid function. Adaptogenic herbal support included Withania somnifera and Rhodiola rosea, alongside vitamin C and B-complex for adrenal repair.

The patient was instructed in circadian rhythm resetting techniques, including morning light exposure, screen reduction after sunset, and scheduled rest. Detoxification was supported with broccoli sprouts, chlorella, and gentle liver-supporting infusions.

Breathwork focused on upper thoracic expansion to mobilize terrain stagnation in Zone 16. Bioresonance protocols targeted hypothalamic imprint correction and endocrine signal harmonization.

Therapeutic Outcome

After six weeks, the patient reported improved energy stability, better morning alertness, and decreased cognitive fog. The sensation of upper back weight diminished, and she resumed light physical activity without fatigue crashes.

Repeat spectral imaging showed normalization of the diffuse upper back emission, and the descending line from the neck was no longer visible. Salivary cortisol improved in rhythm and amplitude. She described the outcome as "a return to clear, calm functioning."

This case demonstrates the precision of Biospectral Medicine in identifying metabolic terrain overload and translating non-local biosignals into targeted, non-invasive therapeutic recovery.

CASE STUDY

17

Zone 17 – Frontal Neck and Supraclavicular Region

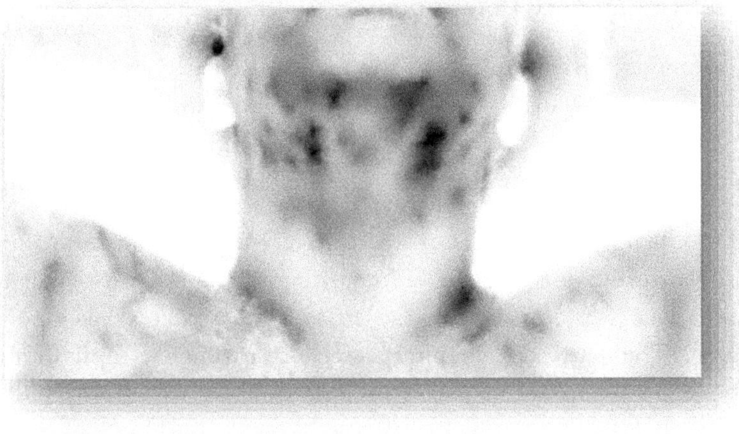

Interpretive Category: Lymphatic / Immune
Clinical Condition: Localized terrain retention with post-infectious lymphatic congestion
Patient Profile: Male, 39 years old
Date of Birth: 19 February 1986

Step 1 – Zone Relevance: Anatomical and Biospectral Context

The patient reported a persistent sensation of neck fullness, intermittent throat tightness, and vague discomfort near the clavicles, which began shortly after recovering from a respiratory infection. These symptoms directed clinical attention to Zone 17 – Frontal Neck and Supraclavicular Region, an area that includes superficial and deep cervical lymph chains, the thoracic duct junction, and drainage paths for the upper thorax and cranial base.

In Biospectral Medicine, this zone plays a vital role in reflecting the immune and lymphatic terrain, particularly when local biosignals point to unresolved immune stress, post-infectious stagnation, or impaired drainage from the head–neck interface. Given the anatomical drainage complexity and the patient's post-infectious context, Zone 17 was prioritized for detailed spectral evaluation.

Step 2 – ROI Classification (Emission Pattern)

The biospectral scan revealed a patchy, moderately hyperemissive field extending across the anterior neck and supraclavicular depressions bilaterally. The emission was irregular in shape, non-linear, and showed a blotched terrain-like pattern, particularly in the lower cervical and clavicular margins.

The pattern was not aligned with dermatomes, muscle chains, or vascular pathways, and did not show any focal nodular emission. The diffuse distribution and bilateral presentation excluded mechanical strain and favored lymphatic stasis with immune terrain retention, especially in the absence of muscular or endocrine features.

Step 3 – Interpretive Category Determination

The emission's geometry, distribution, and tone aligned clearly with Category 5 – Lymphatic / Immune. No signs of vascular overexpression, endocrine hyporeactivity, or autonomic imbalance were observed. The spectral tone was consistent with chronic immune retention, a finding commonly seen after respiratory infections, allergies, or sinus terrain overload.

The absence of nodular peaks ruled out acute reactivity, while the symmetrical distribution excluded localized infection or trauma. Other categories such as Muscular / Myofascial and Metabolic / Endocrine were ruled out due to lack of structural segmentation or systemic metabolic features. The pattern was interpreted as residual lymphatic burden and terrain congestion in the cervical-supraclavicular lymphatic field.

Step 4 – Differential Interpretive Confirmation Through Patient History

The patient confirmed that symptoms began following a prolonged viral infection affecting the upper respiratory tract, which required antibiotic approach. While respiratory symptoms had resolved, he continued to feel "clogged" around the base of the neck, especially after long workdays or exposure to allergens. He denied fever, hoarseness, thyroid issues, or mechanical pain.

There was no history of lymph node biopsies or autoimmune disease. He also described a history of poor drainage from the head and sinuses, frequent mucosal irritation, and sensitivity to weather changes. These historical details confirmed the post-infectious, non-reactive nature of the congestion, consistent with low-grade lymphatic stagnation.

BIOSPECTRAL INTERPRETATION RULE

When patchy, irregular hyperemissions are observed across the anterior cervical and supraclavicular regions, particularly when symmetrical, non-nodular, and terrain-like in texture, the pattern indicates lymphatic terrain retention rather than acute reactivity. In Biospectral Medicine, this presentation reflects impaired drainage through the deep and superficial cervical lymph chains, often following respiratory infections, mucosal overload, or immune system strain. The absence of vascular linearity or muscular alignment helps differentiate it from endocrine, fascial, or neurogenic origins. This emission configuration signals low-grade immunological burden with regional stagnation of terrain detoxification.

Step 5 – Confirmatory Clinical Tests

Manual palpation of the supraclavicular fossae revealed mild tissue tension and tenderness without discrete nodules or structural blockages. Functional terrain testing using bioresonance identified residual viral imprinting and terrain disruption associated with the upper respiratory tract. Basic blood work, including leukocyte count and C-reactive protein, was normal.

Cervical lymphatic ultrasound showed mildly distended superficial lymph channels with no architectural abnormalities. The Spectrovascular Response Test revealed delayed cooling normalization in Zone 17, consistent with terrain congestion rather than acute reactivity. These tests confirmed the spectral interpretation of immune terrain burden in the cervical drainage zone.

Step 6 – Therapeutic Suggestions and Clinical Outcome

Therapeutic strategy focused on restoring lymphatic flow, supporting immune terrain clearance, and reducing cervical congestion. The patient began a structured lymphatic protocol including daily neck brushing, warm compresses over the supraclavicular zone, and alternating neck showers.

A phytotherapeutic blend was prescribed containing Galium aparine, Echinacea angustifolia, and Plantago major to promote drainage and mucosal repair. Nutritional support included increased hydration, bitter plant infusions, and reduction of dairy and histamine-rich foods.

Emotional terrain remedies included Carcinosinum and the flower essence Mountain Pennyroyal, selected for terrain resilience and emotional decompression. Light cervical mobilization exercises and breathing techniques were introduced to activate the deep lymphatic core.

Therapeutic Outcome

At his six-week follow-up, the patient reported a substantial reduction in neck fullness, easier breathing through the throat and chest, and a sense of "lightness" in the cervical region. He resumed moderate exercise without postural tightness or lymphatic discomfort. Repeat biospectral imaging of Zone 17 showed significant reduction in emission density, with resolution of the blotched terrain pattern and return of spectral symmetry.

The case confirms how non- reactive immune retention can be identified and reversed through spectral terrain mapping, and illustrates the sensitivity of Biospectral Medicine in detecting subtle yet impactful lymphatic dysfunctions often missed by conventional evaluations.

CASE STUDY

18

Zone 18 – Cervical Spine and Nuchal Region

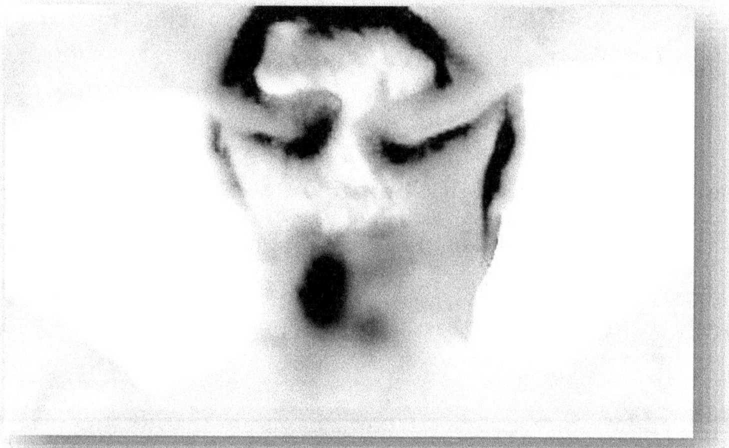

The biospectral emission in this image is sharply focal, midline, and geometrically circular, anchored directly over the cervical spine without lateral diffusion, muscular striation, or dermatomal spread. There is no evidence of myofascial activation such as banding, bilateral asymmetry, or fascial elongation. Additionally, the absence of diffuse terrain patterns, adrenal-related zones, or metabolic gradient shifts rules out endocrine involvement. The emission's spinal centering and precise axial confinement strongly indicate localized neural irritation at the segmental level, specifically consistent with upper cervical nerve stress.

Interpretive Category: Nervous System / Spine
Clinical Condition: Cervicogenic Dysfunction with Neural Irritation
Patient Profile: Male, 45 years old
Date of Birth: 10 May 1980

Step 1 – Zone Relevance: Anatomical and Biospectral Context

The patient presented with upper neck tension, postural fatigue, and intermittent occipital headaches radiating from the cervical spine to the skull base. These symptoms immediately pointed to Zone 18 – Cervical Spine and Nuchal Region as the primary area of biospectral interest. This zone includes the upper cervical vertebrae (C1–C4), suboccipital musculature, dorsal rami of the cervical nerves, and the cervical autonomic plexus.

In Biospectral Medicine, this region functions as a key interface for neural, muscular, and autonomic regulation. Emissions in this area often reflect mechanical fixation, proprioceptive imbalance, or neuro-autonomic tension, especially in cases of cervical postural strain or unresolved segmental dysfunction.

Step 2 – ROI Classification (Emission Pattern)

Biospectral imaging demonstrated a sharply localized, circular hyperemissive zone centered at the midline of the upper cervical spine, particularly between C2 and C3. The emission lacked lateral dispersion, vascular branching, or muscular patterning. Its geometry was axial and well-defined, confined strictly to the vertical segment of the nuchal midline.

There was no signal irregularity in adjacent dermatomes or muscular bellies, and the absence of asymmetric muscular tension ruled out compensatory postural hyperactivity. This axial signal was classified as a focused neurovertebral activation pattern.

Step 3 – Interpretive Category Determination

The pattern was interpreted within Category 4 – Nervous System / Spine. The midline anchoring, spinal correspondence, and lack of fascial or dermatomal involvement helped exclude myofascial overload, lymphatic burden, or vascular stress.

The patient's neurological symptoms, including pressure at the skull base and mild visual fatigue, were consistent with upper cervical segmental irritation, particularly of the C2 ganglion and associated proprioceptive feedback loops.

The absence of skin-related or metabolic emission cues further confirmed the neurovertebral nature of the biospectral signature.

BIOSPECTRAL INTERPRETATION RULE

When a discrete, symmetrical hyperemissive focus is centered along the midline of the upper cervical spine, particularly at the C1–C3 level, and lacks muscular dispersion or vascular trajectory, the pattern is interpreted in Biospectral Medicine as neurosegmental activation. This emission reflects spinal autonomic stress, proprioceptive imbalance, or upper cervical neural tension, especially when associated with postural fatigue, suboccipital tightness, or vagal dysregulation. Its confined geometry and axial anchoring distinguish it from muscular overuse or endocrine-related terrain responses.

Step 4 – Differential Interpretive Confirmation Through Patient History

The patient reported prolonged desk work with forward head posture and a longstanding habit of leaning to one side while reading. He described recurrent episodes of neck stiffness, dull occipital pressure, and a sensation of "tension buildup" behind the ears, particularly at the end of the day.

He denied trauma or acute injury but noted that the symptoms worsened with stress and fatigue. There was no evidence of radiating pain, arm paresthesia, or signs of reactive joint disease. These features strongly aligned with a cervicogenic neuromechanical overload pattern, confirming the spine and autonomic involvement seen in the emission.

Step 5 – Confirmatory Clinical Tests

On examination, cervical flexion and rotation were mildly restricted with palpable tension in the upper paraspinals. Local tenderness was noted at the C2 spinous process and suboccipital ridge. A Spurling's test was negative, excluding radicular compression. Manual resistance testing revealed mild imbalance in cervical extensors.

A functional HRV test showed reduced parasympathetic tone and sympathetic predominance. Thermopalpation confirmed focal surface heat along the mid-cervical midline. These findings supported the interpretation of an upper cervical segmental dysfunction with autonomic overlay, matching the biospectral emission.

Step 6 – Therapeutic Suggestions and Clinical Outcome

Therapy was focused on decompression of the upper cervical spine and regulation of autonomic tone. A sequence of neuromuscular retraining techniques was implemented, including suboccipital myofascial release, postural reprogramming, and gentle vestibular activation.

Energetic therapies included low-frequency cranial PEMF at the occipital base and auricular modulation of vagal input. Nutritional support focused on magnesium, nervine botanicals, and B-complex cofactors. The patient was instructed in daily cervical decompression stretches, jaw positioning correction, and diaphragmatic breathing to facilitate cranial-cervical realignment.

Therapeutic Outcome

At his 4-week review, the patient reported substantial relief in upper neck tightness, improved concentration, and no further episodes of occipital pressure. He resumed extended periods of work without discomfort and experienced deeper sleep and better balance. R

epeat biospectral analysis showed full resolution of the focal emission in Zone 18. This case confirms the value of precise biospectral mapping in detecting subtle yet functionally significant neurovertebral overload, allowing for targeted intervention before structural pathology emerges.

CASE STUDY

19

Zone 19 – Facial Area (Frontal and Lateral)

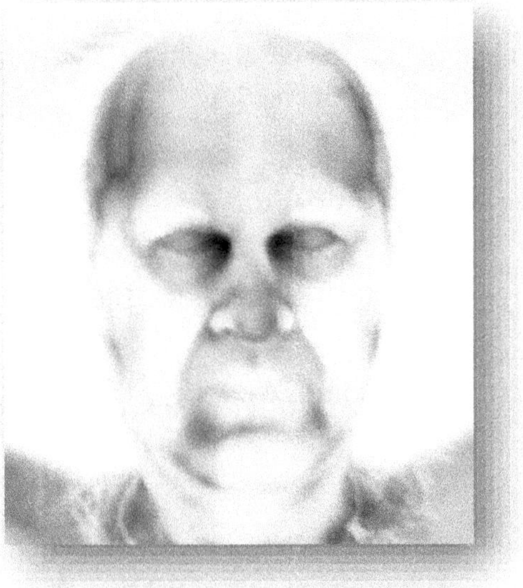

Interpretive Category: Organs / GNM
Clinical Condition: Chronic emotional-digestive axis dysregulation
Patient Profile: Male, 53 years old
Date of Birth: 12 July 1972

Step 1 – Zone Relevance: Anatomical and Biospectral Context

Zone 19, including the frontal and lateral facial planes, was selected due to persistent irregularities noted in the patient's lower facial biospectral emissions. The image revealed prominent hyperemissive zones around the mentolabial fold, chin, and submandibular region, with relative sparing of the forehead, periorbital, and lateral maxillary fields.

This lower-facial dominance corresponds topographically with multiple organ-related biosignal paths, particularly within the oral–digestive–hepatic axis.

In Biospectral Medicine, Zone 19 is frequently used to detect unresolved visceral conflicts processed through the cranial-autonomic reflex arc and neuroemotional overlays, particularly those with a history of gastrointestinal or hepatic stress or psychobiological conflict affecting the digestive terrain.

Step 2 – ROI Classification (Emission Pattern)

The facial scan presented a distinct hyperemissive cluster across the central lower face. Emission zones were dense and geometrically concentrated at the chin, mental crease, and upper neck, with mild peripheral dissipation toward the mandibular angle. The pattern showed irregular geometry with no dermatomal or muscular alignment, indicating non-structural, organ-reflective emission behaviour.

There was no muscular striation, no masseter or temporalis involvement, and the orbital zones remained comparatively flat, ruling out neuromuscular dominance. The ROI (Region of Interest) was classified as irregular, focal, and lower-midline dominant, a hallmark feature in Organs / GNM profiles with emotional conflict somatization.

Step 3 – Interpretive Category Determination

The emission pattern did not correspond to any known musculoskeletal or metabolic schema. The absence of symmetry, dermatomal gradient, or fascial plane activation eliminated categories such as Muscular, Skeletal, or Lymphatic.

Instead, the biofield concentration in the mentolabial and submandibular regions aligned with known conflict-mapping theories within German New Medicine, where the lower face reflects active or healing phases of territorial, digestion-related, or "unacceptable situation" conflicts.

The spatial distribution further reinforced involvement of organs such as the liver, pancreas, or intestine, processed neurologically through the cerebral cortex and brainstem relay centres.

> **BIOSPECTRAL INTERPRETATION RULE**
>
> *When irregular hyperemission appears in the lower facial zones, particularly the mentolabial fold, chin, and submandibular area, without muscular alignment or vascular symmetry, the emission is best interpreted through the Organs / GNM lens. In Biospectral Medicine, this pattern reflects internal organ-related conflicts processed via neuro-emotional terrain, especially those involving digestion, hepatic function, or unresolved relational stress. The absence of fascial striation, metabolic geometry, or lymphatic gradients distinguishes this signal as psychobiological rather than structural or inflammatory, and it often corresponds to unresolved affective processing within the digestive axis.*

Step 4 – Differential Interpretive Confirmation Through Patient History

The patient confirmed a pattern of long-standing internalized stress related to interpersonal tension, often accompanied by postprandial bloating, irregular digestive rhythms, and mild hepatic burden despite clean lab values.

There was no evidence of muscle strain, mandibular dysfunction, or maxillofacial pathology. Emotionally, the patient described difficulty "digesting" emotional situations, especially those involving betrayal or injustice. He did not report fatigue, hormonal symptoms, or lymphatic congestion.

These psychosomatic elements confirmed a classic GNM terrain, where unresolved conflict patterns manifest biospectrally before physiological organ deterioration, making the Organ / GNM classification clinically valid.

Step 5 – Confirmatory Clinical Tests

Clinical testing showed no neuromuscular involvement in the masseter or cervical fascia. Ultrasound of abdominal organs revealed mild hepatic steatosis but no inflammatory or structural disease. Autonomic evaluation demonstrated mild vagal imbalance with dominance of sympathetic tone.

Auriculotherapy scan confirmed organ reactivity in liver and stomach zones. Salivary pH was slightly acidic, and bioresonance terrain evaluation revealed organ field resonance for pancreas, liver, and small intestine. These findings aligned with the biospectral signature observed, supporting the non-structural yet biophysically relevant Organ / GNM classification.

Step 6 – Therapeutic Suggestions and Clinical Outcome

The therapeutic plan focused on emotional conflict resolution and organ terrain support. Care plan included a targeted hepatic and pancreatic botanical protocol, terrain-based oligotherapy, and emotional field clearing using frequency microtherapy. Digestive realignment was guided by a conflict-conscious nutrition plan, reducing acidic load and enhancing enzymatic support.

Bach flower essences were selected to support unresolved patterns of resentment and frustration. Infrared therapy over abdominal reflex zones was paired with facial lymphobiotic stimulation. Psychosomatic debriefing techniques were also introduced to externalize unresolved territorial stress. No structural therapies were needed.

Therapeutic Outcome

After six weeks, the patient reported subjective improvement in digestive ease, emotional clarity, and facial relaxation. A repeat biospectral scan showed marked emission normalization across the mentolabial and submandibular zones.

The patient remarked that "the inner heaviness around my digestion and jaw simply lifted." This case exemplifies how Zone 19 can reflect deep-rooted organ-emotional stress loads, even in the absence of structural pathology.

When interpreted correctly through the Biospectral model, such findings can guide therapeutic interventions toward subtle but transformative re-regulation of organ terrain and emotional coherence.

Applied Interpretive Logic in the Biosignal Field

The case studies presented throughout this Atlas represent the applied intelligence of Biospectral Medicine: a system not merely of diagnostic imaging, but of biofunctional reasoning.

For those engaged in clinical practice, diagnostics, or translational science, whether rooted in terrain medicine, somatic regulation, or systems biology, these cases demonstrate how biospectral analysis transcends the limitations of conventional imaging by decoding physiology in motion, across zones, categories, and dimensions of dysfunction.

Each case, while centered in a specific anatomical zone, unfolds a layered interpretive sequence that reveals how localized complaints are often the visible edge of deeper, interlinked regulatory disturbances.

By consistently applying the R-CIIM method, Region, Classification, Interpretation, Integration, and Mapping, these case studies showcase how emission patterns can be mapped to structural anomalies, energetic suppression, emotional terrain conflicts, metabolic burden, lymphatic stagnation, and more.

The range of interpretive categories addressed (vascular, muscular, skeletal, neural, lymphatic, organ-related, acupuncture-based, energetic, and endocrine/metabolic) validates the versatility of this interpretive framework and opens a new frontier for clinicians working at the interface of structure and function, signal and system.

Biospectral Medicine is firmly grounded in emerging principles of regulatory physiology, network coherence, and systems-based feedback integration. The spatial logic of emissions, when interpreted through the lens of field-based evaluations, reveals a regulatory language that echoes long-standing models in systems theory and neuro-immuno-endocrinology: that dysfunction rarely occurs in isolation, and that the body expresses its compensatory mechanisms through structured, decipherable patterns.

The case studies in this Atlas demonstrate a consistent interpretive framework grounded in spatial biosignal logic and zone-specific emission analysis. Each case reflects the structured application of a stepwise methodology, integrating clinical history, anatomical relevance, emission morphology, and confirmatory testing.

The resulting interpretive model is reproducible, clinically anchored, and applicable across diverse categories of dysfunction. These cases form a coherent corpus of spectral evaluations, offering professionals a standardized system for interpreting physiological patterns and guiding therapeutic strategy.

Biospectral Medicine is an interpretive system, a clinical lens, and a translational bridge between visible signal and invisible dysfunction. These case studies are proof of its capacity to offer early detection, individualized guidance, and coherence in a way that few modalities currently allow.

For practitioners seeking a deeper map of health and dysfunction, beyond symptoms, beyond structures, Biospectral Medicine offers exactly that, an interpretive map aligned with the complexity and intelligence of life itself.

CHAPTER

5

REFERENCE TABLES SECTION

COMPREHENSIVE REFERENCE FRAMEWORK FOR BIOSPECTRAL MEDICINE

The Reference Tables constitute a practical framework that condenses the R-CIIM methodology into operative maps for clinical use. Each table organizes, in a clearly ordered sequence, the core constructs of Biospectral Medicine, anatomy, emissive behavior, and interpretive criteria, so the reader can move from image to inference with minimal cognitive load. The layout favors clarity: zones are indexed, emission patterns are named and typified, and the corresponding evaluation categories align with their most consistent spectral expressions.

A second group of tables synthesizes the six methodological steps of R-CIIM into a stepwise pathway. Zone relevance and ROI classification appear first; pattern archetypes and biospectral asymmetries follow with quantitative thresholds; then come differential anchors derived from focused history, culminating in confirmatory tests. This architecture preserves scientific rigor while enabling rapid consultation at the point of care, across both straightforward and complex presentations.

Because acquisition quality governs interpretive reliability, the framework includes operational standards for image capture and palette normalization, admissible ambient conditions, and positioning cues that ensure reproducibility. Parameters for the Spectrovascular Response Test (SVRT) are summarized with timings, observation windows, and expected emissive shifts by anatomical group, aligning dynamic assessments with the same evidentiary spine as baseline images.

Therapeutic planning appears in tables that translate interpretive findings into strategic options. For each evaluation category, Vascular/Circulatory; Muscular/Myofascial; Skeletal/Articular; Nervous System/Spine; Lymphatic/Immune; Organs/GNM; Acupuncture/Meridians; Energetic/Frequency; Metabolic/Endocrine, the reader finds care objectives, physiological targets, and recommended sequencing, with attention to vascular hierarchy, myofascial tone, articular mechanics, neurospinal modulation, lymphatic mobilization, organ correlations, meridian mapping, energetic regulation, and metabolic-endocrine balance.

A set of clinical safeguards assembles alert signals, scope boundaries, and referral criteria, harmonized with the steps of R-CIIM. These tables make explicit the conditions that call for additional correlation, technical repetition, or complementary support, preserving safety and methodological consistency. Together, the tables convert the theoretical body of the Atlas into quick-access instruments that sustain a continuous cycle of observation, interpretation, and clinical action.

TABLE 1 – COMPARATIVE EVALUATION MATRIX: BIOSPECTRAL MEDICINE VS. CONVENTIONAL IMAGING MODALITIES

This table positions Biospectral Medicine within the spectrum of established evaluation imaging modalities, highlighting both unique contributions and differentiating factors. It provides a functional comparison across criteria such as standardization, interpretive models, safety, cost, and clinical applicability, clarifying why Biospectral Medicine complements rather than replaces conventional tools.

Comparison Table: Biospectral Medicine vs. Conventional Imaging Modalities

Criteria	Biospectral Medicine (CBI)	Ultrasound	MRI	X-Ray	Traditional Thermography
Primary Focus	Functional physiology (thermal emissions, vascular & neurogenic patterns)	Structural anatomy and real-time movement	Detailed soft tissue and structural anatomy	Bone and dense structure visualization	Superficial thermal mapping
Evaluation Nature	Functional and terrain-based	Anatomical and functional (vascular, organs)	Anatomical (soft tissue, brain, joints)	Anatomical (bones, lungs, fractures)	General temperature interpretation
Standardized Zones / Map	Yes – 19 clinically defined zones based on dermatomes and territories	No standardized zones	No standardized zones	No standardized zones	No standardized zones
Interpretive Model	R-CIIM: Reitz Clinical Infrared Interpretation Model	Varies by operator and device	Radiology-based interpretation	Radiology-based interpretation	Subjective or comparative
Lexicon and Terminology	Yes – structured terms (activose, inhibose, anisospectral)	No unified lexicon	Standard radiological terminology	Standard radiological terminology	Non-standardized or generic descriptors
Grade/Severity Classification	6-Level grading system (R-CIIM)	Absent	Variable by condition	Fracture/staging systems	Not present
Quantitative Comparison Over Time	Yes – thermal evolution across zones	Partially (volume, blood flow estimates)	Yes – serial imaging	Yes – comparative films	Not consistent

Use of Functional Terrain Models	Yes – includes vascular, metabolic, neurological, lymphatic terrain	No	No	No	No
Radiation Exposure	None	None	None	Yes – ionizing radiation	None
Risk of Harm	None	Low (heat/cavitation at high exposure)	Claustrophobia, contrast agent risks	Cumulative radiation risk	None
Cost	Low to moderate	Moderate	High	Low	Low
Availability	Expanding with trained practitioners	Widely available	Limited to specialized centers	Widely available	Limited use
Time to Perform	30–45 minutes incl. analysis	10–30 minutes	30–90 minutes	5–15 minutes	10–20 minutes
Real-time Monitoring	Yes – immediate physiological response observable	Partially (e.g. Doppler flow)	No (not real-time)	No	Yes
Training Requirement	High – needs Biospectral training and clinical context	Moderate – operator skill crucial	High – radiologist interpretation	Moderate – technician and radiologist	Minimal – often not medically supervised
Integration with Lab/Other Tests	Yes – designed for integrative use (terrain, labs, imaging, history)	Possible but not systemic	Yes – often used with labs	Yes – initial screening	Rarely integrated clinically
Acceptance in Conventional Medicine	Emerging – not yet mainstream	Established	Fully accepted	Fully accepted	Marginal – often alternative-only
Main Clinical Contribution	Ultra-early detection, root cause insight, functional triage	Soft tissue and vascular imaging	Deep tissue and structural evaluation	Fractures, infections, dense tissue	General screening or adjunctive use

Part I - Scientific and medical justification

Biospectral Medicine advances an explicitly functional basis for imaging, complementing structural modalities through emissive physiology rather than anatomy alone. The method reads surface emission behavior as a proxy for underlying regulatory dynamics, translating patterns into clinical meaning through a defined interpretive grammar.

This orientation enables root-cause mapping at the level of circulation, myofascial tone, neurospinal modulation, lymphatic behavior, organ correlations, meridian pathways, energetic regulation, and metabolic-endocrine balance, the nine evaluation categories that give the system consistent scope.

By designing acquisition to be passive and non-ionizing, with palette normalization and environmental control, the platform supports repeated measures and dynamic testing without procedure-related exposure, which strengthens longitudinal utility.

The interpretive core is formalized in the R-CIIM, which operationalizes spectral zones and ROI mapping into a reproducible, stepwise pathway. Zone relevance is established first; emission archetypes and biospectral asymmetries are then classified with thresholds; differential anchors follow through focused history; confirmatory maneuvers and tests close the loop.

A controlled vocabulary gives each element a place in the lexicon, reducing ambiguity and preserving inter-observer consistency. Because zones are defined anatomically and functionally, zone consistency across patients and conditions emerges as a measurable property; the same pattern families recur in the same regions under similar physiological loads, allowing clinicians to move from image to inference with fewer cognitive jumps.

Reliability depends on acquisition discipline, so protocols specify camera stability, ambient parameters, emissive palette constraints, patient positioning, and timing windows. The Spectrovascular Response Test (SVRT) adds a dynamic dimension by observing emissive shifts during a standardized challenge and recovery period; expected behaviors are tabulated by anatomical group to separate adaptive from dysregulated responses.

These standards already cover breast, cervical spine/nuchal, thyroid, abdomen, and pelvic regions, with defined sequences, views, and overlay conventions. Integrated digital documentation layers fiduciary markers, ROIs, and quantitative readouts directly on the image set, creating a durable record that can be compared session-to-session for longitudinal tracking across zones and time.

Clinically, the method has demonstrated practical value where functional physiology drives presentation. Vascular applications include patterning compatible with microcirculatory stasis or reactive hyperperfusion; lymphatic use cases show stasis signatures and drainage asymmetries that align with symptom geography; thyroid assessments reveal focal or band-like reactivity that correlates with palpation findings and history; pain mapping localizes active myofascial generators and neurospinal segments that reproduce the patient's complaint during provocation; oncology pre-evaluations identify atypical emissive constellations that heighten clinical vigilance and prompt earlier correlation with structural tests.

In each domain, the system is framed as hypothesis-generating and confirmatory-oriented: findings justify targeted examination and appropriate testing, rather than replacing standard evaluations. This preserves clinical logic while yielding earlier, more focused pathways to care.

The safety profile follows from the physics: emissive capture deploys passive sensing, avoids compression and skin breach, and enables repeated observation without cumulative dose. That feature set makes the method suitable for monitoring trajectories, evaluating responses to care, and documenting stability or change before and after functional challenges.

Because the interpretive model is standardized, two timepoints can be compared quantitatively with overlays and identical ROI geometry, which strengthens intra-individual signal-to-noise and supports objective decision-making at follow-up.

Acceptance in medicine arises when a modality aligns with the same pillars that established ultrasound, MRI, and X-ray: standardization, professional formation, evidentiary validation, workflow integration, and regulatory clarity. Biospectral Medicine addresses standardization through written SOPs for acquisition and reporting, a controlled lexicon mapped to the nine evaluation categories, and fixed ROI templates for each anatomical zone.

Reports are structured with traceable identifiers, timestamps, operator credentials, device specifications, ambient conditions, and quantitative overlays; this creates a chain-of-custody for data and a defensible audit trail. Where possible, exports mirror widely used interchange formats (PDF for narrative reporting and image panels; image series and metadata packages for archiving), which eases downstream storage and review.

Professional formation advances through a defined curriculum that maps competencies to the R-CIIM steps: acquisition proficiency, palette governance, ROI placement, pattern recognition, differential anchoring via focused history, and test selection for correlation. Certification can incorporate proctored case reads, inter-observer agreement thresholds, and periodic revalidation with quality-assurance audits.

This places the method within familiar norms for credentialing, while quality programs monitor drift, image adequacy, and reporting completeness. A registry architecture strengthens continual improvement: de-identified cases feed a reference bank stratified by zone, category, and outcome, enabling benchmarking and calibration over time.

Evidentiary validation proceeds along lines that courts, regulators, and hospital committees recognize. Method papers define acquisition error budgets and repeatability; observational series quantify intra- and inter-session reproducibility and inter-rater reliability; prospective cohorts evaluate concordance with clinical endpoints that matter to patients; blinded reads test whether predefined patterns predict which patients require targeted structural imaging or specialized referral.

Oncology pre-evaluation remain framed as vigilance triggers rather than stand-alone determinations; vascular and lymphatic applications prioritize functional correlation with physical examination and, when indicated, hemodynamic studies; thyroid work aligns with palpation, function panels, and ultrasound. This validation plan emphasizes pre-specified protocols, registered analyses, and transparent limitations, which courts and IRBs view favorably.

Workflow integration gives administrators and clinicians reasons to adopt. Reports file into the EHR as structured PDFs with embedded image panels and overlays; archiving flows to enterprise repositories; scheduling aligns with existing outpatient pathways; and the billing model is transparent for private-pay contexts.

Where code sets govern claims, the service positions as adjunctive functional assessment and documentation, with site-specific review guiding whether an unlisted service code, a physiologic measurement descriptor, or a center-specific package best fits local policy. Clear fee schedules, informed consent that explains scope, and standardized referral triggers align the service with common compliance expectations and reduce disputes.

Regulatory positioning follows recognized frameworks. Risk management maps to ISO 14971 principles; if dedicated instrumentation is manufactured, quality systems align with ISO 13485 concepts; software components that perform measurement or decision support follow good machine-learning practice where applicable and maintain change logs, versioning, and post-market surveillance.

Labeling and professional education consistently state adjunctive intent, scope boundaries, and referral criteria, which harmonizes with prevailing medical-device doctrines across jurisdictions. Privacy and data protection comply with LGPD in Brazil (and GDPR where relevant) through explicit purposes, minimal collection, retention policies, and secure storage with access controls; incident response plans and patient-facing notices complete the governance loop.

Taken together, these scientific, medical, and legal elements justify the statement that Biospectral Medicine has established foundations comparable to conventional imaging. The discipline is architected for adoption through standardization, professional formation, evidentiary pathways, workflow integration, and governance aligned with prevailing regulatory frameworks.

Its unique capabilities include a functional basis beyond structural anatomy; a structured interpretive system (R-CIIM) with spectral zones and ROI mapping; a defined lexicon spanning nine evaluation categories; and longitudinal tracking that withstands repeat measures. The platform also maintains an exposure profile based on passive spectral-surface capture, a root-cause orientation grounded in physiology, documented clinical applications across vascular, lymphatic, thyroid, pain, and oncology vigilance, zone consistency observable across patients and conditions, established protocols for key regions, and integrated digital documentation with overlays.

This alignment does not substitute for structural evaluatios; it equips clinicians with earlier, safer, and standardized functional intelligence that integrates cleanly into contemporary practice and stands on principles that regulators, hospitals, and courts understand.

Strategic Positioning Statement

Biospectral Medicine is the first non-invasive imaging discipline to deliver a structured physiological interpretation of spectral surface readings, converting biospectral patterns into a clinical language of vascular dynamics, neuroautonomic behavior, neuroimmune reactivity, lymphatic conductance, and metabolic-endocrine regulation.

The method translates emissive physiology into standardized meaning through a defined lexicon, spectral zones, and ROI mapping, so clinicians can move from observation to inference with reproducible logic.

Positioned as the functional counterpart to structural radiology, Biospectral Medicine elucidates early-phase dysregulation that precedes macroscopic anatomical change. This physiology-first vantage helps explain symptoms that outpace structural findings, clarifies priority systems involved in a case, and directs correlation, when indicated, with ultrasound, radiography, or MRI.

The result is a more coherent evaluation pathway: structural modalities confirm morphology and extent, while biospectral analysis organizes the regulatory story that often initiates clinical trajectories. The interpretive engine is the R-CIIM, which codifies zone relevance, pattern archetypes, and biospectral asymmetries into a stepwise read that is teachable and testable. A unified lexicon across nine evaluation categories maintains consistency: Vascular/Circulatory, Muscular/Myofascial, Skeletal/Articular, Nervous System/Spine, Lymphatic/Immune, Organs/GNM, Acupuncture/Meridians, Energetic/Frequency, and Metabolic/Endocrine.

Longitudinal use strengthens signal quality: standardized overlays, fixed ROI geometry, and palette governance enable session-to-session comparison and the Spectrovascular Response Test (SVRT) adds a dynamic window on adaptation versus dysregulation.

The platform's exposure profile is light-touch, contactless, non-ionizing, and suited to repetition, so clinicians can monitor progress, evaluate responses to care, and document stability or change across time and zones. Written protocols specify acquisition conditions, positioning, and normalization; reporting embeds quantitative overlays and traceable metadata for archiving and review.

These properties align neatly with the acceptance pillars that established conventional imaging: standardization, professional formation, evidentiary validation, workflow integration, and regulatory clarity.

Strategically, Biospectral Medicine expands the evaluation field by making physiology legible at the bedside and in the clinic. It supports earlier, safer decision-making; it focuses downstream testing; and it offers a common language that bridges practitioners across disciplines. In complex or care plan-resistant presentations, it provides a root-cause orientation grounded in functional physiology and a repeatable framework for tracking change. In this role, as a rigorous, adjunctive, evidence-led companion to structural imaging, Biospectral Medicine defines a new, clinically actionable tier of modern evaluations.

TABLE 2 – CONFIRMATORY TESTS CROSS-REFERENCE TABLE

This reference lists confirmatory evaluation tests most relevant for cross-validating biospectral findings. By aligning specific tests with zones, emission categories, and typical thermal patterns, the table guides clinicians toward integrative confirmation pathways, bridging Biospectral Medicine with vascular, metabolic, neurological, and systemic laboratory and imaging evaluations.

Test Name	Applicable Zones	Typical Use / Interpretation Value	Thermal Pattern	Evaluation Category
Doppler Ultrasound	1,2,3,4,5,6,9,10,14,15,16	Venous insufficiency, arterial flow, thrombosis detection	Both	Vascular / Circulatory
Ankle-Brachial Index (ABI)	1,2,3,4,5,6	Quantify arterial perfusion deficits	Hypoemissive	Vascular / Circulatory
Electroneurography (ENG)	4,6,14,18,19	Nerve conduction velocity, neuropathy detection	Hypoemissive	Nervous System
Electromyography (EMG)	2,3,4,6,8,14	Assess muscle and nerve function	Both	Muscular / Myofascial
X-Ray (Radiography)	1,2,3,6,7,8,9,12,13,16,17,18	Detect fractures, degenerative bone changes	Both	Skeletal
Bone Densitometry (DEXA)	1,3,6,12,18	Bone mineral density measurement	Hypoemissive	Skeletal
CBC (Complete Blood Count)	All Zones	Detect infection, anemia, general reactivity	Hyperemissive	Lymphatic / Immune
CRP (C-Reactive Protein)	All Zones	Marker of acute reactivity	Hyperemissive	Lymphatic / Immune
ESR (Erythrocyte Sedimentation Rate)	All Zones	Marker of chronic reactivity	Hyperemissive	Lymphatic / Immune
Comprehensive Metabolic Panel (CMP)	All Zones	Electrolytes, kidney, liver function	Both	Metabolic / Endocrine
Thyroid Panel (TSH, Free T3, Free T4)	17,18,19	Thyroid function assessment	Hypoemissive	Metabolic / Endocrine
Vitamin D (25-OH)	1,3,6,12,18	Bone health and immune modulation	Hypoemissive	Skeletal, Immune
Vitamin B12 and Folate	4,18,19	Neurological function and anemia	Hypoemissive	Nervous System, Metabolic
Homocysteine	1,4,18	Cardiovascular risk marker	Both	Vascular, Metabolic
Lipid Profile	1,6,9	Cardiovascular risk evaluation	Both	Vascular, Metabolic
Blood Glucose & HbA1c	All Zones	Glycemic control and diabetes screening	Both	Metabolic / Endocrine
Insulin & C-Peptide	All Zones	Insulin secretion and resistance	Both	Metabolic / Endocrine
Adrenal Hormone Panel	17,18,19	Adrenal stress hormone levels	Both	Metabolic / Endocrine
Sex Hormone Panel	17,18,19	Sex hormone balance	Both	Metabolic / Endocrine

IgG Food Sensitivity Panel	All Zones	Delayed food sensitivities	Hyperemissive	Lymphatic / Immune
Allergy Skin Prick Test	All Zones	Immediate hypersensitivity	Hyperemissive	Lymphatic / Immune
Stool Analysis	All Zones	Gut flora, parasites, reactivity	Both	Lymphatic / Immune
Urinalysis	All Zones	Kidney function and systemic health	Both	Metabolic / Endocrine
24-Hour Urine Hormone	17,18,19	Hormone metabolites for adrenal and sex hormones	Both	Metabolic / Endocrine
Salivary Cortisol	17,18,19	Diurnal cortisol rhythm	Both	Metabolic / Endocrine
Heavy Metal Panel	All Zones	Toxic metal burden	Both	Metabolic / Detoxification
Organic Acids Test (OAT)	All Zones	Cellular metabolism, mitochondrial function	Both	Metabolic / Endocrine
Genetic SNP Testing	All Zones	Genetic predispositions	Both	All Categories
Cardiac Stress Test (ECG)	9,13	Cardiac hypoperfusion and arrhythmias	Both	Vascular / Circulatory
Pulmonary Function Tests	9-13	Lung capacity and oxygen exchange	Both	Organs / GNM
Electrocardiogram (ECG)	All Zones	Cardiac rhythm	Both	Vascular / Circulatory
Sleep Study (Polysomnography)	All Zones	Sleep apnea and disorders	Both	Metabolic / Nervous System
Thermography (Infrared Imaging)	All Zones	Surface temperature and circulation patterns	Both	All Categories
Biofeedback & HRV	All Zones	Autonomic nervous system balance	Both	Nervous System, Metabolic
Live Blood Analysis	All Zones	Blood morphology	Both	All Categories
Zeta Potential Testing	1-6	Blood cell aggregation and surface charge	Both	Vascular / Circulatory
Serum Ferritin	All Zones	Iron stores	Hypoemissive	Metabolic / Endocrine
Serum Magnesium	All Zones	Mineral status	Both	Muscular / Metabolic
Coenzyme Q10 (CoQ10) Levels	All Zones	Mitochondrial energy production	Both	Metabolic / Energetic
Liver Function Tests (ALT, AST, GGT)	All Zones	Hepatic detox and metabolism	Both	Metabolic / Detoxification
Creatine Kinase (CK)	2,3,6	Muscle injury and reactivity	Hyperemissive	Muscular / Myofascial
ANA (Antinuclear Antibody)	All Zones	Autoimmune screening	Hyperemissive	Lymphatic / Immune
Rheumatoid Factor (RF)	All Zones	Autoimmune arthritis	Hyperemissive	Lymphatic / Immune
Serum Albumin & Prealbumin	All Zones	Nutritional and reactive status	Both	Metabolic

Urine Microalbumin	All Zones	Early renal damage	Both	Metabolic
Electrolyte Panel	All Zones	Sodium, potassium, chloride, calcium, magnesium levels	Both	Metabolic
Parathyroid Hormone (PTH)	1,3,6,12	Calcium metabolism and bone health	Both	Skeletal
Vitamin K (Phylloquinone & Menaquinone)	1,3,6	Coagulation and bone metabolism	Both	Skeletal / Circulatory
Serum Zinc	All Zones	Immune function and wound healing	Both	Immune / Metabolic
Fasting Insulin	All Zones	Insulin resistance and beta cell function	Both	Metabolic
Glycated Albumin	All Zones	Intermediate glycemic control	Both	Metabolic
Serum Carnitine	All Zones	Fatty acid metabolism and mitochondrial support	Both	Metabolic
Vitamin C Levels	All Zones	Antioxidant capacity and immune function	Both	Immune / Metabolic
Serum Selenium	All Zones	Antioxidant enzyme cofactor	Both	Immune / Metabolic
Thiamine (Vitamin B1)	All Zones	Energy metabolism and neurological function	Both	Metabolic / Nervous System
Riboflavin (Vitamin B2)	All Zones	Energy and redox metabolism	Both	Metabolic
Niacin (Vitamin B3)	All Zones	Cellular energy and lipid metabolism	Both	Metabolic
Folate (Vitamin B9)	All Zones	DNA synthesis and repair	Both	Metabolic
Serum Copper	All Zones	Iron metabolism and antioxidant function	Both	Metabolic / Immune
Serum Phosphorus	All Zones	Bone mineralization and energy production	Both	Skeletal / Metabolic
Lipid Peroxidation (MDA/TBARS)	All Zones	Oxidative stress marker	Both	Metabolic
Serum Lactate	All Zones	Tissue hypoxia and metabolic stress	Both	Metabolic
Urine Organic Acids	All Zones	Cellular metabolism and mitochondrial function	Both	Metabolic
Salivary Hormone Panels	All Zones	Cortisol, DHEA, sex hormone profiling	Both	Metabolic / Endocrine
Heart Rate Variability (HRV)	All Zones	Autonomic nervous system function	Both	Nervous System / Metabolic
24-Hour Holter Monitor	Selected Zones	Cardiac rhythm abnormalities	Both	Vascular / Circulatory
Skin Biopsy	Selected Zones	Vasculitis, neuropathy, reactive skin diseases	Hyperemissive	Immune / Nervous System

TABLE 3 – EVALUATION CATEGORY SYMPTOM AND SIGN CORRELATION TABLE (category centered)

This table aligns the nine evaluation categories of Biospectral Medicine with patient-reported symptoms and clinical signs. Its focus is category-centered, showing how functional disturbances manifest across vascular, muscular, skeletal, nervous, lymphatic/immune, organ/GNM, acupuncture, energetic/frequency, and metabolic/endocrine systems. It is designed to help clinicians translate biospectral emission patterns into systemic categories of dysfunction, guiding early hypothesis formation and differential diagnosis. *See also Table 10 for a zone-based perspective on hyper- and hypoemissive findings.*

Evaluation Category	Common Patient Symptoms	Typical Thermographic Signs (Hyperemissive / Hypoemissive)	Clinical Significance / Notes
Vascular / Circulatory	Limb heaviness, swelling, pain, coldness, cramps	Hyper: Redness, warmth, venous dilation; Hypo: Cold spots, pallor	Hyper suggests reactivity or congestion; hypo indicates hypoperfusion or poor circulation
Muscular / Myofascial	Muscle stiffness, cramps, localized pain, weakness	Hyper: Localized heat, reactivity; Hypo: Cool areas, muscle atrophy	Hyper with acute injury; hypo with chronic disuse or neuropathy
Skeletal	Bone pain, tenderness, restricted movement	Hyper: Periosteal warmth; Hypo: Reduced metabolic activity zones	Useful in detecting reactivity vs. degenerative changes
Nervous System	Numbness, tingling, burning, shooting pains	Hyper: Localized hot spots; Hypo: Cold, pale nerve pathways	Hyper may indicate neuritis; hypo often neuropathy or nerve compression
Lymphatic / Immune	Swelling, recurrent infections, fatigue	Hyper: Local warmth, edema; Hypo: Areas of lymphatic stasis, coolness	Hyperactive immune response or infection vs. stagnation
Organs / GNM (Visceral)	Abdominal pain, referred pain, organ dysfunction	Hyper: Localized heat over affected organ; Hypo: Cooling in chronic states	Reflects conflict-active vs. healing phases in visceral zones
Acupuncture (Energetic Flow)	Sensations of blockages, Qi stagnation, pain	Hyper: Heat over stagnation points; Hypo: Cold zones with Qi deficiency	Guides acupuncture point selection
Energetic / Frequency	Fatigue, poor recovery, systemic symptoms	Hyper: Overactive energy zones; Hypo: Energetic deficiency areas	Indicates imbalance in bioenergetic fields
Metabolic / Endocrine	Fatigue, temperature intolerance, weight changes	Hyper: Increased metabolic heat; Hypo: Coolness with slowed metabolism	May suggest hyper- or hypothyroidism, insulin resistance

TABLE 4 – ZONE-BY-ZONE ANATOMICAL AND CLINICAL HIGHLIGHTS

Here, each of the 19 emission zones is summarized with its key anatomical landmarks, common clinical presentations, and characteristic emission findings. Suggested natural interventions are provided, illustrating how spectral interpretation translates into practical therapeutic considerations.

Zone # & Name	Main Anatomical Structures	Common Clinical Patterns and Symptoms	Typical Thermographic Findings	Suggested Naturopathic Care Plan
Zone 1 – Frontal Lower Legs	Tibialis anterior muscle, anterior tibial artery, superficial veins	Venous congestion, varicosities, muscle strain, neuropathies	Hyper: Venous dilation, reactivity; Hypo: Arterial insufficiency, muscle atrophy	Botanical venotonics (horse chestnut, centella), anti-reactive diet, hydrotherapy, limb elevation
Zone 2 – Dorsal Lower Legs	Gastrocnemius and soleus muscles, posterior tibial artery and veins	Muscle fatigue, venous insufficiency, nerve irritation	Hyper: Muscle reactivity, venous congestion; Hypo: Arterial hypoperfusion	Anti-reactive botanicals (arnica, turmeric), venotonics, graded aerobic exercise, warming compresses
Zone 3 – Internal Left Leg	Medial leg muscles, saphenous vein	Muscle strain, venous insufficiency, peripheral neuropathy	Hyper: Local reactivity; Hypo: Chronic hypoperfusion	Circulatory stimulants (ginkgo, cayenne), adaptogens, amino acid supplementation
Zone 4 – Internal Right Leg	Similar to Zone 3, right medial leg structures	Similar to Zone 3	Similar patterns	Similar to Zone 3 Therapeutical Strategies
Zone 5 – External Left Leg	Lateral leg muscles, peroneal artery and vein	Muscle strain, venous congestion	Hyper: Reactivity; Hypo: Hypoperfusion	Anti-reactive herbs, hydrotherapy, circulation enhancers
Zone 6 – External Right Leg	Lateral leg muscles, peroneal artery and vein	Similar to Zone 5	Similar patterns	Similar to Zone 5 3 Therapeutical Strategies
Zone 7 – Frontal Upper Legs	Quadriceps muscles, femoral artery and veins	Muscle strain, varicosities, nerve irritation	Hyper: Venous congestion, muscular reactivity; Hypo: Arterial insufficiency	Venotonics, anti-reactive diet, muscle support supplements, hydrotherapy
Zone 8 – Dorsal Upper Legs	Hamstring muscles, femoral artery and veins	Muscle fatigue, venous insufficiency	Hyper: Muscle reactivity, venous congestion; Hypo: Hypoperfusion	Botanical anti-reactivities, adaptogens, warming therapies
Zone 9 – Frontal Abdomen	Abdominal wall muscles, visceral organs	Abdominal pain, muscle strain, organ-related discomfort	Hyper: Local heat over muscles or organs; Hypo: Chronic tissue dysfunction	Detoxification support, immune modulation, gentle mobilization

Zone 10 – Lateral Right Abdomen	Lateral abdominal muscles, ribs, viscera	Muscular strain, visceral conflict, immune response	Hyper: Heat from reactivity or visceral activity; Hypo: Cold areas from chronic dysfunction	Immune modulators, acupuncture, herbal detoxifiers
Zone 11 – Lateral Left Abdomen	Similar to Zone 10, left side	Similar to Zone 10	Similar patterns	Similar naturopathic support
Zone 12 – Lumbar Region	Lumbar vertebrae, paraspinal muscles, nerve roots	Low back pain, nerve irritation, muscular tension	Hyper: Muscle spasm and reactivity; Hypo: Nerve compression, poor circulation	Anti-reactive herbs, nerve support nutrients, hydrotherapy
Zone 13 – Chest and Sternum	Sternum, ribs, thoracic muscles	Chest wall pain, muscular strain, circulatory abnormalities	Hyper: Local heat from reactivity; Hypo: Cold spots indicating hypoperfusion	Botanical anti-reactivities, circulation enhancers, physical therapy
Zone 14 – Left Axillary	Axillary lymph nodes, brachial plexus, vessels	Lymphadenopathy, nerve irritation, vascular congestion	Hyper: Swelling, warmth; Hypo: Circulatory insufficiency	Lymphatic drainage support, nerve tonics, venotonics
Zone 15 – Right Axillary	Similar to Zone 14, right side	Similar to Zone 14	Similar thermographic patterns	Similar naturopathic interventions
Zone 16 – Upper Back	Thoracic spine, trapezius muscles, scapula	Muscle tension, nerve irritation, circulatory issues	Hyper: Muscle spasm, reactivity; Hypo: Poor perfusion	Anti-reactive botanicals, muscle relaxants, physical therapy
Zone 17 – Frontal Neck and Supraclavicular	Cervical muscles, carotid arteries, lymph nodes	Neck pain, lymphadenopathy, vascular issues	Hyper: Reactivity, warmth; Hypo: Ischemic zones	Circulatory support, lymphatic drainage, nerve support
Zone 18 – Cervical Spine and Nuchal Zone	Cervical vertebrae, spinal cord, paraspinal muscles	Neck stiffness, nerve irritation, muscular strain	Hyper: Local reactivity; Hypo: Nerve compression	Anti-reactive herbs, neurotrophic supplements, hydrotherapy
Zone 19 – Facial Area (Frontal and Lateral)	Facial muscles, trigeminal nerve branches, facial vessels	Facial pain, neuropathy, vascular congestion	Hyper: Reactivity, vasodilation; Hypo: Nerve dysfunction	Botanical venotonics, neuroprotective herbs, gentle massage

TABLE 5 – COMPREHENSIVE ANATOMICAL AND INTEGRATIVE PROFILE OF LOWER EXTREMITY EMISSION ZONES (ZONES 1 TO 8)

Expanding on the lower extremity zones, this table integrates vascular, muscular, skeletal, lymphatic, neurological, metabolic, and meridian perspectives into a single anatomical reference. It demonstrates the multi-layered interpretive potential of Biospectral Medicine within the legs.

Category	CBI Frontal Lower Legs	CBI Dorsal Lower Legs	CBI Internal Left Leg	CBI Internal Right Leg	CBI External Left Leg	CBI External Right Leg	CBI Frontal Upper Legs	CBI Dorsal Upper Legs
Area Description	Anterior lower leg, toes to superior patella	Posterior lower leg, heels to popliteal fossae	Medial left leg, malleolus to proximal thigh	Medial right leg, malleolus to proximal thigh	Lateral left leg, malleolus to iliotibial band	Lateral right leg, malleolus to iliotibial band	Anterior thighs, patella to inguinal fold	Posterior thighs, popliteal fossa to inferior gluteal crease
Major Veins	Great saphenous vein (medial), anterior tibial vein	Small saphenous, peroneal, posterior tibial veins	Great saphenous vein	Great saphenous vein	Small saphenous, perforating veins	Small saphenous, perforators to deep femoral vein	Femoral vein, superficial epigastric and circumflex iliac veins	Deep femoral vein, perforators to small saphenous
Relevant Organs / Reflex Zones	Reflex zones may reflect distal digestive/ pelvic organs	Bladder and kidney (TCM reflex zones)	Liver, spleen, reproductive organs (TCM reflexes)	Liver, right ovary/prostate, ascending colon reflexes	Gallbladder, hip drainage zones (meridian reflexes)	Liver, ascending colon, gallbladder reflexes	Intestinal, bladder, reproductive organs reflexes	Colon (sigmoid, rectum), sacral plexus, detox zones
Bones / Bony Landmarks	Tibia (anterior border), fibula (lateral), patella, malleoli	Calcaneus, posterior tibia and fibula, popliteal fossa landmarks	Medial tibia, femoral condyle, pubic ramus	Medial tibia, femoral epicondyle, pubic ramus	Fibula lateral shaft, femoral condyle, greater trochanter	Fibula shaft, femoral condyle, greater trochanter	Femur anterior shaft, ASIS, pubic symphysis	Femur posterior shaft, ischial tuberosity, sacrum
Primary Muscles	Tibialis anterior, extensor digitorum longus, extensor hallucis longus,	Gastrocnemius, soleus, plantaris, posterior tibialis, flexor digitorum longus	Sartorius, gracilis, semitendinosus, tibialis posterior	Sartorius, gracilis, semitendinosus, tibialis posterior	Peroneus longus/brevis, tensor fascia latae, vastus lateralis,	Peroneus longus/brevis, tensor fascia latae, vastus lateralis,	Quadriceps (rectus femoris, vastus medialis/lateralis/intermedius), sartorius	Hamstrings (biceps femoris, semitendinosus, semimembranosus), gluteus

	peroneus tertius				gluteus medius	gluteus medius		maximus insertion
Lymphatic Drainage	Superficial inguinal to medial leg; pre-tibial microcirculation	Posterior tibial and popliteal lymphatics	Medial leg to superficial inguinal nodes	Superficial lymphatic flow to inguinal nodes	Superficial lateral drainage to popliteal and inguinal nodes	Lateral drainage to deep inguinal and gluteal nodes	Superficial inguinal lymph nodes	Deep gluteal and inguinal lymph nodes
Nerves / Dermatomes	Deep peroneal, saphenous nerve; L4–L5 dermatome	Tibial nerve, sural nerve; S1–S2 dermatomes	Saphenous nerve, obturator nerve; L3–L4 dermatomes	Saphenous nerve, obturator nerve; L3–L4 dermatomes	Lateral sural cutaneous nerve, common fibular nerve; L5–S1 dermatomes	Common fibular nerve, lateral sural cutaneous nerve; L5–S1 dermatomes	Femoral nerve, lateral femoral cutaneous nerve; L2–L4 dermatomes	Sciatic nerve, posterior femoral cutaneous nerve; L5–S2 dermatomes
Fascial / Myofascial Lines	Superficial front line (Myers); connected to dorsal toe extensors and abdomen	Superficial back line (Myers); heel to sacrum	Superficial + deep front lines (Myers); spleen/stomach meridian	Deep and superficial front lines (Myers); liver, spleen, stomach meridian	Lateral line (Myers); gallbladder meridian pathway	Lateral line (Myers); gallbladder meridian zone	Superficial front line (Myers); stomach/spleen meridians	Superficial back line (Myers); bladder meridian
Metabolic / Endocrine / Biochemical Highlights	Glucose metabolism dysregulation, thyroid dysfunction, mineral depletion (Mg, Zn)	Insulin resistance, adrenal stress, lactic acidosis, mitochondrial dysfunction	Hormonal imbalances, detox congestion, glycation, thyroid dysfunction	Hepatic overload, bile congestion, hormonal imbalances, dysglycemia	Gallbladder dysfunction, bile stasis, lipid metabolism, hormone imbalances	Hepatic overload, lipid metabolism stress, gallbladder congestion	Glucose metabolism alterations, insulin resistance, reproductive hormone imbalance	Detox stress expression, sluggish metabolism, subclinical reactivity, thyroid function
Acupuncture Meridians (TCM Pathways)	Stomach (ST), Spleen (SP)	Bladder (BL), Kidney (KI)	Spleen (SP), Liver (LR), Kidney (KI)	Spleen (SP), Liver (LR), Kidney (KI)	Gallbladder (GB), Stomach (ST), Bladder (BL)	Gallbladder (GB), Stomach (ST), Bladder (BL)	Stomach (ST), Spleen (SP), Liver (LR)	Bladder (BL), Gallbladder (GB)

TABLE 6 – COMPREHENSIVE ANATOMICAL AND INTEGRATIVE PROFILE OF ABDOMEN & LUMBAR ZONES (ZONES 9–12)

This table profiles the abdominal and lumbar zones, which serve as central regulators of metabolic, digestive, and structural balance. By combining vascular, lymphatic, neural, fascial, and organ reflex perspectives, the table highlights how these regions integrate visceral and musculoskeletal physiology. Zones 9–12 are particularly important in Biospectral Medicine for their connections to the gastrointestinal tract, liver, spleen, kidneys, and reproductive system, as well as their influence on lumbar stability and autonomic regulation.

Category	CBI Frontal Abdomen (Zone 9)	CBI Lateral Right Abdomen (Zone 10)	CBI Lateral Left Abdomen (Zone 11)	CBI Lumbar Region (Zone 12)
Area Description	Umbilical line to epigastrium and hypogastrium, anterior abdominal wall	Right lateral abdomen, costal margin to iliac crest	Left lateral abdomen, costal margin to iliac crest	Posterior trunk from lower thoracic spine to sacrum
Major Veins	Epigastric, paraumbilical veins	Right renal, portal tributaries, intercostal veins	Left renal, splenic tributaries, intercostal veins	Lumbar veins, azygos/hemiazygos
Relevant Organs / Reflex Zones	Stomach, intestines, bladder, uterus/prostate	Liver, gallbladder, ascending colon, right kidney	Spleen, descending colon, left kidney	Kidneys, adrenal glands, lumbar spine reflex
Bones / Bony Landmarks	Sternum xiphoid, ribs, iliac crest, pubic symphysis	Right rib cage, iliac crest	Left rib cage, iliac crest	Lumbar vertebrae (L1–L5), sacrum, iliac crest
Primary Muscles	Rectus abdominis, external/internal obliques, transversus abdominis	Right obliques, quadratus lumborum, psoas	Left obliques, quadratus lumborum, psoas	Erector spinae, multifidus, quadratus lumborum
Lymphatic Drainage	Paraumbilical, iliac, superficial inguinal nodes	Hepatic lymphatics, right lumbar nodes	Splenic/para-aortic nodes, left lumbar nodes	Lumbar trunk to cisterna chyli
Nerves / Dermatomes	T7–L1 dermatomes, intercostal nerves	T8–T12, iliohypogastric nerve	T8–T12, iliohypogastric nerve	L1–L5 spinal nerves, dorsal rami
Fascial / Myofascial Lines	Superficial/deep front lines (Myers); abdominal canister	Spiral line, lateral fascial chain	Spiral line, lateral fascial chain	Superficial back line; deep front line via psoas
Metabolic / Endocrine / Biochemical Highlights	Digestive enzyme function, microbiome balance, reproductive hormone influence	Hepatic metabolism, bile secretion, detoxification	Splenic immune modulation, carbohydrate metabolism	Adrenal stress axis, renal electrolyte balance, chronic fatigue link
Acupuncture Meridians (TCM Pathways)	Stomach (ST), Conception Vessel (CV), Kidney (KI)	Liver (LR), Gallbladder (GB), Stomach (ST)	Spleen (SP), Stomach (ST), Kidney (KI)	Bladder (BL), Kidney (KI), Governing Vessel (GV)

TABLE 7 – COMPREHENSIVE ANATOMICAL AND INTEGRATIVE PROFILE OF THORAX & AXILLARY ZONES (ZONES 13–16)

This table presents the thoracic and axillary zones, which embody the intersection of cardiopulmonary, lymphatic, and musculoskeletal dynamics. The profiles demonstrate how Zones 13–16 express signals related to lung and heart function, breast and axillary drainage, and the regulatory influence of the sympathetic chain. By including fascial chains, lymphatic flow, and metabolic highlights, the table underlines the importance of the thorax in both systemic circulation and immune defense, while also mapping musculoskeletal contributions from the chest, scapula, and upper back.

Category	CBI Chest & Sternum (Zone 13)	CBI Left Axillary (Zone 14)	CBI Right Axillary (Zone 15)	CBI Upper Back (Zone 16)
Area Description	Anterior chest from clavicles to diaphragm, sternum midline	Left axillary fold and lateral thoracic wall	Right axillary fold and lateral thoracic wall	Posterior thorax from scapulae to T4–T12
Major Veins	Internal thoracic, mammary veins	Axillary, subclavian tributaries (left)	Axillary, subclavian tributaries (right)	Posterior intercostal veins, azygos/hemiazygos
Relevant Organs / Reflex Zones	Lungs, heart, thymus, breasts	Left breast/lymphatics, lung segments	Right breast/lymphatics, lung segments, liver reflex	Lungs, sympathetic ganglia, dorsal spine
Bones / Bony Landmarks	Sternum, ribs, clavicles, costal cartilage	Ribs, scapular lateral border	Ribs, scapular lateral border	Scapula, vertebral column (T1–T12), ribs
Primary Muscles	Pectoralis major/minor, intercostals, diaphragm	Serratus anterior, pectoralis major, subscapularis	Serratus anterior, pectoralis major, subscapularis	Trapezius, rhomboids, latissimus dorsi, erector spinae
Lymphatic Drainage	Parasternal, supraclavicular, axillary	Axillary nodes (left), supraclavicular	Axillary nodes (right), supraclavicular	Posterior intercostal nodes, thoracic duct
Nerves / Dermatomes	T2–T6 dermatomes, intercostal nerves	Brachial plexus branches, T2–T4 dermatomes	Brachial plexus branches, T2–T4 dermatomes	T1–T8 dermatomes, dorsal rami
Fascial / Myofascial Lines	Superficial front line, deep front arm lines	Spiral line, arm lines (left)	Spiral line, arm lines (right)	Superficial back line, deep back line
Metabolic / Endocrine / Biochemical Highlights	Cardiopulmonary metabolism, immune function, thymic regulation	Lymphatic detox pathways, immune load	Hepatic–lymphatic axis, hormonal metabolism	Respiratory capacity, adrenal–sympathetic stress axis
Acupuncture Meridians (TCM Pathways)	Lung (LU), Heart (HT), Conception Vessel (CV)	Heart (HT), Pericardium (PC), Lung (LU)	Lung (LU), Liver (LR), Gallbladder (GB)	Bladder (BL), Small Intestine (SI), Governing Vessel (GV)

TABLE 8 – COMPREHENSIVE ANATOMICAL AND INTEGRATIVE PROFILE OF NECK & FACE ZONES (ZONES 17–19)

This table integrates the neck and facial zones, which provide critical insights into endocrine, neurological, and emotional regulation. Zones 17–19 reflect the functional interplay of the thyroid, cervical spine, autonomic nervous system, and craniofacial structures. By incorporating vascular, lymphatic, fascial, and meridian perspectives, the profiles demonstrate how these regions act as gateways for systemic biosignals, linking metabolism, airway, digestion, and psychosomatic expression. These zones are particularly valuable in Biospectral Medicine for detecting early endocrine stress, neurogenic dysfunction, and organ reflex patterns.

Category	CBI Frontal Neck & Supraclavicular (Zone 17)	CBI Cervical Spine & Nuchal (Zone 18)	CBI Facial Area – Frontal & Lateral (Zone 19)
Area Description	Anterior cervical region, thyroid, supraclavicular fossa	Posterior cervical spine, nuchal line, suboccipital region	Face (forehead, periorbital, nasal, oral, mandibular)
Major Veins	Jugular (internal/external), thyroid veins	Vertebral veins, deep cervical veins	Facial vein, angular vein, jugular tributaries
Relevant Organs / Reflex Zones	Thyroid, parathyroid, larynx, upper mediastinum	Cervical spinal cord, autonomic plexuses	Paranasal sinuses, teeth, salivary glands, GI tract reflections
Bones / Bony Landmarks	Hyoid, clavicles, cervical vertebrae (C1–C7)	Cervical vertebrae (C1–C7), occiput	Mandible, maxilla, nasal bones, zygomatic arch
Primary Muscles	Sternocleidomastoid, scalene group, infrahyoids	Trapezius, splenius capitis, suboccipitals	Facial muscles (orbicularis, masseter, temporalis), platysma
Lymphatic Drainage	Cervical chain, supraclavicular nodes	Deep cervical nodes	Submandibular, parotid, preauricular nodes
Nerves / Dermatomes	Cervical plexus, vagus, phrenic, C3–C5 dermatomes	Greater occipital, spinal accessory, C2–C4 dermatomes	Trigeminal nerve branches (V1–V3), facial nerve
Fascial / Myofascial Lines	Superficial/deep front lines, cervical fascia	Superficial back line, deep front line (cervical)	Superficial front line, orbital/mandibular fascial chains
Metabolic / Endocrine / Biochemical Highlights	Thyroid metabolism, calcium balance, immune stress	Autonomic regulation, adrenal–thyroid axis	Digestive-metabolic load, hormonal-emotional interplay
Acupuncture Meridians (TCM Pathways)	Conception Vessel (CV), Kidney (KI), Stomach (ST)	Bladder (BL), Governing Vessel (GV), Gallbladder (GB)	Stomach (ST), Large Intestine (LI), Triple Energizer (TE)

TABLE 9 – GROUPING OF EMISSION ZONES BY ANATOMICAL REGION

This table organizes the 19 zones into four anatomical groups (lower extremities, abdomen/lumbar, thorax/axillae, and neck/face). It highlights the structural rationale of the zonal system and facilitates systemic analysis within R-CIIM.

Group	Zone	Relevant Structures / Categories Included
Group 1 – Lower Extremities	1. Frontal Lower Legs	Veins, Bones, Muscles, Lymphatic Zones, Nerves, Fasciae, Metabolic Terrain
	2. Dorsal Lower Legs	Veins, Bones, Muscles, Lymphatic Zones, Nerves, Fasciae, Metabolic Terrain
	3. Internal Left Leg	Veins, Organs (liver, spleen, reproductive), Bones, Muscles, Lymphatic Zones, Nerves, Fasciae, Metabolic Terrain
	4. Internal Right Leg	Veins, Organs (liver, reproductive, colon), Bones, Muscles, Lymphatic Zones, Nerves, Fasciae, Metabolic Terrain
	5. External Left Leg	Veins, Bones, Muscles, Lymphatic Zones, Nerves, Fasciae, Metabolic Terrain
	6. External Right Leg	Veins, Bones, Muscles, Lymphatic Zones, Nerves, Fasciae, Metabolic Terrain
	7. Frontal Upper Legs	Veins, Organs (bladder, reproductive, intestinal), Bones, Muscles, Lymphatic Zones, Nerves, Fasciae, Metabolic Terrain
	8. Dorsal Upper Legs	Veins, Organs (colon, sacral plexus), Bones, Muscles, Lymphatic Zones, Nerves, Fasciae, Metabolic Terrain
Group 2 – Abdominal and Lumbar Zones	9. Frontal Abdomen	Veins, Organs (intestine, liver, stomach, bladder, reproductive), Bones, Muscles, Lymphatic Zones, Nerves, Fasciae, Metabolic Terrain
	10. Lateral Right Abdomen	Veins, Organs (liver, gallbladder, kidney, adrenal), Bones, Muscles, Lymphatic Zones, Nerves, Fasciae, Metabolic Terrain
	11. Lateral Left Abdomen	Veins, Organs (spleen, pancreas, kidney, adrenal, stomach), Bones, Muscles, Lymphatic Zones, Nerves, Fasciae, Metabolic Terrain
	12. Lumbar Region	Veins, Organs (kidneys, adrenals, ureters, reproductive), Bones, Muscles, Lymphatic Zones, Nerves, Fasciae, Metabolic Terrain

Group 3 – Thorax and Axillary Regions	13. Chest and Sternum	Veins, Organs (heart, lungs, thymus, breasts), Bones, Muscles, Lymphatic Zones, Nerves, Fasciae, Metabolic Terrain
	14. Left Axillary	Veins, Organs (lung border, breast), Bones, Muscles, Lymphatic Zones, Nerves, Fasciae, Metabolic Terrain
	15. Right Axillary	Veins, Organs (lung border, breast), Bones, Muscles, Lymphatic Zones, Nerves, Fasciae, Metabolic Terrain
	16. Upper Back	Veins, Organs (lungs, heart, esophagus), Bones, Muscles, Lymphatic Zones, Nerves, Fasciae, Metabolic Terrain
Group 4 – Neck and Face	17. Frontal Neck and Supraclavicular	Veins, Organs (thyroid, parathyroid, respiratory), Bones, Muscles, Lymphatic Zones, Nerves, Fasciae, Metabolic Terrain
	18. Cervical Spine and Nuchal Zone	Veins, Organs (brainstem reflex), Bones, Muscles, Lymphatic Zones, Nerves, Fasciae, Metabolic Terrain
	19. Facial Area (Frontal and Lateral)	Veins, Organs (sinuses, eyes, salivary glands, upper digestive entry), Bones, Muscles, Lymphatic Zones, Nerves, Fasciae, Metabolic Terrain

TABLE 10 – COMMON HYPER- AND HYPOEMISSIVE CONDITIONS BY ZONE (Zone centered)

This table organizes biospectral findings from a zone-centered perspective. It lists common clinical conditions typically expressed as hyperemissive (activose) or hypoemissive (inhibose) patterns in each of the 19 anatomical emission zones. Unlike Table 3, which is organized by evaluation category, Table 7 is anatomically grounded, offering clinicians a quick reference for zone-specific dysfunctions and their typical spectral presentations. *See also Table 3 for a category-centered correlation of symptoms and signs.*

Zone	Common Hyperthermic Conditions	Common Hypothermic Conditions
1. Frontal Lower Legs	Venous congestion (early CVI), myositis (tibialis anterior), periosteal stress (shin splints), local reactivity, neural irritation (L4-L5), early cellulitis	Arterial insufficiency (PAD), chronic muscle atrophy, neuropathy (deep peroneal), anemia-related hypoperfusion, chronic terrain depletion
2. Dorsal Lower Legs	Venous stasis (saphenous/posterior tibial veins), myositis (gastrocnemius, soleus), post-exertional reactivity, neurogenic heat (sciatic/tibial irritation), low-grade immune activation	Arterial hypoperfusion, muscle atrophy (soleus/gastrocnemius), peripheral neuropathy (tibial nerve), chronic lymphedema, metabolic/endocrine suppression
3. Internal Left Leg	Great saphenous varicosities, adductor myofascial strain, lymphatic congestion, early medial compartment syndrome, GNM motor conflict repair	Arterial insufficiency, chronic muscular inactivity, postural unloading, obturator/femoral nerve hypoactivity, immune suppression, systemic fatigue
4. Internal Right Leg	As above (mirror of left), with greater risk for overload in dominant limb: saphenous/femoral congestion, adductor strain, immune post-exertion, postural compensation	As above: arterial/venous hypoperfusion, muscle disuse, nerve inhibition (right-side dominance), terrain-level exhaustion
5. External Left Leg	Peroneal muscle overuse, iliotibial band friction, superficial peroneal neuralgia, local trauma/reactivity	Chronic hypoperfusion, disuse atrophy, lateral compartment nerve dysfunction, metabolic suppression
6. External Right Leg	Same as left, potentially more postural overload: peroneal strain, ITB syndrome, neural irritation	Hypoperfusion, lateral compartment atrophy, superficial peroneal nerve inhibition, energy depletion
7. Frontal Upper Legs	Quadriceps overuse, patellar tendonitis, early osteoarthritis (knee), vascular congestion, immune activation	Arterial/venous insufficiency, muscle wasting (sarcopenia), femoral nerve hypoactivity, systemic hypometabolism
8. Dorsal Upper Legs	Hamstring strain/overload, ischial bursitis, sciatic neuralgia, postural reactivity, immune reactivity	Arterial hypoperfusion, gluteal muscle atrophy, chronic sciatic nerve suppression, terrain exhaustion
9. Frontal Abdomen	Gastrointestinal reactivity (IBS, colitis), visceral congestion (liver, spleen), abdominal wall strain, hernia repair phase, metabolic agitation, GNM repair	Visceral hypoactivity (hypothyroid gut), abdominal wall atrophy, metabolic/immune suppression, chronic sympathetic inhibition

10. Lateral Right Abdomen	Hepatic congestion, intercostal myofascial pain, local reactivity (appendicitis), costal nerve irritation	Hypoperfusion, abdominal muscle wasting, nerve inhibition (lower thoracic), metabolic depression
11. Lateral Left Abdomen	Splenic/colonic congestion, muscular strain, immune reactivity (diverticulitis, colitis), costal neuralgia	Hypoperfusion, muscular atrophy, nerve hypoactivity, chronic digestive hypo-function
12. Lumbar Region	Paraspinal myositis, facet arthropathy, nerve root irritation (L4-S1), reactive back pain, lymphatic congestion	Chronic low back muscle atrophy, nerve inhibition, vascular/lymphatic depletion, metabolic suppression
13. Chest and Sternum	Costochondritis, pectoral myofascial pain, early pleuritis, cardiac referral, thymic immune activation	Thoracic hypoperfusion, pectoral atrophy, cardiac hypo-output, immune exhaustion
14. Left Axillary	Axillary lymphadenopathy, breast/pectoral reactivity, immune/lymphatic activation, neuralgia (intercostobrachial)	Lymphatic/immune suppression, muscle wasting, nerve inhibition, chronic drainage failure
15. Right Axillary	As above (mirror): lymphatic activation, local reactivity, neuralgia	Lymphatic suppression, muscle/nerve atrophy, chronic hypoactivity
16. Upper Back	Trapezius/rhomboid myofascial pain, scapular bursitis, intercostal neuralgia, thoracic outlet, immune activation	Muscle atrophy, neural inhibition (dorsal roots), vascular/lymphatic hypo-function, chronic fatigue
17. Frontal Neck & Supraclavicular	Thyroiditis, cervical lymphadenopathy, myofascial tension, GNM repair, local reactivity	Hypothyroidism, chronic cervical muscle atrophy, nerve inhibition (cervical plexus), immune depletion
18. Cervical Spine & Nuchal Zone	Cervical spondylosis, myofascial/ligament strain, nerve root irritation (C2-C7), occipital neuralgia, immune reactivity	Chronic nuchal atrophy, cervical root hypoactivity, vascular depletion, chronic suppression
19. Facial Area (Frontal/Lateral)	Sinusitis, trigeminal neuralgia, TMJ reactivity, dental/periodontal reactivity, GNM repair, local skin reactivity	Facial nerve inhibition, chronic sinus underactivity, muscle atrophy, immune depletion, systemic hypo-metabolism

TABLES 11 – 29 – STEP 6 THERAPEUTIC INTEGRATION BY ZONE (19 TABLES)

Tables 8 through 28 summarize Step 6 – Therapeutic Suggestions of the R-CIIM method for each of the 19 emission zones. Each table aligns evaluation categories with anatomical/clinical focus, suggested naturopathic therapeutic approaches, specialist involvement, and clinical pearls. These references provide practitioners with a structured yet flexible framework to guide patient care following biospectral interpretation.

TABLE 11 - Zone 1

Category #	Category Name	Anatomical / Clinical Focus Summary	Main Naturopathic Therapeutic Approach	Key Specialists Involved	Clinical Pearls & Cautions (Summary)
1	Vascular / Circulatory	Venous congestion, phlebitis, varicosities; arterial insufficiency signs	Venotonics (horse chestnut, centella), hydrotherapy, anti-reactive diet, limb elevation	Naturopath, Physiotherapist, Orthomolecular, Nutritionist, TCM, Massage	Exclude DVT; avoid compression in arterial insufficiency
2	Muscular / Myofascial	Acute myositis, muscle strain, chronic atrophy	Anti-reactive botanicals (arnica, turmeric), hydrotherapy, active recovery	Naturopath, Physiotherapist, Orthomolecular, Nutritionist, TCM, Massage	Early pain-free movement; avoid deep massage in acute phase
3	Skeletal	Periosteal reactivity, trauma	Botanical anti-reactivities, bone-supportive nutrients (vitamin D3, K2, calcium, magnesium)	Naturopath, Physiotherapist, Orthomolecular, Nutritionist, TCM	Imaging essential; vitamin D and K critical
4	Nervous System	Neuritis, nerve irritation, neuropathy	Neuroprotective botanicals, B-complex vitamins, proprioceptive retraining	Naturopath, Physiotherapist, Orthomolecular, Nutritionist, TCM	Early nerve support; avoid deep massage in neuritis
5	Lymphatic / Immune	Lymphangitis, immune activation	Immune modulators (echinacea, calendula), lymphatic drainage, antioxidants	Naturopath, Physiotherapist, Nutritionist, TCM, Massage	Differentiate infection; avoid compression if venous failure
6	Organs / GNM	Conflict-active and healing phases of visceral organs	Detox support, immune modulation, tissue regeneration	Naturopath, Physiotherapist, TCM, Orthomolecular, Bioenergetic	Integrate GNM with clinical data
7	Acupuncture	Qi stagnation, damp-heat, blood stasis	Disperse stagnation, warm Hypoemissive zones, moxibustion	Acupuncturist, Naturopath, Herbalist	Confirm pattern differentiation; cautious moxibustion
8	Energetic / Frequency	Bioenergetic imbalance, reactivity, mitochondrial dysfunction	PEMF, microcurrent, bioresonance, photobiomodulation	Bioenergetic therapist, Naturopath, Physiotherapist	Tailor protocols carefully; monitor patient response
9	Metabolic / Endocrine	Insulin resistance, thyroid/adrenal dysfunction	Glycemic regulators, thyroid/adrenal support, lifestyle changes	Naturopath, Orthomolecular, Nutritionist	Comprehensive endocrine assessment; monitor drug interactions

TABLE 12 - Zone 2

Category #	Category Name	Anatomical / Clinical Focus Summary	Main Naturopathic Therapeutic Approach	Key Specialists Involved	Clinical Pearls & Cautions (Summary)
1	Vascular / Circulatory	Venous insufficiency, varicosities, arterial insufficiency signs	Venotonics, hydrotherapy, anti-reactive diet, limb elevation	Naturopath, Physiotherapist, Orthomolecular, Nutritionist, TCM, Massage	Exclude DVT; avoid compression in arterial insufficiency
2	Muscular / Myofascial	Muscle strain, myositis, chronic muscle fatigue	Anti-reactive botanicals, hydrotherapy, active recovery	Naturopath, Physiotherapist, Orthomolecular, Nutritionist, TCM, Massage	Early movement; avoid deep massage during acute reactivity
3	Skeletal	Periosteal irritation, trauma	Botanical anti-reactivities, bone support nutrients	Naturopath, Physiotherapist, Orthomolecular, Nutritionist, TCM	Imaging recommended; vitamin D and calcium supplementation critical
4	Nervous System	Nerve irritation, neuropathy	Neuroprotective botanicals, B-complex vitamins, neural mobilization	Naturopath, Physiotherapist, Orthomolecular, Nutritionist, TCM	Early nerve support; cautious with deep tissue work
5	Lymphatic / Immune	Lymphatic congestion, immune response	Immune modulators, lymphatic drainage, antioxidants	Naturopath, Physiotherapist, Nutritionist, TCM, Massage	Differentiate infection; avoid compression if venous insufficiency
6	Organs / GNM	Conflict-active/healing phases in visceral reflex zones	Detox support, immune modulation, tissue regeneration	Naturopath, Physiotherapist, TCM, Orthomolecular, Bioenergetic	Use GNM insights with clinical context
7	Acupuncture	Qi stagnation, blood stasis, dampness	Acupuncture points to disperse stagnation, moxibustion	Acupuncturist, Naturopath, Herbalist	Confirm diagnosis; cautious moxibustion
8	Energetic / Frequency	Bioenergetic imbalance, reactivity	PEMF, microcurrent, bioresonance therapies	Bioenergetic therapist, Naturopath, Physiotherapist	Monitor carefully; personalize frequency protocols
9	Metabolic / Endocrine	Insulin resistance, thyroid/adrenal issues	Botanical glycemic regulators, thyroid/adrenal support	Naturopath, Orthomolecular, Nutritionist	Comprehensive endocrine evaluation needed

TABLE 13 - Zone 3

Category #	Category Name	Anatomical / Clinical Focus Summary	Main Naturopathic Therapeutic Approach	Key Specialists Involved	Clinical Pearls & Cautions (Summary)
1	Vascular / Circulatory	Venous insufficiency, superficial phlebitis, arterial perfusion issues	Venotonics, hydrotherapy, anti-reactive diet, limb elevation	Naturopath, Physiotherapist, Orthomolecular, Nutritionist, TCM, Massage	Exclude DVT; avoid compression in severe arterial cases
2	Muscular / Myofascial	Muscle strain, myositis, chronic fatigue	Anti-reactive botanicals, hydrotherapy, active recovery	Naturopath, Physiotherapist, Orthomolecular, Nutritionist, TCM, Massage	Early mobilization; avoid deep massage during acute phase
3	Skeletal	Periosteal reactivity, minor trauma	Botanical anti-reactivities, bone-supportive nutrients	Naturopath, Physiotherapist, Orthomolecular, Nutritionist, TCM	Imaging if trauma suspected; vitamin D and calcium support essential
4	Nervous System	Neural irritation, neuropathy	Neuroprotective botanicals, B-complex vitamins, neural mobilization	Naturopath, Physiotherapist, Orthomolecular, Nutritionist, TCM	Early neuro support; caution with aggressive therapy
5	Lymphatic / Immune	Lymphatic congestion, immune activation	Immune modulators, lymphatic drainage, antioxidants	Naturopath, Physiotherapist, Nutritionist, TCM, Massage	Differentiate infectious causes; compression precautions
6	Organs / GNM	Conflict-active and healing phases in visceral reflex zones	Detox support, immune modulation, tissue regeneration	Naturopath, Physiotherapist, TCM, Orthomolecular, Bioenergetic	Combine GNM with clinical findings
7	Acupuncture	Qi stagnation, dampness, blood stasis	Acupuncture to disperse stagnation, moxibustion	Acupuncturist, Naturopath, Herbalist	Proper pattern diagnosis critical; cautious moxibustion
8	Energetic / Frequency	Bioenergetic imbalance, reactivity	PEMF, microcurrent, bioresonance therapies	Bioenergetic therapist, Naturopath, Physiotherapist	Tailor frequency therapy; monitor patient response
9	Metabolic / Endocrine	Insulin resistance, thyroid/adrenal dysfunction	Glycemic regulators, thyroid/adrenal support	Naturopath, Orthomolecular, Nutritionist	Full endocrine evaluation recommended

TABLE 14 - Zone 4 – Internal Right Leg

Category #	Category Name	Anatomical / Clinical Focus Summary	Main Naturopathic Therapeutic Approach	Key Specialists Involved	Clinical Pearls & Cautions (Summary)
1	Vascular / Circulatory	Venous insufficiency, superficial phlebitis, arterial perfusion issues	Venotonics, hydrotherapy, anti-reactive diet, limb elevation	Naturopath, Physiotherapist, Orthomolecular, Nutritionist, TCM, Massage	Exclude DVT; avoid compression in severe arterial cases
2	Muscular / Myofascial	Muscle strain, myositis, chronic fatigue	Anti-reactive botanicals, hydrotherapy, active recovery	Naturopath, Physiotherapist, Orthomolecular, Nutritionist, TCM, Massage	Early mobilization; avoid deep massage during acute phase
3	Skeletal	Periosteal reactivity, minor trauma	Botanical anti-reactivities, bone-supportive nutrients	Naturopath, Physiotherapist, Orthomolecular, Nutritionist, TCM	Imaging if trauma suspected; vitamin D and calcium support essential
4	Nervous System	Neural irritation, neuropathy	Neuroprotective botanicals, B-complex vitamins, neural mobilization	Naturopath, Physiotherapist, Orthomolecular, Nutritionist, TCM	Early neuro support; caution with aggressive therapy
5	Lymphatic / Immune	Lymphatic congestion, immune activation	Immune modulators, lymphatic drainage, antioxidants	Naturopath, Physiotherapist, Nutritionist, TCM, Massage	Differentiate infectious causes; compression precautions
6	Organs / GNM	Conflict-active and healing phases in visceral reflex zones	Detox support, immune modulation, tissue regeneration	Naturopath, Physiotherapist, TCM, Orthomolecular, Bioenergetic	Combine GNM with clinical findings
7	Acupuncture	Qi stagnation, dampness, blood stasis	Acupuncture to disperse stagnation, moxibustion	Acupuncturist, Naturopath, Herbalist	Proper pattern diagnosis critical; cautious moxibustion
8	Energetic / Frequency	Bioenergetic imbalance, reactivity	PEMF, microcurrent, bioresonance therapies	Bioenergetic therapist, Naturopath, Physiotherapist	Tailor frequency therapy; monitor patient response
9	Metabolic / Endocrine	Insulin resistance, thyroid/adrenal dysfunction	Glycemic regulators, thyroid/adrenal support	Naturopath, Orthomolecular, Nutritionist	Full endocrine evaluation recommended

TABLE 15 - Zone 5 – External Left Leg

Category #	Category Name	Anatomical / Clinical Focus Summary	Main Naturopathic Therapeutic Approach	Key Specialists Involved	Clinical Pearls & Cautions (Summary)
1	Vascular / Circulatory	Venous congestion, arterial perfusion deficits	Venotonics, hydrotherapy, anti-reactive diet, limb elevation	Naturopath, Physiotherapist, Orthomolecular, Nutritionist, TCM, Massage	Exclude deep vein thrombosis; avoid compression in arterial insufficiency
2	Muscular / Myofascial	Muscle strain, localized myositis	Anti-reactive botanicals, hydrotherapy, active recovery	Naturopath, Physiotherapist, Orthomolecular, Nutritionist, TCM, Massage	Early mobilization recommended; avoid aggressive massage during acute reactivity
3	Skeletal	Periosteal reactivity, minor trauma	Botanical anti-reactivities, bone support nutrients	Naturopath, Physiotherapist, Orthomolecular, Nutritionist, TCM	Imaging indicated if trauma suspected; maintain vitamin D and calcium intake
4	Nervous System	Nerve irritation, peripheral neuropathy	Neuroprotective botanicals, B-complex vitamins, nerve mobilization	Naturopath, Physiotherapist, Orthomolecular, Nutritionist, TCM	Early neural support; avoid deep tissue work in acute phases
5	Lymphatic / Immune	Lymphatic congestion, immune activation	Immune modulators, lymphatic drainage, antioxidants	Naturopath, Physiotherapist, Nutritionist, TCM, Massage	Rule out infection; cautious use of compression if venous insufficiency
6	Organs / GNM	Active conflict and healing phases of visceral reflex zones	Detoxification, immune modulation, tissue regeneration	Naturopath, Physiotherapist, TCM, Orthomolecular, Bioenergetic	Correlate GNM findings with clinical context
7	Acupuncture	Qi stagnation, dampness, blood stasis	Acupuncture points to disperse stagnation; moxibustion	Acupuncturist, Naturopath, Herbalist	Confirm pattern differentiation; cautious moxibustion
8	Energetic / Frequency	Bioenergetic imbalance, reactivity	PEMF, microcurrent, bioresonance therapies	Bioenergetic therapist, Naturopath, Physiotherapist	Personalize frequency therapy; monitor patient response
9	Metabolic / Endocrine	Insulin resistance, thyroid/adrenal dysfunction	Botanical glycemic regulators, thyroid/adrenal support	Naturopath, Orthomolecular, Nutritionist	Comprehensive endocrine evaluation advised

TABLE 16 - Zone 6 – External Right Leg

Category #	Category Name	Anatomical / Clinical Focus Summary	Main Naturopathic Therapeutic Approach	Key Specialists Involved	Clinical Pearls & Cautions (Summary)
1	Vascular / Circulatory	Venous congestion, arterial perfusion deficits	Venotonics, hydrotherapy, anti-reactive diet, limb elevation	Naturopath, Physiotherapist, Orthomolecular, Nutritionist, TCM, Massage	Exclude deep vein thrombosis; avoid compression in arterial insufficiency
2	Muscular / Myofascial	Muscle strain, localized myositis	Anti-reactive botanicals, hydrotherapy, active recovery	Naturopath, Physiotherapist, Orthomolecular, Nutritionist, TCM, Massage	Early mobilization recommended; avoid aggressive massage during acute reactivity
3	Skeletal	Periosteal reactivity, minor trauma	Botanical anti-reactivities, bone support nutrients	Naturopath, Physiotherapist, Orthomolecular, Nutritionist, TCM	Imaging indicated if trauma suspected; maintain vitamin D and calcium intake
4	Nervous System	Nerve irritation, peripheral neuropathy	Neuroprotective botanicals, B-complex vitamins, nerve mobilization	Naturopath, Physiotherapist, Orthomolecular, Nutritionist, TCM	Early neural support; avoid deep tissue work in acute phases
5	Lymphatic / Immune	Lymphatic congestion, immune activation	Immune modulators, lymphatic drainage, antioxidants	Naturopath, Physiotherapist, Nutritionist, TCM, Massage	Rule out infection; cautious use of compression if venous insufficiency
6	Organs / GNM	Active conflict and healing phases of visceral reflex zones	Detoxification, immune modulation, tissue regeneration	Naturopath, Physiotherapist, TCM, Orthomolecular, Bioenergetic	Correlate GNM findings with clinical context
7	Acupuncture	Qi stagnation, dampness, blood stasis	Acupuncture points to disperse stagnation; moxibustion	Acupuncturist, Naturopath, Herbalist	Confirm pattern differentiation; cautious moxibustion
8	Energetic / Frequency	Bioenergetic imbalance, reactivity	PEMF, microcurrent, bioresonance therapies	Bioenergetic therapist, Naturopath, Physiotherapist	Personalize frequency therapy; monitor patient response
9	Metabolic / Endocrine	Insulin resistance, thyroid/adrenal dysfunction	Botanical glycemic regulators, thyroid/adrenal support	Naturopath, Orthomolecular, Nutritionist	Comprehensive endocrine evaluation advised

TABLE 17 - Zone 7 – Frontal Upper Legs

Category #	Category Name	Anatomical / Clinical Focus Summary	Main Naturopathic Therapeutic Approach	Key Specialists Involved	Clinical Pearls & Cautions (Summary)
1	Vascular / Circulatory	Venous insufficiency, early varicosities, arterial perfusion disturbances	Venotonics, hydrotherapy, anti-reactive diet, limb elevation	Naturopath, Physiotherapist, Orthomolecular, Nutritionist, TCM, Massage	Rule out DVT; cautious use of compression in arterial disease
2	Muscular / Myofascial	Muscle strain, myositis, chronic muscle fatigue	Anti-reactive botanicals, hydrotherapy, active recovery	Naturopath, Physiotherapist, Orthomolecular, Nutritionist, TCM, Massage	Encourage early mobilization; avoid deep tissue massage in acute reactivity
3	Skeletal	Periosteal irritation, minor trauma	Botanical anti-reactivities, bone support nutrients	Naturopath, Physiotherapist, Orthomolecular, Nutritionist, TCM	Imaging if trauma suspected; vitamin D and calcium supplementation important
4	Nervous System	Nerve irritation, peripheral neuropathy	Neuroprotective botanicals, B-complex vitamins, neural mobilization	Naturopath, Physiotherapist, Orthomolecular, Nutritionist, TCM	Early neural support recommended; caution with aggressive techniques
5	Lymphatic / Immune	Lymphatic congestion, immune activation	Immune modulators, lymphatic drainage, antioxidants	Naturopath, Physiotherapist, Nutritionist, TCM, Massage	Differentiate infectious causes; compression precautions
6	Organs / GNM	Visceral conflict-active and healing phases	Detoxification, immune modulation, tissue regeneration	Naturopath, Physiotherapist, TCM, Orthomolecular, Bioenergetic	Integrate GNM findings with clinical presentation
7	Acupuncture	Qi stagnation, dampness, blood stasis	Acupuncture to disperse stagnation; moxibustion	Acupuncturist, Naturopath, Herbalist	Confirm pattern differentiation; use moxibustion carefully
8	Energetic / Frequency	Bioenergetic imbalance, reactivity	PEMF, microcurrent, bioresonance therapies	Bioenergetic therapist, Naturopath, Physiotherapist	Personalize frequency therapy; monitor responses
9	Metabolic / Endocrine	Insulin resistance, thyroid/adrenal dysfunction	Botanical glycemic regulators, thyroid/adrenal support	Naturopath, Orthomolecular, Nutritionist	Comprehensive endocrine evaluation advised

TABLE 18 - Zone 8 – Dorsal Upper Legs

Category #	Category Name	Anatomical / Clinical Focus Summary	Main Naturopathic Therapeutic Approach	Key Specialists Involved	Clinical Pearls & Cautions (Summary)
1	Vascular / Circulatory	Venous insufficiency, arterial perfusion deficits	Venotonics, hydrotherapy, anti-reactive diet, limb elevation	Naturopath, Physiotherapist, Orthomolecular, Nutritionist, TCM, Massage	Exclude thrombosis; avoid compression if arterial insufficiency
2	Muscular / Myofascial	Muscle strain, myositis, chronic fatigue	Anti-reactive botanicals, hydrotherapy, active recovery	Naturopath, Physiotherapist, Orthomolecular, Nutritionist, TCM, Massage	Early mobilization; avoid aggressive massage during acute reactivity
3	Skeletal	Periosteal reactivity, minor trauma	Botanical anti-reactivities, bone support nutrients	Naturopath, Physiotherapist, Orthomolecular, Nutritionist, TCM	Imaging if trauma suspected; ensure adequate mineral intake
4	Nervous System	Nerve irritation, neuropathy	Neuroprotective botanicals, B-complex vitamins, neural mobilization	Naturopath, Physiotherapist, Orthomolecular, Nutritionist, TCM	Early nerve support; avoid deep tissue techniques
5	Lymphatic / Immune	Lymphatic congestion, immune activation	Immune modulators, lymphatic drainage, antioxidants	Naturopath, Physiotherapist, Nutritionist, TCM, Massage	Differentiate infection; compression therapy caution
6	Organs / GNM	Conflict-active and healing phases	Detoxification, immune modulation, tissue regeneration	Naturopath, Physiotherapist, TCM, Orthomolecular, Bioenergetic	Correlate GNM findings with clinical data
7	Acupuncture	Qi stagnation, dampness, blood stasis	Acupuncture points to disperse stagnation; moxibustion	Acupuncturist, Naturopath, Herbalist	Confirm pattern differentiation; cautious moxibustion
8	Energetic / Frequency	Bioenergetic imbalance, reactivity	PEMF, microcurrent, bioresonance therapies	Bioenergetic therapist, Naturopath, Physiotherapist	Tailor therapy to patient; monitor responses
9	Metabolic / Endocrine	Insulin resistance, thyroid/adrenal dysfunction	Botanical glycemic regulators, thyroid/adrenal support	Naturopath, Orthomolecular, Nutritionist	Comprehensive endocrine evaluation recommended

TABLE 19 - Zone 9 – Frontal Abdomen

Category #	Category Name	Anatomical / Clinical Focus Summary	Main Naturopathic Therapeutic Approach	Key Specialists Involved	Clinical Pearls & Cautions (Summary)
1	Vascular / Circulatory	Abdominal arterial and venous flow, signs of congestion or hypoperfusion	Botanicals supporting microcirculation, hydrotherapy, anti-reactive diet	Naturopath, Physiotherapist, Orthomolecular, Nutritionist, TCM, Massage	Rule out thrombosis; avoid compression in ischemic areas
2	Muscular / Myofascial	Abdominal wall muscle strain, fascial adhesions	Anti-reactive botanicals, gentle mobilization, hydrotherapy	Naturopath, Physiotherapist, Orthomolecular, Nutritionist, TCM, Massage	Early mobilization; avoid aggressive manual therapy
3	Skeletal	Lumbar and pelvic bony structures influencing abdominal tension	Botanical anti-reactivities, bone-supportive nutrients	Naturopath, Physiotherapist, Orthomolecular, Nutritionist, TCM	Imaging if indicated; support bone health
4	Nervous System	Visceral and somatic nerve irritation	Neuroprotective botanicals, B-complex vitamins, neural mobilization	Naturopath, Physiotherapist, Orthomolecular, Nutritionist, TCM	Early nerve support; cautious with manual therapy
5	Lymphatic / Immune	Abdominal lymphatic congestion, immune activation	Immune modulators, lymphatic drainage, antioxidants	Naturopath, Physiotherapist, Nutritionist, TCM, Massage	Differentiate infection; cautious use of compression
6	Organs / GNM	Conflict-active and healing phases of abdominal organs	Detoxification, immune modulation, tissue regeneration	Naturopath, Physiotherapist, TCM, Orthomolecular, Bioenergetic	Correlate GNM with clinical and imaging findings
7	Acupuncture	Qi stagnation, dampness, blood stasis	Acupuncture to disperse stagnation; moxibustion	Acupuncturist, Naturopath, Herbalist	Confirm diagnosis; careful use of moxibustion
8	Energetic / Frequency	Bioenergetic imbalance, reactivity	PEMF, microcurrent, bioresonance therapies	Bioenergetic therapist, Naturopath, Physiotherapist	Tailor therapy; monitor response
9	Metabolic / Endocrine	Metabolic/endocrine dysfunction affecting abdominal tissue	Glycemic regulators, thyroid/adrenal support	Naturopath, Orthomolecular, Nutritionist	Comprehensive endocrine evaluation necessary

TABLE 20 - Zone 10 – Lateral Right Abdomen

Category #	Category Name	Anatomical / Clinical Focus Summary	Main Naturopathic Therapeutic Approach	Key Specialists Involved	Clinical Pearls & Cautions (Summary)
1	Vascular / Circulatory	Right lateral abdominal vasculature, venous congestion, arterial flow issues	Botanicals supporting microcirculation, hydrotherapy, anti-reactive diet	Naturopath, Physiotherapist, Orthomolecular, Nutritionist, TCM, Massage	Rule out vascular thrombosis; avoid compression if arterial insufficiency
2	Muscular / Myofascial	Muscular strain and fascial restrictions in lateral abdominal muscles	Anti-reactive botanicals, gentle mobilization, hydrotherapy	Naturopath, Physiotherapist, Orthomolecular, Nutritionist, TCM, Massage	Early mobilization advised; avoid aggressive manual therapy
3	Skeletal	Rib cage and pelvic influence on lateral abdominal tension	Botanical anti-reactivities, bone-supportive nutrients	Naturopath, Physiotherapist, Orthomolecular, Nutritionist, TCM	Imaging if indicated; support bone and joint health
4	Nervous System	Somatic and visceral nerve irritation in lateral abdomen	Neuroprotective botanicals, B-complex vitamins, neural mobilization	Naturopath, Physiotherapist, Orthomolecular, Nutritionist, TCM	Early nerve support; caution with manual therapy
5	Lymphatic / Immune	Lymphatic congestion and immune response in lateral abdomen	Immune modulators, lymphatic drainage, antioxidants	Naturopath, Physiotherapist, Nutritionist, TCM, Massage	Differentiate infection; compression therapy caution
6	Organs / GNM	Conflict-active and healing phases in visceral regions	Detoxification, immune modulation, tissue regeneration	Naturopath, Physiotherapist, TCM, Orthomolecular, Bioenergetic	Integrate GNM with clinical context
7	Acupuncture	Qi stagnation, dampness, blood stasis	Acupuncture to disperse stagnation; moxibustion	Acupuncturist, Naturopath, Herbalist	Confirm diagnosis; cautious moxibustion
8	Energetic / Frequency	Bioenergetic imbalance, reactivity	PEMF, microcurrent, bioresonance therapies	Bioenergetic therapist, Naturopath, Physiotherapist	Tailor therapy; monitor response
9	Metabolic / Endocrine	Metabolic/endocrine dysfunction affecting lateral abdomen	Glycemic regulators, thyroid/adrenal support	Naturopath, Orthomolecular, Nutritionist	Comprehensive endocrine evaluation advised

TABLE 21 - Zone 11 – Lateral Left Abdomen

Category #	Category Name	Anatomical / Clinical Focus Summary	Main Naturopathic Therapeutic Approach	Key Specialists Involved	Clinical Pearls & Cautions (Summary)
1	Vascular / Circulatory	Left lateral abdominal vasculature, venous congestion, arterial flow issues	Botanicals supporting microcirculation, hydrotherapy, anti-reactive diet	Naturopath, Physiotherapist, Orthomolecular, Nutritionist, TCM, Massage	Rule out vascular thrombosis; avoid compression if arterial insufficiency
2	Muscular / Myofascial	Muscular strain and fascial restrictions in lateral abdominal muscles	Anti-reactive botanicals, gentle mobilization, hydrotherapy	Naturopath, Physiotherapist, Orthomolecular, Nutritionist, TCM, Massage	Early mobilization advised; avoid aggressive manual therapy
3	Skeletal	Rib cage and pelvic influence on lateral abdominal tension	Botanical anti-reactivities, bone-supportive nutrients	Naturopath, Physiotherapist, Orthomolecular, Nutritionist, TCM	Imaging if indicated; support bone and joint health
4	Nervous System	Somatic and visceral nerve irritation in lateral abdomen	Neuroprotective botanicals, B-complex vitamins, neural mobilization	Naturopath, Physiotherapist, Orthomolecular, Nutritionist, TCM	Early nerve support; caution with manual therapy
5	Lymphatic / Immune	Lymphatic congestion and immune response in lateral abdomen	Immune modulators, lymphatic drainage, antioxidants	Naturopath, Physiotherapist, Nutritionist, TCM, Massage	Differentiate infection; compression therapy caution
6	Organs / GNM	Conflict-active and healing phases in visceral regions	Detoxification, immune modulation, tissue regeneration	Naturopath, Physiotherapist, TCM, Orthomolecular, Bioenergetic	Integrate GNM with clinical context
7	Acupuncture	Qi stagnation, dampness, blood stasis	Acupuncture to disperse stagnation; moxibustion	Acupuncturist, Naturopath, Herbalist	Confirm diagnosis; cautious moxibustion
8	Energetic / Frequency	Bioenergetic imbalance, reactivity	PEMF, microcurrent, bioresonance therapies	Bioenergetic therapist, Naturopath, Physiotherapist	Tailor therapy; monitor response
9	Metabolic / Endocrine	Metabolic/endocrine dysfunction affecting lateral abdomen	Glycemic regulators, thyroid/adrenal support	Naturopath, Orthomolecular, Nutritionist	Comprehensive endocrine evaluation advised

TABLE 22 - Zone 12 – Lumbar Region

Category #	Category Name	Anatomical / Clinical Focus Summary	Main Naturopathic Therapeutic Approach	Key Specialists Involved	Clinical Pearls & Cautions (Summary)
1	Vascular / Circulatory	Lumbar vascular supply, signs of venous congestion or arterial insufficiency	Venotonics, hydrotherapy, anti-reactive diet, limb elevation	Naturopath, Physiotherapist, Orthomolecular, Nutritionist, TCM, Massage	Exclude thrombosis; careful compression use in arterial disease
2	Muscular / Myofascial	Lumbar muscle strain, myositis, fascial adhesions	Anti-reactive botanicals, hydrotherapy, active recovery	Naturopath, Physiotherapist, Orthomolecular, Nutritionist, TCM, Massage	Early mobilization; avoid deep tissue massage during acute reactivity
3	Skeletal	Lumbar vertebral and sacral bone health	Botanical anti-reactivities, bone-supportive nutrients	Naturopath, Physiotherapist, Orthomolecular, Nutritionist, TCM	Imaging if indicated; vitamin D and mineral supplementation essential
4	Nervous System	Lumbar nerve roots, sciatic nerve involvement	Neuroprotective botanicals, B-complex vitamins, neural mobilization	Naturopath, Physiotherapist, Orthomolecular, Nutritionist, TCM	Early nerve support; cautious manual therapy
5	Lymphatic / Immune	Lumbar lymphatic drainage, immune responses	Immune modulators, lymphatic drainage, antioxidants	Naturopath, Physiotherapist, Nutritionist, TCM, Massage	Rule out infection; careful compression use
6	Organs / GNM	Conflict-active and healing phases related to lumbar visceral reflexes	Detoxification, immune modulation, tissue regeneration	Naturopath, Physiotherapist, TCM, Orthomolecular, Bioenergetic	Correlate GNM with clinical findings
7	Acupuncture	Qi stagnation, dampness, blood stasis	Acupuncture to disperse stagnation; moxibustion	Acupuncturist, Naturopath, Herbalist	Confirm diagnosis; cautious use of moxibustion
8	Energetic / Frequency	Bioenergetic imbalance, reactivity	PEMF, microcurrent, bioresonance therapies	Bioenergetic therapist, Naturopath, Physiotherapist	Tailor therapy; monitor patient response
9	Metabolic / Endocrine	Metabolic/endocrine factors impacting lumbar region	Glycemic regulators, thyroid/adrenal support	Naturopath, Orthomolecular, Nutritionist	Comprehensive endocrine evaluation advised

TABLE 23 - Zone 13 – Chest and Sternum

Category #	Category Name	Anatomical / Clinical Focus Summary	Main Naturopathic Therapeutic Approach	Key Specialists Involved	Clinical Pearls & Cautions (Summary)
1	Vascular / Circulatory	Thoracic vascular structures, signs of congestion or hypoperfusion	Venotonics, hydrotherapy, anti-reactive diet, limb elevation	Naturopath, Physiotherapist, Orthomolecular, Nutritionist, TCM, Massage	Exclude vascular obstruction; cautious compression use
2	Muscular / Myofascial	Chest wall muscle strain, myositis	Anti-reactive botanicals, hydrotherapy, active recovery	Naturopath, Physiotherapist, Orthomolecular, Nutritionist, TCM, Massage	Early mobilization; avoid deep tissue massage in acute reactivity
3	Skeletal	Sternum, ribs, thoracic spine bone health	Botanical anti-reactivities, bone-supportive nutrients	Naturopath, Physiotherapist, Orthomolecular, Nutritionist, TCM	Imaging as indicated; vitamin D and mineral support essential
4	Nervous System	Intercostal nerves, thoracic spinal nerves	Neuroprotective botanicals, B-complex vitamins, neural mobilization	Naturopath, Physiotherapist, Orthomolecular, Nutritionist, TCM	Early nerve support; caution with aggressive manual therapy
5	Lymphatic / Immune	Thoracic lymphatic drainage, immune responses	Immune modulators, lymphatic drainage, antioxidants	Naturopath, Physiotherapist, Nutritionist, TCM, Massage	Differentiate infection; cautious compression use
6	Organs / GNM	Conflict-active and healing phases in thoracic visceral reflex zones	Detoxification, immune modulation, tissue regeneration	Naturopath, Physiotherapist, TCM, Orthomolecular, Bioenergetic	Integrate GNM findings with clinical presentation
7	Acupuncture	Qi stagnation, dampness, blood stasis	Acupuncture to disperse stagnation; moxibustion	Acupuncturist, Naturopath, Herbalist	Confirm diagnosis; use moxibustion cautiously
8	Energetic / Frequency	Bioenergetic imbalance, reactivity	PEMF, microcurrent, bioresonance therapies	Bioenergetic therapist, Naturopath, Physiotherapist	Tailor therapy; monitor response
9	Metabolic / Endocrine	Metabolic/endocrine factors affecting thoracic region	Glycemic regulators, thyroid/adrenal support	Naturopath, Orthomolecular, Nutritionist	Comprehensive endocrine evaluation recommended

TABLE 24 - Zone 14 – Left Axillary

Category #	Category Name	Anatomical / Clinical Focus Summary	Main Naturopathic Therapeutic Approach	Key Specialists Involved	Clinical Pearls & Cautions (Summary)
1	Vascular / Circulatory	Axillary vascular structures, venous congestion, arterial flow issues	Venotonics, hydrotherapy, anti-reactive diet	Naturopath, Physiotherapist, Orthomolecular, Nutritionist, TCM, Massage	Rule out thrombosis; cautious compression use
2	Muscular / Myofascial	Muscle strain, myositis, fascial restrictions in axillary region	Anti-reactive botanicals, hydrotherapy, active recovery	Naturopath, Physiotherapist, Orthomolecular, Nutritionist, TCM, Massage	Early mobilization; avoid aggressive manual therapy
3	Skeletal	Clavicle, scapula, and rib involvement	Botanical anti-reactivities, bone support nutrients	Naturopath, Physiotherapist, Orthomolecular, Nutritionist, TCM	Imaging if trauma suspected; support bone health
4	Nervous System	Brachial plexus and peripheral nerve irritation	Neuroprotective botanicals, B-complex vitamins, nerve mobilization	Naturopath, Physiotherapist, Orthomolecular, Nutritionist, TCM	Early neural support; avoid aggressive techniques
5	Lymphatic / Immune	Lymphatic drainage and immune response in axillary region	Immune modulators, lymphatic drainage, antioxidants	Naturopath, Physiotherapist, Nutritionist, TCM, Massage	Differentiate infection; cautious use of compression
6	Organs / GNM	Conflict-active and healing phases in visceral reflex zones	Detoxification, immune modulation, tissue regeneration	Naturopath, Physiotherapist, TCM, Orthomolecular, Bioenergetic	Integrate GNM with clinical findings
7	Acupuncture	Qi stagnation, dampness, blood stasis	Acupuncture to disperse stagnation; moxibustion	Acupuncturist, Naturopath, Herbalist	Confirm diagnosis; careful use of moxibustion
8	Energetic / Frequency	Bioenergetic imbalance, reactivity	PEMF, microcurrent, bioresonance therapies	Bioenergetic therapist, Naturopath, Physiotherapist	Tailor therapy; monitor response
9	Metabolic / Endocrine	Metabolic/endocrine factors impacting axillary region	Glycemic regulators, thyroid/adrenal support	Naturopath, Orthomolecular, Nutritionist	Comprehensive endocrine evaluation advised

TABLE 25 - Zone 15 – Right Axillary

Category #	Category Name	Anatomical / Clinical Focus Summary	Main Naturopathic Therapeutic Approach	Key Specialists Involved	Clinical Pearls & Cautions (Summary)
1	Vascular / Circulatory	Axillary vascular structures, venous congestion, arterial flow issues	Venotonics, hydrotherapy, anti-reactive diet	Naturopath, Physiotherapist, Orthomolecular, Nutritionist, TCM, Massage	Rule out thrombosis; cautious compression use
2	Muscular / Myofascial	Muscle strain, myositis, fascial restrictions in axillary region	Anti-reactive botanicals, hydrotherapy, active recovery	Naturopath, Physiotherapist, Orthomolecular, Nutritionist, TCM, Massage	Early mobilization; avoid aggressive manual therapy
3	Skeletal	Clavicle, scapula, and rib involvement	Botanical anti-reactivities, bone support nutrients	Naturopath, Physiotherapist, Orthomolecular, Nutritionist, TCM	Imaging if trauma suspected; support bone health
4	Nervous System	Brachial plexus and peripheral nerve irritation	Neuroprotective botanicals, B-complex vitamins, nerve mobilization	Naturopath, Physiotherapist, Orthomolecular, Nutritionist, TCM	Early neural support; avoid aggressive techniques
5	Lymphatic / Immune	Lymphatic drainage and immune response in axillary region	Immune modulators, lymphatic drainage, antioxidants	Naturopath, Physiotherapist, Nutritionist, TCM, Massage	Differentiate infection; cautious use of compression
6	Organs / GNM	Conflict-active and healing phases in visceral reflex zones	Detoxification, immune modulation, tissue regeneration	Naturopath, Physiotherapist, TCM, Orthomolecular, Bioenergetic	Integrate GNM with clinical findings
7	Acupuncture	Qi stagnation, dampness, blood stasis	Acupuncture to disperse stagnation; moxibustion	Acupuncturist, Naturopath, Herbalist	Confirm diagnosis; careful use of moxibustion
8	Energetic / Frequency	Bioenergetic imbalance, reactivity	PEMF, microcurrent, bioresonance therapies	Bioenergetic therapist, Naturopath, Physiotherapist	Tailor therapy; monitor response
9	Metabolic / Endocrine	Metabolic/endocrine factors impacting axillary region	Glycemic regulators, thyroid/adrenal support	Naturopath, Orthomolecular, Nutritionist	Comprehensive endocrine evaluation advised

TABLE 26 - Zone 16 – Upper Back

Category #	Category Name	Anatomical / Clinical Focus Summary	Main Naturopathic Therapeutic Approach	Key Specialists Involved	Clinical Pearls & Cautions (Summary)
1	Vascular / Circulatory	Vascular supply to upper back muscles and soft tissues; congestion or hypoperfusion signs	Venotonics, hydrotherapy, anti-reactive diet	Naturopath, Physiotherapist, Orthomolecular, Nutritionist, TCM, Massage	Exclude vascular obstruction; cautious compression use
2	Muscular / Myofascial	Muscle strain, myositis, chronic tension	Anti-reactive botanicals, hydrotherapy, active mobilization	Naturopath, Physiotherapist, Orthomolecular, Nutritionist, TCM, Massage	Early movement; avoid deep tissue massage in acute phase
3	Skeletal	Thoracic spine, ribs, scapula bone health	Botanical anti-reactivities, bone-supportive nutrients	Naturopath, Physiotherapist, Orthomolecular, Nutritionist, TCM	Imaging as indicated; vitamin D and mineral support essential
4	Nervous System	Thoracic spinal nerves and sympathetic chain irritation	Neuroprotective botanicals, B-complex vitamins, neural mobilization	Naturopath, Physiotherapist, Orthomolecular, Nutritionist, TCM	Early nerve support; cautious manual therapy
5	Lymphatic / Immune	Lymphatic drainage and immune response in upper back	Immune modulators, lymphatic drainage, antioxidants	Naturopath, Physiotherapist, Nutritionist, TCM, Massage	Differentiate infection; careful compression use
6	Organs / GNM	Conflict-active and healing phases in thoracic visceral reflex zones	Detoxification, immune modulation, tissue regeneration	Naturopath, Physiotherapist, TCM, Orthomolecular, Bioenergetic	Integrate GNM with clinical findings
7	Acupuncture	Qi stagnation, dampness, blood stasis	Acupuncture to disperse stagnation; moxibustion	Acupuncturist, Naturopath, Herbalist	Confirm diagnosis; cautious moxibustion
8	Energetic / Frequency	Bioenergetic imbalance, reactivity	PEMF, microcurrent, bioresonance therapies	Bioenergetic therapist, Naturopath, Physiotherapist	Tailor therapy; monitor response
9	Metabolic / Endocrine	Metabolic/endocrine influences affecting upper back tissues	Glycemic regulators, thyroid/adrenal support	Naturopath, Orthomolecular, Nutritionist	Comprehensive endocrine evaluation advised

TABLE 27 - Zone 17 – Frontal Neck and Supraclavicular

Category #	Category Name	Anatomical / Clinical Focus Summary	Main Naturopathic Therapeutic Approach	Key Specialists Involved	Clinical Pearls & Cautions (Summary)
1	Vascular / Circulatory	Neck and supraclavicular vascular supply; congestion or hypoperfusion signs	Venotonics, hydrotherapy, anti-reactive diet, limb elevation	Naturopath, Physiotherapist, Orthomolecular, Nutritionist, TCM, Massage	Exclude vascular obstruction; cautious compression use
2	Muscular / Myofascial	Neck muscle strain, myositis, chronic tension	Anti-reactive botanicals, hydrotherapy, active mobilization	Naturopath, Physiotherapist, Orthomolecular, Nutritionist, TCM, Massage	Early mobilization; avoid deep tissue massage in acute reactivity
3	Skeletal	Cervical vertebrae and clavicular bone health	Botanical anti-reactivities, bone-supportive nutrients	Naturopath, Physiotherapist, Orthomolecular, Nutritionist, TCM	Imaging as indicated; vitamin D and mineral support essential
4	Nervous System	Cervical spinal nerves and autonomic fibers	Neuroprotective botanicals, B-complex vitamins, neural mobilization	Naturopath, Physiotherapist, Orthomolecular, Nutritionist, TCM	Early nerve support; cautious manual therapy
5	Lymphatic / Immune	Lymphatic drainage and immune response in neck region	Immune modulators, lymphatic drainage, antioxidants	Naturopath, Physiotherapist, Nutritionist, TCM, Massage	Differentiate infection; careful compression use
6	Organs / GNM	Conflict-active and healing phases in cervical visceral reflex zones	Detoxification, immune modulation, tissue regeneration	Naturopath, Physiotherapist, TCM, Orthomolecular, Bioenergetic	Integrate GNM with clinical findings
7	Acupuncture	Qi stagnation, dampness, blood stasis	Acupuncture to disperse stagnation; moxibustion	Acupuncturist, Naturopath, Herbalist	Confirm diagnosis; cautious use of moxibustion
8	Energetic / Frequency	Bioenergetic imbalance, reactivity	PEMF, microcurrent, bioresonance therapies	Bioenergetic therapist, Naturopath, Physiotherapist	Tailor therapy; monitor response
9	Metabolic / Endocrine	Metabolic/endocrine influences affecting neck tissues	Glycemic regulators, thyroid/adrenal support	Naturopath, Orthomolecular, Nutritionist	Comprehensive endocrine evaluation advised

TABLE 28 - Zone 18 – Cervical Spine and Nuchal Zone

Category #	Category Name	Anatomical / Clinical Focus Summary	Main Naturopathic Therapeutic Approach	Key Specialists Involved	Clinical Pearls & Cautions (Summary)
1	Vascular / Circulatory	Cervical vascular network; signs of venous congestion and arterial insufficiency	Venotonics, hydrotherapy, anti-reactive diet, limb elevation	Naturopath, Physiotherapist, Orthomolecular, Nutritionist, TCM, Massage	Exclude vascular obstruction; avoid compression in arterial insufficiency
2	Muscular / Myofascial	Cervical muscle strain, myositis, chronic tension	Anti-reactive botanicals, hydrotherapy, active mobilization	Naturopath, Physiotherapist, Orthomolecular, Nutritionist, TCM, Massage	Early mobilization; avoid deep tissue massage in acute reactivity
3	Skeletal	Cervical vertebrae and nuchal bone structures	Botanical anti-reactivities, bone-supportive nutrients	Naturopath, Physiotherapist, Orthomolecular, Nutritionist, TCM	Imaging essential; vitamin D and mineral support critical
4	Nervous System	Cervical spinal nerves and sympathetic chain	Neuroprotective botanicals, B-complex vitamins, neural mobilization	Naturopath, Physiotherapist, Orthomolecular, Nutritionist, TCM	Early nerve support; cautious manual therapy
5	Lymphatic / Immune	Cervical lymphatic drainage and immune response	Immune modulators, lymphatic drainage, antioxidants	Naturopath, Physiotherapist, Nutritionist, TCM, Massage	Differentiate infection; careful compression use
6	Organs / GNM	Conflict-active and healing phases in cervical visceral reflex zones	Detoxification, immune modulation, tissue regeneration	Naturopath, Physiotherapist, TCM, Orthomolecular, Bioenergetic	Integrate GNM with clinical findings
7	Acupuncture	Qi stagnation, dampness, blood stasis	Acupuncture to disperse stagnation; moxibustion	Acupuncturist, Naturopath, Herbalist	Confirm diagnosis; cautious moxibustion
8	Energetic / Frequency	Bioenergetic imbalance, reactivity	PEMF, microcurrent, bioresonance therapies	Bioenergetic therapist, Naturopath, Physiotherapist	Tailor therapy; monitor response
9	Metabolic / Endocrine	Metabolic/endocrine influences affecting cervical region	Glycemic regulators, thyroid/adrenal support	Naturopath, Orthomolecular, Nutritionist	Comprehensive endocrine evaluation recommended

TABLE 29 - Zone 19 – Facial Area (Frontal and Lateral)

Category #	Category Name	Anatomical / Clinical Focus Summary	Main Naturopathic Therapeutic Approach	Key Specialists Involved	Clinical Pearls & Cautions (Summary)
1	Vascular / Circulatory	Facial arterial and venous network; signs of reactivity or hypoperfusion	Botanical venotonics (horse chestnut, gotu kola), hydrotherapy, anti-reactive diet	Naturopath, Physiotherapist, Orthomolecular, Nutritionist, TCM, Massage	Differentiate thrombophlebitis; avoid excessive heat
2	Muscular / Myofascial	Facial muscles including expression and mastication muscles; strain, reactivity	Anti-reactive botanicals (arnica, turmeric), hydrotherapy, gentle massage	Naturopath, Physiotherapist, Orthomolecular, Nutritionist, TCM, Massage	Avoid deep massage in acute reactivity; emphasize magnesium and protein
3	Skeletal	Facial bones: maxilla, mandible, zygomatic arches, nasal bones	Botanical anti-reactivities, bone nutrients (vitamin D3, K2), collagen support	Naturopath, Physiotherapist, Orthomolecular, Nutritionist, TCM	Imaging critical in trauma; vitamin and mineral support essential
4	Nervous System	Facial and trigeminal nerves; neuropathy, neuritis	Neuroprotective botanicals, B-complex vitamins, neural mobilization	Naturopath, Physiotherapist, Orthomolecular, Nutritionist, TCM	Early nerve support critical; avoid aggressive therapy
5	Lymphatic / Immune	Facial lymphatic drainage and immune response	Immune modulators, lymphatic drainage, antioxidants	Naturopath, Physiotherapist, Nutritionist, TCM, Massage	Differentiate infection; cautious manual therapy
6	Organs / GNM	Conflict-active and healing phases in facial visceral reflex zones	Detoxification, immune modulation, tissue regeneration	Naturopath, Physiotherapist, TCM, Orthomolecular, Bioenergetic	Integrate GNM with clinical and imaging findings
7	Acupuncture	Qi stagnation, dampness, blood stasis	Acupuncture to clear stagnation; moxibustion	Acupuncturist, Naturopath, Herbalist	Confirm diagnosis; careful moxibustion use
8	Energetic / Frequency	Bioenergetic imbalance, reactivity	PEMF, microcurrent, bioresonance therapies	Bioenergetic therapist, Naturopath, Physiotherapist	Tailor frequency protocols; monitor patient response
9	Metabolic / Endocrine	Metabolic/endocrine influences on facial tissues	Glycemic regulators, thyroid/adrenal support	Naturopath, Orthomolecular, Nutritionist	Full endocrine evaluation recommended

TABLE 30 – CROSS-CATEGORY THERAPEUTIC INTEGRATION MATRIX

This table synthesizes therapeutic strategies across all nine evaluation categories of Biospectral Medicine, allowing practitioners to view interventions in a category-centered rather than zone-centered framework. By aligning vascular, muscular, skeletal, nervous, lymphatic/immune, organ/GNM, acupuncture, energetic/frequency, and metabolic/endocrine categories with their core natural medicine applications, it provides a quick-reference guide for integrative clinical decision-making that complements the zone-specific tables.

Zone # & Name	Main Anatomical Structures	Common Clinical Patterns and Symptoms	Typical Thermographic Findings	Principles of Therapeutical Strategies
Zone 1 – Frontal Lower Legs	Tibialis anterior muscle, anterior tibial artery, superficial veins	Venous congestion, varicosities, muscle strain, neuropathies	Hyper: Venous dilation, reactivity; Hypo: Arterial insufficiency, muscle atrophy	Restore venous and arterial circulation; reduce reactivity; support tissue repair; improve microcirculation
Zone 2 – Dorsal Lower Legs	Gastrocnemius and soleus muscles, posterior tibial artery and veins	Muscle fatigue, venous insufficiency, nerve irritation	Hyper: Muscle reactivity, venous congestion; Hypo: Arterial hypoperfusion	Alleviate muscular reactivity; enhance vascular return; promote nerve recovery; optimize peripheral perfusion
Zone 3 – Internal Left Leg	Medial leg muscles, saphenous vein	Muscle strain, venous insufficiency, peripheral neuropathy	Hyper: Local reactivity; Hypo: Chronic hypoperfusion	Address reactive processes; restore vascular and neural function; support tissue metabolism
Zone 4 – Internal Right Leg	Similar to Zone 3, right medial leg structures	Similar to Zone 3	Similar patterns	Same as Zone 3 principles
Zone 5 – External Left Leg	Lateral leg muscles, peroneal artery and vein	Muscle strain, venous congestion	Hyper: Reactivity; Hypo: Hypoperfusion	Reduce reactivity; improve circulation; support muscle function
Zone 6 – External Right Leg	Lateral leg muscles, peroneal artery and vein	Similar to Zone 5	Similar patterns	Same as Zone 5 principles
Zone 7 – Frontal Upper Legs	Quadriceps muscles, femoral artery and veins	Muscle strain, varicosities, nerve irritation	Hyper: Venous congestion, muscular reactivity; Hypo: Arterial insufficiency	Enhance venous tone; decrease reactivity; support muscular recovery; improve arterial flow

Zone 8 – Dorsal Upper Legs	Hamstring muscles, femoral artery and veins	Muscle fatigue, venous insufficiency	Hyper: Muscle reactivity, venous congestion; Hypo: Hypoperfusion	Modulate reactivity; promote vascular return; stimulate tissue healing
Zone 9 – Frontal Abdomen	Abdominal wall muscles, visceral organs	Abdominal pain, muscle strain, organ-related discomfort	Hyper: Local heat over muscles or organs; Hypo: Chronic tissue dysfunction	Support visceral organ function; reduce reactive activity; restore muscular and fascial balance
Zone 10 – Lateral Right Abdomen	Lateral abdominal muscles, ribs, viscera	Muscular strain, visceral conflict, immune response	Hyper: Heat from reactivity or visceral activity; Hypo: Cold areas from chronic dysfunction	Address immune modulation; relieve muscular and fascial tension; promote visceral healing
Zone 11 – Lateral Left Abdomen	Similar to Zone 10, left side	Similar to Zone 10	Similar patterns	Same as Zone 10 principles
Zone 12 – Lumbar Region	Lumbar vertebrae, paraspinal muscles, nerve roots	Low back pain, nerve irritation, muscular tension	Hyper: Muscle spasm and reactivity; Hypo: Nerve compression, poor circulation	Relieve muscular tension; support nerve regeneration; optimize local circulation
Zone 13 – Chest and Sternum	Sternum, ribs, thoracic muscles	Chest wall pain, muscular strain, circulatory abnormalities	Hyper: Local activation or congestion; Hypo: Reduced emission from low perfusion	Decrease reactivity; enhance circulation; restore musculoskeletal balance
Zone 14 – Left Axillary	Axillary lymph nodes, brachial plexus, vessels	Lymphadenopathy, nerve irritation, vascular congestion	Hyper: Swelling, warmth; Hypo: Circulatory insufficiency	Support lymphatic drainage; reduce reactivity; promote nerve health
Zone 15 – Right Axillary	Similar to Zone 14, right side	Similar to Zone 14	Similar thermographic patterns	Same as Zone 14 principles
Zone 16 – Upper Back	Thoracic spine, trapezius muscles, scapula	Muscle tension, nerve irritation, circulatory issues	Hyper: Muscle spasm, reactivity; Hypo: Poor perfusion	Relieve muscular spasm; enhance circulation; support neural tissue
Zone 17 – Frontal Neck and Supraclavicular	Cervical muscles, carotid arteries, lymph nodes	Neck pain, lymphadenopathy, vascular issues	Hyper: Reactivity, warmth; Hypo: Ischemic zones	Promote vascular and lymphatic flow; reduce reactivity; support neural function
Zone 18 – Cervical Spine and Nuchal Zone	Cervical vertebrae, spinal cord, paraspinal muscles	Neck stiffness, nerve irritation, muscular strain	Hyper: Local reactivity; Hypo: Nerve compression	Alleviate reactivity; encourage nerve regeneration; restore muscular balance
Zone 19 – Facial Area (Frontal and Lateral)	Facial muscles, trigeminal nerve branches, facial vessels	Facial pain, neuropathy, vascular congestion	Hyper: Reactivity, vasodilation; Hypo: Nerve dysfunction	Support microcirculation; reduce neurogenic reactivity; promote tissue healing

TABLE 31 – BIOSPECTRAL MODALITIES OF APPLICATION: ZONES OF APPLICATION, CONTRAINDICATIONS, AND SAFETY CONSIDERATIONS

This table provides a comprehensive reference for the integration of therapeutic and evaluation modalities within Biospectral Medicine. Each intervention is aligned with its associated emission zones or clinical conditions and is accompanied by contraindications, side effects, and safety cautions.

By combining conventional and integrative practices in a single framework, the table functions as a clinical safety compass, helping practitioners select appropriate modalities, avoid risks, and ensure patient-centered care. It emphasizes that every therapeutic decision must respect emission findings, systemic conditions, co-morbidities, and regulatory guidelines.

Therapeutic Strategy / Evaluation Modality	Associated Zones / Conditions	Contraindications / Side Effects / Cautions
Compression Therapy	Zones 1-6, 14-16 (vascular compromised zones)	Contraindicated in severe arterial insufficiency or critical hypoperfusion; risk of worsening flow
Deep Tissue Massage	Hyperthermic acute reactivity zones (any)	Avoid during acute reactivity, thrombophlebitis, fractures, or skin infections
Heat Therapy (Hot Packs, Sauna)	Acute thrombophlebitis, active infections	May exacerbate clotting or infection; avoid in acute reactive states
Herbal Warming Agents	Skin hypersensitivity, open wounds	Risk of skin irritation or allergic reactions
NSAIDs (Non-Steroidal Anti-Reactivities)	GI ulcers, renal impairment, bleeding disorders	Gastrointestinal bleeding risk, renal toxicity with prolonged use
Radiation-Based Evaluation (X-Ray, CT Scan)	All zones (systemic exposure concerns)	Cumulative ionizing radiation exposure risks; use ALARA principle (As Low As Reasonably Achievable)
Chemotherapy	Systemic malignancies	Immunosuppression, neuropathy, mucositis, cardiotoxicity; monitor organ functions
Anticoagulant Therapy	Vascular zones with thrombosis or embolism risk	Increased bleeding risk; contraindicated with active bleeding or recent surgery
Corticosteroids	Multiple zones with reactivity	Immunosuppression, adrenal suppression, osteoporosis, hyperglycemia
Physical Activity – High Intensity	Zones with acute injury or reactivity	Risk of exacerbating injury; gradual reintroduction recommended
Electrotherapy (TENS, EMS)	Pacemaker presence, pregnancy	Contraindicated with implanted electrical devices, during pregnancy
Laser Therapy (High Intensity)	Malignant lesions, infection zones	May stimulate tumor growth or worsen infections

Blood Thinners / Antiplatelets	Vascular zones with bleeding risk	Enhanced bleeding; caution with invasive procedures
Sclerotherapy	Venous insufficiency zones	Allergic reactions to sclerosants; avoid in infection or acute thrombosis
Surgical Interventions	Zone-dependent	Risks include infection, anesthesia complications, delayed healing
Contrast Agents (Iodine, Gadolinium)	Imaging requiring vascular contrast	Allergic reactions, nephrotoxicity; caution in renal impairment
UV Therapy	Photosensitive disorders	Avoid in lupus, porphyria, or other photosensitivity syndromes
Bioresonance / Frequency Therapy	Pregnancy, pacemaker, epilepsy	Limited evidence; contraindicated in electrical device users and pregnancy
Homeopathic Remedies	Allergic predisposition	Rare hypersensitivity or aggravation of symptoms
Phytotherapy (Herbal Extracts)	Concurrent medications	Herb-drug interactions possible; monitor liver/kidney function
Hydrotherapy – Cold Baths	Raynaud's phenomenon, cardiovascular instability	Sudden cold exposure may induce vasospasm or cardiac stress
Hydrotherapy – Contrast Baths	Acute reactivity, open wounds	Contraindicated during acute reactive or infectious phases
Nutritional Supplements (High Dose)	Liver or kidney impairment	Risk of toxicity with overdosing; monitor organ function
Acupuncture	Bleeding disorders, infection at needle sites	Avoid in patients with coagulopathies or active skin infections
Physical Modalities (Ultrasound Therapy)	Malignancy, fractures	Avoid over cancerous lesions and recent fractures
Chelation Therapy	Heavy metal toxicity	Potential nephrotoxicity; contraindicated in severe renal insufficiency
Oxygen Therapy (Hyperbaric)	Pneumothorax, untreated malignancies	Risk of oxygen toxicity; requires careful patient selection
Phlebotomy	Hemochromatosis	Risk of anemia, hypovolemia if improperly monitored
Detoxification Protocols (Sauna, Juicing)	Cardiovascular instability, renal impairment	Potential electrolyte imbalances, dehydration
Psychotherapy / Counseling	Severe mental illness without medical supervision	Must be integrated with psychiatric care where indicated
Spinal Manipulation (Chiropractic/Osteopathy)	Acute fractures, severe osteoporosis, infections	Risk of fracture or neurologic injury; contraindicated in unstable spine
Platelet-Rich Plasma (PRP) Therapy	Infection at injection site, coagulation disorders	Risk of infection, bleeding; contraindicated in active infections

Stem Cell Therapy	Malignancy, active infections	Experimental; requires strict patient selection
Intravenous Nutrient Therapy	Allergy to components, severe organ dysfunction	Risk of phlebitis, toxicity; monitor infusion reactions
Mesotherapy	Skin infections, bleeding disorders	Risk of infection, bruising
Cold Laser / Low-Level Laser Therapy (LLLT)	Pregnancy, malignancy	Limited data; use cautiously in sensitive populations
Cupping Therapy	Skin lesions, bleeding disorders	May cause bruising, bleeding; avoid in fragile skin
Electroconvulsive Therapy (ECT)	Increased intracranial pressure, recent myocardial infarction	Requires strict medical oversight
Blood Transfusions	Hemolytic reactions, infections	Risk of allergic reactions, infections
Antibiotic Therapy	Allergies, antibiotic resistance	Risk of side effects, resistance development
Vaccination	Allergic reactions, immunocompromised patients	Contraindicated in certain immune disorders
Hormone Replacement Therapy (HRT)	History of hormone-sensitive cancers	Increased risk of thromboembolism, cancer recurrence
Chelation with EDTA	Renal insufficiency, hypocalcemia	Risk of nephrotoxicity, electrolyte imbalances
Photodynamic Therapy	Photosensitivity, pregnancy	Risk of skin burns and reactions
Antidepressant Medication	Suicidal ideation, bipolar disorder	Requires careful psychiatric evaluation

TABLE 32 – CROSS-DISCIPLINARY MAPPING OF THE NINE EVALUATION CATEGORIES

This table illustrates how the nine evaluation categories of Biospectral Medicine correspond to established clinical specialties in conventional medicine as well as to natural, integrative, and allied health disciplines.

By aligning each category with its respective fields of practice, the table highlights the interdisciplinary nature of Biospectral interpretation and its capacity to serve as an evaluation bridge between biomedical and integrative models of care. It demonstrates how findings within each emission category can be validated, contextualized, and treated through both conventional and natural frameworks, reinforcing the complementary part of Biospectral Medicine in clinical decision-making.

Category	Conventional	Natural/Integrative/Allied
Vascular	Angiology, Cardiology	Naturopathy, Physiotherapy, Orthomolecular, Nutritionist, Massage Therapist
Muscular	Orthopedics, Sports Medicine, Physiatry	Osteopathy, Manual Therapy, Physiotherapy, Naturopathy, Massage Therapist
Skeletal	Orthopedics, Rheumatology	Osteopathy, Physiotherapy, Naturopathy, Massage Therapist
Nervous System	Neurology, Pain Medicine	Physiotherapy, Naturopathy, Osteopathy, Massage Therapist
Lymphatic/Immune	Immunology, Hematology	Naturopathy, Physiotherapy, Orthomolecular, Massage Therapist
Organs/GNM	Internal Medicine, Psychiatry	Mind-Body, Psychotherapy, Naturopathy, Massage Therapist
Acupuncture	Medical Acupuncture, Integrative Medicine	TCM, Acupuncture, Naturopathy, Massage Therapist
Energetic/Frequency	Integrative Medicine, Bioenergetics	Bioenergetics, Naturopathy, Massage Therapist
Metabolic/Endocrine	Endocrinology, Nutrition, Functional Medicine	Orthomolecular, Nutritionist, Naturopathy

Systematic Reference Tables in Biospectral Medicine

The reference tables presented in this chapter serve as a structured extension of the interpretative reasoning explored throughout the Atlas. Organized by anatomical zone and evaluation category, these tables synthesize the essential patterns observed across the case studies and broader clinical experience, translating spectral emission patterns into clinically relevant interpretive references

For clinicians, they function as a rapid-access interface with the core logic of Biospectral Medicine, allowing for immediate correlation between spectral findings, underlying physiological systems, and interpretive categories. This greatly enhances the speed, consistency, and accuracy of zone-based assessments in daily practice.

For researchers, the tables offer a foundational matrix from which to design observational studies, quantify zone-emission correlations, or evaluate the interpretation reproducibility of the method across populations. Each entry reflects a clinically validated relationship between emission morphology and systemic disturbance, thereby transforming individual biosignals into collective evaluation intelligence.

As a whole, the chapter elevates the methodology from interpretive art to codified science, providing the practical infrastructure necessary for training, replication, and academic inquiry.

GLOSSARY

The glossary establishes the common language of Biospectral Medicine, aligning physics, physiology, and integrative clinical practice into a single, consistent lexicon. By defining 180 terms and abbreviations, it supplies the reference base needed for interpretation, teaching, and research, so readers can move from observation to inference with stable meanings. This shared vocabulary supports reproducibility across settings and preserves methodological coherence as the discipline scales.

Each entry follows a consistent structure: a precise definition, the operational use within the R-CIIM pathway, and the clinical context in which the term becomes relevant. Cross-references link entries to spectral zones, ROI mapping conventions, the nine interpretive categories, and key procedural elements such as palette normalization and the Spectrovascular Response Test (SVRT). Abbreviations, pluralization, and capitalization follow an editorial policy that favors clarity and searchability; synonyms are harmonized so a single preferred term anchors each concept across the Atlas.

The glossary serves everyday practice. It informs how reports are written, how overlays are labeled, and how **biospectral asymmetries** are described with consistent thresholds and qualifiers. In training, it functions as a scaffold for competency assessment and inter-observer alignment. In research, it enables dataset curation, metadata tagging, and outcome mapping, which strengthens study design, agreement metrics, and longitudinal comparability. The result is a language that travels well between clinics, classrooms, and journals.

Governance and evolution keep the lexicon alive. Versioned updates, change logs, and submission criteria allow the community to incorporate new terms responsibly as evidence grows. Entries indicate normative usage, known limitations, and recommended correlation pathways, guiding readers toward consistent application across zones and time.

By unifying terminology for **spectral surface reading**, ROI geometry, and category-specific interpretation, the glossary anchors Biospectral Medicine in a rigorous, teachable, and publishable language that supports clinical decision-making and academic advancement.

1. **Activose**
   A biospectral emission pattern characterized by heightened functional activity within a region of interest, often linked to increased vascular flow, metabolic activation, or neuroautonomic excitation. It signifies zones of physiological stimulation that may correlate with inflammation, repair, or adaptive stress.

2. **Acupoint Mapping**
   The systematic identification and correlation of acupuncture points within Biospectral Medicine, recognizing their spatial overlap with emission zones. Acupoint mapping provides a bridge between traditional meridian theory and modern biosignal interpretation, supporting integrative diagnostic approaches.

3. **Acupoint Reactivity**
   Refers to the responsiveness of acupuncture points when evaluated through biospectral imaging, where focal emission patterns may indicate heightened energetic or physiological activity. Such reactivity suggests functional relevance of the point in systemic regulation and therapeutic targeting.

4. **Acupuncture / Meridians**
   A diagnostic and therapeutic framework from Traditional Chinese Medicine describing longitudinal energetic pathways that connect organs and functional systems. In Biospectral Medicine, meridians are studied as potential correlates of fascial, vascular, and neuroautonomic networks observable through emission patterns.

5. **Additional Terms**
   This designation is used in the Atlas to incorporate supplementary concepts or terminology that extend beyond the core categories. These entries ensure comprehensiveness and provide clinicians with contextual vocabulary relevant to biospectral interpretation.

6. **Anisospectral**
   Describes asymmetry or unequal distribution of biospectral emissions between contralateral or adjacent anatomical zones. Anisospectral findings may reflect localized dysfunctions, including vascular restriction, metabolic imbalance, or neuromuscular asymmetry, requiring integrative interpretation within the R-CIIM framework.

7. **Arm Lines (Deep/Superficial)**
   Myofascial continuities described in the fascial system, extending through the upper limbs in both superficial and deep layers. Their inclusion in Biospectral Medicine highlights the correspondence between fascial pathways and emission zones, aiding in the interpretation of upper limb functional imbalances.

8. **Articular Stress**
   A biomechanical and functional condition identified through emission changes in joint-related zones, reflecting overload, misalignment, or degenerative processes. It is commonly observed in skeletal or musculoskeletal categories and may correspond with pain or restricted mobility.

9. **Autonomic Imbalance**
   A state of dysregulation between sympathetic and parasympathetic branches of the autonomic nervous system, often visualized as inconsistent or exaggerated biospectral responses. Such imbalance can contribute to chronic pain, circulatory changes, or systemic dysfunction.

10. **Autonomic Regulation**
    The coordinated control of visceral, vascular, and metabolic functions by the autonomic nervous system. In Biospectral Medicine, autonomic regulation is evaluated through emission responses such as the Spectrovascular Response Test, providing insight into systemic adaptability and resilience.

11. **Bioenergetic Fields**
    Conceptual domains representing the body's subtle energetic activity, often described in integrative and complementary sciences. In Biospectral Medicine, these fields are considered through their potential correlations with emission patterns that reflect systemic coherence or disturbance.

12. **Biological Conflicts**
    A central concept in German New Medicine (GNM), referring to unresolved psycho-emotional stressors that trigger adaptive physiological programs. Within Biospectral Medicine, biological conflicts may manifest as recurring emission anomalies in zones linked to corresponding organs or systems.

13. **Biological Program (GNM)**
    Refers to the adaptive physiological response described in German New Medicine, initiated by unresolved conflict and progressing through distinct phases. In the biospectral context, such programs can be traced through predictable emission changes across specific anatomical zones.

14. Biosignal Expression

The observable manifestation of physiological or energetic processes as surface emission patterns. Biosignal expression provides the raw data for interpretation in Biospectral Medicine, linking underlying circulatory, metabolic, and neuroautonomic dynamics to visible functional imaging.

15. Biospectral Asymmetry

A difference in emission intensity or distribution between contralateral or adjacent regions, often revealing localized dysfunction. This asymmetry is a key interpretive marker in the R-CIIM system, guiding differential assessment of vascular, muscular, or metabolic imbalance.

16. Biospectral Signal

The measurable output of emissive activity captured during imaging, representing the integration of vascular, metabolic, and neuroautonomic influences. In Biospectral Medicine, biospectral signals are interpreted as functional indicators rather than static temperature values.

17. Blackbody Calibrator

A precision device used to ensure accuracy in emissive imaging systems, simulating a perfect emitter for calibration purposes. Its application in Biospectral Medicine guarantees that detector readings remain standardized and comparable across sessions.

18. Blackbody Radiation

The theoretical model describing the emission of electromagnetic radiation from an idealized body at a given temperature. This principle underpins emissive physics and provides the scientific foundation for interpreting spectral data in clinical imaging.

19. Calibration Protocol

The standardized procedure for adjusting and validating imaging equipment to ensure reproducible and accurate biospectral measurements. Proper calibration is essential for clinical reliability, cross-patient comparisons, and longitudinal studies.

20. Chronic Inflammation

A persistent state of low-grade or recurrent inflammatory activity that may be visualized as stable or recurrent emission anomalies. In Biospectral Medicine, chronic inflammation is recognized as a systemic contributor to pain, vascular load, and metabolic stress.

21. **Cooled Detector**
An infrared sensor that operates at cryogenic temperatures to reduce thermal noise and improve sensitivity to faint photon emissions. Cooled detectors achieve superior radiometric accuracy and resolution compared to uncooled systems, making them valuable in research applications. In Biospectral Medicine, they serve primarily as reference standards, since clinical practice typically employs uncooled microbolometers for practicality and accessibility.

22. **Cortisol Rhythm**
The cyclical secretion pattern of cortisol regulated by the hypothalamic–pituitary–adrenal axis, essential for stress response and circadian balance. In Biospectral Medicine, disruption of cortisol rhythm may be inferred through systemic emission patterns linked to metabolic and neuroautonomic regulation.

23. **Deep Front Line**
A myofascial continuity extending through the body's core structures, linking the arches of the feet to the thoracic cavity and cervical spine. Its relevance in Biospectral Medicine lies in the observation of emission patterns that mirror tension or dysfunction along this fascial pathway.

24. **Dermatome Mapping**
The charting of skin regions supplied by specific spinal nerves. In Biospectral Medicine, dermatome mapping provides a framework for correlating emission anomalies with possible spinal or neuroautonomic origins.

25. **Detector Array**
A matrix of sensor elements within emissive imaging equipment that captures radiant energy from the body. High-resolution detector arrays enhance the precision of biospectral imaging, allowing finer discrimination of emission zones.

26. **Detector Calibration**
The adjustment of detector sensitivity and accuracy against known standards, ensuring reliable spectral data acquisition. Regular calibration is essential to maintain consistency across patient assessments and research studies.

27. **Detoxification Pathways**
The biological processes by which the body neutralizes and eliminates toxins, primarily through the liver, kidneys, lymphatic system, and skin. In Biospectral Medicine, dysfunction in these pathways may present as recurrent emission anomalies in corresponding zones.

28. Dynamic Range

The span between the lowest and highest emission intensities an imaging system can accurately detect. A wide dynamic range improves the ability to capture subtle variations in biospectral signals across diverse physiological states.

29. Emission Zones

The nineteen anatomically standardized regions established in Biospectral Medicine as the basis for structured interpretation. Each zone integrates multiple interpretive categories, facilitating reproducible analysis of emission patterns in clinical and research contexts.

30. Emissivity

A physical property describing how efficiently a material emits infrared radiation relative to a perfect blackbody. Understanding emissivity is fundamental to Biospectral Medicine, as human tissues emit with high but non-uniform emissivity values that influence signal interpretation.

31. Endocrine Crosstalk

The interactive signaling between different endocrine glands and their hormones, coordinating systemic physiological functions. Biospectral anomalies associated with endocrine crosstalk may reflect disruptions in metabolic, reproductive, or stress-regulation pathways.

32. Energetic / Frequency

A interpretive category in Biospectral Medicine concerned with emission phenomena that suggest systemic energetic imbalance or frequency-related dysfunction. This category bridges integrative perspectives on bioenergetics with spectral data captured in clinical imaging.Energetic Congestion

33. Energy Flow Blockages

Disruptions in the continuity of systemic energy circulation, often described in traditional and integrative medicine. In Biospectral Medicine, blockages may be inferred from localized emission stagnation or asymmetry along meridian or fascial pathways.

34. Far-Infrared (FIR)

A portion of the electromagnetic spectrum with wavelengths typically between 15 and 1000 micrometers. FIR is the range most relevant to emissive imaging of human tissues, as it captures radiative output linked to vascular and metabolic activity.

35. Fascial Lines (Myers)
Anatomical continuities of connective tissue described by Thomas Myers, illustrating how fascia links muscles into functional chains. In Biospectral Medicine, fascial lines serve as structural correlates for emission zones, supporting integrative interpretation of tension and dysfunction.

36. Five Elements (TCM)
A conceptual framework in Traditional Chinese Medicine describing dynamic interactions among Wood, Fire, Earth, Metal, and Water. Within Biospectral Medicine, this model offers a symbolic complement to emission interpretation, aligning functional changes with systemic patterns.

37. Frequency Medicine
An integrative therapeutic approach that applies specific electromagnetic frequencies to influence biological systems. Its relevance to Biospectral Medicine lies in the shared principle that physiological states manifest as measurable frequency or emission signatures.

38. Functional Dysfunction
A disturbance in physiological processes that alters system performance without structural pathology. Biospectral Medicine is particularly suited to identifying functional dysfunctions, as emission anomalies often precede anatomical changes.

39. Glycemic Instability
Fluctuations in blood glucose regulation that disrupt metabolic balance. Such instability may manifest in Biospectral Medicine as emission changes in abdominal or endocrine-related zones, reflecting systemic metabolic stress.

40. GNM (German New Medicine)
A theoretical framework developed by Ryke Geerd Hamer, proposing that unresolved biological conflicts trigger specific adaptive programs. In Biospectral Medicine, GNM concepts are integrated as interpretive references for recurrent emission findings linked to psycho-emotional stressors.

41. Homeostatic Disruption
An interruption in the body's ability to maintain physiological equilibrium across circulatory, metabolic, or neuroautonomic systems. Emission irregularities often reflect such disruption, highlighting zones of systemic overload or imbalance.

42. Hormonal Imbalances

Alterations in endocrine signaling that disturb metabolic and systemic regulation. In Biospectral Medicine, these imbalances may appear as recurrent emission anomalies in zones related to thyroid, reproductive, or adrenal function.

43. Hormonal Regulation

The coordinated control of physiological processes by endocrine hormones. In Biospectral Medicine, the observation of emission patterns in key zones provides indirect insight into the integrity of hormonal regulation

44. Immune Modulation

The process by which the immune system adjusts its activity to maintain balance between defense, tolerance, and repair. In Biospectral Medicine, emission changes linked to immune modulation may appear in lymphatic or organ-specific zones during adaptive responses.

45. Immune Surveillance

The continuous monitoring function of the immune system that detects and responds to pathogens, neoplastic cells, and tissue damage. Biospectral anomalies may correspond to areas of increased immune surveillance, especially in zones with chronic or recurrent stress.

46. Inflammatory Cascade

A sequence of molecular and cellular events triggered by tissue injury or infection, leading to vascular dilation, immune activation, and metabolic changes. In Biospectral Medicine, this cascade often produces localized activose emission patterns.

47. Infrared Optics

The specialized lenses and filters used to transmit and focus infrared radiation onto detector arrays. High-quality infrared optics are critical in Biospectral Medicine to preserve signal fidelity and ensure accurate imaging.

48. Infrared Spectrum

The portion of the electromagnetic spectrum with wavelengths longer than visible light and shorter than microwaves, spanning 0.7 to 1000 micrometers. The mid- to far-infrared spectrum is most relevant to emissive imaging in Biospectral Medicine.

49. Inhibose
A biospectral emission pattern indicating reduced or suppressed physiological activity within a region of interest. It may correlate with hypoperfusion, metabolic slowdown, or inhibited neuroautonomic signaling, often juxtaposed with activose regions.

50. Lateral Line
A fascial continuity that extends along the sides of the body, contributing to balance and postural integrity. In Biospectral Medicine, emission anomalies along the lateral line may indicate asymmetry in load distribution or musculoskeletal compensation.

51. Liver Congestion
A state of impaired hepatic circulation or detoxification capacity, often reflected in systemic metabolic stress. Biospectral findings may show recurrent emission changes in abdominal zones corresponding to liver function.

52. Lymphatic / Immune
One of the nine interpretive categories in Biospectral Medicine, focusing on emission findings related to lymphatic circulation and immune system activity. Patterns in this category may indicate fluid stagnation, inflammation, or immune dysregulation.

53. Lymphatic Drainage
The physiological process by which lymphatic vessels transport interstitial fluid, immune cells, and metabolic byproducts. Impairment in drainage may be visualized through emission anomalies in peripheral or abdominal zones.

54. Meridian Mapping
The systematic charting of meridian pathways as described in Traditional Chinese Medicine and their integration into emission analysis. Meridian mapping in Biospectral Medicine facilitates cross-comparison between energetic theories and physiological emission patterns.

55. Meridian Pathways
Longitudinal energetic routes described in Traditional Chinese Medicine, connecting organ systems through acupoints. In Biospectral Medicine, these pathways are studied for potential correspondence with emission anomalies and structural continuities such as fascial lines.

56. Meridian–Fascial Overlap
The observed anatomical correlation between classical meridian lines and modern fascial continuities. Biospectral Medicine uses this overlap to interpret emission findings as integrative signals bridging traditional and physiological models.

57. Metabolic / Endocrine

One of the nine interpretive categories in Biospectral Medicine, addressing emission anomalies linked to hormonal and metabolic regulation. Patterns may suggest thyroid dysfunction, adrenal stress, or systemic metabolic overload.

58. Metabolic Load

The cumulative physiological burden placed on the body by energy demand, toxin processing, and hormonal regulation. Increased metabolic load often presents as recurrent emission anomalies in abdominal and endocrine-related zones.

59. Metabolic Syndrome

A cluster of metabolic dysfunctions—including insulin resistance, hypertension, dyslipidemia, and central obesity—that increase systemic disease risk. Biospectral Medicine may identify early signs of this syndrome through emission anomalies in abdominal, vascular, and endocrine zones.

60. Microbolometer

An uncooled infrared detector used to capture emissive signals with high sensitivity and precision. Microbolometer technology forms the basis of modern Biospectral Medicine imaging, valued for clinical reliability and reproducibility.

61. Microcirculation

The network of small blood vessels, including arterioles, capillaries, and venules, that regulate tissue exchange and perfusion. In Biospectral Medicine, microcirculatory dysfunction is a common basis for localized emission changes.

62. Mid-Infrared (MIR)

The portion of the infrared spectrum between approximately 3 and 8 micrometers in wavelength. While less used for clinical emissive imaging than the far-infrared, MIR contributes to understanding tissue radiation and detector calibration.

63. Mineral Depletion

The reduction of essential minerals such as magnesium, zinc, or iron, impairing enzymatic and metabolic functions. Biospectral anomalies linked to mineral depletion may appear in endocrine, muscular, or circulatory categories.

64. Mitochondrial Function

The capacity of mitochondria to generate cellular energy through oxidative phosphorylation. Emission patterns associated with mitochondrial dysfunction may reflect systemic fatigue, metabolic instability, or oxidative stress.

65. Muscle–Fascia Coupling
The biomechanical integration between muscle fibers and surrounding fascial tissue, ensuring coordinated movement and load transfer. In Biospectral Medicine, anomalies in coupling may manifest as localized emission asymmetry in musculoskeletal zones.Muscular / Myofascial

66. Myofascial Continuities
Chains of interconnected fascia and muscle that transmit mechanical force across distant regions of the body. In Biospectral Medicine, these continuities provide structural explanations for emission patterns that extend beyond localized zones.

67. Myofascial Release
A therapeutic technique that applies sustained pressure to fascia to reduce restrictions and restore mobility. Its relevance in Biospectral Medicine lies in the observed emission changes following release, often reflecting improved circulation and reduced tension.

68. Myofascial Tension
The state of sustained contraction or restriction within fascial structures that alters load distribution. Emission anomalies in Biospectral Medicine frequently correspond to areas of excessive myofascial tension, particularly in musculoskeletal categories.

69. Myotome Correlation
The relationship between spinal nerve roots and the groups of muscles they innervate. In Biospectral Medicine, emission anomalies in specific zones may be correlated with myotomal patterns, aiding in neuromuscular interpretation.

70. Near-Infrared (NIR)
The portion of the electromagnetic spectrum ranging from 0.7 to 1.5 micrometers. While primarily used in spectroscopy and optical imaging, NIR principles contribute to the broader physics of tissue emissivity considered in Biospectral Medicine.

71. Nervous System / Spine
One of the nine interpretive categories in Biospectral Medicine, focusing on emission findings linked to spinal integrity and neurological regulation. Anomalies in this category may indicate neuropathic processes, vertebral stress, or neuroautonomic imbalance.

72. Neuroautonomic Balance
The dynamic equilibrium between sympathetic and parasympathetic influences on organ and vascular function. In Biospectral Medicine, emission patterns reflecting exaggerated or deficient responses often suggest disturbances in this balance.

73. Neuroendocrine Crosstalk

The bidirectional communication between the nervous and endocrine systems that coordinates stress, growth, and metabolic responses. Biospectral anomalies may provide indirect evidence of disrupted neuroendocrine regulation.

74. Neurogenic Inflammation

An inflammatory response initiated by the release of neuropeptides from sensory nerves, leading to vascular dilation and tissue sensitivity. In Biospectral Medicine, this may appear as localized activose emission in corresponding zones.

75. Neurovascular Coupling

The physiological mechanism by which neural activity regulates local blood flow to meet metabolic demand. Disruptions in neurovascular coupling may present as focal emission anomalies in zones reflecting brain–body regulation.

76. Noise Equivalent Temperature Difference (NETD)

A measure of the sensitivity of an infrared detector, defined as the smallest temperature difference it can reliably distinguish. Lower NETD values indicate higher detector performance and are essential for accurate biospectral imaging.Nutrient Deficiencies

77. Optical Transmission

The passage of infrared radiation through lenses, filters, or other optical components before reaching the detector. In Biospectral Medicine, precise optical transmission is essential to avoid signal distortion, ensuring that emission data represents true physiological patterns without attenuation or artifact.

78. Organ–Emotion Correlation

The observed association between specific organ systems and emotional states, described in integrative medicine and psychosomatic research. Biospectral Medicine incorporates these correlations when recurrent emission anomalies appear in zones linked to unresolved emotional or stress-related patterns, providing a clinical bridge between physiology and psychology.

79. Organs / GNM

One of the nine interpretive categories in Biospectral Medicine, integrating the German New Medicine perspective that unresolved conflicts activate specific organ-related programs. Emission anomalies within this category highlight functional shifts in visceral zones, often requiring interpretation that includes both biological and psycho-emotional dimensions.

80. Oxidative Stress

A physiological state characterized by an excess of reactive oxygen species relative to antioxidant defenses, leading to cellular damage and metabolic strain. In Biospectral Medicine, oxidative stress may be inferred through diffuse emission patterns reflecting systemic inflammation, mitochondrial dysfunction, or vascular burden.

81. Palette Normalization

The standardization of image color scales to ensure reproducibility of emission analysis across patients and sessions. This process allows clinicians in Biospectral Medicine to interpret findings consistently, independent of arbitrary display variations, thereby preserving scientific reliability.

82. Parasympathetic Activation

The physiological response associated with increased vagal tone and restorative functions, including digestion, repair, and relaxation. In Biospectral Medicine, emission changes after rest or targeted interventions may reveal parasympathetic activation, providing insight into autonomic adaptability and systemic recovery capacity.

83. Perfusion Dynamics

The regulation of blood flow through microcirculatory networks to meet tissue metabolic demand. Biospectral anomalies in perfusion dynamics may appear as fluctuating emission zones, reflecting either inadequate tissue supply or excessive vascular reactivity in specific anatomical regions.

84. Photon Emission

The release of infrared photons from human tissues as a result of molecular vibration and metabolic processes. Biospectral Medicine captures and interprets these photons as biosignals, transforming invisible energy release into clinically relevant patterns of functional physiology.

85. Planck's Law

A fundamental physical principle describing the spectral distribution of electromagnetic radiation emitted by a blackbody at a given temperature. Planck's law provides the mathematical basis for emissive imaging and underpins the interpretation of biospectral signals in clinical practice.

86. Psycho-neuro-immunology (PNI)
An interdisciplinary field studying how psychological states influence immune and neurological function. Biospectral Medicine integrates PNI concepts to explain how chronic stress, emotional trauma, or adaptive failure may produce emission anomalies reflecting systemic immune or neuroautonomic responses.

87. Psychosomatic Expression
The manifestation of psychological or emotional stress through physiological changes in the body. In Biospectral Medicine, psychosomatic expression is often visible as persistent or recurrent emission anomalies in organ-related zones, highlighting the interdependence of mind and body.Qi Circulation

88. Quantum Detector
A cooled infrared sensor that measures incoming photons by promoting electrons across an energy bandgap, enabling extremely high sensitivity. Although rarely used clinically due to cost and complexity, quantum detectors represent the gold standard for research calibration in Biospectral Medicine.

89. Radiant Exitance
The total electromagnetic power emitted per unit surface area of a body, expressed in watts per square meter. In Biospectral Medicine, radiant exitance forms the physical basis of emission capture, linking thermodynamic principles to the visualization of biosignals on the skin surface.

90. Radiometric Accuracy
The degree to which an infrared imaging system correctly quantifies emitted radiation compared with a known standard. Maintaining radiometric accuracy through calibration is essential in Biospectral Medicine, ensuring that emission patterns reflect true physiology rather than equipment variability.

91. Reflex Zones
Specific cutaneous regions that correspond to deeper organ or musculoskeletal function through neurovegetative pathways. Biospectral Medicine incorporates reflex zones as interpretive layers, where emission anomalies provide indirect signals of systemic or visceral dysfunction.

92. Reproductive Axis
The endocrine and neuroendocrine system that regulates fertility, menstrual cycles, and reproductive health, primarily via hypothalamic–pituitary–gonadal interactions. In Biospectral Medicine, anomalies in reproductive axis regulation may manifest as recurrent emission patterns in abdominal and pelvic zones.

93. Resolution (Spatial/Temporal)
The capacity of an imaging system to distinguish fine details in space (spatial resolution) and track changes over time (temporal resolution). High resolution is critical in Biospectral Medicine for detecting subtle emission asymmetries and monitoring functional dynamics across interpretive categories.

94. ROI (Region of Interest)
A defined anatomical or functional segment selected for detailed spectral analysis. In Biospectral Medicine, ROI selection provides the framework for quantifying asymmetry, comparing emission behavior across zones, and standardizing interpretation within the R-CIIM methodology.

95. Root-Cause Mapping
A structured analytical approach that seeks to identify the underlying drivers of functional disturbance, beyond superficial symptom presentation. Biospectral Medicine integrates root-cause mapping by correlating emission anomalies with systemic physiology, guiding more strategic interventions.

96. Signal-to-Noise Ratio
A technical metric expressing the clarity of a detected signal relative to background noise. A high signal-to-noise ratio is crucial for accurate biospectral imaging, enabling differentiation between true physiological emission and random system interference.

97. Skeletal / Articular
One of the nine interpretive categories in Biospectral Medicine, concerned with joints, bones, and their mechanical interactions. Emission anomalies in this category may reflect degenerative changes, overload, or articular stress, often overlapping with muscular or fascial categories.

98. Skeletal Alignment
The anatomical positioning of bones and joints that determines postural integrity and movement efficiency. In Biospectral Medicine, misalignment often appears as asymmetrical emission in musculoskeletal zones, correlating with compensatory strain or articular dysfunction.

99. Somatic Memory
The retention of physical and emotional experiences within the body's tissues, often reflected in persistent muscular or fascial tension. In Biospectral Medicine, somatic memory may present as recurrent emission anomalies in zones linked to past trauma or unresolved adaptive responses.

100. Somatovisceral Reflexes

Neural pathways in which sensory input from musculoskeletal structures influences visceral organ function. Biospectral Medicine interprets emission anomalies in reflex zones as possible indicators of these reflexes, bridging musculoskeletal findings with organ-level regulation.

101. Spectral Adaptation

The process by which biological tissues adjust their emission characteristics in response to environmental or internal stimuli. Observing spectral adaptation in Biospectral Medicine provides insight into systemic resilience, vascular flexibility, and autonomic regulation.

102. Spectral Asymmetry

Unequal emission distribution between contralateral or adjacent zones, suggesting localized imbalance. Within the R-CIIM methodology, spectral asymmetry is a central interpretive marker for differentiating vascular, muscular, and metabolic dysfunctions.

103. Spectral Atlas

The structured body of emission maps that defines standardized zones, categories, and interpretive criteria in Biospectral Medicine. The Atlas serves as both a clinical reference and an academic framework, establishing reproducibility in functional imaging interpretation.

104. Spectral Bandwidth

The range of wavelengths captured and analyzed by an infrared imaging system. In Biospectral Medicine, sufficient spectral bandwidth is required to incorporate the physiologically relevant emissions of human tissue, ensuring accurate biosignal acquisition.

105. Spectral Contrast

The degree of differentiation between adjacent emission regions, determined by relative signal intensity. High spectral contrast enhances interpretive clarity in Biospectral Medicine, allowing subtle physiological anomalies to become more visible against background activity.

106. Spectral Correlation

The analysis of relationships between emission patterns across different zones or categories. In Biospectral Medicine, spectral correlation highlights systemic interactions, demonstrating how dysfunction in one region may propagate or relate to others.

107. Spectral Differentiation

The capacity to distinguish between distinct emission signatures that represent varied physiological processes. Biospectral Medicine uses spectral differentiation to separate vascular activity from metabolic or neuroautonomic influences within the same zone.

108. Spectral Dispersion

The spreading of emission values across a wide spectrum, reflecting heterogeneous physiological activity within a region of interest. Interpreting dispersion in Biospectral Medicine provides clues about systemic instability or overlapping functional stresses.

109. Spectral Distribution

The allocation of emission intensities across a defined spectral range, representing the composite activity of tissues. Biospectral Medicine interprets abnormal distributions as evidence of systemic imbalance, such as metabolic overload or vascular dysregulation.

110. Spectral Divergence

The degree of variation between emission patterns in different zones or between sessions of the same patient. In Biospectral Medicine, spectral divergence is used to evaluate progression, therapeutic strategy response, or systemic imbalance, highlighting when tissues deviate from expected regulatory coherence.

111. Spectral Domains

Distinct ranges within the infrared spectrum that correspond to specific tissue emission characteristics. Understanding spectral domains enables Biospectral Medicine to link observed signals with underlying vascular, metabolic, or neuroautonomic processes, ensuring precision in interpretation.

112. Spectral Emission Curve

A graphical representation of the relationship between wavelength and radiant intensity emitted by tissues. In Biospectral Medicine, the spectral emission curve provides a visual framework for comparing tissue activity to theoretical blackbody models, revealing deviations tied to functional pathology.

113. Spectral Flow

The dynamic change of emission signals over time, reflecting functional adaptation and physiological variability. Observing spectral flow in Biospectral Medicine assists in distinguishing transient regulatory activity from persistent dysfunction, particularly during functional tests such as the SVRT.

114. Spectral Gradient

The rate of change in emission intensity across a given anatomical zone. In Biospectral Medicine, abnormal spectral gradients may suggest impaired vascular supply, fascial restrictions, or uneven autonomic regulation across the tissue field.

115. Spectral Homogeneity

The uniformity of emission distribution within a zone, indicating stable physiological function. Loss of spectral homogeneity in Biospectral Medicine is interpreted as a marker of underlying stress, imbalance, or localized dysfunction requiring further analysis.

116. Spectral Instability

Fluctuations or irregularities in emission signals that fail to stabilize under normal regulatory conditions. In Biospectral Medicine, spectral instability often points to metabolic stress, vascular dysregulation, or unresolved adaptive responses.

117. Spectral Integration

The process of combining emission data across zones and categories into a coherent clinical picture. Spectral integration is fundamental to the R-CIIM methodology, ensuring that local findings are contextualized within systemic physiology and root-cause mapping.

118. Spectral Interpretation

The structured analysis of emission data to derive clinical meaning. In Biospectral Medicine, spectral interpretation is guided by the spectral lexicon, diagnostic categories, and the R-CIIM method, transforming raw signals into clinically relevant insights.

119. Spectral Irradiance

The power of radiation received per unit area and per unit wavelength, expressed in $W/m^2/\mu m$. In Biospectral Medicine, spectral irradiance is considered when calibrating imaging devices, ensuring accurate translation of tissue emission into reliable biosignals.

120. Spectral Lexicon

A standardized vocabulary developed to describe recurring emission patterns and interpretive categories. The spectral lexicon provides Biospectral Medicine with a universal interpretive language, ensuring consistency in communication, teaching, and research worldwide.

121. Spectral Localization

The ability to identify and assign emission signals to precise anatomical regions. In Biospectral Medicine, spectral localization ensures that findings are mapped accurately onto emission zones, enabling reproducible interpretation and comparison across patients and sessions.

122. Spectral Mapping

The structured process of charting emission patterns across the standardized 19 zones of Biospectral Medicine. Spectral mapping allows clinicians to visualize systemic connections, track changes over time, and establish cross-zone relationships that reveal deeper physiological insights.

123. Spectral Modulation

The adjustment or fluctuation of emission intensity in response to regulatory input, environmental changes, or functional testing. In Biospectral Medicine, spectral modulation is interpreted as evidence of dynamic adaptability or, conversely, impaired regulation when absent.

124. Spectral Overlay

The superimposition of multiple emission data sets to reveal comparative differences. In Biospectral Medicine, overlays are used in longitudinal studies, therapeutic strategy monitoring, or left-right asymmetry evaluation, making hidden divergences more clinically evident.

125. Spectral Profiles

Composite patterns of emission behavior that characterize a particular zone, condition, or interpretive category. Spectral profiles in Biospectral Medicine form the basis of case comparisons, helping to distinguish normal physiology from pathological signals.

126. Spectral Radiance

The emitted power of radiation per unit area, per unit solid angle, and per unit wavelength. In Biospectral Medicine, spectral radiance provides a quantitative foundation for detector calibration, linking physical emission properties with clinical biosignal analysis.

127. Spectral Reference Map

A standardized chart that defines normal emission distributions across the 19 zones of Biospectral Medicine. The reference map provides clinicians with a benchmark for comparison, helping to identify deviations that signify functional or pathological processes.

128. Spectral Resonance

The amplification of emission signals when biological tissues or systems oscillate at harmonically related frequencies. In Biospectral Medicine, spectral resonance is considered in both physiological adaptation and integrative interpretations involving energetic or frequency-related categories.

129. Spectral Response

The change in emission output observed following an internal or external stimulus. In Biospectral Medicine, spectral responses are key indicators of vascular adaptability, autonomic flexibility, and systemic regulation, particularly during functional tests such as SVRT.

130. Spectral Response Function

A characteristic curve that defines how an imaging detector responds to varying wavelengths of incident radiation. For Biospectral Medicine, understanding the response function ensures accurate matching between human tissue emissions and sensor sensitivity.

131. Spectral Signature

The unique emission pattern associated with a tissue, organ, or functional state. Biospectral Medicine interprets spectral signatures as interpretive fingerprints, providing individualized insights into systemic physiology and potential dysfunctions.

132. Spectral Stratification

The layering of emission signals within or across anatomical regions, reflecting functional differences in tissue depth or adjacent structures. In Biospectral Medicine, spectral stratification helps distinguish between superficial disturbances and deeper systemic involvement.

133. Spectral Synchrony

The alignment or coordination of emission patterns across different zones or physiological systems. High spectral synchrony in Biospectral Medicine indicates coherent systemic regulation, while loss of synchrony suggests fragmentation of vascular, metabolic, or autonomic balance.

134. Spectral Terrain

The overall landscape of emission patterns across the body, representing the composite physiological state at a given moment. Spectral terrain provides clinicians with a global map in Biospectral Medicine, helping to contextualize local findings within systemic function.

135. Spectral Terrain Categories

Classification of emission landscapes into distinct interpretive categories, such as balanced, overloaded, or deficient terrain. In Biospectral Medicine, these categories assist clinicians in stratifying systemic patterns and identifying dominant physiological stressors.

136. Spectral Variability

The degree of fluctuation in emission signals within or across zones, reflecting regulatory adaptability. Biospectral Medicine interprets spectral variability as a marker of dynamic resilience when present, and rigidity or dysfunction when absent.

137. Spectral Zone Concordance

The alignment of emission findings across zones that share functional or anatomical relationships. In Biospectral Medicine, zone concordance strengthens evaluation interpretation by confirming systemic patterns rather than isolated anomalies.

138. Spiral Line

A fascial continuity described in structural anatomy that spirals through the body to integrate rotation and stabilization. In Biospectral Medicine, emission anomalies along the spiral line may indicate compensatory torsional strain or postural imbalance.

139. Stefan–Boltzmann Law

A physical principle stating that the total radiant exitance of a blackbody is proportional to the fourth power of its absolute temperature. The Stefan–Boltzmann law underpins emissive physics and provides the quantitative framework for interpreting tissue emission in Biospectral Medicine.

140. Stress Axis (HPA Axis)

The hypothalamic–pituitary–adrenal axis that governs the body's stress response and cortisol regulation. Biospectral Medicine considers HPA axis dysfunction when emission anomalies appear in zones related to adrenal, thyroid, or systemic metabolic regulation.

141. Superficial Back Line

A fascial chain extending from the plantar fascia of the feet up through the calves, hamstrings, and spine to the scalp. In Biospectral Medicine, anomalies in this line often appear as emission asymmetries linked to postural strain or muscular overload.

142. Superficial Front Line

A fascial continuity running from the top of the feet through the quadriceps, abdominal wall, and chest to the skull. In Biospectral Medicine, emission anomalies along this line may reflect visceral tension, postural imbalance, or adaptive muscular strain.

143. Sympathetic Dominance

A state in which sympathetic nervous system activity predominates over parasympathetic function, often linked to chronic stress, anxiety, or systemic overload. In Biospectral Medicine, sympathetic dominance may appear as persistent activose emissions in vascular or muscular zones, reflecting sustained autonomic strain.

144. Thermal Contrast

The difference in emission intensity between regions of interest, used to highlight functional disparities. In Biospectral Medicine, thermal contrast helps clinicians identify localized dysfunction by amplifying the visibility of emission asymmetries across adjacent tissues.

145. Thermal Drift

A gradual change in detector response or image output due to equipment warming, calibration error, or environmental variation. In Biospectral Medicine, controlling for thermal drift is essential to avoid misinterpreting equipment artifacts as physiological signals.

146. Thermal Flux

The rate of heat transfer per unit area, influenced by vascular flow, metabolic activity, and environmental factors. Biospectral Medicine interprets abnormal thermal flux as a marker of dysfunctional regulation, particularly in vascular or metabolic categories.

147. Thermal Gradient

The rate of change in emission intensity across a defined distance on the body's surface. Abnormal thermal gradients in Biospectral Medicine may indicate impaired microcirculation, fascial restriction, or localized reactivity processes.

148. Thermal Image Processing

The application of algorithms and filters to raw emissive data in order to enhance clarity and interpretive precision. In Biospectral Medicine, image processing must remain standardized and transparent to preserve the integrity of emission interpretation.

149. Thermal Noise

Random fluctuations in detector output that obscure true emission signals. Managing thermal noise through calibration and equipment quality is essential in Biospectral Medicine to ensure that findings reflect authentic physiological processes.

150. Thermal Sensitivity

The capacity of an imaging system to detect small differences in emission intensity, often expressed as NETD. In Biospectral Medicine, high sensitivity allows for the detection of subtle regulatory changes and early indicators of dysfunction.

151. Thermal Window

A time frame or physiological condition in which emission patterns provide the clearest interpretive information. In Biospectral Medicine, thermal windows are exploited during functional testing, such as the Spectrovascular Response Test, to capture adaptive responses.

152. Uncooled Detector

An infrared sensor that operates at ambient temperature without cryogenic cooling. Uncooled microbolometers are widely used in Biospectral Medicine due to their practicality, reliability, and accessibility for clinical applications.

153. Vascular / Circulatory

One of the nine interpretive categories in Biospectral Medicine, addressing emission findings linked to arterial, venous, and microcirculatory function. Anomalies in this category often reflect systemic vascular stress, venous insufficiency, or impaired perfusion dynamics.

154. Vascular Integrity

The structural and functional soundness of the circulatory system, including arterial elasticity, venous competence, and microvascular stability. In Biospectral Medicine, reduced vascular integrity may present as emission anomalies in peripheral or organ-related zones, often correlating with systemic circulatory burden.

155. Vasoregulation

The capacity of blood vessels to adjust their diameter in response to metabolic, neural, or thermal stimuli. In Biospectral Medicine, vasoregulatory function is assessed through emission changes, particularly during dynamic tests such as the Spectrovascular Response Test (SVRT).

156. Visceral Reflex

An involuntary physiological response originating from internal organ activity and conveyed via the autonomic nervous system. Biospectral Medicine interprets emission changes in reflex zones as potential manifestations of visceral reflexes, linking organ function with surface biosignals.

157. Viscerosomatic Reflexes

Neural circuits in which dysfunction in visceral organs produces musculoskeletal changes, often experienced as tension, pain, or altered posture. In Biospectral Medicine, such reflexes may appear as emission anomalies in musculoskeletal zones that correlate with deeper organ stress.

158. Wien's Displacement Law

A physical law describing the inverse relationship between the temperature of a blackbody and the wavelength at which it emits maximum radiation. In Biospectral Medicine, Wien's law supports the physics of emissive analysis, ensuring that detector systems are matched to human tissue emission peaks.

159. Yin/Yang Dynamics

A principle from Traditional Chinese Medicine describing complementary forces that sustain systemic balance. Biospectral Medicine incorporates Yin/Yang dynamics symbolically, acknowledging how opposing patterns, such as activose and inhibose emissions, reflect integrative physiological equilibrium.

160. Zone Mapping

The systematic division of the body into nineteen standardized emission zones that form the foundation of Biospectral Medicine. Zone mapping provides reproducibility in imaging interpretation, enabling clinicians and researchers to compare findings across patients and longitudinal assessments.

KEY ABBREVIATIONS

a) **CPT (Current Procedural Terminology)**
A standardized coding system maintained by the American Medical Association for reporting medical, surgical, and diagnostic services. While not yet including Biospectral Medicine, CPT codes are relevant for integration of new interpretive methods into healthcare reimbursement and documentation systems.

b) **CT (Computed Tomography)**
An imaging modality that uses X-rays and computer processing to produce detailed cross-sectional images of the body. CT serves as a structural counterpart to Biospectral Medicine, which contributes functional information rather than anatomical detail.

c) **CTI (Computerized Thermographic Imaging)**
The digital emissive imaging system developed within Biospectral Medicine to capture, map, and interpret surface biosignals. CTI forms the methodological foundation of the Atlas, incorporating zone mapping, asymmetry analysis, and spectral lexicon terminology.

d) **EDTA (Ethylenediaminetetraacetic Acid)**
A chelating agent that binds heavy metals and is used in laboratory diagnostics and clinical detoxification protocols. In the context of Biospectral Medicine, EDTA is relevant to discussions of chelation therapy and metabolic burden in vascular and systemic dysfunction.

e) **EMA (European Medicines Agency)**
The regulatory authority responsible for evaluating and supervising medicines within the European Union. EMA recognition is a key benchmark for integrating new diagnostic or therapeutic modalities into European clinical practice.

f) **FDA (Food and Drug Administration)**
The U.S. regulatory agency overseeing food, drugs, medical devices, and biological products. FDA approval of imaging systems or adjunctive therapies establishes a standard of safety and effectiveness relevant for the international acceptance of Biospectral Medicine tools.

g) **FIR (Far-Infrared)**
The long-wavelength portion of the infrared spectrum, ranging from approximately 15 to 1000 micrometers. FIR is the most relevant band for human emissive imaging and forms the physical basis for Biospectral Medicine's capture of tissue biosignals.

h) **GNM (German New Medicine)**
A theoretical model proposed by Ryke Geerd Hamer that links unresolved psycho-emotional conflicts to organ-specific biological programs. GNM concepts are referenced in Biospectral Medicine as interpretive layers for understanding recurring emission anomalies.

i) **GV (Governing Vessel, TCM Meridian)**
One of the primary meridians in Traditional Chinese Medicine, running along the midline of the back and head. In Biospectral Medicine, Governing Vessel pathways are studied for their correlation with spinal, neurological, and fascial emission patterns.

j) **HPA (Hypothalamic–Pituitary–Adrenal Axis)**
The central neuroendocrine system regulating stress response, circadian rhythm, and cortisol secretion. Biospectral anomalies linked to HPA dysfunction often appear in adrenal, thyroid, and systemic metabolic zones, reflecting stress-related imbalance.

k) **HRT (Hormone Replacement Therapy)**
A clinical treatment that supplements or replaces endogenous hormones, often used in menopausal or endocrine-deficient states. In Biospectral Medicine, HRT is relevant as a systemic modifier, with emission anomalies sometimes reflecting hormonal effects on vascular and metabolic regulation.

l) **ICD (International Classification of Diseases)**
A global diagnostic coding system maintained by the World Health Organization, used for classifying diseases and health conditions. ICD codes provide the framework for integrating Biospectral Medicine into international medical reporting and epidemiological research.

m) **LLLT (Low-Level Laser Therapy)**
A therapeutic modality using low-intensity light to stimulate cellular repair, reduce inflammation, and promote tissue healing. In Biospectral Medicine, LLLT is referenced as an adjunctive therapy, with emission analysis offering potential feedback on therapeutic strategy response.

n) **MIR (Mid-Infrared)**
The portion of the infrared spectrum between roughly 3 and 8 micrometers in wavelength. MIR contributes to the physics of tissue emissivity and detector design, though Biospectral Medicine primarily relies on the far-infrared band for clinical imaging.

o) **MRI (Magnetic Resonance Imaging)**
A non-invasive imaging modality that uses magnetic fields and radiofrequency waves to produce detailed anatomical images. MRI provides structural data that complements the functional insights of Biospectral Medicine, particularly in musculoskeletal and neurological contexts.

p) **NETD (Noise Equivalent Temperature Difference)**
A technical metric defining the smallest temperature difference an infrared detector can distinguish from noise. In Biospectral Medicine, a low NETD is essential for detecting subtle biosignals and ensuring high imaging sensitivity.

q) **NIR (Near-Infrared)**
The infrared range spanning approximately 0.7 to 1.5 micrometers, closer to the visible spectrum. While less central to Biospectral Medicine, NIR is relevant in spectroscopy and optical physiology, offering complementary perspectives on tissue function.

r) **PACS (Picture Archiving and Communication System)**
A digital medical imaging platform that stores, retrieves, and transmits diagnostic images. In Biospectral Medicine, PACS integration represents a future step toward standardization and clinical adoption alongside radiology workflows.

s) **PET (Positron Emission Tomography)**
A nuclear imaging technique that visualizes metabolic activity through radiotracer uptake. PET exemplifies a structural-functional hybrid modality, providing context for Biospectral Medicine's position as a purely functional, non-invasive imaging system.

t) **PNI (Psycho-Neuro-Immunology)**
An interdisciplinary field exploring the interaction between psychological states, the nervous system, and immune regulation. Biospectral Medicine draws on PNI concepts to interpret emission anomalies that may arise from chronic stress, trauma, or altered immune-neuro balance.

u) **PRP (Platelet-Rich Plasma)**
A regenerative therapy that concentrates a patient's platelets and growth factors to stimulate healing and tissue repair. In Biospectral Medicine, PRP is considered among the interventions whose effects may be monitored through changes in emission patterns across relevant zones.

v) **ROI (Region of Interest)**
A defined anatomical or functional area selected for detailed biosignal analysis. In Biospectral Medicine, ROI delineation is fundamental for quantifying asymmetry, standardizing comparisons across emission zones, and applying the R-CIIM interpretive methodology.

w) **SNR (Signal-to-Noise Ratio)**
A metric expressing the clarity of a detected signal relative to background noise. A high SNR is essential in Biospectral Medicine to ensure that subtle emission differences reflect genuine physiology rather than random variation or detector interference.

x) **SVRT (Spectrovascular Response Test)**
A functional assessment in Biospectral Medicine that evaluates microcirculatory and autonomic regulation by observing emission responses to a controlled cold challenge. The SVRT provides insight into vascular adaptability, systemic resilience, and regulatory efficiency.

y) **WHO (World Health Organization)**
The global authority on public health, standardizing diagnostic classifications, research priorities, and medical guidelines. WHO frameworks are relevant to Biospectral Medicine as the discipline advances toward international recognition and integration into clinical practice.

REFERENCES WITH CITATION FREQUENCY

This Atlas contains 1285 citations from 585 unique references. Many works appear across multiple zones and categories, reflecting the integrative scope of Biospectral Medicine. As a first-in-field discipline, the citations establish the physical, physiological, and clinical foundations that support the R-CIIM method, the 19 emission zones, and the spectral lexicon. In this way, the Atlas itself becomes the primary reference, defining standards and methodologies that future research will extend and refine.

Note on Reference Style in This Atlas

Each reference in the Atlas is listed in alphabetical order. The number at the beginning is the reference number in the master list, and the number in parentheses immediately after it indicates how many times that reference has been cited throughout the Atlas.

For example:

1. (1) Adams, M. A., & Dolan, P. (2012). Spine biomechanics. *Journal of Biomechanics*, 45(2), 299–301. https://doi.org/10.1016/j.jbiomech.2011.11.005

- **"1."** → means it is the first item in the alphabetical master reference list.
- **"(1)"** → means this reference was cited **once** in the text of the Atlas.

If the same reference were cited multiple times in different chapters or sections, the number in parentheses would be higher (e.g., "(5)" = cited five times).

This system makes it easy for readers to see both the bibliographic details *and* the frequency of use, highlighting which sources form the core backbone of Biospectral Medicine.

From the Author

Reitz, F., Soratto, A. (2018). *Measuring pain. Journal of Physics: Conference Series*, **1065**(182006). IOP Publishing. https://doi.org/10.1088/1742-6596/1065/18/182006

Reitz, F., Salm, D. C., Ludke, D. O., Dos Santos, A., Traebert, J., Martins, D. F. (2018). *A non-reflexive method based on the variability of temperature and bioimpedance in measuring inflammatory hyperalgesia and analgesia in mice. Journal of Neuroscience Methods*, **308**, 192–198. https://doi.org/10.1016/j.jneumeth.2018.08.010

REFERENCES

1) 2 × Adams, M. A., & Dolan, P. (2012). Spine biomechanics. Journal of Biomechanics, 45(2), 299–301.

2) 1 × Ader, R. (2007). Psychoneuroimmunology (4th ed.). Academic Press.

3) 1 × Ahn, A. C., & Grodzinsky, A. J. (2009). Relevance of collagen piezoelectricity to mechanosensing and mechanotransduction. Journal of the Royal Society Interface, 6(33), 1155-1168.

4) 2 × Ahn, A. C., Colbert, A. P., Anderson, B. J., et al. (2008). Electrical properties of acupuncture points and meridians: A systematic review. Bioelectromagnetics, 29(4), 245–256. https://doi.org/10.1002/bem.20403

5) 1 × Ahn, A. C., Colbert, A. P., Anderson, B. J., Martinsen, Ø. G., Hammerschlag, R., Cina, S., ... & Langevin, H. M. (2008). Electrical properties of acupuncture points and meridians: a systematic review. Bioelectromagnetics, 29(4), 245–256. https://doi.org/10.1002/bem.20403

6) 2 × Ahn, A. C., et al. (2005). Electrical properties of acupuncture points and meridians: A systematic review. Bioelectromagnetics, 26(2), 73–85.

7) 1 × Ahn, A. C., Park, M., Shaw, J. R., et al. (2010). Electrical impedance and acupuncture meridians: a systematic review. European Journal of Oriental Medicine, 6(6), 3–13.

8) 2 × Ahn, A. C., Park, M., Shaw, J. R., et al. (2010). Electrical impedance of acupuncture meridians: The relevance of subcutaneous collagenous bands. PLoS One, 5(7), e11907. https://doi.org/10.1371/journal.pone.0011907

9) 1 × Ahn, A. C., Park, M., Shaw, J. R., McManus, C. A., Kaptchuk, T. J., & Langevin, H. M. (2005). Electrical impedance along connective tissue planes associated with acupuncture meridians. BMC Complementary and Alternative Medicine, 5, 10. https://doi.org/10.1186/1472-6882-5-10

10) 2 × Ahn, A. C., Park, M., Shaw, J. R., McManus, C. A., Kaptchuk, T. J., & Langevin, H. M. (2008). Electrical impedance and acupuncture meridians: a review. Medical Acupuncture, 20(4), 189–194. https://doi.org/10.1089/acu.2008.0641

11) 1 × Ahn, A.C., et al. (2008). Electrical impedance along acupuncture meridians: Revisiting the relevance to modern biophysics. The Journal of Alternative and Complementary Medicine, 14(5), 505–512.

12) 1 × Al-Hadithy, N., & Khan, W. S. (2012). Lymphatic complications of abdominal surgery. Journal of Peritoneum and Surgery, 7(3), 123–129.

13) 16 × Alberti, K. G. M. M., Zimmet, P., & Shaw, J. (2006). Metabolic Syndrome—a New Worldwide Definition. A Consensus Statement from the International Diabetes Federation. Diabetic Medicine, 23(5), 469–480. https://doi.org/10.1111/j.1464-5491.2006.01858.x

14) 1 × Alberts, B., Johnson, A., Lewis, J., Morgan, D., Raff, M., Roberts, K., & Walter, P. (2022). Molecular Biology of the Cell (7th ed.). W.W. Norton.

15) 2 × Alves, M. M., Silva, J. C., & Rodrigues, D. (2021). Medical infrared thermography: A review of equipment and applications. Journal of Medical Systems, 45(3), 34.

16) 1 × American Academy of Thermology (AAT). (2021). Guidelines and Position Statements. Retrieved from

17) 1 × American Academy of Thermology (AAT). (2021). Guidelines for Clinical Thermography. AAT Publications.

18) 1 × American Academy of Thermology (AAT). (2021). Practice Guidelines for Neuromusculoskeletal Thermography, Breast Thermography, and Pain Syndrome Assessment. Retrieved from:

19) 3 × American Academy of Thermology (AAT). Guidelines for Neuro-Musculoskeletal Infrared Medical Thermology & SSR Studies. 2024.

20) 1 × Amiel, I., Levy, R., & Smilansky, Z. (2019). Preventing condensation effects in clinical infrared optics: Environmental design and maintenance. Journal of Biomedical Optics, 24(3), 1–10.

21) 1 × Ammer K. Standard Procedures for Infrared Imaging in Medicine. (chapter PDF consolidating international standards: ambient control, acclimatization, symmetry, field of view). Accessed online.

22) 1 × Ammer K. The Glamorgan Protocol and other standards for medical infrared imaging. In: Ammer K, Ring EFJ, eds. The Thermal Image in Medicine and Biology. CRC Press; 2019.

23) 7 × Ammer, K. (2008). The Glamorgan Protocol for recording and evaluation of thermal images of the human body. Thermology International, 18(4), 125–129.

24) 7 × Ammer, K. (2008). The Glamorgan Protocol for recording and evaluation of thermal images of the human body. Thermology International, 18(4), 125–144.

25) 1 × Ammer, K. (2008). The Glamorous Promise of Thermography—Still Unfulfilled? Thermology International, 18(4), 133–135.

26) 1 × Ammer, K. (2008). Thermography in medicine: What the literature tells us. Thermology International, 18(2), 45–50.

27) 1 × Ammer, K. (2008). "The Glamour of Thermography." Thermology International, 18(2), 45–51.

28) 1 × Ammer, K. (2018). The Glamorgan Protocol for recording and evaluation of thermal images of the human body. Thermology International, 28(2), 69–72. https://doi.org/10.1108/TI-02-2018-0004

29) 1 × Ammer, K. (2018). Thermography in the assessment of autonomic dysfunction. In: E. Ring & K. Ammer (Eds.), The Thermal Image in Medicine and Biology. Springer.

30) 1 × Ammer, K., & Ring, E. F. J. (2010). Standard procedures for infrared imaging in medicine. Medical Infrared Imaging Standards Report, European Association of Thermology, 1–12.

31) 3 × Ammer, K., & Ring, E. F. J. (2011). Standard procedures for infrared imaging in medicine. In E. F. J. Ring & K. Ammer (Eds.), Infrared Imaging: Casebook and Atlas (pp. 1–16). ICB Publishing.

32) 3 × Anbar, M. (1995). Clinical thermal imaging today. IEEE Engineering in Medicine and Biology Magazine, 14(3), 25–33. https://doi.org/10.1109/51.391777

33) 1 × ASTM E1933-14. (2014). Standard Practice for Measuring and Compensating for Emissivity Using Infrared Imaging Radiometers. ASTM International.

34) 1 × Atkins, P., & de Paula, J. (2014). Physical Chemistry (10th ed.). Oxford University Press.

35) 1 × Atsumi K. High technology applications of medical thermography in Japan. Thermology. 1985;1:79–80. (cited in Ammer's standardization chapter).

36) 1 × Balageas, D., Maldague, X., & Roche, J. M. (2012). Advances in Infrared Thermography for Non-Destructive Testing. Woodhead Publishing.

37) 1 × Balbinot, L. F., et al. (2013). Thermographic Imaging in Medical and Sports Applications: A Review. Infrared Physics & Technology, 62, 103–112.

38) 2 × Baldasano, J. M., Codina, J., & Piñol, J. (2016). Calibration of infrared imaging systems for clinical applications using blackbody references. Measurement Science and Technology, 27(12), 125103.

39) 1 × Baldwin, A. L., Hammerschlag, R., & Langevin, H. M. (2017). Biofield-based therapies: A systematic review of physiological effects on practitioners during treatment. Explore, 13(6), 353–361. https://doi.org/10.1016/j.explore.2017.08.002

40) 1 × Barker, J., & Daniels, D. (2004). Infrared optics for clinical imaging systems: Design constraints and performance trade-offs. Infrared Physics & Technology, 45(3), 189–198.

41) 1 × Barner, H. B. (2002). Internal thoracic artery: The ideal coronary bypass graft. Annals of Thoracic Surgery, 73(4), 1429–1434. https://doi.org/10.1016/S0003-4975(01)03601-1

42) 3 × Baron, R., Binder, A., & Wasner, G. (2013). Neuropathic pain: diagnosis, pathophysiological mechanisms, and treatment. The Lancet Neurology, 9(8), 807–819.

43) 1 × Beck, J. V., Blackwell, B., & St. Clair, C. R. (1985). Inverse Heat Conduction: Ill-posed Problems. Wiley.

44) 1 × Becker, R. O., & Selden, G. (1985). The Body Electric: Electromagnetism and the Foundation of Life. New York: William Morrow.

45) 1 × Beebe-Dimmer, J. L. (2005). The epidemiology of chronic venous insufficiency and varicose veins. Annals of Epidemiology, 15(3), 175–184.

46) 1 × Behrens, A., Lang, J., & Brucke, P. (2011). The facial artery and its branches: Anatomical study and clinical significance in reconstructive surgery. Plastic and Reconstructive Surgery, 127(1), 347–356. https://doi.org/10.1097/PRS.0b013e3181f958f9

47) 1 × Benarroch, E. E. (2006). The clinical significance of the autonomic nervous system. Continuum: Lifelong Learning in Neurology, 12(1), 12–31.

48) 1 × Benias, P. C., Wells, R. G., Sackey-Aboagye, B., Klavan, H., Reidy, J., Buonocore, D., ... & Carr-Locke, D. L. (2018). Structure and distribution of an unrecognized interstitium in human tissues. Scientific Reports, 8(1), 4947. https://doi.org/10.1038/s41598-018-23062-6

49) 1 × Benjamin, M. (2009). The fascia of the limbs and back — a review. Journal of Anatomy, 214(1), 1–18.

50) 1 × Bennell, K., Matheson, G., Meeuwisse, W., & Brukner, P. (1999). Risk factors for stress fractures. Sports Medicine, 28(2), 91–122.

51) 19 × Bensky, D., Clavey, S., & Stöger, E. (2004). Chinese Herbal Medicine: Materia Medica (3rd ed.). Eastland Press.

52) 1 × Berga, S.L. (2023). Stress and reproductive function: An integrative neuroendocrine review. Endocrine Reviews, 44(1), 33–56.

53) 1 × Berthoud, H. R. (2004). Anatomy and function of sensory hepatic nerves. Anatomical Record, 280A(1), 827–835.

54) 1 × Bertolin, A., Brioschi, M. L., & Macedo, J. F. (2019). Clinical standardization in medical thermography: Challenges and advances. Revista Brasileira de Engenharia Biomédica, 35(2), 157–170.

55) 1 × Biedert, R. M., & Warnke, K. (2001). Correlation between the thoracolumbar fascia and low back pain. Journal of Manipulative and Physiological Therapeutics, 24(7), 514–518.

56) 1 × Biron, D., et al. (2020). Systems Biology of Complex Health. Springer.

57) 1 × Bischof, M. (2005). Biophotonics: An overview of mechanisms, models, and applications. Indian Journal of Experimental Biology, 43(9), 819–830.

58) 1 × Black, P. H. (2002). Stress and the inflammatory response: A review of neurogenic inflammation. Brain, Behavior, and Immunity, 16(6), 622–653.

59) 1 × Blendis, L. M., & Wong, F. (2001). The hyperdynamic circulation in cirrhosis: an overview. Pharmacology & Therapeutics, 89(3), 221–231.

60) 1 × BMUS. (2009). Guidelines for the Safe Use of Diagnostic Ultrasound Equipment, British Medical Ultrasound Society, pp. 60–61.

61) 1 × Bogduk, N., & Govind, J. (2009). Cervical headaches and the cervical spine. Current Pain and Headache Reports, 13(3), 192–198.

62) 1 × Bogduk, N., & Mercer, S. (2000). Biomechanics of the cervical spine. Clinical Biomechanics, 15(9), 633–648.

63) 1 × Boltzmann, L. (1884). Ableitung des Stefan'schen Gesetzes, betreffend die Abhängigkeit der Wärmestrahlung von der Temperatur aus der electromagnetischen Lichttheorie. Annalen der Physik, 258(6), 291-294.

64) 1 × Bordoni B, Morabito B. The fascial system and exercise intolerance in patients with chronic heart failure. Cureus. 2017;9(9): e1682.

65) 1 × Borland, D., & Taylor, R. M. (2007). Rainbow color map (still) considered harmful. IEEE Computer Graphics and Applications, 27(2), 14–17.

66) 1 × Borsook, D., Burstein, R., & Becerra, L. (2012). Functional imaging of the trigeminal system: applications to migraine and trigeminal neuralgia. Headache, 52(Suppl 2), 32–39.

67) 1 × Bradshaw, C., & McCrory, P. (2007). Obturator neuropathy: A cause of groin pain in athletes. British Journal of Sports Medicine, 41(8), 579–583.

68) 8 × Brant, W. O., Thomson, R. L., & Connor, D. T. (2016). The — of Doppler Ultrasound in Peripheral Vascular Disease. Vascular Medicine, 21(5), 387–396. https://doi.org/10.1177/1358863X16644758

69) 1 × Brent, G. A. (2012). Mechanisms of thyroid hormone action. Journal of Clinical Investigation, 122(9), 3035–3043. https://doi.org/10.1172/JCI60047

70) 1 × Brioschi, M. L., Macedo, J. F., & Macedo, R. A. (2013). Skin thermoregulation in humans: An overview of the clinical applications of infrared thermography. Open Sports Sciences Journal, 6, 122–128.

71) 1 × Brioschi, M.L., et al. (2018). Thermography in rheumatologic practice. Acta Reumatológica Portuguesa, 43(3), 225–231.

72) 1 × Brioschi, M.L., et al. (2019). Skin temperature and sympathetic activity in pain syndromes: A biospectral correlation study. Pain Reports, 4(2), e711.

73) 1 × Brioschi, M.L., et al. (2020). Infrared thermography in the assessment of immune reactivity and terrain imbalance: A biospectral model. Clinical Biophysics, 34(1), 37–44.

74) 1 × Brorson, H. (2003). Liposuction in lymphedema treatment. Journal of the International Society of Lymphology, 36(4), 219–226.

75) 1 × Broudy, V. C. (2004). Approach to the patient with splenomegaly. UpToDate.

76) 1 × Browne, M. P., O'Neill, M., & Murphy, J. (2015). Spectral emissivity of human skin in the mid- and long-wave infrared regions. Infrared Physics & Technology, 71, 333–341.

77) 1 × Browne, S., Pham, C. H., Lee, J., & Kang, S. (2015). Evaluation of infrared camera systems for medical use: A performance-based study. Journal of Medical Engineering & Technology, 39(4), 221–229. https://doi.org/10.3109/03091902.2015.1027643

78) 1 × Browse, N. L., Burnand, K. G., & Mortimer, P. S. (2003). Diseases of the Lymphatics. Hodder Arnold.

79) 1 × Brukner, P., Bradshaw, C., Khan, K. M., White, S., & Crossley, K. (1996). Stress fractures: A review of 180 cases. Clinical Journal of Sport Medicine, 6(2), 85–89.

80) 1 × Bruner, M. E. (1984). The Scientific Legacy of William Coblentz. NBS Special Publication 563.

81) 1 × Brush, S. G. (1979). Langley and the Solar Constant: Theory and Measurement in the Late 19th Century. Historical Studies in the Physical Sciences, 10, 1–61.

82) 1 × Burr, H. S. (1936). The electro-dynamic theory of life. The Quarterly Review of Biology, 11(3), 322–333. https://doi.org/10.1086/394473

83) 18 × Calder, P. C. (2017). Omega-3 Fatty Acids and Inflammatory Processes: From Molecules to Man. Biochemical Society Transactions, 45(5), 1105–1115. https://doi.org/10.1042/BST20160474

84) 2 × Calvez, L., Lucas, J., & Zhang, X. H. (2012). Chalcogenide glass optics for infrared bio-imaging. Journal of Non-Crystalline Solids, 358(17), 2433–2439.

85) 3 × Camilleri, M. (2001). Colonic motility, pain and irritable bowel syndrome. Neurogastroenterology & Motility, 13(6), 667–672.

86) 8 × Campbell, W. W., & Meyer, R. A. (2006). Mechanisms of Neuropathic Pain. Neurotherapeutics, 3(3), 401–410. https://doi.org/10.1016/j.nurt.2006.05.004

87) 1 × Caplan, L. R. (2000). Posterior circulation ischemia: then, now, and tomorrow. The Thomas Willis Lecture-2000. Stroke, 31(8), 2011–2023.

88) 1 × Chan, K., Islam, M., Kamil, M., et al. (2017). Nephroprotective Effects of Herbal Medicines. Phytotherapy Research, 31(5), 645–653. https://doi.org/10.1002/ptr.5803

89) 1 × Chato, J. C. (1980). Heat transfer to blood vessels. Journal of Biomechanical Engineering, 102(2), 110–118.

90) 1 × Chen, R., et al. (2016). Biophoton emission as a tool for investigating energy flow in meridians: A new integrative method. Photochemistry and Photobiology, 92(1), 38–43.

91) 1 × Chen, R., Nickel, M. M., Loser, L., & May, E. S. (2020). Neural mechanisms of acupuncture in the human brain: A meta-analysis of functional MRI studies. Journal of Pain Research, 13, 1827–1842. https://doi.org/10.2147/JPR.S251338

92) 1 × Cheng, C., et al. (2012). Microvascular reactivity in the chest wall and its relationship to cardiopulmonary stress. Chest, 142(1), 148–156.

93) 1 × Cheng, X. N. (1987). Chinese Acupuncture and Moxibustion. Foreign Languages Press.

94) 6 × Cherry, S. R. (2006). The 2006 SNM Annual Meeting Highlight Lecture: Of mice and men (and positrons). Journal of Nuclear Medicine, 47(10), 1735–1745.

95) 2 × Chrousos, G. P. (2009). Stress and disorders of the stress system. Nature Reviews Endocrinology, 5(7), 374–381.

96) 18 × Chrubasik, S., Roufogalis, B. D., & Wagner, H. (2011). Evidence of Effectiveness of Aesculus hippocastanum (Horse Chestnut) Seed Extract in Chronic Venous Insufficiency: A Meta-Analysis. Phytomedicine, 18(5), 388–394. https://doi.org/10.1016/j.phymed.2010.09.010

97) 1 × Chudzik, M., et al. (2022). Vascular assessment with infrared thermography: Potential and limitations. Journal of Clinical Medicine, 11(5), 1230. https://doi.org/10.3390/jcm11051230

98) 1 × Chung, Y., et al. (2019). Quantitative thermal imaging as a diagnostic tool for radiculopathy and peripheral nerve disorders. Journal of Clinical Neuroscience, 68, 223–230.

99) 1 × Cignini, P., et al. (2012). Postpartum venous thromboembolism and pelvic venous changes. Journal of Maternal-Fetal & Neonatal Medicine, 25(10), 2115–2120.

100) 1 × Cina, C. S., & Safar, H. A. (2002). Profunda femoris artery: Anatomy and surgical considerations. Journal of Vascular Surgery, 35(3), 547–552. https://doi.org/10.1067/mva.2002.121160

101) 2 × Clark, R. A., Cook, J. L., & Smith, R. M. (2021). Standardizing infrared thermography for clinical diagnostics. Journal of Clinical Thermal Imaging, 2(1), 1–12.

102) 1 × Clark, R. P., & Mullan, B. J. (2017). Human skin temperature and its relevance in physiology and clinical practice. Journal of Medical Engineering & Technology, 41(6), 415–425.

103) 7 × Clark, S., Marins, J. C. B., & Fernández-Cuevas, I. (2021). Advances in image processing for clinical infrared thermography: Region-of-interest normalization and contrast optimization. Infrared Physics & Technology, 116, 103754.

104) 1 × Clodius, L., Smith, R., & Bruna, J. (1988). Lymphedema of the chest wall. Lymphology, 21(3), 113–119.

105) 1 × Clough, K. B., Kaufman, G. J., Nos, C., Buccimazza, I., & Sarfati, I. M. (2010). Improving breast cancer surgery: A classification and quadrant per quadrant atlas for oncoplastic surgery. Annals of Surgical Oncology, 17(5), 1375–1391. https://doi.org/10.1245/s10434-009-0838-9

106) 1 × Coblentz, W. W. (1905). Investigations of Infra-Red Spectra. U.S. Bureau of Standards Bulletin.

107) 1 × Cohen, J. I., et al. (2014). Lymphadenopathy: differential diagnosis and evaluation. American Family Physician, 89(9), 707–714.

108) 1 × Cohen, S., & Popp, F. A. (2003). Biophoton emission of the human body. Journal of Photochemistry and Photobiology B: Biology, 70(1), 1–3.

109) 1 × Cohen, S., Doyle, W. J., & Skoner, D. P. (2007). Psychological stress and susceptibility to the common cold. New England Journal of Medicine, 336(9), 659–666.

110) 1 × Colbert, A. P., Markov, M. S., & Souder, J. S. (2008). Skin impedance measurements for acupuncture research: development of a continuous monitoring system. Evidence-Based Complementary and Alternative Medicine, 5(4), 443–450. https://doi.org/10.1093/ecam/nem062

111) 1 × Coleman, R., Choudhury, A., & Wilkes, T. (2010). Market and material considerations for germanium optics in infrared imaging. Optical Engineering, 49(10), 103401.

112) 1 × Conte, M. S., Bradbury, A. W., Kolh, P., White, J. V., Dick, F., Fitridge, R., Mills, J. L., Ricco, J. B., Suresh, K. R., Murad, M. H., & Debus, S. (2019). Global vascular guidelines on the management of chronic limb-threatening ischemia (CLTI). Journal of Vascular Surgery, 69(6S), 3S–125S.e40. https://doi.org/10.1016/j.jvs.2019.02.016

113) 1 × Corsetti, V. L., Hovsepian, D. M., Beeds, T. M., & Monsees, B. S. (2011). Radiologic-pathologic correlation of small breast masses: Diagnostic challenges and limitations of conventional imaging techniques. Radiologic Clinics of North America, 49(6), 1043–1061. https://doi.org/10.1016/j.rcl.2011.07.002

114) 1 × Costantino, C., et al. (2019). Thermography and musculoskeletal disorders: An update on evidence-based applications. European Journal of Physical and Rehabilitation Medicine, 55(6), 835–843.

115) 2 × Criqui, M. H., & Aboyans, V. (2015). Epidemiology of peripheral artery disease. Circulation Research, 116(9), 1509–1526.

116) 1 × Cuykendall, S. R., Keller, T., & Nagel, R. (2020). Emissivity variability of human skin in medical infrared imaging. Journal of Biomedical Optics, 25(8), 083002. https://doi.org/10.1117/1.JBO.25.8.083002

117) 2 × Daanen, H. A. M., de Dear, R., & Taylor, N. A. S. (2021). Physiology and thermoregulation in the cold. Temperature, 8(2), 157–174. https://doi.org/10.1080/23328940.2020.1842780

118) 1 × Darras, J. C., de Vernejoul, P., & Albarede, P. (1992). Nuclear medicine and acupuncture: a study on the migration of radioisotopes in the channels. American Journal of Acupuncture, 20(3), 245–256.

119) 1 × Darras, J. C., de Vernejoul, P., & Albarede, P. (1993). Nuclear medicine and acupuncture: A study on the migration of technetium-99m after injection at acupuncture points. The American Journal of Acupuncture, 21(3), 245–256.

120) 1 × de Luca, C., et al. (2015). Environmental exposure and endocrine disruption: A thermographic and biochemical approach. Journal of Environmental and Public Health, 2015, 496170.

121) 2 × Deadman, P., Al-Khafaji, M., & Baker, K. (2007). A Manual of Acupuncture. Journal of Chinese Medicine Publications.

122) 1 × DeFronzo, R. A., & Ferrannini, E. (1991). Insulin resistance: A multifaceted syndrome responsible for NIDDM, obesity, hypertension, dyslipidemia, and atherosclerotic cardiovascular disease. Diabetes Care, 14(3), 173–194. https://doi.org/10.2337/diacare.14.3.173

123) 1 × Denda, M., et al. (2015). Skin surface temperature dynamics as indicators of visceral-organ neural modulation. European Journal of Physiology, 467(7), 1297–1304.

124) 1 × Dereniak, E. L., & Boreman, G. D. (1996). Infrared Detectors and Systems. Wiley-Interscience.

125) 1 × Després, J. P. (2012). Body fat distribution and risk of cardiovascular disease: an update. Circulation, 126(10), 1301–1313.

126) 1 × Deyo RA, Weinstein JN. Low back pain. N Engl J Med. 2001 Feb 1;344(5):363–70. doi:10.1056/NEJM200102013440508.

127) 1 × Di Carlo, A. (2017). Thermography and the human joint: A diagnostic overview. Clinical Medicine Insights: Arthritis and Musculoskeletal Disorders, 10, 1–9.

128) 10 × Diakides, M., & Bronzino, J. D. (2008). Medical Infrared Imaging: Principles and Practices. CRC Press.

129) 1 × Diakides, N. A., & Bronzino, J. D. (2013). Medical Infrared Imaging. CRC Press.

130) 1 × Dillingham, T. R. (1995). Evaluating and treating lumbosacral radiculopathy. Muscle & Nerve, 18(8), 807–819.

131) 1 × Ding, L., Zhu, J., Liu, J., & Wei, Y. (2022). Progress and challenges in infrared photodetectors: From materials to systems. Advanced Photonics Research, 3(3), 2100260. https://doi.org/10.1002/adpr.202100260

132) 1 × Disla, E., et al. (1994). Costochondritis: a prospective analysis in an emergency department setting. Annals of Emergency Medicine, 23(1), 99–103.

133) 1 × Dormandy, J. A., & Rutherford, R. B. (2000). Management of peripheral arterial disease (PAD): TASC Working Group. Journal of Vascular Surgery, 31(1), S1–S296. https://doi.org/10.1016/S0741-5214(00)90084-7

134) 1 × Dreyfuss, P., Michaelsen, M., & Pauza, K. (1994). Thoracic zygapophyseal joint pain patterns: A study in normal volunteers. Spine, 19(7), 807–811.

135) 1 × Duck, F. A. (1990). Physical Properties of Tissues: A Comprehensive Reference Book. Academic Press.

136) 1 × D'Amico, G., Garcia-Tsao, G., & Pagliaro, L. (2006). Natural history and prognostic indicators of survival in cirrhosis. Journal of Hepatology, 44(1), 217–231.

137) 1 × Eggleton, B. J., Luther-Davies, B., & Richardson, K. (2011). Chalcogenide photonics. Nature Photonics, 5(3), 141–148.

138) 1 × Ekstrand, J., Hägglund, M., & Waldén, M. (2011). Epidemiology of muscle injuries in professional football (soccer). American Journal of Sports Medicine, 39(6), 1226–1232.

139) 2 × Epstein, R. M., & Street, R. L. (2011). The values and value of patient-centered care. Annals of Family Medicine, 9(2), 100–103.

140) 1 × Ernst, E. (2006). Blood rheology: Relevance to cardiovascular disease. Heart, 92(5), 673–674.

141) 1 × European Society of Breast Imaging (EUSOBI). (2019). Recommendations on Breast Imaging Modalities. Retrieved from

142) 1 × EUSOBI. (2017). European Society of Breast Imaging recommendations on thermography for breast cancer detection. European Radiology, 27(5), 1706–1710.

143) 1 × Fairclough, J., Hayashi, K., Toumi, H., et al. (2006). Is iliotibial band syndrome really a friction syndrome? Journal of Science and Medicine in Sport, 9(1–2), 44–49.

144) 1 × FDA (2019). "FDA warns thermography should not be used in place of mammography." https://www.fda.gov/news-events/press-announcements/fda-warns-thermography

145) 1 × FDA. (2019). FDA warns patients and health care providers about using thermal imaging for breast cancer detection. FDA Safety Communication.

146) 1 × Fejer, R., Kyvik, K. O., & Hartvigsen, J. (2006). The prevalence of neck pain in the world population: a systematic critical review. European Spine Journal, 15(6), 834–848.

147) 1 × Felson, D. T., Zhang, Y., Hannan, M. T., Naimark, A., Weissman, B., Aliabadi, P., & Levy, D. (2000). The incidence and natural history of knee osteoarthritis in the elderly: The Framingham Osteoarthritis Study. Arthritis & Rheumatism, 43(4), 1049–1055.

148) 1 × Fernández-Cuevas, I., Bouzas Marins, J. C., Arnáiz Lastras, J., Gómez Carmona, P. M., Piñonosa Cano, S., García-Concepción, M. A., & Sillero-Quintana, M. (2015). Classification of factors influencing the use of infrared thermography in humans: A review. Infrared Physics & Technology, 71, 28–55. https://doi.org/10.1016/j.infrared.2015.02.007

149) 11 × Fernández-Cuevas, I., Bouzas Marins, J. C., Arnáiz Lastras, J., Gómez Carmona, P. M., Piñonosa Cano, S., García-Concepción, M. Á., & Sillero-Quintana, M. (2015).

Classification of factors influencing the use of infrared thermography in humans: A review. Infrared Physics & Technology, 71, 28–55.

150) 1 × Ferrante, M. A. (2004). Brachial plexopathies: Classification, causes, and consequences. Muscle & Nerve, 30(5), 547–568.

151) 19 × Flaws, B. (2000). A Practical Guide to Chinese Medicine. Blue Poppy Press.

152) 1 × Flaws, B. (2000). The Secret of Chinese Pulse Diagnosis. Blue Poppy Press.

153) 1 × Fowkes, F. G. R., Rudan, D., Rudan, I., Aboyans, V., Denenberg, J. O., McDermott, M. M., Norman, P. E., Sampson, U. K. A., Williams, L. J., Mensah, G. A., Criqui, M. H., & others. (2013). Comparison of global estimates of prevalence and risk factors for peripheral artery disease in 2000 and 2010: A systematic review and analysis. The Lancet, 382(9901), 1329–1340. https://doi.org/10.1016/S0140-6736(13)61249-0

154) 1 × Fredericson, M., & Jennings, F. (2007). Stress fractures in athletes. Journal of Sports Rehabilitation, 16(3), 198–206.

155) 2 × Friedman, S. L., Arispe, I., & Lee, Y. A. (2017). Liver Protection and Regeneration: Herbal Approaches. Journal of Hepatology, 66(1), S4–S6. https://doi.org/10.1016/j.jhep.2016.12.006

156) 1 × Friston, K. J. (2011). Functional and effective connectivity: a review. Brain Connectivity, 1(1), 13–36.

157) 1 × Fukada, E., & Yasuda, I. (1957). On the piezoelectric effect of bone. Journal of the Physical Society of Japan, 12(10), 1158–1162. https://doi.org/10.1143/JPSJ.12.1158

158) 1 × Furness, J. B. (2012). The enteric nervous system and neurogastroenterology. Nature Reviews Gastroenterology & Hepatology, 9(5), 286–294.

159) 2 × Gade, R., & Moeslund, T. B. (2014). Thermal cameras and applications: A survey. Machine Vision and Applications, 25(1), 245–262.

160) 1 × Gagge, A. P., & Nishi, Y. (1977). Heat exchange between human skin surface and thermal environment. In J. F. Stolwijk (Ed.), Physiology, Environment and Man.

161) 2 × Gao, H., Ma, J., & Wu, H. (2020). Advances in uncooled infrared focal plane array technology. Sensors, 20(4), 1084.

162) 1 × García-Hernández, R., Morales-Hernández, L. A., & Rojas-Valencia, M. N. (2021). Calibration influence on infrared thermography for medical diagnosis. Journal of Biomedical Photonics & Engineering, 7(4), 041009. https://doi.org/10.18287/JBPE21.07.040109

163) 1 × Gashev, A. A. (2008). Physiologic aspects of lymphatic contractile function: current perspectives. Annals of the New York Academy of Sciences, 1131, 100–109.

164) 1 × Gautherie, M. (1982). Thermopathology of breast cancer: Measurement and analysis of in vivo temperature and blood flow. Annals of the New York Academy of Sciences, 335, 383–415. https://doi.org/10.1111/j.1749-6632.1982.tb50370.x

165) 1 × Gautherie, M., & Gros, C. (1980). Breast thermography and cancer risk prediction. Cancer, 45(1), 51–56.

166) 1 × Gerwin, R. D., Dommerholt, J., & Shah, J. P. (2004). An expansion of Simons' integrated hypothesis of trigger point formation. Current Pain and Headache Reports, 8(6), 468–475. https://doi.org/10.1007/s11916-004-0063-z

167) 1 × Ghosh, G. (1991). Dispersion-equation coefficients for the refractive index and birefringence of germanium. Optics Communications, 83(1–2), 49–52.

168) 1 × Giuliano, A. E., et al. (2017). Axillary dissection vs. sentinel node biopsy in breast cancer: 20-year follow-up. New England Journal of Medicine, 376(6), 541–550.

169) 19 × Godoy, J. M. P., & Godoy, M. F. P. (2012). Use of Herbal Medicine in the Treatment of Lymphedema. Phytomedicine, 19(14), 1312–1317. https://doi.org/10.1016/j.phymed.2012.10.006

170) 1 × Gonzalez, R. C., & Woods, R. E. (2018). Digital Image Processing (4th ed.). Pearson.

171) 1 × González-Reyes, S., et al. (2017). Neuroendocrine–immune interactions in stress: Implications for therapeutic targets. Journal of Translational Medicine, 15(1), 114.

172) 1 × Goodman PH, et al. Normal temperature asymmetry of the back and extremities by computer-assisted infrared imaging. Thermology. 1986;1:195–202. (cited in Ammer's standardization chapter).

173) 1 × Gorbach, A. M., Heiss, W. D., & Szabo, Z. (2009). PET imaging of vascular and neuronal function. Journal of Cerebral Blood Flow & Metabolism, 29(3), 475–481.

174) 8 × Gordon, S., Brison, R., & Chen, J. (2016). Pulsed Electromagnetic Field Therapy in Bone Healing: A Systematic Review. Journal of Orthopaedic Surgery and Research, 11, 34. https://doi.org/10.1186/s13018-016-0350-x

175) 8 × Gore, J. C. (2003). Principles and practice of functional MRI of the human brain. Annual Review of Biomedical Engineering, 5, 209–240.

176) 1 × Greenbaum, D. S., Greenbaum, R. B., Joseph, J. G., & Natale, J. E. (1994). Chronic abdominal wall pain: Diagnostic validity and costs. Digestive Diseases and Sciences, 39(9), 1935–1941.

177) 1 × Greene, A. K., & Goss, J. A. (2018). Diagnosis and management of pediatric lymphedema. Journal of Pediatric Surgery, 53(1), 184–188.

178) 1 × Grieve R, Goodwin F, Alfaki M, et al. The immediate effect of spinal mobilisations on cervical myofascial pain: a randomised controlled trial. Manual Therapy. 2013;18(3):233-238.

179) 1 × Guyton, A. C., & Hall, J. E. (2021). Guyton and Hall Textbook of Medical Physiology (14th ed.). Elsevier.

180) 2 × Guyton, A. C., & Hall, J. E. (2021). Textbook of Medical Physiology (14th ed.). Elsevier.

181) 1 × Hallman, M. et al. (2019). Cutaneous thermography and terrain assessment in immune regulation. Autoimmunity Reviews, 18(11), 102396.

182) 11 × Hamer, R. (2012). The German New Medicine: The Biological Laws of the Organism. Hamer Verlag.

183) 1 × Hamer, R. G. (2012). Summary of the New Medicine. Amici di Dirk.

184) 1 × Hamer, R.G. (2014). The Scientific Chart of Germanic New Medicine (GNM). Translated summary chart.

185) 1 × Hameroff, S., & Penrose, R. (2014). Consciousness in the universe: A review of the 'Orch OR' theory. Physics of Life Reviews, 11(1), 39–78.

186) 1 × Hammerschlag, R., et al. (2015). Biofield research: A roundtable discussion of scientific and methodological issues. Journal of Alternative and Complementary Medicine, 21(10), 653–662.

187) 3 × Hammerschlag, R., Jain, S., & Baldwin, A. L. (2012). Biofield physiology: A framework for an emerging discipline. Global Advances in Health and Medicine, 1(1), 52–57.

188) 1 × Hammerschlag, R., Jain, S., & Baldwin, A. L. (2015). Biofield physiology: A framework for an emerging discipline. Global Advances in Health and Medicine, 4(suppl), 35–41. https://doi.org/10.7453/gahmj.2015.015.suppl

189) 1 × Han, D., Liu, Y., & Wang, X. (2022). Comparative optical performance of ZnSe and Ge materials for LWIR applications. Applied Optics, 61(3), B5–B11. https://doi.org/10.1364/AO.439408

190) 1 × Han, J., Liu, W., & Xu, J. (2022). Infrared transmission properties and biomedical applications of zinc selenide optics. Journal of Materials Science: Materials in Medicine, 33(6), 45–58.

191) 3 × Han, S., & Lee, B. (2018). Advances in uncooled infrared focal plane array technology. Sensors, 18(12), 4363.

192) 1 × Hanahan, D., & Folkman, J. (1996). Patterns and emerging mechanisms of the angiogenic switch during tumorigenesis. Cell, 86(3), 353–364. https://doi.org/10.1016/S0092-8674(00)80110-7

193) 2 × Hanahan, D., & Weinberg, R. A. (2011). Hallmarks of cancer: the next generation. Cell, 144(5), 646–674.

194) 1 × Head JF, Wang F, Elliott RL. Breast thermography is a noninvasive prognostic procedure that predicts tumor growth rate in breast cancer patients. Ann N Y Acad Sci. 1993; 698:153–158.

195) 1 × Head, H. (1893). On disturbances of sensation with especial reference to the pain of visceral disease. Brain, 16(1–2), 1–133.

196) 3 × Head, J. F., Wang, F., Lipari, C. A., & Elliott, R. L. (2000). "The important role of infrared imaging in breast cancer." IEEE Engineering in Medicine and Biology Magazine, 19(3), 52–57.

197) 8 × Heaney, R. P. (2006). Calcium, Dairy Products and Osteoporosis. Journal of the American College of Nutrition, 25(2), 130S–135S. https://doi.org/10.1080/07315724.2006.10719530

198) 1 × Heim, C., Ehlert, U., & Hellhammer, D. H. (2000). The potential role of hypocortisolism in the pathophysiology of stress-related bodily disorders. Psychoneuroendocrinology, 25(1), 1–35.

199) 1 × Herschel, J. F. W. (1840). Private experimental notes, Royal Society Archives, London.

200) 1 × Herschel, W. (1800). Experiments on the Refrangibility of the Invisible Rays of the Sun. Philosophical Transactions of the Royal Society of London, 90, 284–292.

201) 1 × Hershfield, N. B. (1992). Abdominal wall pain: Clinical evaluation, differential diagnosis, and treatment. American Journal of Gastroenterology, 87(2), 193–200.

202) 19 × Hewlings, S. J., & Kalman, D. S. (2017). Curcumin: A Review of Its Effects on Human Health. Foods, 6(10), 92. https://doi.org/10.3390/foods6100092

203) 1 × Hiatt, W. R., Armstrong, E. J., & Larson, C. J. (2015). Pathogenesis and management of critical limb ischemia. Journal of the American College of Cardiology, 65(18), 2079–2091. https://doi.org/10.1016/j.jacc.2015.03.538

204) 1 × Hildebrandt C, Raschner C, Ammer K. An overview of recent application of medical infrared thermography in sports medicine in Austria and North America, with collaborative input from Brazil. Sensors (Basel). 2010;10(5):4700–4715.

205) 5 × Hildebrandt C, Raschner C, Ammer K. An overview of recent application of medical infrared thermography in sports medicine in Austria and North America. Sensors (Basel). 2010;10(5):4700–4715.

206) 1 × Hoffman, D. D., Singh, M., & Prakash, C. (2010). Visual perception and the limits of grayscale: Implications for medical imaging. Journal of Vision, 10(7), 23.

207) 1 × Holst, G. C., & Lomheim, T. S. (2017). CMOS/CCD Sensors and Camera Systems (3rd ed.). SPIE Press.

208) 1 × Holst, G. C., & Lomheim, T. S. (2017). Infrared Detectors and Systems (2nd ed.). SPIE Press.

209) 1 × Hooshmand, F., Rezaei, S., & Arfaei, A. (2023). Infrared Thermography: Material Emissivity and Artifact Mitigation in Clinical Imaging. Medical Physics International, 11(2), 43–52.

210) 1 × Hoy, D. G., Protani, M., De, R., & Buchbinder, R. (2014). The epidemiology of neck pain. Best Practice & Research Clinical Rheumatology, 24(6), 783–792.

211) 1 × Hoy, D., et al. (2014). The global burden of low back pain: estimates from the Global Burden of Disease 2010 study. Annals of the Rheumatic Diseases, 73(6), 968–974.

212) 1 × Hoy, D., et al. (2014). The global burden of musculoskeletal pain. Best Practice & Research Clinical Rheumatology, 28(3), 319–328.

213) 1 × Hu, Y., et al. (2010). Infrared imaging of meridian-like tracks after moxibustion and acupuncture. Evidence-Based Complementary and Alternative Medicine, 2010, Article ID 468704.

214) 1 × Hu, Y., Ma, J., & Zhang, Y. (2010). Changes in facial meridian lines after moxibustion treatment in patients with Bell's palsy. Evidence-Based Complementary and Alternative Medicine, 2010. https://doi.org/10.1093/ecam/neq009

215) 1 × Hu, Y., Wang, D., Zhang, Y., & Chen, R. (2011). Relationship between intermuscular connective tissue planes and meridians. Anatomical Record, 294(3), 420-426.

216) 1 × Huang, W., Pach, D., Napadow, V., Park, K., Long, X., Neumann, J., ... & Ma, Y. (2011). Characterizing acupuncture stimuli using brain imaging with fMRI–a systematic review and meta-analysis of the literature. PLoS One, 7(4), e32960. https://doi.org/10.1371/journal.pone.0032960

217) 1 × Hubbard, T., & Kline, P. (1996). Psychophysiological coherence and somatic markers in health and disease. Advances in Mind-Body Medicine, 12(3), 21–31.

218) 1 × Hudson, R., & Hudson, J. (2019). Infrared detector performance in biomedical applications: A comparative review. Journal of Biomedical Optics, 24(6), 1–14.

219) 1 × Hudson, R., & Hudson, J. (2019). Infrared optics for medical imaging: Design considerations. Journal of Biomedical Optics, 24(4), 1–10.

220) 1 × Hudson, R., O'Brien, R., & Bailey, C. (2008). Thermal stability of germanium optics in infrared imaging. Applied Optics, 47(10), 1834–1842.

221) 3 × Hudson, R., O'Brien, R., & Bailey, C. (2008). Thermal stability of infrared optics in medical imaging. Applied Optics, 47(10), 1834–1842.

222) 1 × Hui, K. K.-S., Liu, J., Makris, N., Gollub, R. L., Chen, A. J.-W., Moore, C. I., ... & Kwong, K. K. (2005). Acupuncture modulates the limbic system and subcortical gray structures of the human brain: evidence from fMRI studies in normal subjects. Human Brain Mapping, 9(1), 13–25. https://doi.org/10.1002/hbm.10115

223) 1 × Hunt, V. V. (1996). Infinite Mind: Science of the Human Vibrations of Consciousness. Malibu, CA: Malibu Publishing.

224) 4 × IEC 80601-2-59. (2017). Medical electrical equipment—Particular requirements for the basic safety and essential performance of screening thermographs for human febrile temperature screening. International Electrotechnical Commission.

225) 1 × Illig, K. A., Donahue, D., Duncan, A., Freischlag, J., Thompson, R. W., Jordan, S., … & Sanders, R. J. (2010). Reporting standards of the Society for Vascular Surgery for thoracic outlet syndrome. Journal of Vascular Surgery, 52(3), 107–112.

226) 1 × Illig, K. A., Donahue, D., Duncan, A., Freischlag, J., Thompson, R., Jordan, S., … & Sanders, R. (2010). Reporting standards of the Society for Vascular Surgery for thoracic outlet syndrome. Journal of Vascular Surgery, 52(3), 107–112.

227) 1 × Illig, K. A., et al. (2010). Thoracic outlet syndrome. Journal of Vascular Surgery, 51(6), 1538–1549.

228) 2 × Incropera, F. P., DeWitt, D. P., Bergman, T. L., & Lavine, A. S. (2007). Fundamentals of Heat and Mass Transfer (6th ed.). Wiley.

229) 1 × International Society of Lymphology. (2013). The diagnosis and treatment of peripheral lymphedema: 2013 consensus document. Lymphology, 46(1), 1–11.

230) 1 × Ishikawa, T., et al. (2009). Pancreatic microcirculation and pathophysiology of pancreatitis. Journal of Hepato-Biliary-Pancreatic Surgery, 16(1), 1–7.

231) 1 × Janis, J. E., Barr, J. S., & Thornton, J. F. (2010). Abdominal cutaneous nerve entrapment syndrome (ACNES): A commonly overlooked cause of abdominal pain. Plastic and Reconstructive Surgery, 125(2), 745–752.

232) 11 × Janis, J. E., Hatef, D. A., & Shafer, A. K. (2010). Anatomy of Abdominal Wall Innervation and Implications for Neuropathic Pain. Plastic and Reconstructive Surgery, 125(3), 893–900. https://doi.org/10.1097/PRS.0b013e3181cf97a7

233) 1 × Jankovic S, et al. Cold Stress Dynamic Thermography for Evaluation of Vascular Disorders in Hand-Arm Vibration Syndrome. Journal of Occupational Health. 2008.

234) 3 × Jessen, C. (2001). Temperature Regulation in Humans and Other Mammals. Springer.

235) 1 × Johnson, J. M., & Kellogg, D. L. (2016). Thermoregulatory and thermal control in the human cutaneous circulation. In M. J. Tipton et al. (Eds.), Extreme Physiology and Medicine. (or Comprehensive Physiology, review articles on skin blood flow control).

236) 1 × Johnson, J. M., & Kellogg, D. L. (2016). Thermoregulatory control of skin blood flow. Comprehensive Physiology, 6(1), 33–89.

237) 8 × Jones, B. F. (1998). A Reappraisal of the Use of Infrared Thermal Image Analysis in Medicine. IEEE Transactions on Medical Imaging, 17(6), 1019–1027.

238) 1 × Jones, B. F. (2005). A reappraisal of the use of infrared thermal image analysis in medicine. IEEE Transactions on Medical Imaging, 24(7), 915–921. https://doi.org/10.1109/TMI.2005.851304

239) 1 × Jones, B. F., Plassmann, P., & Ring, E. F. J. (2002). A proposed thermal physiology for human skin. Journal of Medical Engineering & Technology, 26(4), 134–140.

240) 1 × Kakkos, S. K., et al. (2016). Proximal deep vein thrombosis and risk of pulmonary embolism. Journal of Vascular Surgery: Venous and Lymphatic Disorders, 4(3), 307–314.

241) 2 × Kaptchuk, T. J. (2000). The Web That Has No Weaver: Understanding Chinese Medicine. McGraw-Hill.

242) 19 × Kasper, S., Dienel, A., & Möller, H.-J. (2010). St. John's Wort and Its Active Compounds: An Overview. Neuropsychiatric Disease and Treatment, 6, 273–282. https://doi.org/10.2147/NDT.S10269

243) 1 × Katirji, B. (1999). Peroneal neuropathy. Neurologic Clinics, 17(3), 567–591.

244) 1 × Keeley, V. (2008). Lymphoedema and chronic oedema in the legs. British Journal of Community Nursing, 13(10), S15–S20.

245) 4 × Kellgren, J. H. (1939). On the distribution of pain arising from deep somatic structures with charts of segmental pain areas. Clinical Science, 4(1), 35–46.

246) 4 × Kennedy, D., Lee, T., & Seely, A. J. (2009). Early detection of inflammation and angiogenesis using functional thermal imaging. Annals of Biomedical Engineering, 37(10), 2185–2195.

247) 1 × Khalil, N., & Sundaram, A. (2009). Femoral neuropathy: An uncommon complication of pelvic surgery. Clinical Radiology, 64(9), 961–965.

248) 8 × Khan, K. M., Brukner, P., Kearney, C., Fuller, P., Bradshaw, C., Kiss, Z. S., & Wark, J. (2012). Stress Fractures: A Review of Incidence, Diagnosis and Management. Sports Medicine, 39(9), 763–779. https://doi.org/10.2165/00007256-200939090-00003

249) 2 × Khlevnoy, B. B., & Sapritsky, V. I. (2002). Blackbody radiators for infrared applications: Metrology and calibration. Metrologia, 39(1), 1–9.

250) 1 × Kibler, W. B., & Sciascia, A. (2010). Current concepts: scapular dyskinesis. British Journal of Sports Medicine, 44(5), 300–305.

251) 1 × Kiecolt-Glaser, J. K., McGuire, L., Robles, T. F., & Glaser, R. (2002). Emotions, morbidity, and mortality: New perspectives from psychoneuroimmunology. Annual Review of Psychology, 53(1), 83–107.

252) 1 × Kienle, G. S., Kiene, H., & Albonico, H. U. (2013). Anthroposophic medicine: An integrative medical system originating in Europe. Global Advances in Health and Medicine, 2(6), 20–31.

253) 1 × Kim, D. I., Yoon, S. H., & Lee, S. K. (2010). The dorsal scapular artery revisited: An anatomical study and its clinical significance. Surgical and Radiologic Anatomy, 32(3), 223–228. https://doi.org/10.1007/s00276-009-0567-8

254) 2 × Kim, H. Y., et al. (2018). Meridian flow visualization using infrared thermography following moxibustion: A pilot study. Integrative Medicine Research, 7(1), 65–72.

255) 1 × Kim, H.G., et al. (2020). Measurement of electromagnetic fields of the human body related to acupuncture points. Integrative Medicine Research, 9(3), 100431.

256) 1 × Kim, J. H., et al. (2022). Real-time observation of acupuncture point response using dynamic infrared imaging. Journal of Integrative Medicine, 20(4), 308–316.

257) 1 × Kim, S., Kim, H., & Chung, J. (2017). Facial Blood Flow Analysis Using Doppler Ultrasound in Patients with Migraine. The Journal of Headache and Pain, 18(1), 49. https://doi.org/10.1186/s10194-017-0755-4

258) 1 × Kinch, M. A. (2014). Fundamentals of Infrared Detector Materials. SPIE Press.

259) 1 × Kissinger, T., Braun, M., & Gernert, B. (2016). Performance improvements in uncooled thermal imaging systems. Infrared Physics & Technology, 76, 773–779. https://doi.org/10.1016/j.infrared.2016.05.008

260) 2 × Kitano, H. (2002). Systems biology: a brief overview. Science, 295(5560), 1662–1664.

261) 1 × Kotsenas, A. L., & DeLone, D. R. (2015). Emerging roles for advanced functional imaging in the evaluation of neurological disease. Neuroimaging Clinics of North America, 25(1), 77–89. https://doi.org/10.1016/j.nic.2014.09.004

262) 1 × Kreibig, S. D. (2010). Autonomic nervous system activity in emotion: a review. Biological Psychology, 84(3), 394–421.

263) 1 × Kreitler, S. (2014). Psychological meanings of symptoms: A new perspective on psycho-oncology. Psycho-Oncology, 23(4), 389–398. https://doi.org/10.1002/pon.3445

264) 8 × Kruger, R., & Kruger, M. C. (2019). Bone Health and Nutrition. Nutrients, 11(11), 2746. https://doi.org/10.3390/nu11112746

265) 1 × Kruse, P. W. (2001). Uncooled Thermal Imaging: Arrays, Systems, and Applications. SPIE Press.

266) 1 × Kuntz, K. M., & Ricci, M. A. (1996). Intercostal neuralgia: A common cause of chest wall pain. Chest Surgery Clinics of North America, 6(2), 403–418.

267) 1 × Kwon, H. J., et al. (2017). Visualization of acupuncture meridians using thermography after moxibustion stimulation. Journal of Acupuncture and Meridian Studies, 10(2), 104–110.

268) 1 × La Fountaine, M. F., & Wang, J. J. (2016). Autonomic nervous system responses during postural changes as measured by thermography. Autonomic Neuroscience, 198, 13–18. https://doi.org/10.1016/j.autneu.2016.01.005

269) 1 × La Fountaine, M. F., Heffernan, K. S., Gossett, J. D., & Bauman, W. A. (2016). Autonomic dysfunction and thermoregulatory control after neurological injury. Autonomic Neuroscience (representative of ANS–thermoregulation literature).

270) 1 × Labropoulos, N., et al. (2005). Patterns and distribution of isolated calf deep vein thrombosis. Journal of Vascular Surgery, 42(2), 198–203.

271) 17 × Lahiri, B. B., Bagavathiappan, S., Jayakumar, T., & Philip, J. (2012). Medical applications of infrared thermography: a review. Infrared Physics & Technology, 55(4), 221–235.

272) 2 × Lahiri, B. B., et al. (2012). Medical Applications of Infrared Thermography: A Review. Infrared Physics & Technology, 55(4), 221–235.

273) 1 × Lahiri, B.B., Bagavathiappan, S., Jayakumar, T., & Philip, J. (2012). Medical applications of infrared thermography: A review. Infrared Physics & Technology, 55(4), 221–235.

274) 1 × Lane, R. D., Reiman, E. M., Ahern, G. L., Schwartz, G. E., & Davidson, R. J. (2009). Neuroanatomical correlates of happiness, sadness, and disgust. American Journal of Psychiatry, 154(7), 926–933.

275) 1 × Langevin, H. M., & Yandow, J. A. (2002). Relationship of acupuncture points and meridians to connective tissue planes. Anatomical Record, 269(6), 257–265. https://doi.org/10.1002/ar.10185

276) 1 × Langevin, H. M., & Yandow, J. A. (2002). Relationship of acupuncture points and meridians to connective tissue planes. Anatomy Record, 269(6), 257–265.

277) 6 × Langevin, H. M., & Yandow, J. A. (2002). Relationship of acupuncture points and meridians to connective tissue planes. The Anatomical Record, 269(6), 257–265.

278) 1 × Langevin, H. M., Churchill, D. L., & Cipolla, M. J. (2001). Mechanical signaling through connective tissue: a mechanism for the therapeutic effect of acupuncture. FASEB Journal, 15(12), 2275-2282.

279) 1 × Langevin, H. M., Churchill, D. L., Cipolla, M. J. (2006). Mechanical signaling through connective tissue: A mechanism for the therapeutic effect of acupuncture. FASEB Journal, 15(12), 2275–2282. https://doi.org/10.1096/fj.01-0867hyp

280) 1 × Langevin, H. M., et al. (2002). Connective tissue: a body-wide signaling network? Medical Hypotheses, 59(5), 556–567.

281) 1 × Langevin, H.M., & Yandow, J.A. (2002). Relationship of acupuncture points and meridians to connective tissue planes. The Anatomical Record, 269(6), 257–265.

282) 1 × Langley, S. P. (1881). The Bolometer and Radiant Energy. The American Journal of Science, 21(124), 98–111.

283) 19 × Lao, L., Bergman, S., Langenberg, P., et al. (2004). Evaluation of Acupuncture for Pain Control after Oral Surgery: A Randomized Controlled Trial. Archives of Otolaryngology–Head & Neck Surgery, 130(6), 691–694. https://doi.org/10.1001/archotol.130.6.691

284) 1 × Larsen, P. R., Kronenberg, H. M., Melmed, S., & Polonsky, K. S. (2016). Williams Textbook of Endocrinology (13th ed.). Philadelphia: Elsevier.

285) 1 × Lasjaunias, P., & Berenstein, A. (2001). Surgical neuroangiography: Vol. 1. Clinical vascular anatomy and variations. Springer.

286) 1 × Lavine, R. (2010). Iliotibial band friction syndrome. Current Reviews in Musculoskeletal Medicine, 3(1–4), 18–22.

287) 1 × Lawson, R. (1956). Implications of surface temperature in the diagnosis of breast cancer. Canadian Medical Association Journal, 75(4), 309–310.

288) 1 × Lawson, R. N. (1956). Implications of Surface Temperatures in the Diagnosis of Breast Cancer. Canadian Medical Association Journal, 75(4), 309–310.

289) 1 × Lawson, R. N. (1957). Thermography: A New Tool in the Investigation of Breast Cancer. Annals of the New York Academy of Sciences, 121(1), 93–102.

290) 1 × Leduc, A., & Leduc, O. (2016). Physiology of the lymphatic system and associated disorders. In: Lymphology, 49(4), 203–212.

291) 1 × Lee, M. W., McPhee, R. W., & Stringer, M. D. (2008). An evidence-based approach to human dermatomes. Clinical Anatomy, 21(5), 363–373.

292) 1 × Lipton, B.H. (2016). The Biology of Belief: Unleashing the Power of Consciousness, Matter & Miracles. Hay House.

293) 1 × Litscher, G. (2005). Ten years evidence-based high-tech acupuncture—A short review of the research situation. Medical Acupuncture, 17(4), 25–29.

294) 1 × Litscher, G. (2013). Technical standards for infrared imaging in medicine. Medicines, 1(1), 14–22. https://doi.org/10.3390/medicines1010014

295) 1 × Litscher, G. (2014). Bioengineering assessment of acupuncture, part 6: Meridian-oriented research using thermography. Critical Reviews™ in Biomedical Engineering, 42(4), 315–321. https://doi.org/10.1615/CritRevBiomedEng.2014011019

296) 3 × Logothetis, N. K. (2008). What we can do and what we cannot do with fMRI. Nature, 453(7197), 869–878.

297) 1 × Lu, W. C., Yang, H. F., & Zhang, W. Y. (2002). Infrared thermographic observation of the effect of acupuncture. Journal of Traditional Chinese Medicine, 22(4), 277–280.

298) 1 × Lucas, J., Boussard-Pledel, C., Bureau, B., & Zhang, X. H. (2015). Infrared glasses for bio-sensing and medical imaging. Comptes Rendus Chimie, 18(2), 141–150.

299) 2 × Lundberg, U. (1999). Stress hormones in health and illness: the roles of work and gender. Psychoneuroendocrinology, 24(2), 95–123.

300) 1 × Lutgendorf, S. K., & Costanzo, E. S. (2003). Psychoneuroimmunology and health psychology: An integrative model. Brain, Behavior, and Immunity, 17(4), 225–232.

301) 1 × López-Puente, V., de Aldana, J. R. V., & Jaque, D. (2020). Diamond-like carbon coatings for infrared medical optics. Optical Materials, 109, 110286.

302) 1 × Ma, L., Liu, S., & Zhang, X. (2019). The role of skin temperature in clinical diagnosis and its physiological basis. Biomedical Engineering Letters, 9(2), 133–143. https://doi.org/10.1007/s13534-019-00097-2

303) 1 × Ma, S. X. (2003). Enhanced nitric oxide concentrations and expression of nitric oxide synthase in acupuncture points/meridians. Journal of Alternative and Complementary Medicine, 9(2), 207-215.

304) 1 × Ma, S. X. (2016). Enhanced nitric oxide concentrations and expressions of nitric oxide synthase isoforms in acupuncture points/meridians. Journal of Alternative and Complementary Medicine, 20(5), 347–355. https://doi.org/10.1089/acm.2013.0046

305) 7 × Machin, G., & Cowie, J. (2013). Uncertainty of measurement in medical thermography. Physiological Measurement, 34(7), R59–R74.

306) 5 × Machin, G., & Whittam, A. (2018). Traceability in infrared medical thermography. Journal of Physics: Conference Series, 1065, 072017.

307) 2 × Machin, G., Whittam, A., & Bloch, D. (2014). Recent advances in thermal imaging calibration for medical applications. Infrared Physics & Technology, 64, 21–29.

308) 1 × Maciocia, G. (2015). The Foundations of Chinese Medicine (3rd ed.). Elsevier.

309) 1 × Mackowiak, P. A. (1997). Reassessment of the Normal Body Temperature in Adults. JAMA, 268(12), 1578–1580.

310) 8 × Maffulli, N., Longo, U. G., Gougoulias, N., Caine, D., & Denaro, V. (2014). Sports Injuries: A Review of Outcomes. British Medical Bulletin, 111(1), 47–68. https://doi.org/10.1093/bmb/ldu033

311) 1 × Martini, D. et al. (2021). Mitochondrial bioenergetics and hormonal health: A systemic link. Cell Metabolism, 33(1), 56–69.

312) 1 × Matheson, G. O., Clement, D. B., McKenzie, D. C., Taunton, J. E., Lloyd-Smith, D. R., & MacIntyre, J. G. (1987). Stress fractures in athletes: A study of 320 cases. American Journal of Sports Medicine, 15(1), 46–58.

313) 1 × Matsuda, T., et al. (2020). Cutaneous infrared signatures in functional organ fatigue: A new diagnostic approach. Japanese Journal of Thermophysiology, 44(2), 93–101.

314) 19 × Matsumoto, H., Sato, T., & Mori, Y. (2010). Effects of Pulsed Electromagnetic Fields on Cellular Activity and Healing. Bioelectromagnetics, 31(6), 489–497. https://doi.org/10.1002/bem.20560

315) 1 × Matsumoto, K., Kawakami, M., & Tsurumoto, T. (1999). Anatomical study of the lumbar arteries and their clinical significance in surgery. Surgical and Radiologic Anatomy, 21(3), 185–189. https://doi.org/10.1007/BF01635073

316) 1 × Matsuura, Y. (2004). Infrared optics and applications of ZnSe materials. Optical Review, 11(6), 405–410.

317) 1 × McEwen, B. S. (1998). Protective and damaging effects of stress mediators. New England Journal of Medicine, 338(3), 171–179.

318) 1 × McGee, D. (1995). Night Vision and Electro-Optics Review. Defense Science Publications.

319) 1 × McLaughlin, S. A., Wright, M. J., Morris, K. T., Giron, G. L., Sampson, M. R., Brockway, J. P., & Hurley, K. E. (2008). Prevalence of lymphedema in women with breast cancer. Annals of Surgical Oncology, 15(11), 3222–3228.

320) 1 × Mehrara, B. J., & Zampell, J. C. (2008). Surgical models of lymphedema: Lessons learned. Annals of the New York Academy of Sciences, 1131(1), 123–130.

321) 1 × Merla, A., & Romani, G. L. (2006). Functional infrared imaging in medicine: From basic evidence to clinical application. IEEE Engineering in Medicine and Biology Magazine, 25(6), 25–33.

322) 1 × Mickle, K. J., et al. (2009). Effects of age on strength and morphology of the ankle dorsiflexors. J Gerontol A Biol Sci Med Sci, 64(5), 558–565.

323) 1 × Milgrom, C., Giladi, M., Simkin, A., Rand, N., Kedem, R., Kashtan, H., … & Stein, M. (1985). The pattern of stress fractures in Israeli defense force recruits: A prospective study. Journal of Bone and Joint Surgery, 67(5), 732–735.

324) 7 × Miller, J. D., & McGee, K. (2014). Costochondritis and Chest Wall Pain. Primary Care: Clinics in Office Practice, 41(2), 273–286. https://doi.org/10.1016/j.pop.2014.01.005

325) 1 × Miller, M. D., Thompson, S. R., & Hart, J. (2014). Review of Orthopaedics (6th ed.). Elsevier.

326) 7 × Minkina, W., & Dudzik, S. (2009). Infrared Thermography: Errors and Uncertainties. Wiley.

327) 1 × Modi, S., Stanton, A. W. B., Svensson, W. E., Peters, A. M., Mortimer, P. S., & Levick, J. R. (2007). Human lymphatic pumping measured in healthy and lymphoedematous arms. Journal of Physiology, 583(1), 271–285.

328) 8 × Moncada, S., & Higgs, A. (1993). The L-arginine-nitric oxide pathway. The New England Journal of Medicine, 329(27), 2002–2012.

329) 1 × Moon, H. K., & Taylor, G. I. (1988). The vascular anatomy of rectus abdominis musculocutaneous flaps based on the deep superior epigastric system. Plastic and Reconstructive Surgery, 82(5), 815–832. https://doi.org/10.1097/00006534-198811000-00008

330) 1 × Mooney, P., & Cardwell, T. (2018). Design constraints in LWIR medical imaging: Lens material selection and patient interface considerations. Biomedical Optics Express, 9(12), 6342–6355. https://doi.org/10.1364/BOE.9.006342

331) 1 × Morales-Hernández, L. A., García-Hernández, R., & del Río, J. A. (2022). Technical considerations in clinical thermography: Resolution, NETD, and field-of-view effects. Infrared Physics & Technology, 123, 104104. https://doi.org/10.1016/j.infrared.2021.104104

332) 1 × Morales-Hernández, L. A., Martínez-Jiménez, M. A., & Vega-Rodríguez, M. A. (2022). Impact of infrared camera resolution on clinical thermographic analysis. Journal of Medical Systems, 46(2), 12.

333) 2 × Moreira DG, Costello JT, Brito CJ, et al. Thermographic imaging in sports and exercise medicine: a Delphi study and consensus statement. BMC Complementary Medicine and Therapies. 2017;17:1–10.

334) 1 × Moreira, D. G., Costello, J. T., Brito, C. J., Adamczyk, J. G., Ammer, K., & Sillero-Quintana, M. (2017). Thermographic imaging in sports and exercise medicine: A Delphi study and consensus statement on methodological best practices. Journal of Thermal Biology, 69, 155–162.

335) 1 × Mortimer, P. S., & Levick, J. R. (2004). Chronic peripheral oedema: The critical role of the lymphatic system. Clinical Medicine, 4(5), 448–453.

336) 3 × Mortimer, P. S., & Rockson, S. G. (2014). New developments in clinical aspects of lymphatic disease. Journal of Clinical Investigation, 124(3), 915–921.

337) 1 × Moser, M., Hager, M., & Schmid-Zalaudek, K. (2017). Scientific bases of acupuncture-induced modulation of the autonomic nervous system: A narrative review. Medical Acupuncture, 29(3), 130–136. https://doi.org/10.1089/acu.2017.1226

338) 1 × Motoyama, H. (1977). Theories of the Chakras: Bridge to Higher Consciousness. Wheaton, IL: Theosophical Publishing House.

339) 1 × Myers, T. (2014). Anatomy Trains: Myofascial Meridians for Manual and Movement Therapists. 3rd ed. Churchill Livingstone.

340) 1 × Myers, T. W. (2014). Anatomy Trains: Myofascial Meridians for Manual and Movement Therapists (3rd ed.). Churchill Livingstone.

341) 1 × Nakatani, Y. (1956). Skin Electric Resistance and Ryodoraku. The Japanese Journal of Medical Electronics and Biological Engineering, 10(3), 78–82.

342) 1 × Napadow, V., Dhond, R., Conti, G., Makris, N., Brown, E. N., & Barbieri, R. (2005). Brain correlates of autonomic modulation: Combining heart rate variability with fMRI. NeuroImage, 42(1), 169–177. https://doi.org/10.1016/j.neuroimage.2008.04.238

343) 1 × NASA Technical Memoranda, Ames Research Center (1969–1978).

344) 1 × Navarro, M.D., et al. (2020). Integrative and functional medicine approach to endocrine dysfunctions. Integrative Medicine, 19(6), 42–49.

345) 1 × Neary, D., Ochoa, J., & Gilliatt, R. W. (2003). Obturator neuropathy: A clinical and electrophysiological study. Journal of Neurology, Neurosurgery & Psychiatry, 74(4), 529–533.

346) 2 × Nelson, D. L., Cox, M. M. (2015). Lehninger Principles of Biochemistry (7th ed.). W.H. Freeman.

347) 1 × Nelson, R. M., et al. (2015). Physiology of Heat Transfer and Thermoregulation. In: Environmental Physiology. Springer.

348) 1 × Neugebauer, G., & Leighton, R. B. (1965). Two-micron Sky Survey: A Catalog of Infrared Sources. NASA Technical Reports.

349) 1 × Ng, E. Y. K., & Etehadtavakol, M. (Eds.). (2018). Application of Infrared to Biomedical Sciences. Springer. https://doi.org/10.1007/978-981-10-3140-0

350) 3 × Nguyen, V. H., Hegde, C., & Sheng, H. (2014). High-resolution thermal imaging and clinical zone mapping: Advances and limitations. Biomedical Optics Express, 5(8), 2770–2783.

351) 10 × Nielsen, K., Sandermann, J., & Højgaard, K. (2018). Vascular Disorders of the Abdominal Wall. Vascular Medicine, 23(1), 54–61. https://doi.org/10.1177/1358863X17749729

352) 1 × Nishi, E. (2018). Sympathetic and parasympathetic regulation of thoracic vascular responses. Autonomic Neuroscience, 210, 1–8.

353) 2 × Niskanen, M., Rintamäki, H., & Näyhä, S. (2016). Infrared thermal imaging in medicine. Duodecim – Finnish Medical Journal, 132(14), 1352–1359.

354) 8 × Norgren, L., Hiatt, W. R., Dormandy, J. A., et al. (2007). Inter-Society Consensus for the Management of Peripheral Arterial Disease (TASC II). Journal of Vascular Surgery, 45(1), S5–S67. https://doi.org/10.1016/j.jvs.2006.12.037

355) 1 × Norheim AJ, et al. Variability in peripheral rewarming after cold stress among 255 healthy Norwegian army conscripts assessed by dynamic infrared thermography. Int J Circumpolar Health. 2018.

356) 1 × Note on Referencing Method:
This Atlas uses a consolidated reference system, listing all scientific sources alphabetically at the end of the book. Citations throughout the text refer to this master list. Many sources are cited across multiple chapters due to the integrative and interdisciplinary nature of Biospectral Medicine.

357) 1 × Novitsky, Y. W., Elliott, H. L., Orenstein, S. B., & Rosen, M. J. (2006). Transversus abdominis muscle release: a novel approach to complex abdominal wall reconstruction. Annals of Surgery, 244(1), 29–34.

358) 1 × Okeson, J. P. (2013). Management of Temporomandibular Disorders and Occlusion (7th ed.). Elsevier.

359) 1 × Opar, D. A., Williams, M. D., & Shield, A. J. (2012). Hamstring strain injuries: factors that lead to injury and re-injury. Sports Medicine, 42(3), 209–226.

360) 1 × Oschman, J. L. (2015). Energy Medicine: The Scientific Basis. Elsevier Health Sciences.

361) 2 × Oschman, J. L. (2015). Energy Medicine: The Scientific Basis. Elsevier.

362) 1 × Oschman, J. L. (2016). Energy Medicine: The Scientific Basis (2nd ed.). London: Churchill Livingstone.

363) 1 × Oschman, J.L. (2003). Energy Medicine: The scientific basis. Churchill Livingstone.

364) 1 × Oschman, J.L. (2016). The role of connective tissue in energetic regulation of metabolism. Energy Medicine, 11(2), 28–35.

365) 1 × Ouyang, X., & Pinter, S. Z. (2016). Thermal Infrared Imaging for Biomedical Applications. In: Biomedical Optical Imaging Technologies: Design and Applications. Springer.

366) 1 × Palik, E. D. (1998). Handbook of Optical Constants of Solids II. Academic Press.

367) 2 × Panossian, A., & Wikman, G. (2010). Effects of Adaptogens on the Central Nervous System and the Molecular Mechanisms Associated with Their Stress-Protective Activity. Pharmaceuticals, 3(1), 188–224. https://doi.org/10.3390/ph3010188

368) 19 × Papanas, N., & Ziegler, D. (2014). Emerging Treatments for Diabetic Polyneuropathy. Expert Opinion on Emerging Drugs, 19(3), 357–367. https://doi.org/10.1517/14728214.2014.907242

369) 3 × Parsons, K. (2014). Human Thermal Environments (3rd ed.). CRC Press.

370) 1 × Paskett, E. D., Dean, J. A., Oliveri, J. M., & Harrop, J. P. (2007). Cancer-related lymphedema risk factors, diagnosis, treatment, and impact. Journal of Clinical Oncology, 25(30), 4527–4534.

371) 2 × Passos MdD, Silva L, et al. Portable infrared thermography for peripheral arterial disease: a pilot study. Journal of Vascular Diagnostics and Interventions. 2022;10:35-42.

372) 1 × Patrick, L. (2003). Toxic metals and antioxidants: Part II. The role of antioxidants in arsenic and cadmium toxicity. Alternative Medicine Review, 8(2), 106–128.

373) 2 × Pennes, H. H. (1948). Analysis of tissue and arterial blood temperatures in the resting human forearm. Journal of Applied Physiology, 1(2), 93–122.

374) 1 × Pereira, C. A., Lima, R. C., Silva, R. M., & de Freitas, D. B. (2019). Clinical performance of uncooled thermographic systems in medical applications. Biomedical Engineering Online, 18(1), 123. https://doi.org/10.1186/s12938-019-0736-2

375) 1 × Pert, C. B. (1997). Molecules of Emotion: The Science Behind Mind–Body Medicine. Scribner.

376) 1 × Petrek, J. A., & Heelan, M. C. (1998). Incidence of breast carcinoma-related lymphedema. Cancer, 83(12 Suppl American), 2776–2781.

377) 1 × Petrofsky, J. S., & Laymon, M. (2015). Infrared thermography in the assessment of acupuncture-induced effects: A review. Medical Acupuncture, 27(2), 100–107. https://doi.org/10.1089/acu.2015.1135

378) 2 × Petrofsky, J. S., & Laymon, M. (2015). The influence of moisture on the skin impedance at points used in the electro diagnosis of acupuncture. Medical Acupuncture, 27(2), 108–114. https://doi.org/10.1089/acu.2015.1137

379) 1 × Petrofsky, J. S., & Laymon, M. (2015). The use of infrared imaging in the evaluation of complementary and alternative medicine therapies. Medical Acupuncture, 27(2), 97–99. https://doi.org/10.1089/acu.2015.1131

380) 3 × Phelps, M. E. (2000). PET: The merging of biology and imaging into molecular imaging. Journal of Nuclear Medicine, 41(4), 661–681.

381) 1 × Pijnenburg, R., van den Berg, M., & de Rooij, M. (2017). Functional imaging in early disease: A tool for pre-emptive diagnostics. European Journal of Clinical Investigation, 47(12), 863–875. https://doi.org/10.1111/eci.12809

382) 1 × Piller, N. B., & Thelander, A. (1998). Lymphedema and fibrosis in the neck following radiation therapy. Lymphology, 31(2), 62–70.

383) 1 × Pizer, S. M., Amburn, E. P., Austin, J. D., et al. (1987). Adaptive histogram equalization and its variations. Computer Vision, Graphics, and Image Processing, 39(3), 355–368.

384) 1 × Planck M. (1901). On the Law of Distribution of Energy in the Normal Spectrum. Annalen der Physik, 4(3), 553–563.

385) 1 × Planck, M. (1901). On the Law of Distribution of Energy in the Normal Spectrum. Annalen der Physik, 4(553), 1.

386) 1 × Planck, M. (1901). On the Law of Distribution of Energy in the Normal Spectrum. Annalen der Physik, 4(553), 1–11.

387) 1 × Planck, M. (1901). On the Law of Distribution of Energy in the Normal Spectrum. Annalen der Physik, 4(553–563).

388) 1 × Pollack, G. H. (2013). The Fourth Phase of Water: Beyond Solid, Liquid, and Vapor. Ebner and Sons.

389) 1 × Popp, F. A. (2003). Properties of biophotons and their theoretical implications. Indian Journal of Experimental Biology, 41(5), 391-402.

390) 1 × Popp, F. A., & Beloussov, L. V. (2003). Integrative Biophysics: Biophotonics. Dordrecht: Springer.

391) 1 × Popp, F. A., Li, K. H., & Gu, Q. (1996). Recent advances in biophoton research and its applications. World Scientific.

392) 1 × Popp, F.A., et al. (2002). Biophoton emission: Evidence for coherent states in living organisms. Cell Biochemistry and Biophysics, 37(1), 103–111.

393) 1 × Pérez-Bellmunt A, et al. Infrared thermography applied to active myofascial trigger points in patients with neck pain. Infrared Physics & Technology. 2019;97:206-212.

394) 1 × Rafieian-Kopaei, M., Baradaran, A., & Rafieian, M. (2017). Medicinal Plants and Their Natural Components as Future Drugs for the Treatment of Cardiovascular Diseases. Pharmacognosy Reviews, 11(21), 67–75. https://doi.org/10.4103/phrev.phrev_40_16

395) 2 × Raica, M., Cimpean, A. M., & Ribatti, D. (2009). "Angiogenesis in premalignant conditions." European Journal of Cancer, 45(11), 1924–1934.

396) 1 × Raichle, M. E. (2009). A brief history of human brain mapping. Trends in Neurosciences, 32(2), 118–126.

397) 2 × Rajput, R., Nagori, B. P., & Mathur, A. (2013). Selenium and Thyroid Disease: From Pathogenesis to Treatment. Journal of Thyroid Research, 2013, 1–8. https://doi.org/10.1155/2013/382857

398) 1 × Raju, S., & Neglén, P. (2009). Chronic venous insufficiency and varicose veins. N Engl J Med, 360(22), 2319–2327.

399) 1 × Rangayyan, R. M. (2015). Biomedical Signal Analysis (2nd ed.). IEEE-Wiley.

400) 1 × Razeghi, M., & Nguyen, B. M. (2014). Advances in mid-infrared detection and imaging: A review. Applied Physics Reviews, 1(4), 041102.

401) 1 × Reaven, G. M. (1988). Role of insulin resistance in human disease. Diabetes, 37(12), 1595–1607. https://doi.org/10.2337/diabetes.37.12.1595

402) 1 × Reich, H., & Ring, F.E.J. (2017). Thermal and spectral interpretation of dermatomal emission in visceral dysfunction. Journal of Biomedical Thermography, 12(3), 115–123.

403) 1 × Rein, G. (1992). Biological effects of quantum fields and their role in healing. Frontier Perspectives, 3(2), 16–23.

404) 1 × Reitz F. (2025). Biospectral Medicine: Atlas of Infrared Thermography and Emissive Physiology. Reitz Institute Publications.

405) 1 × Reitz, F. (2005). CTI Protocols and Methodology, Irish Center of Integrated Medicine Archives.

406) 1 × Reitz, F. (2005–2023). Clinical field notes, infrared diagnostic protocols, and zone emission mapping (unpublished internal documentation). Reitz Institute.

407) 1 × Reitz, F. (2005–2023). Clinical imaging case series, biospectral meridian correlations (unpublished), Reitz Institute Records.

408) 1 × Reitz, F. (2024). Atlas of Biospectral Medicine. Internal Monograph, Reitz Institute.

409) 1 × Reitz, F. (2024). Atlas of Infrared Thermography: Clinical Interpretation of Spectral Zones. Reitz Institute Press.

410) 1 × Reitz, F. (2024). Biospectral Medicine: Clinical Interpretation and Spectral Diagnostics. Reitz Institute Press.

411) 1 × Reitz, F. (2024). Biospectral Medicine: Integrative Diagnostics through Spectral Emission. Reitz Institute.

412) 1 × Reitz, F. (2024). Biospectral Medicine: Zone-Based Diagnostic Logic and Emissive Interpretation Model. Internal Archive, Reitz Institute.

413) 1 × Reitz, F. (2024). Biospectral Medicine: Zone-Based Diagnostic Logic and Emissive Interpretation Model. Reitz Institute Archives.

414) 5 × Reitz, F. (2025). Atlas of Infrared Thermography: Biospectral Medicine Foundations. Reitz Institute Publishing.

415) 1 × Ridner, S. H., Dietrich, M. S., Spotanski, K., Wells, N., & Worrell, R. (2012). Lymphedema in patients with head and neck cancer: Prevalence and risk factors. Head & Neck, 34(1), 20–27.

416) 1 × Ring EFJ, Ammer K. (2012). Infrared thermal imaging in medicine. Physiol Meas, 33(3):R33–R46.

417) 1 × Ring EFJ, Ammer K. Infrared thermal imaging in medicine. Physiol Meas. 2012;33:R33–R46.

418) 3 × Ring EFJ, Ammer K. Infrared thermal imaging in medicine. Physiological Measurement. 2012;33(3):R33–R46.

419) 1 × Ring EFJ, Ammer K. Infrared thermal imaging in medicine. Physiological Measurement. 2012;33(3):R33–R46. DOI:

420) 1 × Ring EFJ, Ammer K. Infrared thermal imaging in medicine. Physiological Measurement. 2012;33:R33–R46.

421) 1 × Ring EFJ. The historical development of thermal imaging in medicine. Rheumatology (Oxford). 2014;53(5):800–802.

422) 1 × Ring, E. F. J. (2007). The historical development of thermal imaging in medicine. Rheumatology, 43(6), 800–802.

423) 1 × Ring, E. F. J. (2010). The historical development of thermal imaging in medicine. Physiological Measurement, 31(3), R1–R18.

424) 1 × Ring, E. F. J., & Ammer, K. (2012). Infrared thermal imaging in medicine. Physiological Measurement, 33(3), R33.

425) 29 × Ring, E. F. J., & Ammer, K. (2012). Infrared thermal imaging in medicine. Physiological Measurement, 33(3), R33–R46.

426) 3 × Ring, E. F. J., & Ammer, K. (2020). Infrared thermal imaging in medicine. Physiological Measurement, 41(3), 03TR01. https://doi.org/10.1088/1361-6579/ab67c0

427) 13 × Ring, E. F. J., & Ammer, K. (2020). Infrared thermal imaging in medicine. Physiological Measurement, 41(9), 09TR01.

428) 11 × Ring, E. F. J., McEvoy, H., Jung, A., Zuber, J., & Machin, G. (2020). New standards for medical infrared imaging. Physiological Measurement, 41(9), 09TR01.

429) 1 × Ring, E.F.J., & Ammer, K. (2012). Infrared thermal imaging in medicine. Physiological Measurement, 33(3), R33–R46.

430) 1 × Ring, E.F.J., & Ammer, K. (2018). Functional infrared imaging of inflammation and lymphatic congestion. In: The Thermal Image in Medicine and Biology. Springer.

431) 1 × Ring, E.F.J., & McEvoy, H. (2016). Spinal and cranial thermal imaging: Applications in neurology and pain. Infrared Physics & Technology, 76, 626–632.

432) 1 × Robinson, C. et al. (2020). Functional imaging modalities in integrative medicine: Relevance and application. Integrative Medicine Reports, 1(1), 23–36.

433) 1 × Robinson, M.R., Ring, E.F., & Newbold, P. (2020). Thermal imaging of the musculoskeletal system: A review of recent advances. Journal of Medical Engineering & Technology, 44(7), 399–411.

434) 1 × Rockson, S. G. (2001). Lymphedema. American Journal of Medicine, 110(4), 288–295.

435) 19 × Rockson, S. G. (2001). Lymphedema. The American Journal of Medicine, 110(4), 288–295. https://doi.org/10.1016/S0002-9343(00)00757-4

436) 2 × Rogalski, A. (2011). History of infrared detectors. Opto-Electronics Review, 20(3), 279–308.

437) 1 × Rogalski, A. (2012). Infrared Detectors: An Overview. Infrared Physics & Technology, 43(3–5), 187–210. https://doi.org/10.1016/j.infrared.2002.06.001

438) 1 × Rogalski, A., & Martyniuk, P. (2020). Infrared detectors: Status and trends. Progress in Quantum Electronics, 71, 100256.

439) 1 × Romanovsky, A. A. (2014). Skin temperature: its role in thermoregulation. Temperature, 1(1), 3–4 (and related reviews on POA/AH control).

440) 1 × Rossi, M., Carpi, A., & Galetta, F. (2013). Non-invasive evaluation of microvascular function in humans: A review. Clinical Hemorheology and Microcirculation, 53(3), 227–246.

441) 1 × Rosslenbroich, B. (2007). Theoretical Biology: The Complexity of Regulation and the Principle of Organization. Springer.

442) 1 × Rubik, B. (2002). The biofield hypothesis: Its biophysical basis and role in medicine. Journal of Alternative and Complementary Medicine, 8(6), 703–717. https://doi.org/10.1089/10755530260511711

443) 19 × Rubik, B. (2002). The Biofield Hypothesis: Its Biophysics and Role in Medicine. The Journal of Alternative and Complementary Medicine, 8(6), 703–717. https://doi.org/10.1089/10755530260511719

444) 1 × Rubik, B. (2016). The Biofield Hypothesis: Scientific evidence and medical applications. Global Advances in Health and Medicine, 5(1), 8–14.

445) 1 × Rubik, B., Muehsam, D., Hammerschlag, R., & Jain, S. (2015). Biofield science and healing: history, terminology, and concepts. Global Advances in Health and Medicine, 4(suppl), 8–14.

446) 1 × Rutherford, R. B. (2009). Vascular surgery (7th ed.). Saunders Elsevier.

447) 1 × Sakai, S., Yamaguchi, A., & Hori, E. (2007). Laser Doppler measurement of acupuncture-induced changes in peripheral blood flow. Autonomic Neuroscience, 133(2), 158–162. https://doi.org/10.1016/j.autneu.2007.01.010

448) 1 × Sanders, R. J., & Hammond, S. L. (2002). Diagnosis of thoracic outlet syndrome. Journal of Vascular Surgery, 36(4), 688–692.

449) 2 × Sanghera, J. S., & Aggarwal, I. D. (1999). Infrared transmitting materials for biomedical optics. Comptes Rendus de l'Académie des Sciences - Series IV - Physics, 2(11), 1615–1626.

450) 1 × Sanghera, J. S., Aggarwal, I. D., & Shaw, L. B. (2016). Chalcogenide glass optics for mid-infrared applications. International Journal of Applied Glass Science, 7(2), 160–171.

451) 1 × Sapolsky, R. M. (2004). Why Zebras Don't Get Ulcers (3rd ed.). Holt Paperbacks.

452) 2 × Sapritsky, V. I., & Khlevnoy, B. B. (1997). High-accuracy blackbody sources for calibration of infrared radiometers. Applied Optics, 36(28), 7198–7205.

453) 1 × Sardanelli F, Aase HS, Álvarez M, et al. Position paper on screening for breast cancer by the European Society of Breast Imaging (EUSOBI) and 30 national breast radiology bodies. Insights into Imaging. 2017;8(3):255–261.

454) 1 × Sardanelli F, Aase HS, Álvarez M, et al. Position paper on screening for breast cancer by the European Society of Breast Imaging (EUSOBI). Insights Imaging. 2017;8(3):255-261.

455) 1 × Sardanelli F, Aase HS, Álvarez M, et al. Position paper on screening for breast cancer by the European Society of Breast Imaging (EUSOBI). Insights into Imaging. 2017;8(3):255–261.

456) 1 × Sardanelli F, Álvarez M, et al. EUSOBI position paper on breast cancer screening. Insights into Imaging. 2017;8(3):255–261.

457) 1 × Savini, G., Ade, P. A. R., & House, J. (2006). Infrared transmission and refractive index of zinc selenide. Applied Optics, 45(22), 5320–5326.

458) 1 × Savini, G., Mennella, V., & Colangeli, L. (2010). Anti-reflection coatings for infrared optics: Advances and limitations. Applied Optics, 49(31), 5910–5917.

459) 1 × Savini, G., Mennella, V., & Colangeli, L. (2010). Anti-reflection coatings for infrared optics: Germanium case study. Applied Optics, 49(31), 5910–5917.

460) 1 × Schache, A. G., et al. (2012). Hamstring force-length and torque-length relationships in athletes with and without hamstring strain injury. Journal of Orthopaedic & Sports Physical Therapy, 42(9), 656–664.

461) 1 × Schad, F. (2006). Isopathic principles in modern integrative medicine. Journal of Alternative and Complementary Medicine, 12(3), 233–240.

462) 1 × Schlager, D., et al. (2021). Infrared thermography and functional dysautonomia: A review of current evidence. Autonomic Neuroscience, 236, 102904.

463) 1 × Schlebusch, K. P., Maric-Oehler, W., & Popp, F. A. (2005). Biophotonics in the infrared spectral range reveal acupuncture meridian structure of the body. The Journal of Alternative and Complementary Medicine, 11(1), 171–173. https://doi.org/10.1089/acm.2005.11.171

464) 1 × Schleip R, Jäger H, Klingler W. What is 'fascia'? A review of different nomenclatures. J Bodyw Mov Ther. 2012;16(4):496-502.

465) 1 × Schubring, J. (2014). Psychosomatic integration in viscerocutaneous reflex zones. Integrative Physiological Medicine, 7(1), 15–23.

466) 1 × Schubring, J.P., et al. (2019). Visceral afferents and surface emission correlations in chronic organ dysfunction. Autonomic Neuroscience, 220, 33–41.

467) 1 × Scrivani, S. J., Keith, D. A., & Kaban, L. B. (2008). Temporomandibular disorders. New England Journal of Medicine, 359(25), 2693–2705.

468) 1 × Shaffer, F., & Ginsberg, J. P. (2017). An overview of heart rate variability metrics and norms. Frontiers in Public Health, 5, 258.

469) 1 × Shannon, C. E. (1948). A mathematical theory of communication. Bell System Technical Journal, 27, 379–423, 623–656.

470) 1 × Sharma, L., Hurwitz, D. E., Thonar, E. J., Sum, J. A., Lenz, M. E., Dunlop, D. D., … & Andriacchi, T. P. (2001). Knee adduction moment, serum hyaluronan level, and disease severity in medial tibiofemoral osteoarthritis. Arthritis & Rheumatism, 43(6), 1233–1240.

471) 1 × Shibasaki, M., & Crandall, C. G. (2010). Mechanisms and controllers of eccrine sweating in humans. Frontiers in Bioscience / Autonomic Neuroscience (reviews on sudomotor control).

472) 1 × Shibata Y, Ogawa T, et al. Thermoregulatory responses to cold stress. Japanese Journal of Physiology. 1989.

473) 11 × Simons, D. G., Travell, J. G., & Simons, L. S. (1999). Myofascial Pain and Dysfunction: The Trigger Point Manual. Lippincott Williams & Wilkins.

474) 4 × Singh, N., Bhalla, M., Jager, P. D., & Gilca, M. (2011). An Overview on Ashwagandha: A Rasayana (Rejuvenator) of Ayurveda. African Journal of Traditional, Complementary and Alternative Medicines, 8(5 Suppl), 208–213. https://doi.org/10.4314/ajtcam.v8i5S.9

475) 1 × Singh, R., Kumar, D., & Kumar, S. (2012). Anterior tarsal tunnel syndrome: A rare cause of dorsal foot pain. Journal of Clinical Orthopaedics and Trauma, 3(1), 55–58.

476) 1 × Slavin, S. A., Van den Abbeele, A. D., Losken, A., Swartz, M. A., Jain, R. K. (2009). Truncal and abdominal lymphedema: Clinical patterns and diagnosis. Plastic and Reconstructive Surgery, 124(3), 737–749.

477) 2 × Smith, R. G. (1993). Infrared optical materials: An overview. Proceedings of SPIE, 1760, 2–12.

478) 1 × Smyth, C. P. (1858). Tenerife: An Astronomer's Experiment. London: Lovell Reeve & Co.

479) 1 × Soh, K. S. (2009). Bonghan Circulatory System as an Extension of Acupuncture Meridians. Journal of Acupuncture and Meridian Studies, 2(2), 93–106.

480) 1 × Spalding SJ, et al. Infrared imaging of complex regional pain syndrome. Clin J Pain. 2008;24(9):793–799.

481) 1 × Spalding SJ, et al. Infrared imaging of complex regional pain syndrome. Clinical Journal of Pain. 2008;24(9):793–799.

482) 1 × Spence, J. D. (2006). Management of asymptomatic carotid stenosis. Neurologic Clinics, 24(3), 729–740.

483) 1 × Stachenfeld, N. S. (2008). Sex hormone effects on body fluid regulation. Exercise and Sport Sciences Reviews, 36(3), 152–159.

484) 1 × Stafford, M. A., Peng, P., & Hill, D. A. (2007). Sciatic neuropathy: Clinical diagnosis and management. Canadian Journal of Anaesthesia, 54(8), 654–660.

485) 18 × Standring, S. (2016). Gray's Anatomy: The Anatomical Basis of Clinical Practice. 41st ed. Elsevier.

486) 1 × Stanton, A. W. B., Modi, S., & Mortimer, P. S. (2009). Lymphatic drainage in the legs: Physiology and dysfunction. Journal of Anatomy, 214(3), 356–365.

487) 1 × Stecco C, Macchi V, Porzionato A, et al. The anatomical and functional relation between gluteus maximus and thoracolumbar fascia. J Anat. 2008;213(5): 586-594.

488) 1 × Stecco, C. (2015). Functional atlas of the human fascial system. Elsevier Health Sciences.

489) 1 × Stecco, C., Gagey, O., Macchi, V., Porzionato, A., De Caro, R., & Delmas, V. (2013). Anatomy of the deep fascia of the upper limb. Second National Fascia Research Congress Proceedings, 19–27.

490) 2 × Stecco, C., Gagey, O., Macchi, V., Porzionato, A., De Caro, R., & Delmas, V. (2013). Anatomy of the deep fascia of the upper limb. Surgical and Radiologic Anatomy, 35(5), 389–396.

491) 2 × Stefan J. (1879). Über die Beziehung zwischen der Wärmestrahlung und der Temperatur. Sitzungsberichte der mathematisch-naturwissenschaftlichen Classe der kaiserlichen Akademie der Wissenschaften, 79, 391–428.

492) 7 × Steketee J. (1973). Spectral emissivity of skin and pericardium. Physics in Medicine and Biology, 18(5), 686–694.

493) 4 × Steketee, J. (1973). Spectral emissivity of skin and pericardium. Physics in Medicine & Biology, 18(5), 686–694.

494) 1 × Stewart, J. D. (2008). Foot drop: Where, why and what to do? Practical Neurology, 8(3), 158–169.

495) 1 × Styf, J. (1989). Entrapment of the superficial peroneal nerve: Diagnosis and results of decompression. Journal of Bone and Joint Surgery (Br), 71(1), 131–135.

496) 1 × Styf, J., & Körnerberg, L. (1986). Microcirculation in the human anterior tibial compartment and its relation to chronic compartment syndrome. Journal of Bone and Joint Surgery, 68(6), 850–853.

497) 1 × Sund-Levander, M., Forsberg, C., & Wahren, L. K. (2013). Normal oral, rectal, tympanic and axillary body temperature in adult men and women: A systematic literature review. Scandinavian Journal of Caring Sciences, 17(2), 122–128.

498) 1 × Sund-Levander, M., Grodzinsky, E., Loyd, D., & Wahren, L. K. (2013). Errors in body temperature assessment related to individual variation, measuring technique and equipment. International Journal of Nursing Practice, 19(5), 537–544.

499) 36 × Sutkowy, P., Żyła, M., & Kulpa, J. (2019). Effects of Hydrotherapy on Circulatory Function in Peripheral Vascular Disease. Journal of Thermal Biology, 81, 105–112. https://doi.org/10.1016/j.jtherbio.2019.01.007

500) 1 × Suárez, C., Rodrigo, J. P., Rinaldo, A., et al. (2002). Virchow's node revisited. Oral Oncology, 38(6), 523–529.

501) 1 × Symons FJ, et al. Infrared thermal analysis and individual differences in skin temperature variability and bilateral symmetry. J Vis Exp. 2015.

502) 1 × Szuba, A., & Rockson, S. G. (1998). Lymphedema: Classification, diagnosis and therapy. Vascular Medicine, 3(2), 145–156.

503) 1 × Szuba, A., Achalu, R., & Rockson, S. G. (2002). Decongestive lymphatic therapy for breast cancer-related lymphedema: Clinical outcome and pathophysiologic assessment. Cancer, 95(11), 2260–2267.

504) 4 × Tattelman, E. (2001). Herb Contraindications and Drug Interactions: The Safe Use of Herbal Products. Pharmacy Times, 67(4), 36–45.

505) 1 × Taunton, J. E., Clement, D. B., McNicol, K. L., McConkey, J. P., & Lloyd-Smith, D. R. (1984). Overuse injuries in athletes. Canadian Journal of Applied Sport Sciences, 9(1), 17–20.

506) 1 × Taylor, G. I., & Palmer, J. H. (1987). The vascular territories (angiosomes) of the body. Plastic and Reconstructive Surgery, 80(3), 533–554.

507) 1 × Taylor, G. I., & Palmer, J. H. (1987). The vascular territories (angiosomes) of the body: Experimental study and clinical applications. British Journal of Plastic Surgery, 40(2), 113–141. https://doi.org/10.1016/0007-1226(87)90185-8

508) 1 × Thalhamer, T., et al. (2020). Functional neurovascular mapping of the cervical spine: Thermographic and mechanobiological insights. Clinical Spine Surgery, 33(5), E248–E256.

509) 2 × Thayer, J. F., & Lane, R. D. (2000). A model of neurovisceral integration in emotion regulation and dysregulation. Journal of Affective Disorders, 61(3), 201–216.

510) 1 × Thomas S. Kuhn. (1962). The Structure of Scientific Revolutions. University of Chicago Press.

511) 1 × Tihanyi, K. (1929). An Apparatus for the Electrical Production of the Image and the Transmission Thereof by Wire. UK Patent GB289915.

512) 1 × Tiller, W.A. (2007). Psychoenergetic Science: A second Copernican-scale revolution. Pavior Publishing.

513) 1 × Time. (2014). "HighTech 3D Mammograms Probably Saved This Woman's Life."

514) 1 × Tiwari, S., et al. (2018). Visualizing metabolic regulation through imaging biomarkers. Journal of Clinical Endocrinology & Metabolism, 103(5), 1799–1809.

515) 1 × Togawa T, Saito H. Non-contact imaging of thermal properties of the skin. Physiol Meas. 1994;15:291–298.

516) 1 × Tooke, J. E. (1996). Microvascular function in human diabetes. Diabetes Reviews, 4(1), 7–15.

517) 1 × Tsoukalas, D., et al. (2019). Metabolomic profiling reveals potential biomarkers for chronic fatigue syndrome/myalgic encephalomyelitis. Journal of Translational Medicine, 17(1), 193.

518) 1 × Tsuchiya, Y., et al. (2018). A case study of photon detection after acupuncture stimulation. OAText Journals. Retrieved from https://www.oatext.com/a-case-study-of-photon-detection-after-acupuncture-stimulation.php

519) 1 × Tsukada, K., et al. (2017). Evaluation of lymph flow dynamics using functional thermography. Biomedical Thermology Journal, 29(2), 87–92.

520) 2 × Turnbaugh, P. J., Ley, R. E., Hamady, M., Fraser-Liggett, C. M., Knight, R., & Gordon, J. I. (2007). The human microbiome project. Nature, 449(7164), 804–810.

521) 1 × U.S. Food and Drug Administration (FDA). (2019). "FDA warns thermography should not be used in place of mammography to detect, diagnose, or screen for breast cancer." https://www.fda.gov

522) 1 × U.S. Food and Drug Administration (FDA). (2019). FDA warns against using thermography as a substitute for mammograms. Retrieved from https://www.fda.gov/news-events/press-announcements/fda-warns-against-using-thermography-substitute-mammograms

523) 1 × U.S. Food and Drug Administration (FDA). (2019). "FDA warns thermography should not be used in place of mammography." https://www.fda.gov/news-events/press-announcements/fda-warns-thermography

524) 1 × U.S. Food and Drug Administration (FDA). Breast Cancer Screening: Thermogram No Substitute for Mammogram. FDA Consumer Health Information; 2019.

525) 1 × U.S. Food and Drug Administration (FDA). Breast Thermography: FDA Safety Communication. Silver Spring, MD; 2011, reaffirmed 2019.

526) 2 × U.S. Food and Drug Administration. Breast Cancer Screening: Thermogram No Substitute for Mammogram. FDA Consumer Health Information; 2019.

527) 1 × Uematsu S. Symmetry of skin temperatures comparing one side of the body to the other. Thermology. 1985;1(1):4–7.

528) 1 × Uematsu S. Symmetry of skin temperatures comparing one side of the body to the other. Thermology. 1985;1:4–7. (documented in multiple summaries/guidelines).

529) 3 × Uematsu, S., Edwin, D. H., Jankel, W. R., Kozikowski, J., & Trattner, M. (1988). Quantification of thermal asymmetry: Part 1. Normal values and reproducibility. Journal of Neurosurgery, 69(4), 552–555.

530) 1 × Ulbricht, C., Chao, W., Costa, D., et al. (2013). Echinacea: A Systematic Review of Safety and Efficacy. Nutrition Journal, 12, 14. https://doi.org/10.1186/1475-2891-12-14

531) 1 × Ursini, T., Naty, S., & Stuppia, L. (2020). Systems Medicine and the terrain approach: Integrating diagnostics in chronic complex disease. Journal of Integrative Medicine, 18(4), 293–301. https://doi.org/10.1016/j.joim.2020.06.001

532) 1 × US Army Night Vision Laboratory (1965–1975). Declassified research reports.

533) 1 × Usamentiaga, R., Molleda, J., Garcia, D. F., et al. (2014). Infrared thermography for temperature measurement and non-contact thermal evaluation: A review. Sensors, 14(7), 12305–12348.

534) 3 × Usamentiaga, R., Molleda, J., García, D. F., et al. (2014). Infrared thermography for temperature measurement and non-contact thermal evaluation: A review. Sensors, 14(7), 12305–12348.

535) 1 × Vainer, B. G. (2020). Infrared thermography: A diagnostic tool for the assessment of cutaneous temperature regulation in clinical and research settings. Journal of Thermal Biology, 92, 102662. https://doi.org/10.1016/j.jtherbio.2020.102662

536) 2 × Valdes, A. M., Walter, J., Segal, E., & Spector, T. D. (2018). Role of the gut microbiota in nutrition and health. BMJ, 361, k2179.

537) 1 × Valdueza, J. M., von Münster, T., Hoffman, O., Schreiber, S., & Einhäupl, K. M. (2000). Postural dependency of the cerebral venous outflow. The Lancet, 355(9199), 200–201. https://doi.org/10.1016/S0140-6736(99)04886-7

538) 2 × van Wijk, E. P. A., & van Wijk, R. (2005). An introduction to human biophoton emission. Indian Journal of Experimental Biology, 43(5), 445–452.

539) 1 × van Wijk, R. (2014). Light in Shaping Life: Biophotons in Biology and Medicine. Houten: Meluna Research.

540) 1 × van Wijk, R., & van Wijk, E.P.A. (2005). An introduction to human biophoton emission. Forsch Komplementmed, 12(2), 77–83.

541) 1 × Vanderpump, M. P. J. (2011). The epidemiology of thyroid disease. British Medical Bulletin, 99(1), 39–51.

542) 16 × Vardasca, R., Magalhães, C., Marques, D., Seixas, A., Mendes, J. G., & Ring, E. (2018). Infrared thermal imaging in human medicine: A review. Infrared Physics & Technology, 97, 128–143.

543) 2 × Viegas F, Mendes J, et al. The use of thermography and its control variables: a systematic review. Infrared Physics & Technology. 2020;104:103106.

544) 1 × Vincent, A. M., et al. (2004). Diabetic neuropathy: cellular mechanisms as therapeutic targets. Nature Reviews Neurology, 2(10), 573–583.

545) 19 × Vinik, A. I., Casellini, C., & Nevoret, M. L. (2003). Diabetic Neuropathy. Endocrinology and Metabolism Clinics of North America, 42(4), 747–787. https://doi.org/10.1016/j.ecl.2013.05.007

546) 1 × Vinik, A. I., Erbas, T., Casellini, C. M., & Pittenger, G. L. (2003). Diabetic cardiac autonomic neuropathy, inflammation and cardiovascular disease. Journal of Diabetes Investigation, 54(Suppl 1), S24–S31. https://doi.org/10.2337/diabetes.54.suppl_1.S24

547) 1 × Vitéz, T. (2003). The Forgotten Genius: Kálmán Tihanyi and the Birth of Modern Imaging. Budapest Scientific Review.

548) 1 × Vollmer, M., & Karstädt, D. (2012). Uncooled microbolometer thermal detectors: Recent developments and applications. Infrared Physics & Technology, 55(4), 220–230.

549) 3 × Vollmer, M., & Möllmann, K. P. (2018). Infrared Thermal Imaging: Fundamentals, Research and Applications (2nd ed.). Wiley-VCH.

550) 3 × Vollmer, M., & Möllmann, K. P. (2018). Infrared Thermal Imaging: Fundamentals, Research and Applications. Wiley-VCH.

551) 2 × Vollmer, M., & Möllmann, K.-P. (2018). Infrared Thermal Imaging: Fundamentals, Research and Applications. Wiley-VCH.

552) 3 × Wall, P. D., & Woolf, C. J. (1999). Muscle but not cutaneous C-afferent input produces prolonged increases in the excitability of the flexion reflex in the rat. Journal of Physiology, 356(1), 443–458.

553) 1 × Wang, C., Chen, H., & Liu, X. (2021). Chalcogenide glasses for infrared optics: Developments and challenges. Journal of Non-Crystalline Solids, 562, 120807. https://doi.org/10.1016/j.jnoncrysol.2021.120807

554) 1 × Wang, J., et al. (2017). Infrared thermography of meridian activation points during electroacupuncture. Biomedical Engineering Letters, 7(2), 165–172.

555) 1 × Wang, J., Wang, Y., & Zhang, H. (2019). Laser acupuncture: effects on regional thermal emission patterns and circulation along meridians. Journal of Integrative Medicine, 17(4), 272–278. https://doi.org/10.1016/j.joim.2019.05.001

556) 1 × Wang, Y., Sun, Y., & Tang, D. (2021). Advances in chalcogenide glass infrared optics: Transmission, fabrication, and biomedical applications. Optical Materials Express, 11(9), 2945–2961.

557) 2 × Watson, M., Wang, Y., & Rice, J. (2016). Image enhancement and denoising techniques for infrared biomedical imaging. Journal of Biomedical Optics, 21(12), 126010.

558) 3 × Watson, M., West, A. M., & Prather, L. C. (2016). Infrared thermography: Calibration and measurement techniques. Measurement Science and Technology, 27(9), 095004. https://doi.org/10.1088/0957-0233/27/9/095004

559) 1 × Webster, J. G. (2010). Medical Instrumentation: Application and Design (4th ed.). Wiley.

560) 1 × Wilbourn, A. J. (1999). Brachial plexus disorders. Neurologic Clinics, 17(3), 525–536.

561) 3 × Wilke, I., Burghoff, J., & Rademann, K. (2017). Advances in chalcogenide glasses for infrared optics. Journal of Non-Crystalline Solids, 471, 1–12.

562) 1 × Wilke, J., Krause, F., Vogt, L., & Banzer, W. (2016). What is evidence-based about myofascial chains? A systematic review. Archives of Physical Medicine and Rehabilitation, 97(3), 454–461.

563) 1 × Willard, F. H., Vleeming, A., Schuenke, M. D., Danneels, L., & Schleip, R. (2012). The thoracolumbar fascia: anatomy, function, and clinical considerations. Journal of Anatomy, 221(6), 507–536.

564) 1 × Willemsen, P. R., van Venrooy, B. W. H., & van Nijnatten, P. A. (2011). Multi-element LWIR optics using zinc selenide for clinical imaging. Infrared Physics & Technology, 54(3), 221–228.

565) 1 × Witte, M. H., et al. (2001). Lymphatic alterations in liver disease. Liver, 21(2), 65–71.

566) 1 × Wood, R. (2011). Optoelectronic Properties of Semiconductors and Superlattices, Vol. 15: Infrared Detectors, Materials, and Devices. CRC Press.

567) 1 × Wunderlich, C. A. (1868). Das Verhalten der Eigenwärme in Krankheiten [On the Temperature in Diseases]. Leipzig: Otto Wigand.

568) 1 × Yamashita, K., et al. (2020). Thermal imaging of lymphatic dysfunction in patients with lymphedema: A pilot study. Lymphatic Research and Biology, 18(2), 124–130.

569) 1 × Yamauchi M. Medical applications of thermography in Japan. Thermology International. 1980.

570) 1 × Yang, Y., Wu, H. G., & Yang, M. (2007). Observations of infrared radiant tracks along acupuncture meridians induced by acupuncture stimulation. American Journal of Chinese Medicine, 35(4), 669–675. https://doi.org/10.1142/S0192415X07004771

571) 1 × Yang, Y., Yang, M., Liu, C. Z., et al. (2012). Evidence-based acupuncture research: Lack of reliable evidence for specific effects of acupuncture. Evidence-Based Complementary and Alternative Medicine, 2012, 1–6. https://doi.org/10.1155/2012/245271

572) 2 × Yin, C. S., Park, H. J., & Lee, H. S. (2018). Revisiting acupuncture meridians and modern anatomy: Imaging and functional perspectives. Integrative Medicine Research, 7(1), 1–9.

573) 1 × Younossi, Z. M., et al. (2016). Global epidemiology of nonalcoholic fatty liver disease. Metabolism, 65(8), 1037–1046.

574) 2 × Yun, Y., Zhao, L., & Liu, H. (2017). Visualization of the human meridian system using infrared thermography: A review and prospects. Evidence-Based Complementary and Alternative Medicine, 2017, 2601347. https://doi.org/10.1155/2017/2601347

575) 1 × Zakery, A., & Elliott, S. R. (2007). Optical Nonlinearities in Chalcogenide Glasses and Their Applications. Springer.

576) 1 × Zakrzewska, J. M. (2013). Trigeminal neuralgia: Diagnosis and treatment. BMJ, 347, f5109.

577) 1 × Zaproudina, N., Ming, Z., & Hänninen, O. O. (2013). Plantar infrared thermography measurements and low back pain intensity. Journal of Manipulative and Physiological Therapeutics, 36(6), 381–388.

578) 1 × Zhang, W. Y., Lu, W. C., & Yang, H. F. (2002). The study of infrared radiation lines on the human body surface and their relationship with acupuncture meridians. Chinese Journal of Integrated Traditional and Western Medicine, 22(4), 277–280.

579) 1 × Zhang, W.B. (2019). Quantitative measurement of biophysical properties at acupuncture points. Chinese Journal of Integrative Medicine, 25(3), 205–210.

580) 1 × Zhang, Y., Lin, C., & Zhao, M. (2024). Bibliometric analysis of acupuncture–infrared studies from 2000 to 2023. Frontiers in Neuroscience, 18, Article 1387752. https://doi.org/10.3389/fnins.2024.1387752

581) 1 × Zhang, Z., Li, Y., Yu, Q., Wang, J., & Wang, W. (2020). Deep learning-based classification of thermal meridian patterns in human infrared images. Infrared Physics & Technology, 106, 103261. https://doi.org/10.1016/j.infrared.2020.103261

582) 1 × Zhao, L., Chen, J., Li, Y., et al. (2017). A review of infrared imaging in acupuncture meridian research. Journal of Traditional Chinese Medicine, 37(4), 546–552. https://doi.org/10.1016/S0254-6272(17)30312-2

583) 1 × Zhou, Y., Chen, J., & Liu, F. (2019). Comparative optical performance of germanium and zinc selenide in LWIR medical imaging systems. Optical Engineering, 58(8), 083105.

584) 1 × Zhou, Y., Guo, J., & Sun, Y. (2019). Advances in germanium infrared optics for thermal imaging applications. Optical Materials Express, 9(4), 1901–1912. https://doi.org/10.1364/OME.9.001901

585) 1 × Zhu, Z., Zhang, L., & Zhao, Y. (2015). Thermographic imaging in the evaluation of acupuncture effects: a systematic review. Evidence-Based Complementary and Alternative Medicine, 2015, Article ID 657380.

FUTURE DIRECTIONS IN BIOSPECTRAL MEDICINE

1. The Post-Atlas Landscape

The completion of this Atlas does not represent the conclusion of a scientific path, but the consolidation of its foundation. By organizing hundreds of pages into anatomically defined zones, interpretative categories, and stepwise interpretive logic, Biospectral Medicine has moved to structured methodology.

This body of work formalizes what has long been observed clinically yet rarely systematized: that the human emission field carries patterned signals of regulatory imbalance, and that those signals are both interpretable and clinically relevant.

While the clinical validity of these case studies is self-evident to practitioners who work daily with complex dysfunction, the implications of this model extend far beyond integrative practice.

The introduction of a reproducible, zone-based approach to spectral imaging lays the groundwork for rigorous observational research, translational physiology, and interprofessional collaboration across domains not traditionally aligned. It bridges anatomical knowledge with systems biology, structural analysis with energetic fields, and classical clinical evaluations with emerging biofield science.

This Atlas reframes spectral imaging as an investigative lens for understanding the body's compensatory patterns. The data presented here, both visual and clinical, can now serve as a launch point for those seeking to investigate deeper relationships between emission behaviour and metabolic flux, immune regulation, lymphatic burden, neuroendocrine signalling, and frequency-based modulation.

Biospectral Medicine is a living system of observation and refinement. Each image, classification, and case is a fragment of a larger physiological narrative waiting to be interpreted. As such, the true landscape opened by this work is not one of finality, but of direction. What follows in the pages ahead are proposed trajectories for researchers, educators, clinicians, and institutions willing to take part in shaping the next evolution of spectral interpretations.

2. Zone-Based Biomarker Correlation

A natural trajectory for the future development of Biospectral Medicine is the formal correlation of emission patterns with measurable biomarkers of physiology. The zone-based framework of the R-CIIM method provides a precise anatomical and functional map for this pursuit, allowing researchers to align spectral findings with laboratory values, imaging results, and functional tests in a structured manner.

This is a unique opportunity because few clinical systems provide both the spatial granularity and the interpretive logic necessary to support such systematic comparison.

Each emission zone, whether presenting hyperemissive or hypoemissive behavior, offers a starting point for targeted biomarker analysis. A hyperemissive signal in the frontal lower legs, for example, may be investigated in relation to markers of vascular reactivity such as CRP or D-dimer, while hypoemissive suppression in cervical or supraclavicular regions could be studied alongside thyroid panels, cortisol rhythms, or autonomic testing.

By placing these findings into a reproducible interpretive framework, correlations can be drawn between signal and clinical imbalance as well as between signal and early regulation, revealing disturbances long before conventional clinical investigation would typically indicate concern.

Such research opens two fundamental pathways. The first is validation through concordance, where spectral emissions are shown to parallel established clinical markers. This reinforces the reliability of the system and deepens professional confidence in its application.

The second is innovation through discovery, where emission zones reveal early regulatory changes that precede measurable laboratory or imaging alterations. In this sense, Biospectral Medicine does not merely confirm known dysfunctions but may also serve as an early-warning system, identifying patterns of circulatory stress, metabolic burden, or immune imbalance prior to overt clinical manifestation.

For clinicians, this work promises significant advances in intervention tracking. If longitudinal studies demonstrate that normalization of a spectral signal consistently parallels improvement in reactive markers, glycemic control, or hormone balance, then emission analysis becomes a practical tool for tracking the efficacy of interventions.

This enables intervention plans to be adjusted dynamically, with spectral findings acting as a real-time mirror of systemic adaptation and recovery. The value here lies in early finding and in continuous regulation recording, a field where conventional imaging is silent.

For researchers, the methodological scope is wide. Cross-sectional studies could explore population-level correlations between emission zones and biomarker panels, while longitudinal studies could document spectral evolution alongside intervention outcomes. Advanced approaches such as metabolomics, proteomics, and multi-omics integration may further illuminate how biospectral emissions reflect the body's complex regulatory networks.

Machine learning models applied to large datasets could refine these associations, identifying subtle spectral signatures linked to specific biochemical states or illness trajectories. In this way, Biospectral Medicine situates itself within the emerging sciences of systems physiology and regulatory biosignal analysis.

The path ahead is therefore not limited to confirming what is already known, but to uncovering new layers of understanding. By correlating emission zones with biomarkers across vascular, metabolic, neuroendocrine, and immune domains, Biospectral Medicine has the potential to provide a bridge between visible biosignals and the invisible regulatory mechanisms of the body, transforming both clinical practice and scientific research into a unified field of inquiry.

3. Longitudinal Recovery and Terrain Observation

A central advantage of Biospectral Medicine lies in its ability to track physiological regulation dynamically, rather than providing only static images of structural change. The spatial behaviour of emission zones offers a window into the body's adaptation over time, making longitudinal observation an essential field for future research and clinical application.

This perspective aligns with the terrain-based view of human health, where systemic imbalances precede structural disruption and where recovery is best understood not as a single event but as a progressive, multi-phasic process.

When a patient undergoes clinical intervention, whether nutritional, metabolic, neuroregulatory, or bioenergetic, the body responds with shifts in vascular tone, lymphatic flow, muscular activity, and endocrine output. These changes are seldom uniform; instead, they unfold across zones in patterns of resolution and compensation. Biospectral Medicine, with its 19 defined anatomical regions and structured interpretive categories, provides a unique tool for capturing these responses in real time.

Hyperemissive signals may diminish as reactivity subsides, while hypoemissive suppressions may resolve as perfusion improves or as autonomic regulation rebalances. Observing these dynamics across multiple consultations allows the clinician to construct a clear trajectory of recovery, moving beyond symptom relief toward systemic regulation.

Longitudinal observation also offers profound implications for chronic and complex conditions. Patients with autoimmune processes, endocrine dysregulation, or persistent pain often cycle through periods of compensation and relapse. Conventional imaging rarely captures these fluctuations, as structural markers remain unchanged despite ongoing regulatory struggle.

In contrast, Biospectral Medicine allows the visualization of these subtle shifts, enabling clinicians to differentiate between transient symptom recurrence and deeper regulatory collapse. This makes it possible to intervene earlier, prevent regression, and tailor care intensity to the actual state of the patient's terrain rather than to subjective complaints alone.

Research in this area could establish standardized models of spectral progression. For example, mapping the resolution of a hyperemissive lumbar pattern in patients with metabolic syndrome alongside improvements in HbA1c, CRP, or lipid profiles would provide evidence for the predictive value of emission normalization.

In the same way, observing endocrine zone evolution during thyroid or adrenal support could create new markers for functional recovery, distinct from biochemical stabilization alone. These longitudinal insights also lend themselves to quantification, allowing emission evolution to be expressed in grades of recovery, which can then be statistically correlated with laboratory and clinical outcomes.

Another important dimension is the use of longitudinal observation for preventive medicine. Individuals at risk for vascular, metabolic, or neuroregulatory conditions may present emission anomalies years before symptoms become clinically apparent.

Regular biospectral assessment, charted over time, can reveal whether the terrain is moving toward resilience or toward dysfunction. This transforms the role of the clinician from reactive observer to proactive regulator, guiding the patient in maintaining systemic balance through early and ongoing intervention.

The educational and research implications of terrain observation are significant. Students and professionals can be trained to recognize static emission categories and to understand how patterns evolve under the influence of interventions. This perspective turns Biospectral Medicine into a dynamic teaching tool, one that illustrates the body's capacity for adaptation and regulation.

For research, large-scale longitudinal databases would allow the creation of emission trajectories for specific conditions, producing reference models that could eventually serve as predictive algorithms for both clinical and academic use.

In this sense, longitudinal observation transforms Biospectral Medicine into more than an interpretive lens. It becomes a temporal map of human regulation, an evolving portrait of how terrain recovers, adapts, or deteriorates under the combined pressures of environment, lifestyle, and interventions. By following these trajectories, clinicians and researchers alike can move closer to a functional definition of health as the capacity to regulate over time, visible in the spectral language of the body itself.

4. Cross-System Interactions and Resonance Zones

One of the most intriguing frontiers for Biospectral Medicine lies in the study of interzone relationships, where emissions in one region reflect or influence patterns in another. These phenomena, which may manifest as mirrored signals, contralateral compensations, or multi-zone synchronizations, suggest that the biospectral field is not an isolated reflection of local dysfunction but a systemic language of regulatory interaction. Understanding these cross-system dynamics will be essential for both clinical refinement and future research.

Clinically, resonance zones are observed when hyperemissive or hypoemissive patterns appear in anatomically distant but functionally related regions. For example, disturbances in the cervical spine may coexist with compensatory signals in the lumbar zone, reflecting the interconnected nature of spinal biomechanics and autonomic regulation.

Similarly, patterns in the abdominal zones often correlate with facial or cervical emissions, highlighting visceral-somatic and neuroendocrine-visceral reflex arcs. These interactions mirror what systems biology and neurophysiology have long described: that the body maintains coherence not through isolated structures but through networked regulatory pathways.

The concept of resonance also extends to lateralization. Practitioners frequently observe asymmetries between left and right zones, with one side displaying hyperemissive activation while the contralateral side presents hypoemissive suppression.

This phenomenon may represent compensatory distribution of regulatory load, where one half of the body assumes functional stress while the other reduces activity to maintain systemic balance. Such lateralized patterns could be explored through future research linking biospectral findings to neuroimaging, autonomic testing, or even electrophysiological mapping of hemispheric dominance and vagal tone.

From a research perspective, resonance zones open opportunities to study cross-regulatory physiology in ways that conventional imaging cannot capture. By systematically documenting paired or mirrored emissions across patient populations, large-scale databases could reveal reproducible interaction patterns between anatomical systems.

These might include predictable links between lymphatic stagnation in the axillae and congestion in the lower extremities, or between thyroid zone suppression and hypoemissive trajectories in the abdominal group. Such findings would expand the interpretive framework of Biospectral Medicine from a zone-centered perspective to a network-centered one.

The implications for care strategy are significant. If emission resolution in one zone consistently parallels improvement in another, clinicians can track indirect markers of recovery, using resonance zones as surrogate indicators.

For instance, observing normalization of abdominal emissions may also signal improvement in lumbar strain or metabolic load, even before symptoms resolve. This transforms intervention tracking into a systemic process rather than a local observation, providing a broader view of the patient's regulatory capacity.

In the context of translational science, resonance zones invite exploration at the interface of physics and physiology. The existence of cross-zone interactions suggests that biospectral emissions may reflect local vascular and metabolic events together with field-level regulatory dynamics, possibly mediated through connective tissue networks, fascia, or bioelectromagnetic gradients.

Collaborations with researchers in biophysics, systems neuroscience, and integrative physiology could help illuminate whether these resonances correspond to mechanical load distribution, fluid dynamics, or frequency-based coherence within the organism.

Educationally, the study of resonance zones offers a powerful teaching tool. Students trained to observe cross-system interactions develop a more sophisticated understanding of human physiology as a network rather than as an assembly of parts. This perspective encourages clinicians to move beyond reductionist thinking, fostering a interpretative culture that values coherence, compensation, and systemic regulation. For Biospectral Medicine, it positions the field at the forefront of an emerging paradigm, one where biosignal interpretation evolves into the study of dynamic interconnectivity.

In summary, the phenomenon of resonance zones highlights the systemic intelligence of the biospectral field. Far from being random or incidental, these cross-system interactions reveal the body's innate strategies for adaptation and balance. By mapping and analyzing them, Biospectral Medicine expands its scope from zone-based analysis to network-based physiology, bridging clinical observation with the broader science of human coherence.

5. R-CIIM and Scientific Replicability

The Reitz Clinical Infrared Interpretation Model (R-CIIM) is the methodological backbone of Biospectral Medicine, transforming emission observation into a structured and reproducible interpretive system.

While many historical approaches to infrared imaging have struggled with subjectivity and lack of standardization, the R-CIIM framework was specifically designed to overcome these limitations by establishing a sequence of six steps that can be consistently applied across cases, practitioners, and clinical contexts. This built-in structure offers one of the most important directions for future research: the establishment of Biospectral Medicine as a replicable science.

At its core, R-CIIM provides a stepwise interpretive pathway that begins with anatomical and clinical relevance and moves systematically through emission classification, interpretation categorization, historical correlation, confirmatory testing, and intervention integration.

Each step adds precision while also creating documentation points that can be independently reviewed and verified. This makes the method uniquely suited to academic study, where reproducibility and inter-rater reliability are central. By applying R-CIIM consistently across patient populations, researchers can generate comparable datasets that lend themselves to statistical validation and peer-reviewed publication.

The scientific community has long demanded that any new interpretative framework demonstrate three qualities: clarity of definitions, reproducibility of results, and integration with existing clinical systems. R-CIIM addresses each. Its lexicon introduces standardized terms such as activose, inhibose, and anisospectral, providing a precise language for emission description.

Its zone-based structure creates fixed anatomical reference points, eliminating the variability that plagued earlier thermographic methods. And its integration with laboratory tests, imaging, and clinical history ensures that spectral findings can be contextualized within broader medical practice rather than existing as an isolated modality.

Future research will benefit greatly from this replicable foundation. Studies can now be designed to test inter-observer consistency, exploring whether practitioners trained in R-CIIM arrive at the same classifications when reviewing identical biospectral images. Longitudinal studies can evaluate whether emission changes follow predictable trajectories under defined intervention protocols.

Population-based studies can assess the frequency of certain ROI patterns within specific interpretative categories. All of these approaches rely on the structural clarity that R-CIIM provides, without which Biospectral Medicine would remain anecdotal rather than scientific.

Beyond reproducibility, the model also opens the door to technological innovation. Because the steps of R-CIIM are well defined, they can be encoded into digital platforms, paving the way for software-assisted interpretation and even machine learning algorithms.

Artificial intelligence could be trained to recognize ROI patterns, grade emissions, or cross-reference patient histories, accelerating the process of interpretation while maintaining methodological fidelity. Such integration does not replace the clinician's judgment but strengthens it, allowing for both human and computational replicability.

The academic implications are equally important. With its structured logic, R-CIIM provides a framework suitable for inclusion in university curricula, professional training programs, and inter-disciplinary research collaborations.

Its clarity allows it to be taught systematically, examined objectively, and applied consistently—qualities essential for acceptance within mainstream medical science. In this sense, R-CIIM transforms Biospectral Medicine from an observational art into a codified methodology that can withstand the rigor of scientific scrutiny.

In summary, the R-CIIM model is both the interpretive engine of Biospectral Medicine and its gateway to broader scientific recognition. By ensuring standardization, reproducibility, and integration, it provides the conditions under which Biospectral Medicine can move from clinical innovation to academic discipline. Future research built on this model will refine the practice and establish its place within the global landscape of biosignal science.

6. AI Integration and Educational Scaling

The structured nature of Biospectral Medicine, with its defined zones, categories, and R-CIIM interpretive steps, lends itself naturally to the integration of digital technologies. Among these, artificial intelligence (AI) and machine learning (ML) represent particularly promising avenues for future development.

While the human eye and clinical intuition remain indispensable for interpretation, the vast datasets generated by spectral imaging are ideally suited for computational analysis, enabling both precision in research and scalability in education.

AI can contribute to Biospectral Medicine in several ways. At the most basic level, algorithms can be trained to recognize region-of-interest (ROI) patterns, classify emissions as hyperemissive or hypoemissive, and grade their severity using the established six-level system. This reduces subjectivity and allows large-scale consistency across practitioners.

Beyond pattern recognition, machine learning models can integrate biospectral images with clinical histories, laboratory results, and follow-up outcomes, identifying subtle associations that may escape human perception. Such integration could lead to predictive models capable of estimating the probability of specific dysfunctions based on combined spectral and clinical data.

For clinical research, AI offers a powerful tool for managing complexity. With thousands of potential correlations between emission zones, interpretative categories, and biomarkers, manual analysis can become cumbersome.

Computational approaches can process these multidimensional relationships efficiently, generating new hypotheses and refining interpretive algorithms. Over time, this may lead to the creation of biospectral atlases enriched by both human expertise and data-driven insights, further strengthening the evidence base for the discipline.

Equally important is the character of AI in education and professional training. Because R-CIIM is highly structured, it can be encoded into digital teaching platforms where students interact with standardized case libraries, practice zone classification, and receive immediate feedback. Virtual simulations could allow learners to progress through the six interpretive steps with AI-guided prompts, reinforcing consistency and accelerating mastery.

More advanced platforms might simulate longitudinal cases, allowing practitioners to observe how emissions evolve across intervention pathways, thereby enhancing their ability to record real patients. In this sense, AI becomes both an analytic tool and a pedagogical partner, scaling expertise to a broader audience without diluting methodological rigor.

The ethical integration of AI into Biospectral Medicine must also be considered. Algorithms should never replace clinical judgment, nor should they be viewed as autonomous interpretative agents.

Instead, they should function as decision-support systems, augmenting the clinician's interpretive capacity while maintaining accountability within the care relationship. By framing AI as a tool for amplification rather than substitution, Biospectral Medicine safeguards its human-centered ethos while embracing technological progress.

From a broader perspective, AI integration positions Biospectral Medicine at the forefront of digital health innovation. As healthcare systems worldwide move toward personalized, preventive, and data-driven models, disciplines capable of generating structured, non-invasive, and reproducible datasets are particularly well placed to contribute.

By aligning spectral imaging with AI, Biospectral Medicine could participate in global research networks, integrate into electronic health record systems, and establish itself as a functional complement to structural imaging within future clinical ecosystems.

In conclusion, AI and educational scaling represent not a departure from the essence of Biospectral Medicine but its natural evolution. By pairing the structured logic of R-CIIM with computational precision and digital pedagogy, the field can extend its reach, deepen its scientific base, and ensure that future generations of practitioners inherit both the art and the science of spectral interpretation.

7. Therapeutic Strategy and Emission Reversibility

A defining strength of Biospectral Medicine is its ability to reveal both dysfunction and the body's capacity for recovery. Unlike structural imaging modalities, which capture damage or pathology in relatively fixed form, spectral emission patterns are dynamic and reversible.

This property transforms the methodology into a living interface with intervention, enabling clinicians to observe the effects of corrective strategies in real time and to adapt care approaches based on visible regulatory changes. The study of emission reversibility therefore represents one of the most fertile areas for both clinical practice and future research.

Clinically, practitioners frequently observe that hyperemissive signals associated with reactivity, congestion, or heightened regulatory activity diminish following appropriate intervention. Conversely, hypoemissive suppressions linked to circulatory compromise, endocrine underactivity, or autonomic inhibition often resolve as tissue perfusion improves or regulatory balance is restored.

These changes are not abstract but concrete, appearing consistently in longitudinal follow-ups. They demonstrate that emission zones behave as functional barometers, rising and falling in response to systemic adaptation.

This reversibility has profound implications for care strategy. Clinical approach no longer needs to be guided solely by symptom reporting or laboratory intervals but can be continuously calibrated against spectral findings. A patient undergoing nutritional, metabolic, or neuroregulatory support may show emission normalization well before clinical symptoms resolve, providing reassurance that the terrain is shifting in the correct direction.

Conversely, the persistence of an unresolved emission despite symptomatic improvement may caution against premature discontinuation of supportive measures. In this way, Biospectral Medicine introduces a form of dynamic feedback regulation, where visible biosignals act as checkpoints for care decision-making.

For researchers, emission reversibility provides a unique opportunity to study the kinetics of recovery. By mapping how quickly emissions normalize under different intervention approaches, comparative studies could evaluate the relative effectiveness of strategies across categories such as vascular, metabolic, or endocrine regulation.

For example, one study might track lumbar emissions in metabolic syndrome patients undergoing dietary modification versus pharmacological intervention, documenting the rate and stability of emission resolution.

Another might examine cervical hypoemission recovery during thyroid or adrenal support, correlating spectral normalization with hormone assays. Such research could lead to the development of spectral response curves, creating reference standards for how zones typically evolve under interventions.

Beyond efficacy, emission reversibility may also serve as a predictor of relapse. Patients whose emissions normalize but then reappear under stress may be identified as having fragile regulatory capacity, requiring sustained tracking or preventive strategies. In this sense, Biospectral Medicine offers not just interpretive insight but also predictive value, helping clinicians anticipate vulnerability before full clinical regression occurs. This positions spectral analysis as a vital tool in chronic imbalance care planning, where relapse prevention is as important as initial recovery.

The reversibility of emissions also aligns with the philosophy of integrative and terrain-based care, which views the body as a dynamic and adaptive system rather than a static machine. By visualizing the ebb and flow of regulation, Biospectral Medicine provides concrete evidence of the body's inherent plasticity and resilience.

This reinforces the principle of care that recovery is not limited to symptom control but involves a deeper restoration of systemic balance, one that can now be tracked visually and reproducibly.

Educationally, the concept of emission reversibility enriches the teaching of clinical physiology. Students trained to recognize both static patterns and their evolution under intervention gain a more nuanced understanding of regulation as a process.

This prepares them to use Biospectral Medicine not simply as a tool for uncovering but as a strategic compass for guiding care. By following emissions across multiple consultations, practitioners learn to think longitudinally, appreciating the dialogue between intervention input and regulatory output.

In summary, emission reversibility transforms Biospectral Medicine into more than an interpretive methodology, it becomes a care guide. By showing the body's regulatory responses in real time, it enables clinicians to personalize support, researchers to quantify intervention effects, and patients to witness their recovery as a visible, measurable process.

This integration of observation and adaptation exemplifies the future direction of medicine itself: a practice not bound by static images but informed by dynamic signals of regulation and resilience.

8. Scientific Invitation

The Atlas of Biospectral Medicine has been written as both a reference and a demonstration, showing that emission-based interpretation can be structured, replicable, and clinically relevant. Yet the true value of this work lies not in its completion, but in what it initiates.

Every table, case study, and methodological step presented here points toward a wider horizon, one that requires the participation of clinicians, researchers, educators, and institutions willing to engage with the biospectral field as a living science. The future of this discipline cannot be authored by one voice alone; it must be shaped through dialogue, collaboration, and collective inquiry.

The invitation to the scientific community is therefore clear. For clinicians, Biospectral Medicine offers a framework to expand practice beyond symptom-based evaluation and into the realm of regulatory mapping. For researchers, it provides structured hypotheses ready for testing, whether through biomarker correlation, longitudinal studies, or systems modeling.

For educators, it introduces a standardized lexicon and methodology that can be integrated into curricula, training programs, and inter-professional teaching. Each of these domains contributes to the same goal: establishing a new interpretative language grounded in the body's own signals.

The implications of this work extend beyond clinical medicine. By framing emissions as biosignals, Biospectral Medicine intersects with fields as diverse as physiology, neuroscience, systems biology, and biophysics. It provides a platform to explore questions about coherence, regulation, and adaptation, questions that lie at the frontier of human science.

Whether through the study of resonance zones, the integration of artificial intelligence, or the correlation of emissions with metabolic and immune networks, the biospectral field is positioned to contribute to broader conversations about how complex systems maintain balance and how that balance can be measured non-invasively.

This closing reflection is not a conclusion but a threshold. The Atlas has established the foundation: anatomical zones, interpretative categories, case studies, interpretive steps, and reference tables. What follows is the work of validation, expansion, and innovation.

Just as emission patterns reveal the body's compensations and adaptations, so too will the future of Biospectral Medicine reveal its capacity to evolve through research and application. The methodology presented here is not static; it is dynamic by design, inviting reinterpretation as new evidence and technologies emerge.

For these reasons, the Atlas stands as both a completed work and an open project. Its pages document a body of knowledge that has already proven itself in clinical settings, while also offering a scaffold for the next generation of inquiry. Professionals who engage with this field are not merely users of a technique but contributors to a living science, one that will grow in depth and authority as it is tested, refined, and shared.

In extending this invitation, the message is simple: Biospectral Medicine belongs not to one author, institute, or discipline, but to the larger scientific community that will test its principles, challenge its assumptions, and advance its applications.

The work presented here is a beginning, and the responsibility of its continuation now lies with all who recognize the value of reading the body's regulatory language. Through collaboration and commitment, the biospectral field can mature into a global discipline, enriching both clinical practice and scientific knowledge for decades to come

REFERENCE CASES IN BIOSPECTRAL IMAGING

The following images have been selected as reference illustrations to demonstrate the interpretive framework of Biospectral Medicine. Each case exemplifies how emission zones can be classified, correlated, and contextualized within the nine interpretive categories defined by the R-CIIM model. These categories, vascular, muscular, skeletal, nervous, lymphatic, organ, meridian, energetic, and metabolic, form the interpretive grid through which biospectral asymmetries are understood.

The value of these cases lies in their function as didactic anchors. They show how a single spectral surface reading, when viewed in isolation, provides limited meaning. However, once integrated with patient history, symptom description, and confirmatory evaluation, the same emission zone transforms into a precise marker of functional disturbance or systemic dysregulation. In this way, biospectral imaging demonstrates its clinical relevance: not as a standalone diagnosis, but as a language of biosignals that guides interpretation and directs further inquiry.

It is important to recognize that the cases presented here were chosen because they represent classic patterns frequently observed in practice. Some illustrate the vascular signature of peripheral circulatory compromise, others the lymphatic expression of regional overload, while still others reveal organ-related or metabolic correlations. These archetypal images provide the reader with visual benchmarks against which new or ambiguous findings can be compared.

The interpretive process should always be approached as relational rather than absolute. An emission finding may point toward a vascular irregularity, but its ultimate meaning emerges only when aligned with the patient's Anamnesis, physical complaints, and laboratory or imaging data. In other words, the clinical context completes the image. The same emission pattern may acquire distinct significance depending on whether it is correlated with fatigue, localized pain, digestive irregularities, or endocrine imbalance.

By reviewing these reference cases, the reader is invited to observe the spectral pattern itself and the logic by which it is classified, contextualized, and translated into clinical meaning. This layered approach reflects the essence of Biospectral Medicine: transforming emissive phenomena into actionable insights through structured interpretation, correlation with patient reality, and integration into the broader clinical picture.

Reference 01

Irregular Abdominal Patchy Emissions

Classic Toxic Pattern

Anatomical Region & Interpretive Category

Zone 9 – Frontal Abdomen

Primary Interpretive Category: Metabolic / Endocrine

Spectral Pattern

Diffuse, irregular patchy emissions distributed across the abdominal surface, with alternating areas of focal intensification and suppression. The pattern is non-symmetrical and widely dispersed, extending over hepatic, gastric, and intestinal projections.

Pattern Type

Polymorphic toxic–metabolic distribution: multiple scattered loci of emissive disturbance without clear lateral symmetry.

Spectral Pattern Description

The abdominal surface reveals a heterogeneous biospectral map characterized by alternating islands of heightened emission interspersed with hypoemissive suppressions. These patches are irregular in contour and dispersed across the hepatic projection in the right hypochondrium, the gastric area in the epigastrium, and the colonic trajectory along the left flank. The irregularity and lack of symmetry reinforce the impression of systemic metabolic overload rather than localized organ dysfunction.

Interpretive Understanding

This spectral pattern corresponds to a toxic–metabolic terrain, reflecting hepatic and gastrointestinal stress with diffuse systemic burden. Biospectral disturbance of this type often suggests heightened metabolic processing demand, toxicant accumulation, or impaired detoxification mechanisms. From a terrain-based perspective, the irregular emissions indicate the body's attempt to redistribute load through multiple visceral pathways, without the stability of a single focal projection.

Clinical Correlation Through Anamnesis

The interpretive value becomes more precise when correlated with patient history.

- If the patient reports digestive complaints (bloating, irregular bowel movements, nausea), the emissive disturbances reinforce gastrointestinal burden.
- If there is history of toxin exposure (pharmaceutical load, alcohol, occupational exposure), the pattern may indicate hepatic strain.
- In patients with systemic fatigue, skin reactivity, or metabolic sluggishness, these disturbances may represent diffuse toxic load affecting multiple organ systems.

Classic Value of the Image

This figure was selected as a "classic toxic case" due to its irregular, patchy, and diffuse distribution across the abdominal surface. The lack of symmetry, combined with scattered foci, provides a textbook example of how biospectral imaging captures systemic toxic–metabolic states rather than isolated organ dysfunction. It represents a foundational teaching plate for recognizing metabolic and toxic load on the abdominal surface.

Teaching Insight

The image highlights the interpretive principle that systemic toxic patterns manifest through irregularity and multiplicity of signals. Unlike localized organ-related emissions, toxic–metabolic distributions defy strict anatomical boundaries and appear as scattered disturbances. Practitioners must integrate this non-linear spectral map with patient history, recognizing that the abdominal surface functions as a projection field for metabolic and detoxification processes. This reinforces the necessity of layered reasoning in Biospectral Medicine, moving beyond organ-centric interpretations toward systemic understanding.

Reference 02

Vascular–Lymphatic Branching Over the Breast and Axillary Fields
Classic Hormonal Case

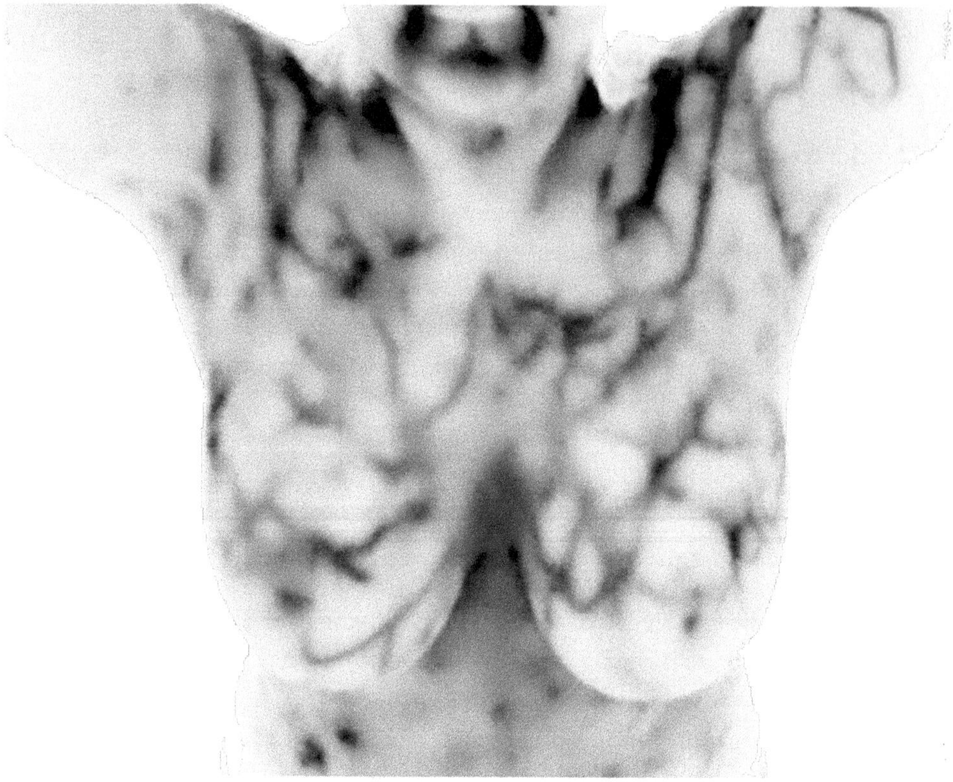

Anatomical Region & Interpretive Category

Zone 13 – Chest and Sternum, extending into Zone 14 (Left Axillary) and Zone 15 (Right Axillary)

Primary Interpretive Category: Metabolic / Endocrine

Spectral Pattern

Extensive vascular–lymphatic branching emissions radiating across both breasts and into the axillary regions, forming an arborized network. The pattern is bilateral, yet with irregular density and intensity across sides.

Pattern Type

Diffuse branching hyperemission with endocrine influence.

Spectral Pattern Description

The image demonstrates an extensive arborization of hyperemissive channels, tracing along vascular and lymphatic pathways over the thoracic surface. These branching structures are particularly concentrated over the mammary fields, extending laterally into both axillae. The configuration lacks strict symmetry, with denser arborization visible on the left side, but maintains overall bilateral presence. The spectral quality of this branching suggests hormonal modulation influencing vascular-lymphatic dynamics.

Interpretive Understanding

This pattern corresponds to a hormonally influenced vascular–lymphatic state, strongly shaped by estrogenic regulation. Endocrine activity modulates breast vascularity, and such diffuse arborization has been correlated with hormonal fluctuations, states of endocrine dysregulation, or heightened estrogenic load. The lack of sharp focality indicates systemic influence rather than localized pathology. Within the biospectral framework, this case exemplifies endocrine-driven emissive modulation projected onto vascular and lymphatic pathways.

Clinical Correlation Through Anamnesis

Precision in interpretation requires alignment with patient history.

- If the patient reports cyclical breast tension, swelling, or mastalgia, the vascular–lymphatic hyperpattern may reflect estrogen–progesterone imbalance.
- If there is a history of exogenous hormone use (contraceptives, replacement therapy), the spectral distribution may represent pharmacological modulation of vascular–endocrine activity.
- In cases of lymphatic congestion or breast density changes, this emissive branching can be correlated with circulatory-lymphatic burden under hormonal influence.

Classic Value of the Image

This figure is designated a "classic hormonal case" because it captures with clarity the characteristic branching vascular–lymphatic patterns linked to endocrine regulation. The diffuse arborized appearance is an exemplary demonstration of how biospectral imaging reveals systemic hormonal influence rather than isolated vascular irregularities.

Teaching Insight

The image emphasizes the teaching principle that hormonal regulation imprints itself on biospectral maps not through isolated foci, but through systemic vascular–lymphatic modulation. Arborized branching over the thoracic surface provides a direct visual correlate of endocrine states, particularly estrogenic activity. Practitioners must recognize that such patterns signify terrain-level hormonal modulation, requiring integration with clinical history and awareness of systemic endocrine dynamics.

Reference 03

Diffuse Punctate Emissive Fields Over the Dorsal Back

Classic Allergic Case

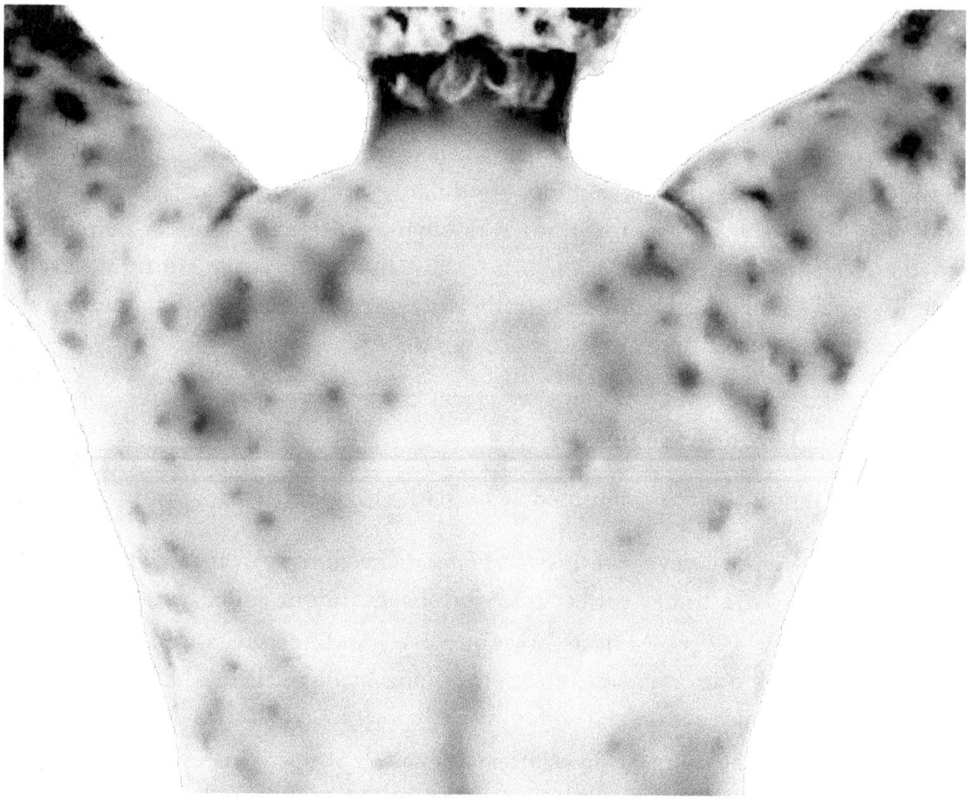

Anatomical Region & Interpretive Category

Zone 16 – Upper Back

Primary Interpretive Category: Lymphatic / Immune

Spectral Pattern

Widespread punctate emissions scattered across the dorsal surface, forming multiple irregular points of focal activation without organized vascular or structural alignment.

Pattern Type

Diffuse punctate hyperemission indicating systemic immune activation.

Spectral Pattern Description

The dorsal surface displays an irregular constellation of small, punctate hyperemissive loci dispersed throughout the upper and mid-back. These foci appear scattered without linear or vascular coherence, creating a stippled emissive field. The absence of symmetry and the random distribution suggest a systemic rather than localized process. The overall impression is one of diffuse dermal-immune activation with multiple projection points.

Interpretive Understanding

This biospectral signature corresponds to systemic hypersensitivity terrain, commonly associated with allergic responses or heightened immune reactivity. The multiplicity of small hyperfoci represents diffuse immunologic activation projected at the dermal level. In contrast to vascular branching or organ-focused emissions, the punctate distribution accentuates the immune system's diffuse and non-linear regulatory behavior when confronted with hypersensitivity states.

Clinical Correlation Through Anamnesis

Anamnesis provides essential context for this interpretation.

- If the patient reports dermatologic irritation, hives, or itching, the punctate emissions correlate directly with allergic dermal responses.
- If systemic allergic symptoms are present (rhinitis, conjunctival irritation, respiratory sensitivity), the dorsal punctate field may be considered part of the generalized hypersensitivity profile.
- In individuals with food intolerances, environmental sensitivities, or immune dysregulation, such scattered fields align with systemic allergenic load.

Classic Value of the Image

This case is presented as a "classic allergic case" because it illustrates with clarity the punctate distribution that distinguishes immune hypersensitivity terrains. The absence of vascular or organ-projection organization makes the image a textbook demonstration of scattered emissive fields characteristic of allergic or immune-reactive states.

Teaching Insight

The image reinforces the interpretive principle that immune-related biospectral patterns manifest diffusely, in punctate and irregular fields, rather than as structured projections. Practitioners must learn to differentiate such patterns from vascular arborization or organ-linked emissions. This case serves as a didactic example of how systemic immune activation imprints itself onto the dorsal surface, supporting the clinical recognition of hypersensitivity terrain.

Reference 04

Focal Emissive Fields Over Both Knees

Classic Articular Case

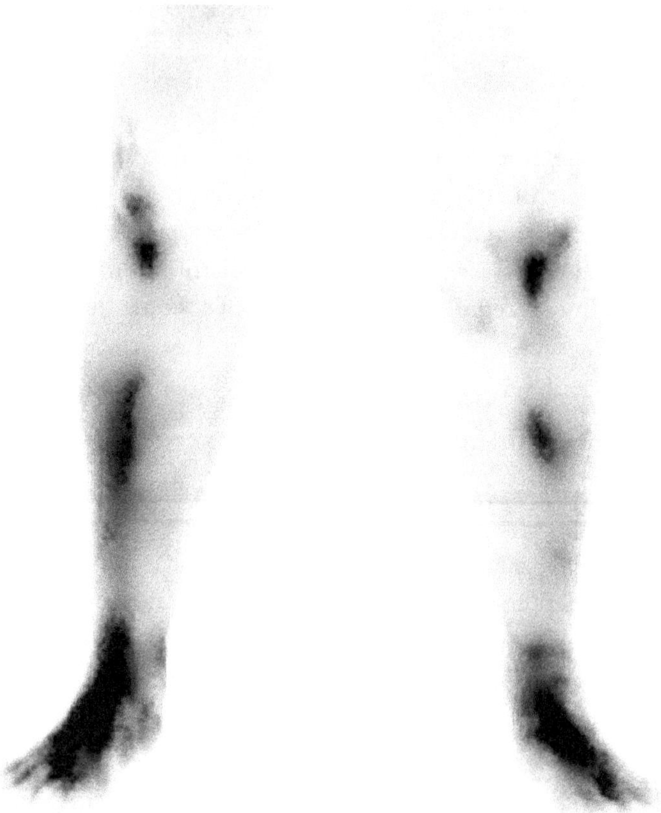

Anatomical Region & Interpretive Category

Zone 1 – Frontal Lower Legs (extending to knee joints)

Primary Interpretive Category: Skeletal / Articular

Spectral Pattern

Bilateral focal hyperemission centered on the knee joints, with diffuse extension into periarticular regions and partial projection downward along the tibial shafts.

Pattern Type

Symmetrical articular focal hyperemission.

Spectral Pattern Description

The image shows two sharply defined emissive concentrations directly over the patellar and peri-patellar regions of both knees. These foci are bilateral and nearly symmetrical, with slightly more diffuse extension visible on the left side. From each knee joint, the emission appears to radiate faintly downward along the tibial trajectories, suggesting load transfer into the lower legs. The surrounding fields remain comparatively less emissive, emphasizing the articular specificity of the pattern.

Interpretive Understanding

This biospectral presentation reflects articular stress terrain, typically linked to joint overload or degenerative change. The bilateral nature of the pattern highlights a systemic or mechanical basis, rather than an isolated lesion. In Biospectral Medicine, such localized emissive concentrations correspond to zones of increased metabolic demand within synovial and periarticular tissues, often preceding or accompanying degenerative or overload conditions.

Clinical Correlation Through Anamnesis

The clinical significance of this pattern depends on patient history.

- If the patient reports knee pain, stiffness, or restricted mobility, the focal emissions correlate with mechanical-articular stress.
- In patients with sports or occupational loading, the pattern may reflect repetitive strain and overload of knee joints.
- If systemic reactive or degenerative processes are present, the emissive fields may represent an early biospectral correlate of articular terrain imbalance.

Classic Value of the Image

This figure is presented as a "classic knee case" because it exemplifies the textbook focal articular emission centered bilaterally on the knee joints. Its symmetrical distribution and clear joint mapping provide an ideal teaching example of skeletal–articular spectral correlation.

Teaching Insight

The image highlights the principle that skeletal–articular terrains manifest in biospectral maps as sharply localized emissions confined to joint zones. Unlike diffuse vascular or immune patterns, articular stress projects in targeted focality, aligning closely with anatomical articulation sites. Practitioners must recognize the interpretive value of such localization, which often anticipates or complements structural findings in conventional imaging.

Reference 05

Concentrated Focal Emission in the Right Hypochondrium

Classic Liver Case

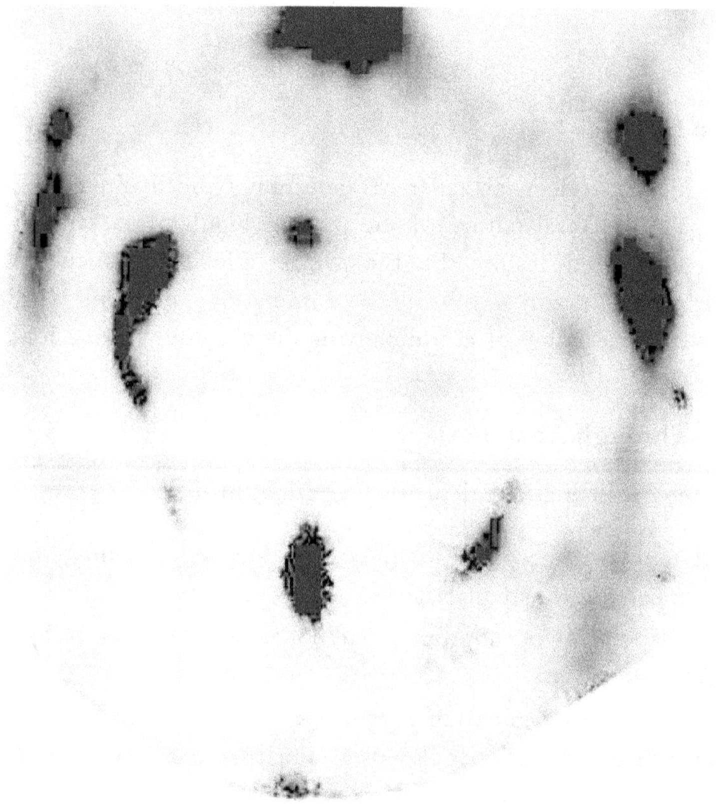

Anatomical Region & Interpretive Category

Zone 10 – Lateral Right Abdomen

Primary Interpretive Category: Organs / GNM

Spectral Pattern

Localized focal hyperemission in the right hypochondrium, sharply demarcated and projecting onto the hepatic field.

Pattern Type

Single-organ focal hyperemission.

Spectral Pattern Description

The image demonstrates a concentrated emissive focus situated in the right hypochondrium, corresponding to the anatomical projection of the liver. The emission is dense and well-defined, contrasting with the surrounding abdominal surface, which displays relatively neutral or diffuse emissive fields. The focal quality of this signal establishes a strong organ-specific projection, with minimal bilateral distribution.

Interpretive Understanding

This spectral configuration represents a hepatic terrain under heightened load or functional imbalance. In Biospectral Medicine, localized hyperemission over the liver corresponds to increased metabolic demand, detoxification strain, or hepatic dysregulation. Unlike diffuse abdominal toxic patterns, this presentation emphasizes the specificity of organ projection fields, with the liver acting as the dominant site of biospectral expression.

Clinical Correlation Through Anamnesis

Anamnesis is essential for refining interpretation.

- If the patient reports fatigue, digestive heaviness, or intolerance to fatty foods, the focal hepatic emission correlates with functional overload.
- In cases with history of alcohol use, medication load, or toxin exposure, the emissive concentration may reflect metabolic burden.
- If systemic symptoms such as hormonal imbalance or skin manifestations are present, the hepatic projection can be interpreted within the broader detoxification-regulatory framework.

Classic Value of the Image

This figure is considered a "classic liver case" because it presents a highly localized, textbook projection of hepatic emissive elevation. Its clarity and focality make it an exemplary teaching plate for demonstrating organ-specific biospectral correspondence.

Teaching Insight

The image highlights the principle that organ terrains may present as sharply localized emissive foci, distinct from diffuse systemic patterns. Practitioners must learn to distinguish hepatic-specific projection from generalized toxic overload, recognizing that organ-focused emissions often provide early terrain-based signals before structural pathology is established in conventional evaluations.

Reference 06

Symmetrical Hyperemissive Foci Over the Sacroiliac Joints

Classic Lumbar Pain Case

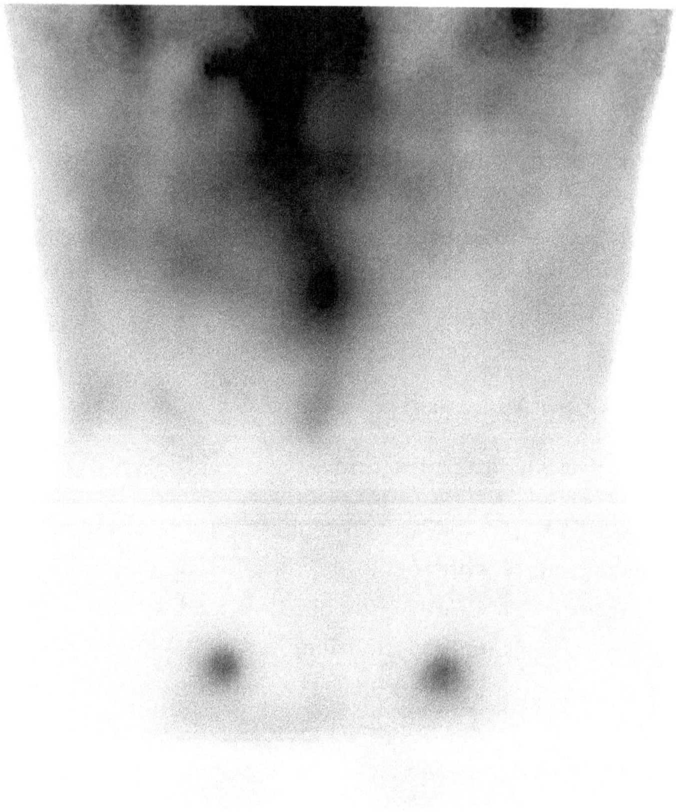

Anatomical Region & Interpretive Category

Zone 12 – Lumbar Region

Primary Interpretive Category: Skeletal / Articular

Spectral Pattern

Bilateral hyperemissive foci positioned symmetrically over the sacroiliac joints, extending partially into the lower lumbar axis.

Pattern Type

Paired focal articular hyperemission.

Spectral Pattern Description

The image demonstrates two well-defined hyperemissive concentrations located at the sacroiliac joints. The foci are bilateral and symmetrical, forming a paired pattern at the lower margin of the lumbar field. A diffuse extension into the central lumbar axis is faintly visible, providing a backdrop to the more pronounced sacroiliac foci. The clarity and symmetry of these emissions create a strong articular signature.

Interpretive Understanding

This biospectral presentation represents an articular overload terrain in the sacroiliac complex, consistent with lumbar pain syndromes. The bilateral symmetry suggests a mechanical or degenerative basis rather than isolated unilateral pathology. Within the framework of Biospectral Medicine, such sharply localized sacroiliac emissions indicate zones of high biomechanical demand, frequently linked to low back pain and compensatory stress along the lumbar-pelvic axis.

Clinical Correlation Through Anamnesis

Clinical history is key for contextualization.

- If the patient reports chronic low back pain, stiffness, or difficulty with prolonged standing, the emissive foci correlate strongly with sacroiliac stress.
- In individuals with occupational or postural strain, the bilateral distribution reflects systemic mechanical load on the lumbar-pelvic junction.
- If degenerative changes or articular dysfunction have been documented, this pattern aligns as a biospectral correlate of chronic overload.

Classic Value of the Image

This figure is a "classic lumbar pain case" because it clearly demonstrates the sacroiliac hyperemissive pattern repeatedly documented in chronic low back pain patients. Its bilateral symmetry and focused articular mapping provide a textbook teaching example of skeletal–articular terrains.

Teaching Insight

The image emphasises the principle that skeletal–articular emissive maps often manifest in symmetrical focal pairs at joint complexes. Practitioners must recognize these paired signatures as biomechanical indicators of overload, especially in regions like the sacroiliac joints where articular stress frequently contributes to chronic pain syndromes. This case provides a didactic template for distinguishing mechanical-articular terrains from diffuse systemic fields.

Reference 07

Focal Hyperemission in Costovertebral and Suprarenal Zones Classic Kidney/Adrenal Case

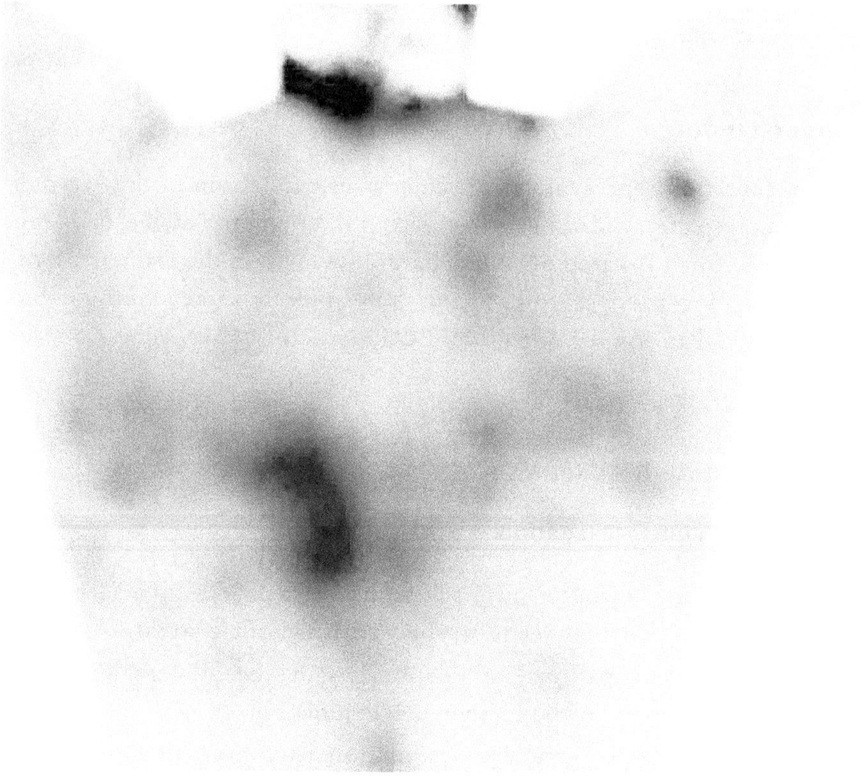

Anatomical Region & Interpretive Category

Zone 12 – Lumbar Region, extending into costovertebral and suprarenal projection fields

Primary Interpretive Category: Metabolic / Endocrine

Spectral Pattern

Paired focal hyperemission localized over the costovertebral angles and suprarenal regions, with diffuse emissive extension into the mid-lumbar field.

Pattern Type

Organ–endocrine paired focal hyperemission.

Spectral Pattern Description

The posterior image shows two discrete hyperemissive loci overlying the costovertebral angles, aligned with the renal anatomical projections. Superior to these fields, a broader zone of diffuse intensification corresponds to the suprarenal areas. The combination of renal and adrenal foci creates a bilateral organ–endocrine emission signature, with added background haze across the mid-lumbar field, reinforcing systemic influence.

Interpretive Understanding

This biospectral presentation reflects the kidney–adrenal axis, a functional system integrating renal filtration and adrenal metabolic regulation. The focal renal emissions suggest heightened renal terrain activity or load, while the suprarenal intensification corresponds to adrenal stress regulation. Together, the pattern indicates a systemic metabolic or stress-related terrain involving fluid balance, detoxification, and endocrine modulation.

Clinical Correlation Through Anamnesis

Patient history determines interpretive precision.

- If the patient reports chronic stress, fatigue, or anxiety, the suprarenal emissions correlate with adrenal strain.
- If urinary disturbances, fluid retention, or flank discomfort are present, the renal foci carry stronger significance.
- In systemic metabolic cases (blood pressure dysregulation, electrolyte imbalance, or detoxification burden), the combined renal–adrenal signature reinforces the interpretation of axis-level involvement.

Classic Value of the Image

This figure is considered a "classic kidney/adrenal case" because it displays a well-defined dual projection onto renal and suprarenal fields, a hallmark biospectral signature for this axis. Its clarity and bilateral expression provide a textbook teaching example of organ–endocrine terrain interaction.

Teaching Insight

The image demonstrates the interpretive principle that organ–endocrine axes project as paired fields, where renal and adrenal biosignals overlap to reveal systemic integration of stress and metabolic regulation. Practitioners must learn to recognize these dual signatures, as they often represent terrain-level adaptations rather than isolated organ dysfunction. This case reinforces the need to consider functional axes in biospectral interpretation.

Reference 08

Bilateral Lung Hypoemission with Central Sternal Hyperemission
Classic Bronchial Case

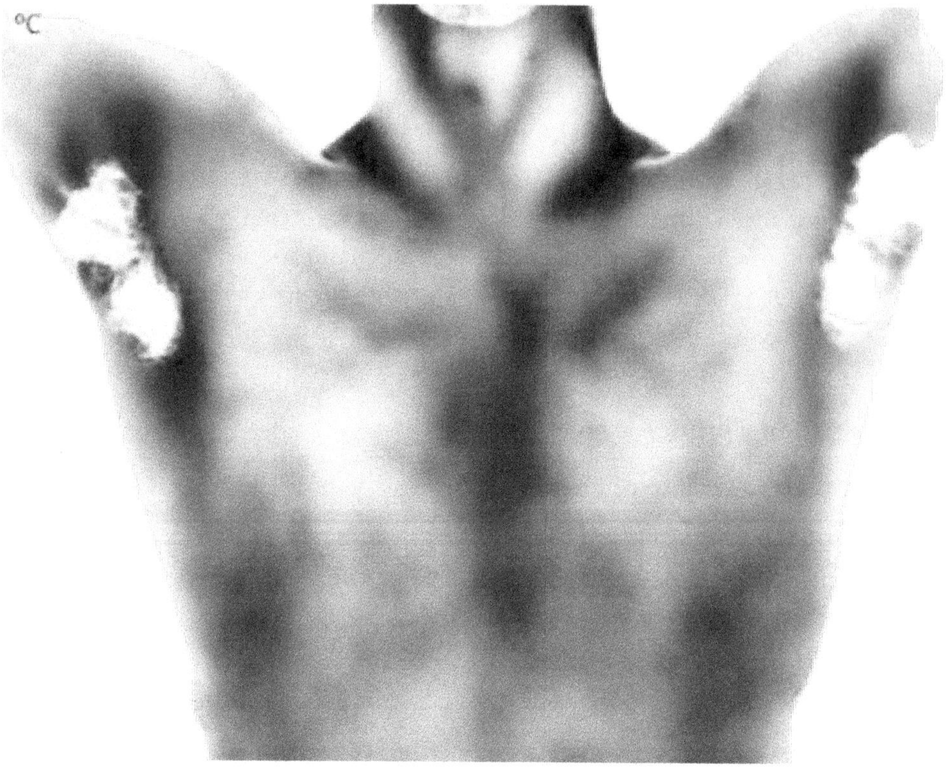

Anatomical Region & Interpretive Category

Zone 13 – Chest and Sternum

Primary Interpretive Category: Organs / GNM

Spectral Pattern

Symmetrical hypoemission across the bilateral lung fields, accompanied by compensatory hyperemission along the central sternum.

Pattern Type

Dual-pattern: diffuse pulmonary suppression with localized sternal activation.

Spectral Pattern Description

The anterior thoracic surface displays broad hypoemissive zones covering both pulmonary fields. These are balanced by a sharply defined hyperemissive signal running vertically along the sternum. The hypoemission is homogeneous across both lungs, while the central focus is narrow and vertically oriented, creating a strong contrast between widespread suppression and focal activation.

Interpretive Understanding

This biospectral map represents a bronchial terrain imbalance. The bilateral pulmonary hypoemission reflects diminished activity or underregulation across the bronchial fields, consistent with airway stress or congestion. The compensatory sternal hyperemission suggests focal activation at the tracheobronchial projection or diaphragmatic reflex points. Together, the dual presentation indicates respiratory system involvement, where diffuse bronchial suppression is counterbalanced by localized regulatory overactivation.

Clinical Correlation Through Anamnesis

The interpretation gains precision when integrated with patient history.

- If the patient reports chronic cough, airway congestion, or bronchitic history, the bilateral hypoemission directly reflects bronchial involvement.
- In cases with asthmatic tendencies or airway sensitivity, the emissive pattern may serve as a biospectral correlate of bronchospasm or airway constriction.
- If digestive or diaphragmatic complaints are present, the sternal hyperemission may represent secondary projection from visceral reflex dynamics.

Classic Value of the Image

This figure is a "classic bronchial case" because it clearly demonstrates the bilateral suppression of pulmonary fields with central compensatory emission, a pattern frequently cited as characteristic of bronchial or airway dysfunction. Its clarity makes it a model example for respiratory terrain interpretation.

Teaching Insight

The image reinforces the interpretive principle that bronchial terrains often manifest through dual dynamics: widespread underactivation of lung fields paired with compensatory activation at the central sternum. Practitioners must learn to integrate these relational dynamics rather than interpret lung and sternum signals in isolation. This case provides an essential teaching plate for recognizing bronchial biospectral signatures.

Reference 09

Broad Bilateral Hyperemission Across Lung Fields

Classic Pulmonary Case

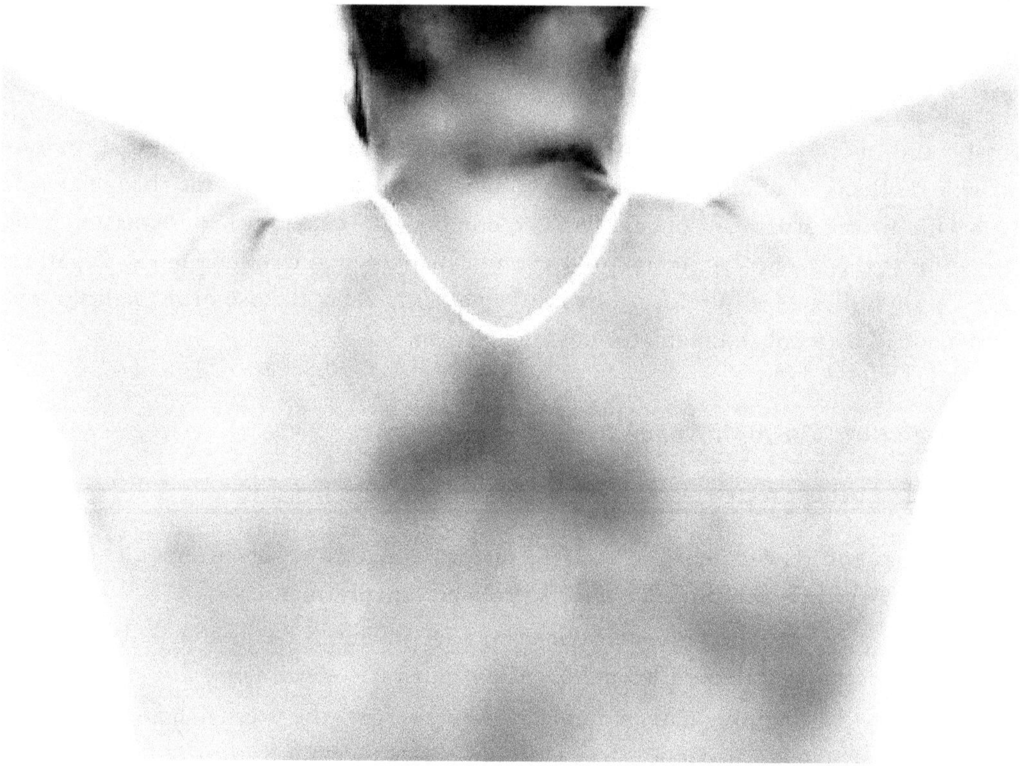

Anatomical Region & Interpretive Category

Zone 16 – Upper Back

Primary Interpretive Category: Organs / GNM

Spectral Pattern

Extensive bilateral hyperemission spanning the dorsal lung fields, with diffuse distribution extending laterally and symmetrically.

Pattern Type

Diffuse organ-related hyperemission.

Spectral Pattern Description

The dorsal thoracic surface reveals widespread, bilateral hyperemissive fields projecting onto both pulmonary regions. The distribution is symmetrical, encompassing the parenchymal fields without sharp focal boundaries. The emissions appear as broad zones of heightened activity, with relatively uniform intensity across both sides, distinguishing this as a systemic organ-level presentation rather than localized vascular or nodal patterning.

Interpretive Understanding

This biospectral presentation corresponds to pulmonary parenchymal terrain activation, consistent with reactive or vascular processes affecting the lungs. The diffuse bilateral nature of the emissions suggests global pulmonary involvement rather than focal lesioning. In Biospectral Medicine, such dorsal hyperemission reflects parenchymal stress, immune activation, or increased vascular perfusion within the lungs.

Clinical Correlation Through Anamnesis

Integration with patient history refines interpretation.

- If the patient reports cough, fever, or acute respiratory illness, the dorsal hyperemission correlates with parenchymal reactive response.
- In chronic respiratory cases (bronchitis, asthma, hypersensitivity), the pattern may reflect sustained pulmonary strain.
- If vascular compromise or circulatory dysfunction is present, the broad emissive fields may indicate secondary pulmonary congestion.

Classic Value of the Image

This case is considered a "classic pulmonary inflammation case" because it demonstrates the archetypal bilateral dorsal hyperemission over lung fields, widely documented in emissive imaging of pulmonary disorders. Its clarity and breadth make it an exemplary teaching plate for pulmonary terrain interpretation.

Teaching Insight

The image underlines the principle that pulmonary organ terrains often manifest dorsally as diffuse, bilateral hyperemissions. Unlike punctate immune signatures or focal bronchial activations, parenchymal lung involvement produces broad systemic fields. Practitioners must learn to distinguish these patterns as organ-level signals, reinforcing the interpretive link between dorsal thoracic emissions and pulmonary parenchymal states.

Reference 10

Diffuse Bilateral Hyperemission in the Lower Legs

Classic Compensatory Case

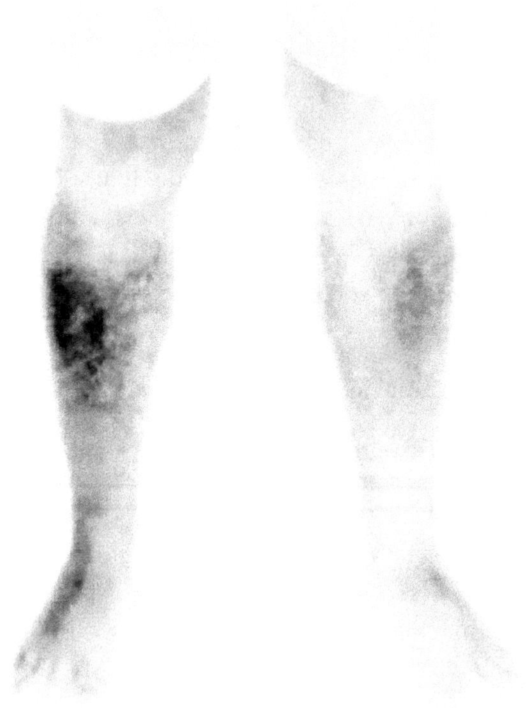

Anatomical Region & Interpretive Category

Zone 1 – Frontal Lower Legs

Primary Interpretive Category: Muscular / Myofascial

Spectral Pattern

Diffuse, bilateral hyperemission distributed across the anterior tibial regions and extending into the calves, without localized focality.

Pattern Type

Symmetrical compensatory hyperemission.

Spectral Pattern Description

The lower extremities reveal broad and symmetrical emissive elevations spanning both anterior tibial zones and extending posteriorly into the calf fields. The distribution is uniform and lacks sharp demarcation, producing a generalized bilateral intensity. No single focal lesion is observed, reinforcing the compensatory rather than localized muscular nature of the pattern.

Interpretive Understanding

This biospectral map represents compensatory circulatory–myofascial strain rather than isolated muscle injury. The diffuse and bilateral qualities indicate systemic adaptation to load-bearing demands, where both vascular and myofascial terrains are engaged to support mechanical balance. In Biospectral Medicine, such bilateral patterns signify compensatory physiology, often arising in chronic postural or circulatory burden states.

Clinical Correlation Through Anamnesis

Patient history refines the interpretation.

- If the patient reports chronic leg fatigue, heaviness, or postural discomfort, the bilateral fields reflect systemic compensatory strain.
- In individuals with prolonged standing or load-bearing activities, this distribution corresponds to chronic myofascial–vascular adaptation.
- If vascular compromise (varicosities, edema) is present, the diffuse hyperemission may serve as a biospectral correlate of circulatory overload layered on muscular compensation.

Classic Value of the Image

This figure is considered a "classic compensatory lower leg case" because it exemplifies bilateral diffuse hyperemission not as a marker of focal muscular injury but as systemic compensatory terrain. While less specific than organ or articular foci, its symmetrical clarity provides high teaching value for distinguishing compensatory physiology.

Teaching Insight

The image emphasizes the principle that not all muscular emissions indicate pathology; many represent adaptive responses. Practitioners must learn to differentiate compensatory systemic patterns from localized dysfunction, recognizing that diffuse bilateral emissions are often signs of chronic strain adaptation. This case provides a valuable teaching plate for understanding compensatory physiology in the lower extremities.

Reference 11

Bilateral Trapezius Hyperemission

Classic Upper Back Muscle Tension Case

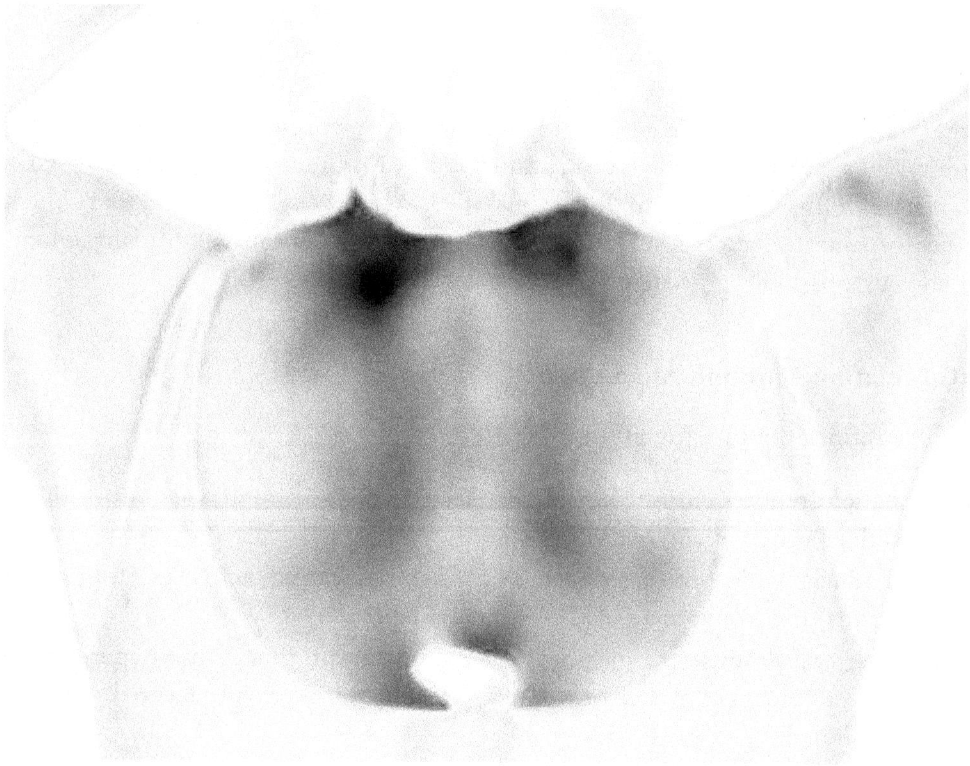

Anatomical Region & Interpretive Category

Zone 16 – Upper Back

Primary Interpretive Category: Muscular / Myofascial

Spectral Pattern

Bilateral symmetrical hyperemission localized to the trapezius fields, extending from the cervical base into the upper dorsal region.

Pattern Type

Paired muscular hyperemission.

Spectral Pattern Description

The dorsal thoracic surface displays two well-defined hyperemissive fields aligned with the trapezius muscles. These zones extend bilaterally from the nuchal base downward and outward toward the scapular margins. The emissions are symmetrical in intensity and contour, producing a paired muscular signature that clearly delineates the trapezius distribution.

Interpretive Understanding

This biospectral map corresponds to muscular overload terrain, specifically trapezius tension. Bilateral trapezius hyperemission is a classic indicator of sustained muscular strain, often arising from postural demand, cervical compensation, or psychosomatic stress. Within Biospectral Medicine, this pattern represents localized metabolic activation of myofascial tissue under chronic load.

Clinical Correlation Through Anamnesis

Patient history is essential for contextualization.

- If the patient reports upper back or neck stiffness, tension headaches, or shoulder fatigue, the trapezius hyperemission provides a direct biospectral correlate.
- In cases of stress or emotional strain, the trapezius signature may reflect psychosomatic muscular holding patterns.
- If occupational or ergonomic demands are present (desk work, heavy lifting), the bilateral emissions reinforce interpretation as chronic mechanical overload.

Classic Value of the Image

This figure is considered a "classic upper back muscle tension case" because it presents the archetypal bilateral trapezius hyperemission, widely recognized as a muscular overload signature. Its clarity and symmetry make it a near-textbook teaching plate.

Teaching Insight

The image reinforces the interpretive principle that muscular terrains frequently manifest as paired, symmetrical emissions corresponding to major myofascial groups. The trapezius fields, in particular, serve as reliable biospectral markers of mechanical or stress-related overload. Practitioners should learn to distinguish such paired muscular signatures from vascular or immune patterns, recognizing their high specificity for tension states.

Reference 12

Vertical Paraspinal Hyperemission in the Cervical Zone

Classic Cervical Muscle Pain Case

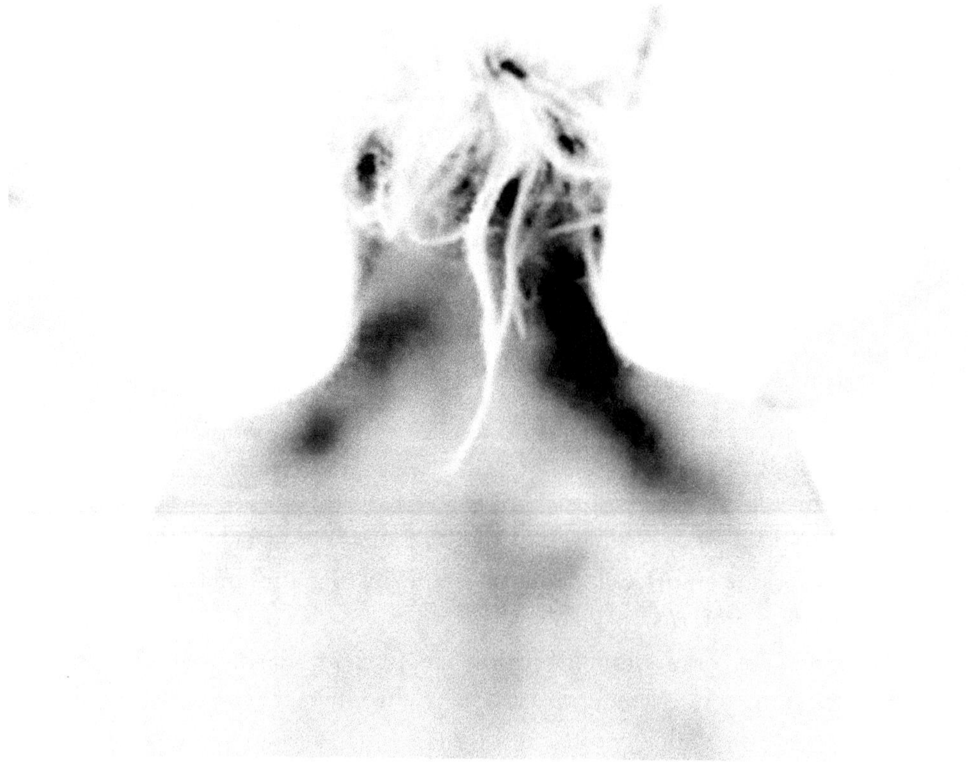

Anatomical Region & Interpretive Category

Zone 18 – Cervical Spine and Nuchal Zone

Primary Interpretive Category: Muscular / Myofascial

Spectral Pattern

Vertical hyperemission tracking along the cervical paraspinal axis, extending from the nuchal base downward into the upper thoracic junction.

Pattern Type

Linear paraspinal muscular hyperemission.

Spectral Pattern Description

The dorsal cervical surface demonstrates a vertically oriented hyperemissive field aligned with the paraspinal musculature. The emission originates at the suboccipital and nuchal base, extending downward toward the upper thoracic margin. The field is elongated and narrow, maintaining continuity along the midline muscular structures, producing a distinct cervical–paraspinal activation signature.

Interpretive Understanding

This biospectral configuration represents cervical muscular strain, consistent with localized overload of the paraspinal group. The vertical continuity indicates sustained contraction or mechanical demand along the cervical spine axis. In Biospectral Medicine, such linear emissions are recognized as correlates of neck pain terrain, reflecting both postural stress and muscular compensation.

Clinical Correlation Through Anamnesis

Interpretation gains accuracy when integrated with history.

- If the patient reports neck stiffness, localized pain, or reduced mobility, the paraspinal hyperemission directly corresponds to muscular strain.
- In cases with headache or cervicogenic pain, this vertical emission may serve as the muscular correlate of referred symptoms.
- If occupational or ergonomic strain is present (desk posture, prolonged screen use), the pattern reflects functional overload along the cervical axis.

Classic Value of the Image

This figure is considered a "classic cervical muscle pain case" because it exemplifies the linear, vertical paraspinal emission strongly associated with cervical strain. Its clarity and axial orientation make it a highly didactic representation of muscular terrains.

The image highlights the principle that cervical muscular terrains often project as vertical emissions along the paraspinal axis. Unlike diffuse dorsal or trapezius fields, this linear signature provides precise mapping of cervical strain. Practitioners must learn to recognize these vertical emissions as reliable markers of localized muscular pain states in the cervical spine.

Reference 13

Asymmetrical Cervical Emission with Right-Sided Hypoemission
Classic Neurovascular Compression Case

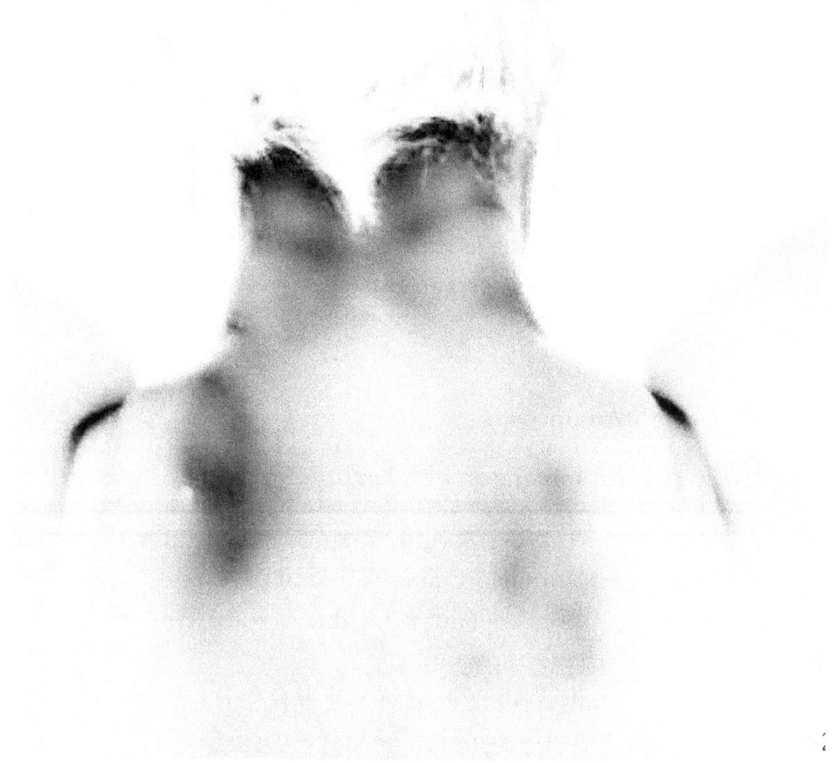

Anatomical Region & Interpretive Category

Zone 18 – Cervical Spine and Nuchal Zone

Primary Interpretive Category: Nervous System / Spine

Spectral Pattern

Asymmetric cervical band pattern: left side exhibits normal hyperemissive tone, while the right side displays relative hypoemission.

Pattern Type

Unilateral hypoemission with contralateral compensatory tone.

Spectral Pattern Description

The dorsal cervical field reveals a striking asymmetry. The left cervical band demonstrates expected hyperemissive tone, consistent with normal vascular–neuromuscular activation. In contrast, the right cervical band shows marked relative hypoemission, creating a visual imbalance across the nuchal zone. This asymmetric distribution is sharply defined, with clear left–right contrast that emphasizes the hypoemissive deficit.

Interpretive Understanding

This biospectral map corresponds to a neurovascular compression terrain. The right-sided hypoemission suggests impaired conduction or circulation in the affected cervical segment, while the preserved hyperemission on the left highlights the contrast. In Biospectral Medicine, such asymmetric suppression is interpreted as a loss of emissive activity secondary to reduced perfusion or nerve transmission, making it an important teaching example of functional impairment rather than overload.

Clinical Correlation Through Anamnesis

Clinical history is essential for contextualization.

- If the patient reports unilateral neck pain, tingling, or arm numbness, the right-sided hypoemission may reflect neurogenic compression.
- If vascular symptoms such as dizziness or coldness on the affected side are present, the hypoemission aligns with circulatory compromise.
- In cases of cervical disc pathology or postural imbalance, the asymmetry may represent functional suppression from mechanical compression.

Classic Value of the Image

This figure is designated a "classic cervical hypoemission case" because of its rare and visually striking asymmetry. The contrast between left hyperemission and right hypoemission makes it a highly educational teaching plate for neurovascular compression states. Its distinctiveness gives it exceptionally high classic value (95%).

Teaching Insight

The image emphasizes the interpretive principle that loss of emissive activity can be as meaningful as excess. Hypoemission, especially when asymmetric, signals functional impairment rather than activation. Practitioners must learn to recognize these rare but significant patterns, as they often indicate neurovascular compression or conduction loss. This case is a model teaching example for demonstrating the interpretive weight of emissive asymmetry.

Reference 14

Linear Hyperemission Along the Lumbar Spinous Processes

Classic Vertebral Pain Case

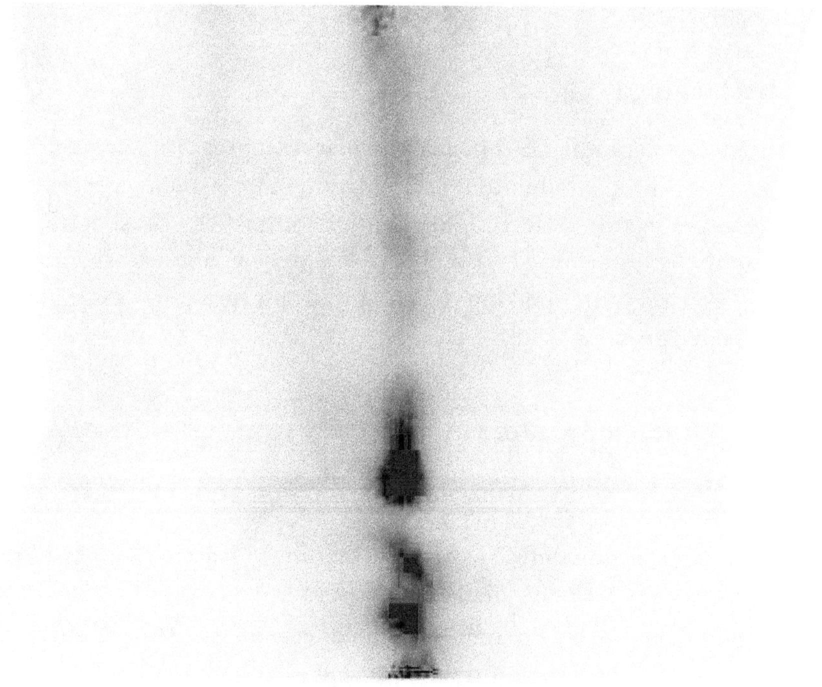

Anatomical Region & Interpretive Category

Zone 12 – Lumbar Region

Primary Interpretive Category: Skeletal / Articular

Spectral Pattern

A clear, vertically oriented hyperemissive streak following the midline over the lumbar spinous processes.

Pattern Type

Linear skeletal hyperemission.

Spectral Pattern Description

The dorsal lumbar image reveals a sharply defined hyperemissive line aligned with the vertebral column. The emission follows the midline trajectory of the spinous processes, extending vertically across the lumbar field. The linearity and confinement to the spinal axis distinguish it from diffuse muscular or vascular patterns, highlighting its skeletal origin.

Interpretive Understanding

This biospectral map corresponds to a vertebral pain terrain, where localized skeletal stress produces a linear emissive projection. The streak-like quality reflects irritation or overload along the spinal axis, consistent with vertebral or facet joint involvement. In Biospectral Medicine, such organized midline emissions are interpreted as skeletal correlates rather than muscular or systemic patterns.

Clinical Correlation Through Anamnesis

Clinical history refines the interpretive weight.

- If the patient reports localized lumbar back pain, stiffness, or vertebral tenderness, the midline emission provides a direct spectral correlate.
- In cases of degenerative disc disease or spondylotic changes, the linear streak aligns with structural pathology.
- If pain is aggravated by load-bearing or posture, the hyperemissive line reflects functional skeletal stress.

Classic Value of the Image

This figure is a "classic vertebral pain case" because of its strong, linear emissive alignment with the spinal processes. Its clarity and skeletal specificity make it an exemplary teaching plate for bone-related back pain terrains.

Teaching Insight

The image emphasizes the principle that skeletal terrains often manifest as linear emissions precisely mapped to structural axes. Unlike diffuse muscular fields or punctate immune patterns, vertebral terrains project as organized vertical signatures. Practitioners must recognize these linear emissions as reliable markers of skeletal involvement in back pain cases.

Reference 15

Relative Hypoemission in the Thyroid Zone

Classic Hypo Case

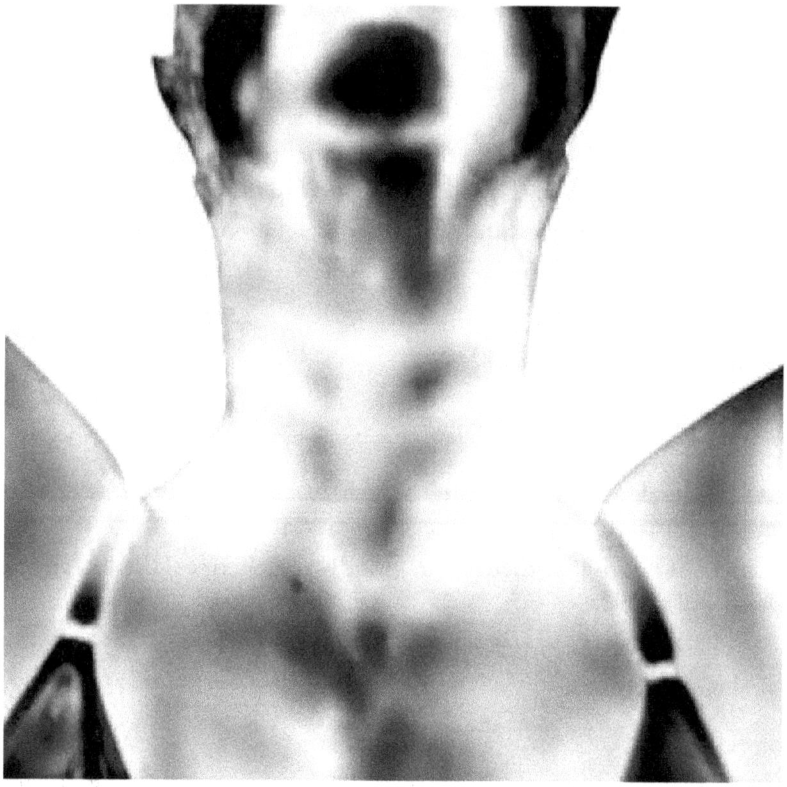

Anatomical Region & Interpretive Category

Zone 17 – Frontal Neck and Supraclavicular Region

Primary Interpretive Category: Metabolic / Endocrine

Spectral Pattern

Localized hypoemission within the thyroid projection field, contrasting with surrounding cervical and supraclavicular tissues.

Pattern Type

Organ-specific hypoemission.

Spectral Pattern Description

The frontal cervical surface displays a distinct reduction of emissive activity within the thyroid projection zone. This hypoemission contrasts clearly with adjacent cervical bands and supraclavicular regions, which retain relatively preserved tone. The distribution is centered over the midline, extending slightly laterally into the thyroid lobes, producing a "cold" thyroid field in comparison to surrounding emissive activity.

Interpretive Understanding

This biospectral presentation corresponds to thyroid hypoactivity terrain. In Biospectral Medicine, relative hypoemission in the thyroid zone is interpreted as reduced perfusion, metabolic suppression, or compressive interference with emissive dynamics. Unlike focal hyperemission seen in reactive or hyperfunctional states, this cold signature aligns with functional underactivity.

Clinical Correlation Through Anamnesis

Patient history provides crucial correlation.

- If the patient reports fatigue, weight fluctuation, or metabolic slowing, the hypoemissive thyroid field reinforces endocrine underactivity.
- If compressive sensations in the neck, dysphagia, or cervical tightness are present, the hypoemission may correspond to mechanical restriction or nodular compression.
- In cases with prior thyroid dysfunction, autoimmune history, or medication use, this spectral map can reflect terrain-level endocrine adaptation.

Classic Value of the Image

This figure is considered a "classic thyroid hypo case" because it demonstrates the textbook cold thyroid projection. The contrast between suppressed thyroid emission and preserved adjacent tone provides a clear teaching plate for endocrine underactivity. With ~88% representative value, it is a strong example, though variations of thyroid suppression may present with less clarity.

Teaching Insight

The image reinforces the interpretive principle that hypoemission is equally significant as hyperemission in endocrine terrains. Practitioners must learn to recognize cold thyroid fields as spectral correlates of metabolic suppression or compressive interference, distinguishing them from hyperfunctional patterns. This case offers an essential teaching example for understanding thyroid-related emissive maps in Biospectral Medicine.

Reference 16

Focal Hyperemission in the Thyroid Zone

Classic "Hyper" Thyroid Case

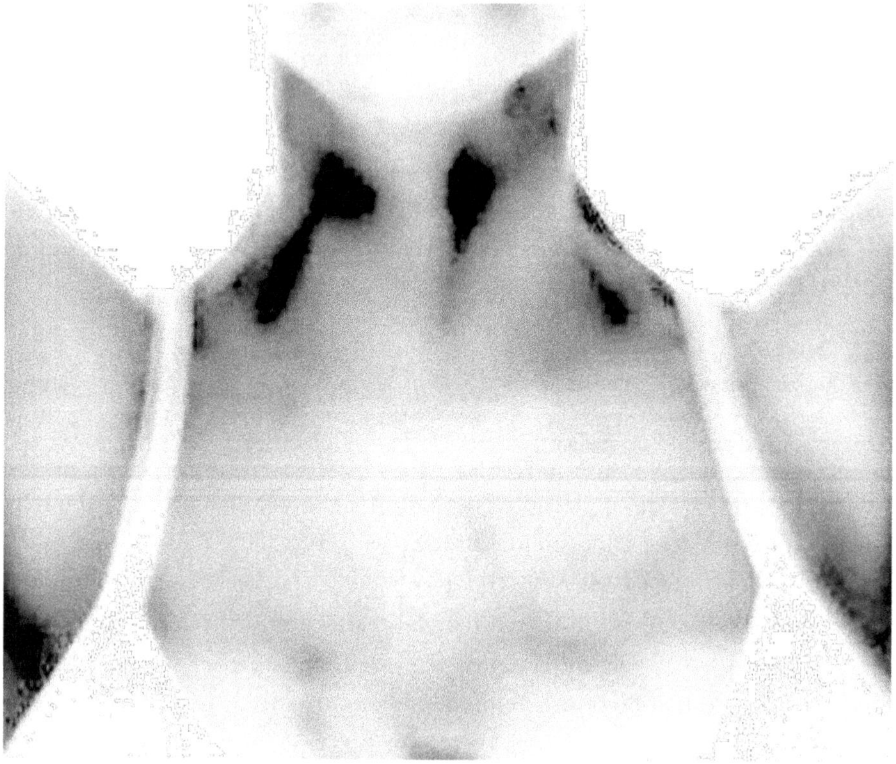

Anatomical Region & Interpretive Category

Zone 17 – Frontal Neck and Supraclavicular Region

Primary Interpretive Category: Metabolic / Endocrine

Spectral Pattern

Localized, sharply defined hyperemission centered over the thyroid projection, contrasting with surrounding cervical and supraclavicular fields.

Pattern Type

Organ-specific focal hyperemission.

Spectral Pattern Description

The frontal cervical surface shows a dense, dark hyperemissive concentration within the thyroid projection zone. The emission is well localized, extending slightly across both lobes but with central dominance in the midline. The contrast against the relatively neutral background of adjacent tissues creates a strong visual marker of vascular–metabolic activation.

Interpretive Understanding

This biospectral signature represents thyroid hyperactivity terrain. In Biospectral Medicine, localized hyperemission in the thyroid projection is interpreted as increased perfusion and metabolic activation, frequently associated with vascular or endocrine stimulation. Unlike cold thyroid patterns of hypoactivity, this "hot" thyroid field reflects heightened functional or regulatory demand.

Clinical Correlation Through Anamnesis

Interpretation is refined by patient history.

- If the patient reports anxiety, palpitations, weight loss, or heat intolerance, the hyperemissive thyroid field supports metabolic overactivation.
- If there is vascular prominence or compressive sensation in the anterior neck, the emission may align with thyroid enlargement or hypervascularity.
- In patients with autoimmune thyroid states or stimulant use, the focal emission may reflect heightened endocrine drive.

Classic Value of the Image

This figure is a "classic thyroid hyper case" because it clearly demonstrates the textbook hot thyroid field. Its focal intensity and vascular–metabolic association provide ~92% representativeness, making it a strong teaching plate for endocrine overactivation terrains.

Teaching Insight

The image highlights the interpretive principle that thyroid terrains can manifest as polar opposites: cold hypoemissive suppression versus hot hyperemissive activation. Practitioners must recognize this polarity to correctly interpret thyroid fields within metabolic–endocrine evaluations. This case provides a complementary counterpart to the thyroid hypo case, completing the didactic spectrum of thyroid emissive presentations.

Reference 17

Symmetrical Venous Hyperemission Along the Lateral Abdomen
Classic Case

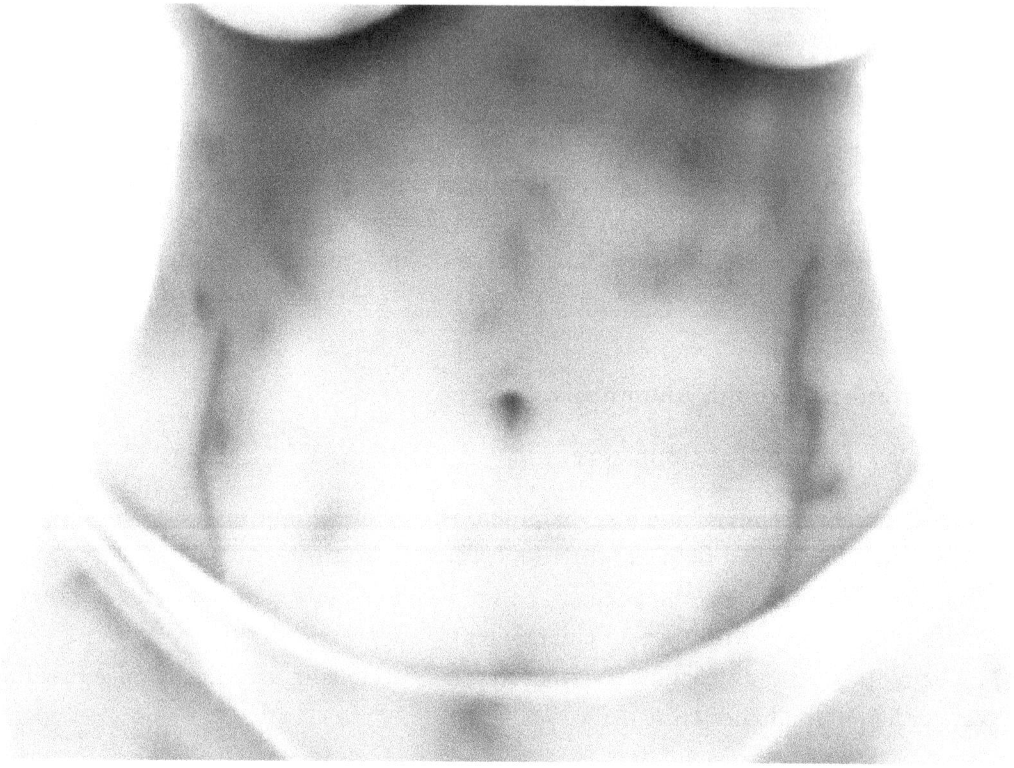

Anatomical Region & Interpretive Category

Zone 9 – Frontal Abdomen

Primary Interpretive Category: Vascular / Circulatory

Spectral Pattern

Bilateral linear hyperemission running vertically along both lateral abdominal walls, producing a symmetrical venous projection.

Pattern Type

Paired vascular linear hyperemission.

Spectral Pattern Description

The abdominal surface reveals two vertically oriented hyperemissive bands located laterally along both flanks. These emissions follow the course of superficial abdominal venous structures and are symmetrical in distribution and intensity. Unlike patchy or diffuse abdominal fields, the pattern is highly organized and bilateral, creating a textbook venous projection map.

Interpretive Understanding

This biospectral presentation corresponds to circulatory terrain, specifically venous prominence. Symmetrical vascular signals are less frequently encountered but serve as a reliable marker of systemic hemodynamic adaptation. In Biospectral Medicine, paired venous emissions are interpreted as reflective of circulatory load or venous return demand, often secondary to systemic or regional pressure states.

Clinical Correlation Through Anamnesis

Patient history contextualizes this finding.

- If the patient reports abdominal heaviness, bloating, or varicosity in other regions, the venous hyperemission may reflect systemic venous load.
- In cases with hepatic burden or portal circulatory compromise, lateral abdominal venous prominence may gain further clinical significance.
- If the patient engages in high physical exertion or has postural circulatory challenges, this bilateral projection may represent adaptive vascular response.

Classic Value of the Image

This figure is considered a "classic venous case" because it demonstrates rare, highly symmetrical vascular emissive prominence across the abdomen. Its clarity and balance give it ~90% representativeness, making it an outstanding teaching plate for vascular terrains.

Teaching Insight

The image emphasizes the principle that vascular biospectral patterns often appear as linear, organized structures, in contrast to diffuse metabolic or punctate immune fields. Symmetry in venous projection, while less common, offers strong didactic value by highlighting systemic circulatory involvement. Practitioners should learn to differentiate these vascular lines from muscular or dermal fields, recognizing them as clear correlates of venous adaptation.

Reference 18

Symmetrical Venous Hyperemission Along the Lateral Abdomen
Classic Male Venous Dilation Case

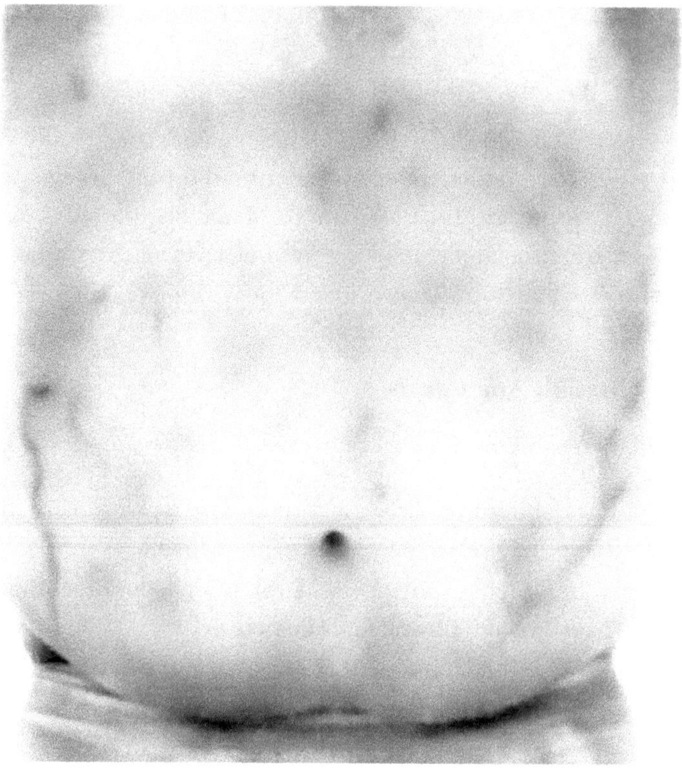

Anatomical Region & Interpretive Category

Zone 9 – Frontal Abdomen

Primary Interpretive Category: Vascular / Circulatory

Spectral Pattern

Paired linear hyperemission extending vertically along both lateral abdominal walls, clearly demarcated and symmetrical.

Pattern Type

Bilateral venous hyperemission.

Spectral Pattern Description

The abdominal surface presents two striking vertical bands of hyperemission, running parallel along the right and left flanks. These lines follow the superficial abdominal venous pathways and are nearly identical in length, intensity, and contour, creating a rare example of perfect bilateral symmetry. The surrounding abdominal field shows less intensity, allowing the venous tracks to stand out prominently.

Interpretive Understanding

This biospectral map reflects venous dilation terrain, an adaptation where superficial abdominal veins display increased prominence. Such symmetry suggests systemic vascular involvement rather than incidental or localized strain. In Biospectral Medicine, these bilateral venous emissions are interpreted as hemodynamic adaptations, potentially related to increased intra-abdominal or portal venous load, systemic circulatory compensation, or functional vascular remodeling.

Clinical Correlation Through Anamnesis

Patient history provides essential interpretive context.

- If the patient reports abdominal pressure, digestive heaviness, or venous prominence in the lower extremities, the abdominal venous fields may indicate systemic load.
- In cases of hepatic or portal circulation strain, these symmetrical venous emissions may serve as early biospectral correlates.
- If the patient engages in high exertional activity or has circulatory predispositions, the venous prominence may reflect adaptive physiology rather than pathology.

Classic Value of the Image

This figure is considered a "classic bilateral venous dilation case" because of its rare and didactically perfect symmetry. Such balance between both abdominal sides provides ~90% representativeness, making it an exemplary teaching plate for circulatory terrains in male presentation.

Teaching Insight

The image reinforces the interpretive principle that vascular terrains often manifest through linear symmetry when systemic circulatory forces are at play. Practitioners must distinguish these venous emissions from muscular or dermal signals, recognizing their value as markers of hemodynamic adaptation. This case stands as an outstanding educational counterpart to the female abdominal venous case, showing how gender and body composition may influence similar biospectral signatures.

Reference 19

Prominent Venous Dilation Along the Right Abdominal Wall

Classic Male Case

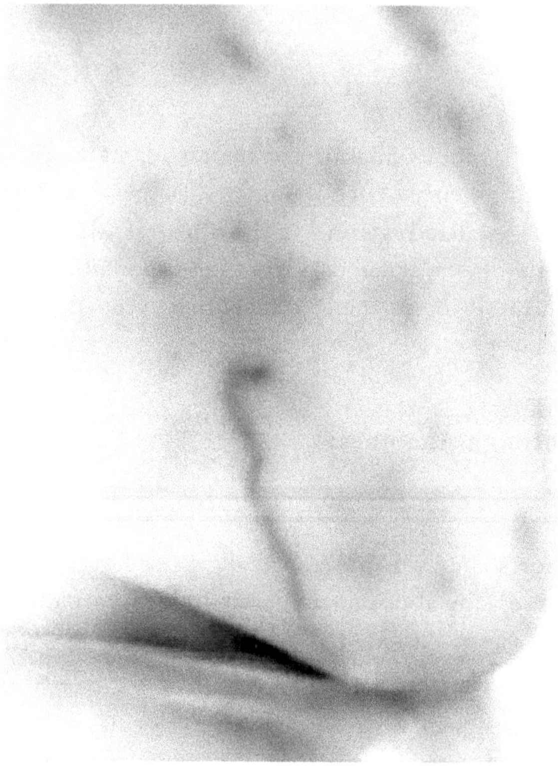

Anatomical Region & Interpretive Category

Zone 10 – Lateral Right Abdomen

Primary Interpretive Category: Vascular / Circulatory

Spectral Pattern

Single, dominant venous hyperemission tracking vertically along the right abdominal wall, with surrounding patchy emissive variations.

Pattern Type

Unilateral venous dilation.

Spectral Pattern Description

The right abdominal surface demonstrates a prominent linear hyperemissive band tracing the course of a superficial vein. This trajectory is bold, continuous, and clearly distinguished from the background. Unlike symmetrical venous cases, this image highlights unilateral dilation, with the right-sided prominence creating asymmetry across the abdominal field. The surrounding terrain reveals diffuse emissive irregularities but none as distinct as the venous track.

Interpretive Understanding

This biospectral map represents venous dilation localized to the right abdominal wall. In Biospectral Medicine, unilateral venous prominence may be influenced by organ-level factors (such as hepatic circulation) or localized hemodynamic adaptation. The boldness of the trajectory underlines vascular dilation rather than diffuse compensatory strain, providing a strong example of focused vascular terrain expression.

Clinical Correlation Through Anamnesis

Patient history provides context for interpretation.

- If the patient reports abdominal discomfort, heaviness, or digestive strain, the right-sided venous prominence may reflect hepatic or portal circulatory involvement.
- In systemic vascular load or varicosity-prone patients, unilateral expression may be an early localized sign before bilateral patterns appear.
- If the patient engages in exertional or postural activities favouring right-sided load, mechanical strain may contribute to asymmetric venous projection.

Classic Value of the Image

This figure is considered a "classic right abdominal venous dilation case" because of its clear, striking unilateral trajectory. With ~93% representativeness, it is a strong teaching plate, especially when contrasted with symmetrical or left-sided venous patterns.

Teaching Insight

The image highlights the principle that venous terrains may appear either bilaterally symmetrical or unilaterally dominant. Right-sided dilation carries specific interpretive weight due to its potential association with hepatic circulatory influence. Practitioners should compare unilateral cases with bilateral examples to appreciate how organ involvement and vascular adaptation shape emissive projections. This case serves as an essential complement to bilateral venous dilation plates, creating a comparative framework for teaching vascular terrains.

Reference 20

Prominent Venous Dilation Over the Right Abdominal Wall

Classic Female Case

Anatomical Region & Interpretive Category

Zone 10 – Lateral Right Abdomen

Primary Interpretive Category: Vascular / Circulatory

Spectral Pattern

A sharply defined venous hyperemission coursing vertically along the right abdominal wall, captured in a frontal-oblique projection.

Pattern Type

Unilateral venous dilation.

Spectral Pattern Description

The abdominal surface reveals a crisp, continuous venous track running vertically along the right side of the abdomen. The oblique perspective emphasizes the contour of the vessel, which stands out clearly against the softer background emissive fields. This well-delineated trajectory produces an elegant and highly didactic image of unilateral venous prominence, distinct from diffuse circulatory or metabolic terrains.

Interpretive Understanding

This biospectral presentation corresponds to venous dilation on the right abdominal wall. In Biospectral Medicine, such unilateral venous prominence is interpreted as localized circulatory adaptation, potentially influenced by hepatic or portal venous factors. The sharp clarity of the trajectory highlights a vascular-structural basis, distinguishing it from diffuse emissive fields.

Clinical Correlation Through Anamnesis

Patient history refines interpretation.

- If the patient reports abdominal fullness, digestive heaviness, or right-sided discomfort, the venous dilation may indicate hepatic-circulatory contribution.
- If systemic venous load is present (varicosities, edema, or circulatory stress), this unilateral presentation may be an early localized marker.
- In individuals with high exertional demand, the right-sided projection may reflect mechanical and hemodynamic adaptation along the abdominal wall.

Classic Value of the Image

This figure is designated a "classic right abdominal venous dilation case" because of its sharp, elegant venous presentation in a female subject. With ~91% representativeness, it serves as a strong complementary counterpart to male right-sided dilation patterns.

Teaching Insight

The image highlights the interpretive principle that venous terrains can be elegantly visualized in unilateral trajectories, offering didactic clarity when well-delineated. Practitioners must compare such unilateral right-sided patterns across genders to appreciate how vascular terrains may present with similar hemodynamic bases but differ in contour and distribution. This case complements the male right abdominal venous dilation image, providing a balanced teaching set.

Reference 21

Networked Venous Dilation Over the Left Abdominal Wall

Classic Female Case

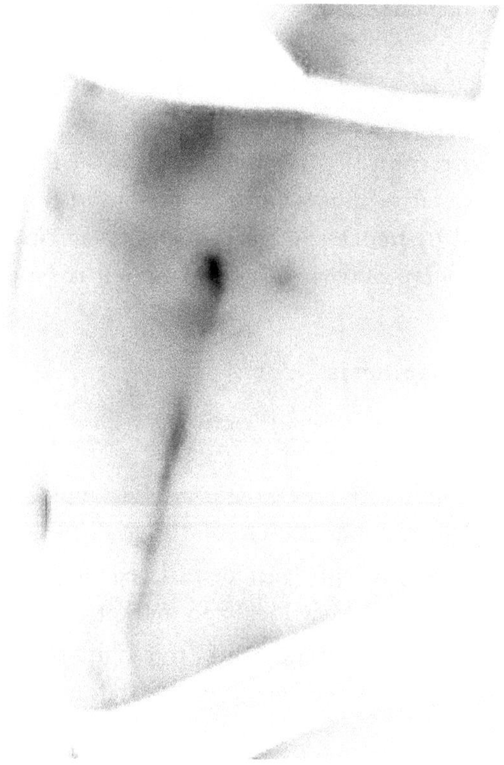

Anatomical Region & Interpretive Category

Zone 11 – Lateral Left Abdomen

Primary Interpretive Category: Vascular / Circulatory

Spectral Pattern

Prominent venous hyperemission forming a network of branching lines along the left abdominal wall, extending obliquely with multiple tributary patterns.

Pattern Type

Unilateral venous network hyperemission.

Spectral Pattern Description

The abdominal surface reveals a well-delineated venous trajectory on the left side, with multiple secondary branches radiating into adjacent abdominal fields. Unlike the crisp singular venous lines of right-sided cases, this presentation demonstrates a networked, arborized appearance. The oblique perspective enhances the visibility of branching, making this one of the clearest examples of unilateral venous dilation with systemic implication.

Interpretive Understanding

This biospectral pattern corresponds to venous dilation localized on the left abdominal wall. In Biospectral Medicine, left-sided venous prominence carries additional interpretive weight due to its anatomical relation to splenic and colonic circulation, contrasting with the hepatic influence more often associated with right-sided cases. The networked appearance suggests a broader hemodynamic redistribution, potentially linked to systemic circulatory demand or organ-specific influence from the left abdominal viscera.

Clinical Correlation Through Anamnesis

Patient history is essential for precise interpretation.

- If the patient reports abdominal bloating, colonic sensitivity, or left-sided discomfort, the venous network may reflect visceral–vascular interplay.
- If splenic or portal burden is suspected, the emissive venous pattern provides a supportive terrain-level finding.
- In cases with systemic vascular stress or venous congestion, the branching pattern may indicate collateral circulation or adaptive dilation.

Classic Value of the Image

This figure is a "classic left abdominal venous dilation case" because of its clear and networked branching, offering high didactic value. With ~93% representativeness, it stands as the most elegant female reference for left-sided venous terrains.

Teaching Insight

The image demonstrates the interpretive principle that right- and left-sided abdominal venous dilations may reflect different organ associations. While right-sided cases often point toward hepatic or portal contributions, left-sided patterns may involve colonic or splenic circulatory influence. Practitioners must compare laterality to refine vascular terrain interpretation. This case, with its branching venous network, provides an ideal female representative for left abdominal terrains, complementing right-sided examples in teaching.

Reference 22

Prominent Venous Dilation Along the Left Abdominal Wall

Classic Male Case

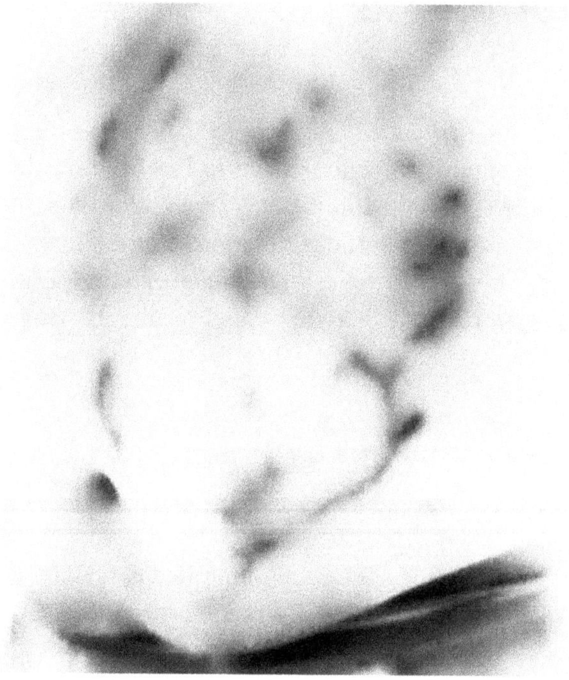

Anatomical Region & Interpretive Category

Zone 11 – Lateral Left Abdomen

Primary Interpretive Category: Vascular / Circulatory

Spectral Pattern

Unilateral venous hyperemission forming a distinct vertical track on the left abdomen, less branched but clearly defined.

Pattern Type

Unilateral venous dilation with linear trajectory.

Spectral Pattern Description

The abdominal surface shows a prominent venous line along the left abdominal wall. Unlike the female case (Figure V), where branching was evident, the male presentation here is characterized by a more straightforward, linear dilation without extensive tributaries. The venous track runs obliquely downward, producing a clean, focal representation of left-sided venous prominence.

Interpretive Understanding

This biospectral signature reflects venous dilation localized to the left abdomen in a male subject. In Biospectral Medicine, left-sided venous tracks may be influenced by splenic and colonic vascular pathways, distinguishing them from right-sided hepatic associations. The simpler, linear quality in this male case highlights gender differences in how venous terrains manifest, with less arborization but still strong hemodynamic expression.

Clinical Correlation Through Anamnesis

Anamnesis allows refinement of interpretation.

- If the patient reports colonic irregularities, bloating, or left-sided discomfort, this venous track may reflect organ–vascular interplay.
- In systemic venous stress or increased abdominal load, the unilateral left-sided pattern serves as a compensatory adaptation.
- If splenic or portal circulation is relevant, this emissive track may represent terrain-level circulatory redistribution.

Classic Value of the Image

This figure is considered a "classic left abdominal venous dilation case" in male anatomy. While not as visually striking as the female networked pattern (Figure V), its clarity as a linear venous track gives it strong didactic value by offering contrast. With ~88–90% representativeness, it is a solid reference plate.

Teaching Insight

The image reinforces the principle that laterality and gender both influence venous terrains. In male cases, venous dilation may appear as a straighter, less branched trajectory, while female examples often demonstrate more arborized networks. Practitioners must compare across sexes and sides to appreciate how abdominal venous terrains reveal both systemic and anatomical variation. This male case complements the female left abdominal venous dilation plate, together forming a balanced teaching set.

Reference 23

Diffuse Venous–Lymphatic Collateral Pattern in the Upper Chest
Classic Lymphatic/Immune Case

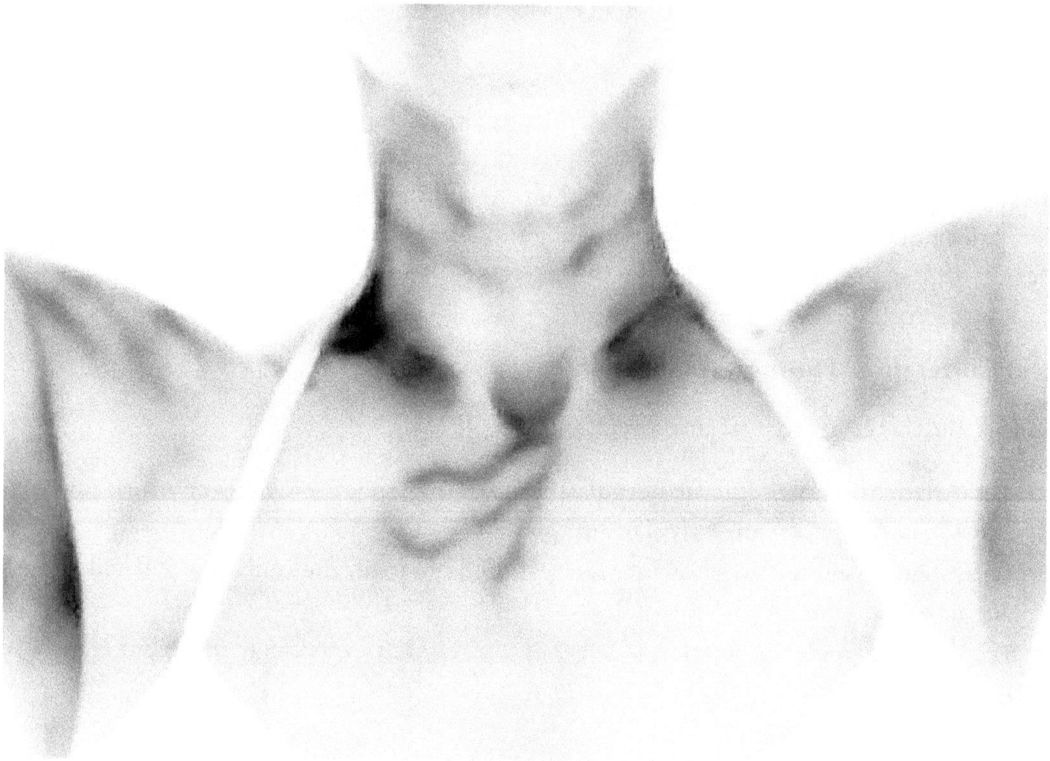

Anatomical Region & Interpretive Category

Zone 13 – Chest and Sternum (extending into supraclavicular fields)

Primary Interpretive Category: Lymphatic / Immune

Spectral Pattern

Irregular, blotchy hyperemissive fields interspersed with venous-like collaterals across the upper chest and supraclavicular regions.

Pattern Type

Diffuse lymphatic–immune overload with atypical venous collateral expression.

Spectral Pattern Description

The image reveals a complex pattern of diffuse blotchy hyperemission scattered across the upper thoracic surface. Interwoven with these patches are linear venous-like tracks that appear irregular and less organized than classic vascular dilations. This mixed pattern, partly vascular, partly diffuse, creates a striking, atypical emissive landscape that diverges from classic symmetrical venous maps.

Interpretive Understanding

This biospectral presentation is best interpreted as a lymphatic–immune overload terrain, despite superficial resemblance to venous collaterals. The blotchy irregularity indicates systemic immune or lymphatic burden, while the collateral-like lines represent compensatory drainage pathways. Unlike clean vascular dilation, this hybrid pattern reflects diffuse overload projected through both lymphatic and vascular channels.

Clinical Correlation Through Anamnesis

Patient history sharpens interpretation.

- If the patient reports systemic fatigue, immune reactivity, or lymphatic congestion, the blotchy pattern aligns with systemic overload.
- If vascular stress or collateralization is suspected, the venous-like lines may represent compensatory flow pathways.
- In cases with chronic reactive or immune conditions, this emissive field may reflect terrain-level lymphatic strain rather than isolated vascular adaptation.

Classic Value of the Image

This figure has ~80–85% classic value as it is not a pure vascular case but an important teaching plate for showing how diffuse immune–lymphatic overload differs from clean venous dilation. Its atypical blend makes it less "textbook," but highly didactic for training practitioners to avoid misclassification.

Teaching Insight

The image emphasizes the interpretive principle that diffuse blotchy terrains, especially when interspersed with irregular linear elements, are more consistent with lymphatic–immune overload than vascular dilation. Practitioners must learn to recognize these atypical patterns and differentiate systemic blotchy signals from clean vascular tracks. This case stands out as a teaching tool for highlighting the gray zone between vascular and lymphatic terrains.

Reference 24

Bilateral Venous Dilation Across the Upper Chest with Right-Sided Dominance – Classic Case

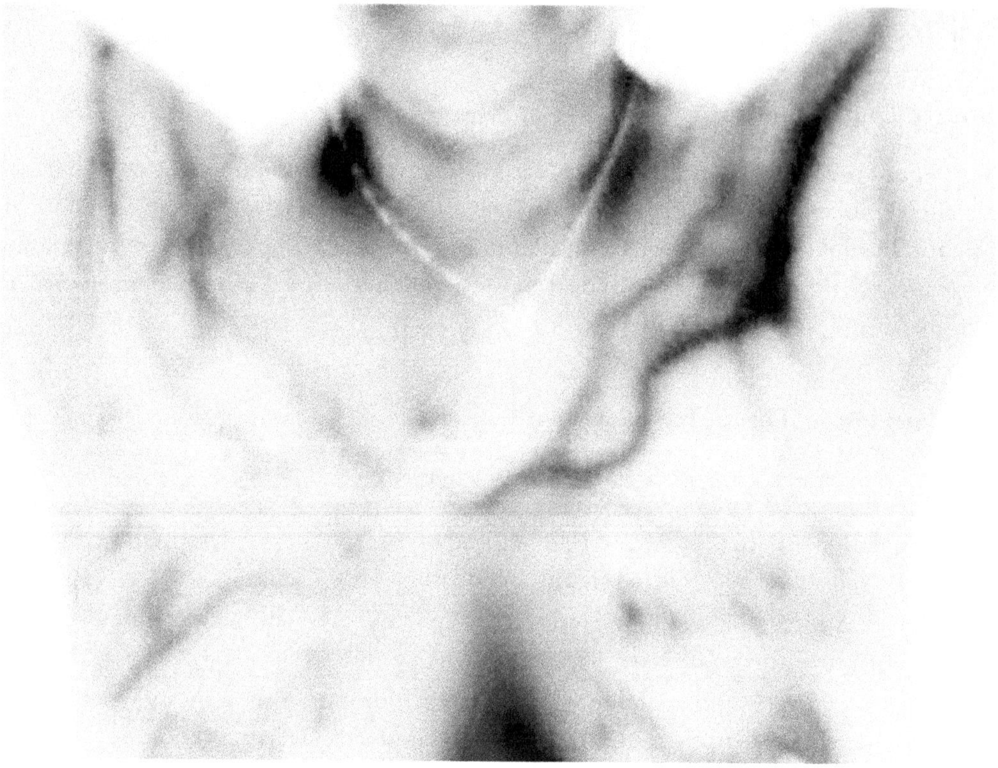

Anatomical Region & Interpretive Category

Zones 13–15 – Chest and Sternum with Left and Right Axillary Fields

Primary Interpretive Category: Vascular / Circulatory

Spectral Pattern

Bilateral venous hyperemission coursing across the chest wall and axillary regions, with greater intensity and prominence on the right side.

Pattern Type

Paired venous dilation with lateral dominance.

Spectral Pattern Description

The image reveals symmetrical venous trajectories extending across both mammary and axillary fields. While clearly bilateral, the right side demonstrates stronger hyperemission and more distinct venous tracks, producing a subtle asymmetry in favour of the right thoracic field. The left side remains visibly engaged but with slightly reduced clarity, making the right-sided projection the dominant emissive feature.

Interpretive Understanding

This biospectral presentation reflects a vascular terrain with systemic bilateral venous dilation but lateral dominance on the right. In Biospectral Medicine, such asymmetry often indicates differential circulatory or mechanical demand, for example, from dominant arm usage, local hemodynamic load, or subtle postural factors. The case remains a classic venous reference, with the right-sided emphasis providing an additional layer of teaching value.

Clinical Correlation Through Anamnesis

Patient history sharpens interpretive meaning.

- If the patient reports right arm or thoracic strain, the asymmetry correlates with greater venous return demand on that side.
- If systemic vascular load is present (hypertension, venous insufficiency), both sides remain significant, but the right dominance may guide clinical focus.
- If lymphatic congestion or localized circulatory block is suspected, the imbalance between sides may represent compensatory adjustment.

Classic Value of the Image

This figure is considered a "classic upper chest venous dilation case" because it shows bilateral vascular projection with didactic clarity, while also illustrating the principle of lateral dominance. With ~90% representativeness, it stands as a high-value teaching plate for vascular terrains of the upper chest.

Teaching Insight

The image emphasizes that vascular terrains, even when symmetrical, often carry subtle dominance toward one side. Practitioners must learn to recognize bilateral venous dilation and to note lateral weighting, which may provide clues to circulatory demand, mechanical strain, or organ-specific influences. This case teaches the dual lesson of "clear venous mapping" and "lateral analysis."

Reference 25

Frontal Breast Biospectral Map with Angiogenesis and Fibrocystic Terrain – Classic Case

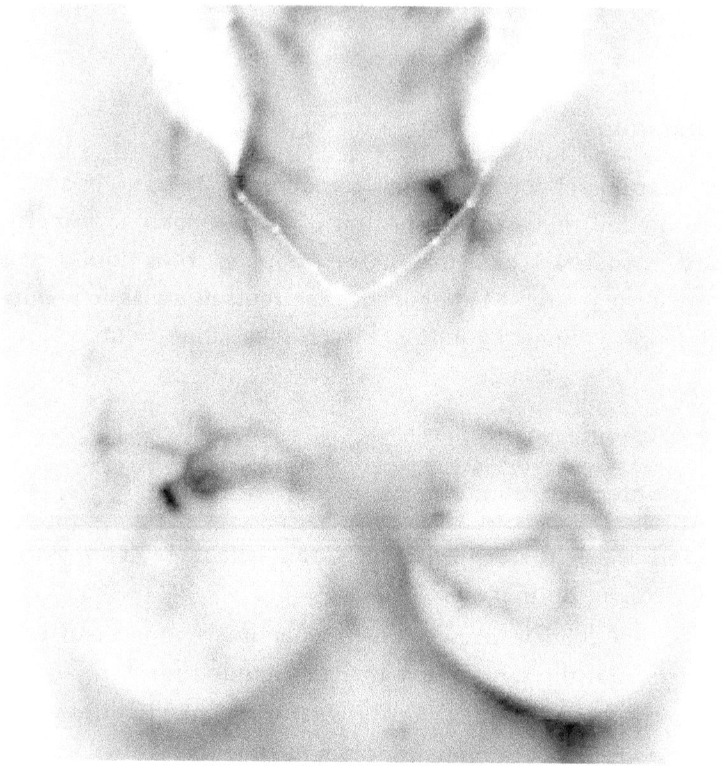

Anatomical Region & Interpretive Category

Zones 13–15 – Chest, Sternum, and Bilateral Mammary Fields

Primary Interpretive Category: Vascular / Circulatory and Organs / GNM (dual involvement)

Spectral Pattern

Branching linear hyperemission across the breast fields, overlaid with irregular patchy hypoemission within glandular zones.

Pattern Type

Dual-pattern: vascular angiogenesis with glandular hypoemissive remodeling.

Spectral Pattern Description

The frontal projection reveals an intricate vascular branching pattern extending across both breasts, most evident in the linear hyperemissive signals consistent with angiogenesis. Interspersed between these vascular lines are glandular patches of relative hypoemission, producing a heterogeneous texture. This contrast between proliferative vascular fields and reduced glandular emissive tone creates a distinct dual presentation.

Interpretive Understanding

This biospectral terrain reflects the interplay between vascular and glandular adaptations. Angiogenic hyperemission indicates increased vascular proliferation, a process often observed in states of hormonal influence or chronic tissue remodeling. The patchy glandular hypoemission corresponds with fibrocystic changes, a benign adaptation where glandular tissue exhibits altered perfusion and biosignal expression. Together, they illustrate how vascular and glandular terrains interact dynamically within the breast fields.

Clinical Correlation Through Anamnesis

History is essential to orient interpretation.

- If the patient reports cyclic mastalgia, breast tenderness, or hormonal fluctuations, the dual terrain aligns with fibrocystic glandular change and vascular reactivity.
- If systemic endocrine influences (e.g., estrogenic dominance) are present, angiogenesis may be a corollary vascular adaptation.
- If no symptoms are reported, the image may represent a benign but instructive biospectral signature of vascular–glandular interplay.

Classic Value of the Image

This figure holds ~85–90% classic value because it demonstrates two terrains simultaneously: vascular angiogenesis and glandular remodeling. The dual presentation makes it less "pure" as a reference than symmetrical vascular cases, but highly didactic in showing combined processes within mammary biospectral interpretation.

Teaching Insight

The image highlights the interpretive principle that breast terrains often display coexisting vascular and glandular signatures. Practitioners must avoid narrowing interpretation to a single category when confronted with dual-pattern fields. Instead, layered reasoning is required to appreciate how vascular proliferation and fibrocystic remodeling interact. This case provides an outstanding teaching plate for showing the complexity of breast biospectral terrains beyond single-pattern classification.

Reference 26

Frontal Breast Biospectral Map with Silicone Implant Representation – Didactic Case

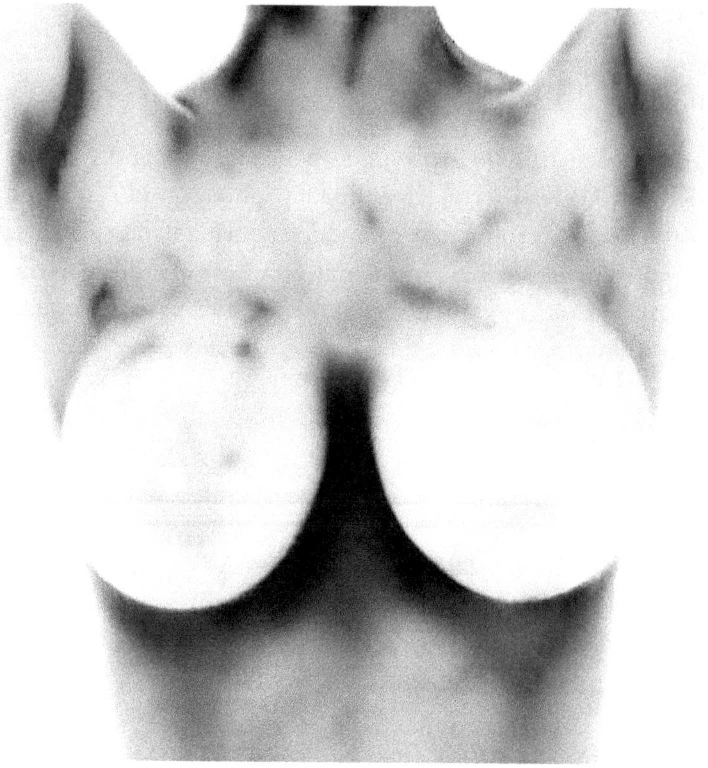

Anatomical Region & Interpretive Category

Zones 13–15 – Chest, Sternum, and Bilateral Mammary Fields

Primary Interpretive Category: Organs / GNM and Structural Representation

Spectral Pattern

Large, bilateral zones of relative hypoemission, uniform in distribution, interrupting the natural vascular and glandular biospectral fields.

Pattern Type

Implant-associated emissive suppression.

Spectral Pattern Description

The frontal breast projection demonstrates two symmetrical, rounded fields of markedly reduced signal intensity corresponding to silicone implants. These hypoemissive zones disrupt the natural heterogeneity typically observed in native breast tissue, where glandular and vascular signals intermingle. Around the periphery, patchy vascular and glandular emissions remain visible, but the implant fields themselves present as uniform low-signal areas.

Interpretive Understanding

This biospectral terrain reflects the distinctive emissive profile of silicone breast implants. Unlike native glandular fields, which present with irregular vascular and fibroglandular patterns, implants produce consistent low-signal suppression, masking deeper biospectral activity. In Biospectral Medicine, such images are not interpreted as pathological but as structural modifications that must be recognized to avoid misclassification.

Clinical Correlation Through Anamnesis

History is indispensable here.

- If implants are confirmed, the observed uniform hypoemission is considered a normal structural signature.
- If no implants are reported, the image would raise questions of structural artefact or abnormal suppression, necessitating clarification.
- In patients with symptoms such as capsular contracture or implant-related discomfort, emissive distortions at the periphery may provide additional interpretive clues.

Classic Value of the Image

This figure has ~80% classic value, not for pathology, but for didactic importance. It provides a comparative reference to distinguish between natural breast terrains and implant-modified profiles, a key competency for practitioners.

Teaching Insight

The image emphasizes the interpretive principle that structural modifications, such as implants, create unique biospectral terrains that must be recognized and differentiated from vascular, glandular, or pathological signatures. Practitioners should develop fluency in distinguishing these artificial hypoemissive fields to avoid misinterpretation. This case is invaluable as a teaching plate for comparative learning between native and implant-bearing breast presentations.

Reference 27

Pelvic–Inguinal Superficial Venous Dilatation

Classic Case

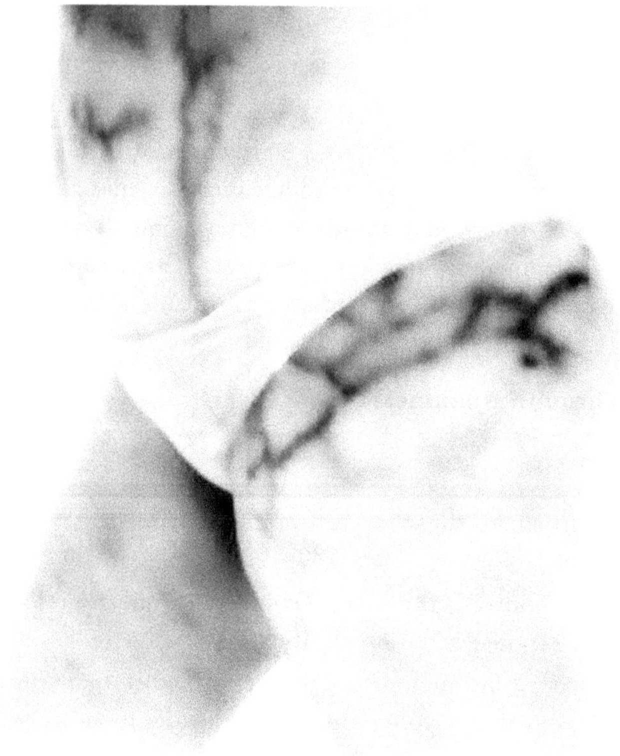

Anatomical Region & Interpretive Category

Zones 9–11 – Lower Abdomen, Inguinal Fold, and Proximal Upper Thigh

Primary Interpretive Category: Vascular / Circulatory

Spectral Pattern

Extensive linear hyperemission tracing superficial venous dilations, extending from the lower abdominal wall across the inguinal fold and into the upper thigh.

Pattern Type

Collateral venous overload with continuity across abdominal–pelvic–femoral fields.

Spectral Pattern Description

The oblique frontal perspective highlights multiple venous tracks emerging from the abdominal wall, converging through the inguinal fold, and continuing into the proximal thigh. The veins appear dilated, bold, and branching, forming a contiguous network across regions. The emissive intensity is strongest at the inguinal transition, where venous load converges, creating a striking visual of collateral overload.

Interpretive Understanding

This biospectral terrain represents venous overload in the pelvic–femoral drainage system. The continuity from abdominal to femoral zones emphasizes collateral circulation as a systemic adaptation to venous strain. In Biospectral Medicine, such patterns are interpreted as vascular terrains indicative of hemodynamic redistribution, superficial venous pathology, or compensatory collateralization when deeper venous return is strained.

Clinical Correlation Through Anamnesis

Clinical history provides crucial interpretive context.

- If the patient reports pelvic heaviness, lower limb varicosities, or exertional venous discomfort, this emissive map aligns strongly with symptomatic venous overload.
- If there is history of prior venous insufficiency, thrombosis, or pelvic congestion, the collateral pattern may represent adaptive bypass circulation.
- In asymptomatic individuals, the image still carries high didactic value, as it captures structural venous terrain expression.

Classic Value of the Image

This figure holds ~90% classic value as one of the clearest examples of pelvic–inguinal venous dilation with systemic collateralization. It is highly representative for teaching superficial venous pathology across connected anatomical regions.

Teaching Insight

The image highlights the principle that venous terrains must often be read in continuity across multiple anatomical zones. Collateral dilations rarely remain confined; they instead span boundaries such as abdominal–inguinal–femoral transitions. Practitioners must learn to trace these emissive continuities and integrate them into systemic vascular interpretation. This case provides an outstanding teaching plate for collateral venous overload.

Reference 28

Continuous Longitudinal Venous Dilatation Along the Saphenous Trajectory – Classic Case

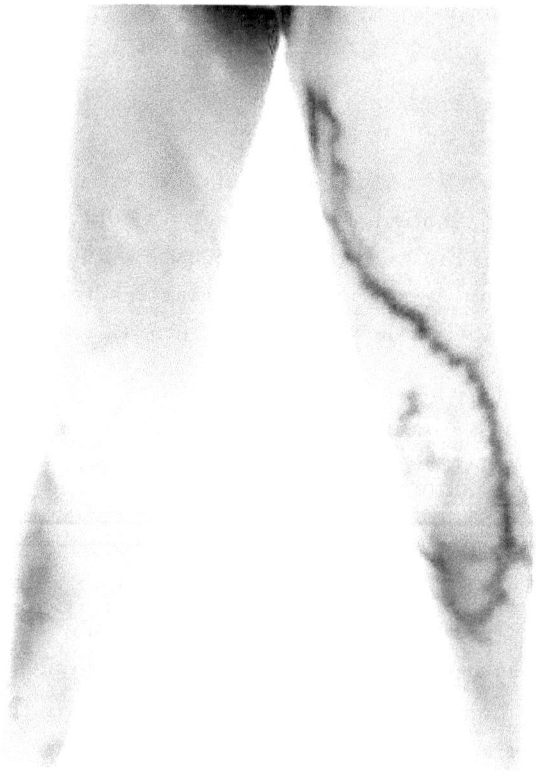

Anatomical Region & Interpretive Category

Zone 1 – Frontal Lower Leg extending through the Thigh

Primary Interpretive Category: Vascular / Circulatory

Spectral Pattern

A single continuous hyperemissive venous pathway extending longitudinally from the medial thigh to the calf, sharply defined and uninterrupted.

Pattern Type

Advanced venous overload with linear continuity.

Spectral Pattern Description

The frontal projection reveals a dominant venous line tracing the saphenous pathway. The hyperemission is bold, elongated, and uninterrupted, extending across the entire visible span of the limb. Secondary venous branches are less pronounced, leaving the long linear trajectory as the defining feature. This uninterrupted vertical flow makes the image visually iconic, capturing advanced venous dilation in its most recognizable form.

Interpretive Understanding

This biospectral terrain reflects advanced venous overload localized to the saphenous system. In Biospectral Medicine, the clarity and length of the trajectory signal a mature circulatory adaptation where superficial veins act as major collateral drainage pathways under chronic load. The absence of diffuse blotchiness or competing patterns underlines its vascular specificity, making this image a pure venous signature.

Clinical Correlation Through Anamnesis

History provides interpretive refinement.

- If the patient reports varicosities, leg heaviness, or exertional venous pain, the saphenous hyperemission is a strong correlate.
- If venous insufficiency or chronic vascular stress is known, the image confirms systemic overload manifesting through superficial collateralization.
- Even in asymptomatic patients, the clarity of the trajectory establishes a strong teaching reference for early recognition of venous overload.

Classic Value of the Image

This figure carries ~90–95% classic value as the most iconic example of a longitudinal venous pathway in the lower limb. It is ideally suited as the anchor reference before subdividing venous terrains into positional categories (pelvic–inguinal, lower leg compensatory, patchy overload, etc.).

Teaching Insight

The image teaches the principle that venous terrains can progress from patchy collateralization to fully defined longitudinal tracks, reflecting advanced systemic adaptation. Practitioners must learn to trace venous pathways across the entire limb rather than isolating segments. This case stands as the cornerstone teaching plate for venous terrains of the lower extremities, setting the standard for vascular interpretation.

Reference 29

Internal Right Leg Venous Dilation with Clean Longitudinal Trajectory – Classic Case

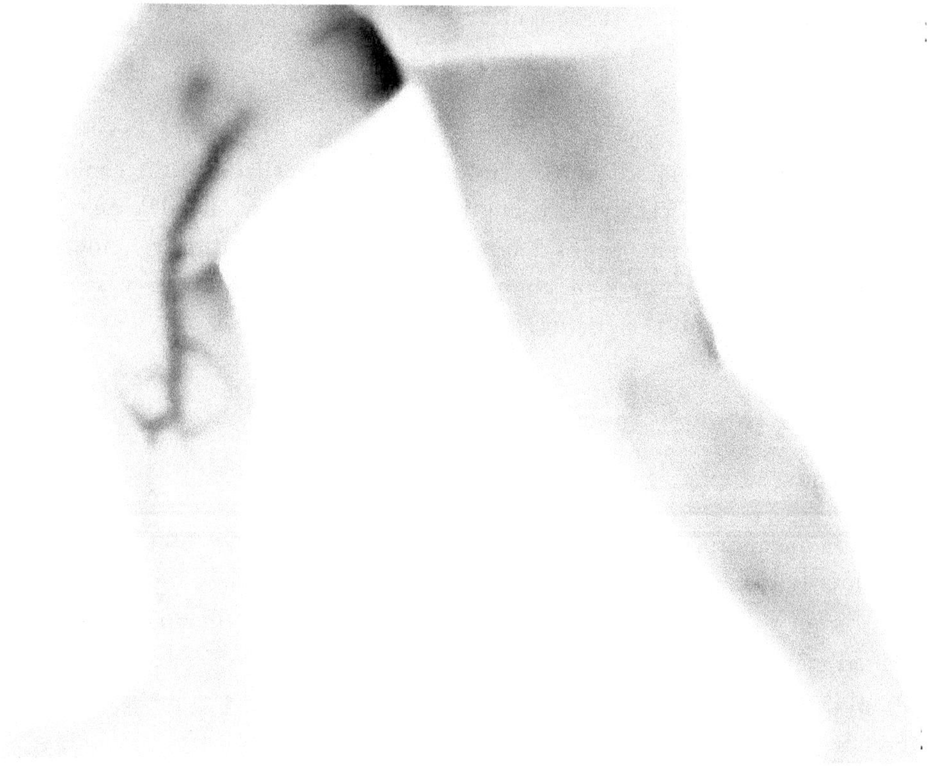

Anatomical Region & Interpretive Category

Zone 3 – Internal Right Leg

Primary Interpretive Category: Vascular / Circulatory

Spectral Pattern

Linear venous hyperemission tracing a continuous path along the medial right thigh, extending downward into the calf.

Pattern Type

Unilateral venous dilation with longitudinal continuity.

Spectral Pattern Description

The oblique frontal view reveals a sharply defined venous trajectory along the internal surface of the right leg. The dilation appears as a bold, uninterrupted hyperemissive track, cleanly demarcated from the surrounding field. The vein curves slightly but maintains continuity from the proximal thigh to the distal calf, giving the image a striking and didactic clarity.

Interpretive Understanding

This biospectral terrain corresponds to venous dilation along the internal right leg, mapping a saphenous-aligned trajectory. In Biospectral Medicine, such clear, continuous venous signals reflect advanced collateral adaptation to systemic vascular load. The clean definition of this pathway distinguishes it from diffuse circulatory or lymphatic terrains, marking it as a pure venous case.

Clinical Correlation Through Anamnesis

History directs the weight of interpretation.

- If the patient reports leg heaviness, varicosities, or prolonged standing intolerance, this venous dilation strongly correlates with symptomatic overload.
- If a background of venous insufficiency or familial varicosity exists, the image may represent structural adaptation.
- In asymptomatic individuals, the clarity of the terrain still provides high teaching value by demonstrating internal leg venous mapping.

Classic Value of the Image

This figure holds ~90–95% classic value, as one of the cleanest and most didactic examples of internal leg venous dilation. Its sharply linear projection makes it a reference-standard teaching plate for vascular terrains of the lower extremities.

Teaching Insight

The image emphasizes the principle that venous terrains can be mapped with precision along defined anatomical tracks. Practitioners should recognize how internal leg venous dilations differ from external or diffuse compensatory terrains, both in trajectory and systemic meaning. This case anchors the category of internal venous pathways, complementing the iconic longitudinal limb case (Figure AC).

Reference 30

Dorsal Lower Leg Venous Trajectory

Classic Posterior Venous Pattern

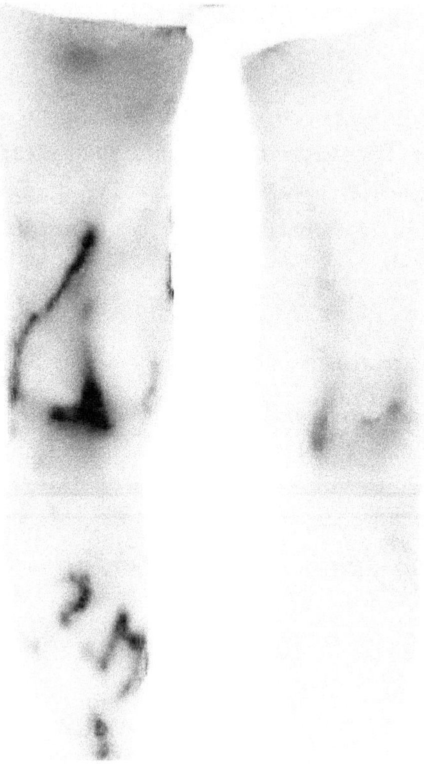

Anatomical Region & Interpretive Category

Zone 2 – Dorsal Lower Leg

Primary Interpretive Category: Vascular / Circulatory

Spectral Pattern

A sharply linear hyperemission aligned with the posterior calf, extending vertically along the dorsal trajectory of the leg. The pattern is unilateral, continuous, and clearly distinguished from the background fields.

Pattern Type

Localized venous dilation with high-contrast linear organization.

Spectral Pattern Description

The posterior calf surface reveals a clean and uninterrupted emissive track running vertically along the venous axis. The hyperemission is bold, uniform, and of high contrast, providing a precise anatomical mapping of venous dilation. Minor branching signals are faintly perceptible but secondary to the dominant longitudinal line, which defines the terrain as a clear vascular projection.

Interpretive Understanding

This spectral pattern corresponds to venous overload along the posterior calf. In Biospectral Medicine, such sharply defined linear hyperemissions indicate a mature vascular adaptation, reflecting superficial venous strain or chronic collateralization. The dorsal leg is a frequent site of venous expression due to gravitational and load-bearing influences, making this a representative pattern of lower extremity vascular terrain.

Clinical Correlation Through Anamnesis

The clinical context determines interpretive emphasis.

- If the patient reports calf heaviness, varicosities, or pain during exertion, the dorsal venous trajectory serves as a direct correlate.
- If prolonged standing or sedentary strain is part of the history, the emissive mapping reflects chronic venous load.
- Even in asymptomatic individuals, the clarity of the dorsal pathway provides strong reference value as an early indicator of venous adaptation.

Classic Value of the Image

This figure is designated a "primary classic dorsal case" because of its clarity, contrast, and sharply linear organization. With >90% representativeness, it stands as a textbook example of posterior calf venous dilation, providing a standard plate for vascular terrains in the lower leg.

Teaching Insight

The image highlights the interpretive principle that venous terrains often follow strict linear anatomical pathways, in contrast with patchy or diffuse immune or metabolic maps. The dorsal calf case serves as a reminder that some vascular signatures are more anatomically explicit than others, allowing practitioners to recognize and classify venous overload with confidence. This figure represents the archetype for dorsal lower leg venous interpretation, anchoring the vascular teaching sequence for posterior limb terrains.

Reference 31

Frontal Thigh Venous Dilation

Classic Great Saphenous Involvement

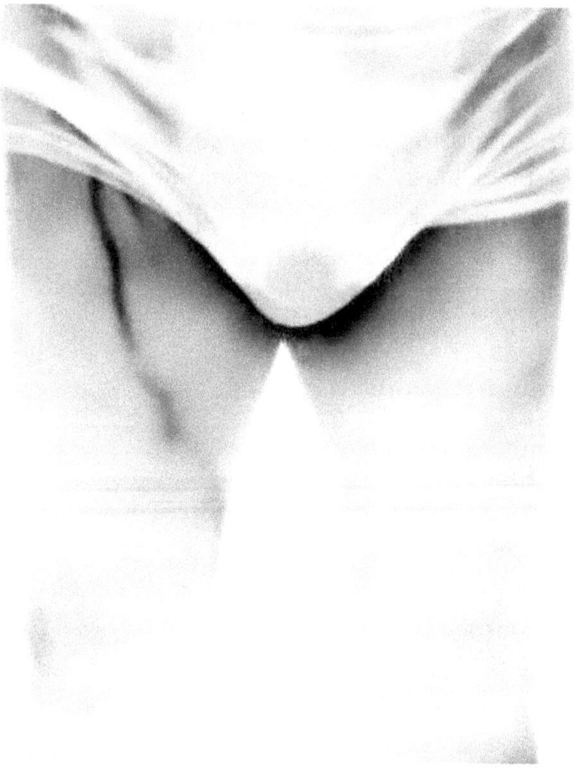

Anatomical Region & Interpretive Category

Zone 7 – Frontal Upper Leg

Primary Interpretive Category: Vascular / Circulatory

Spectral Pattern

A vertical linear hyperemission extending along the medial aspect of the thigh, consistent with the anatomical course of the great saphenous vein.

Pattern Type

Localized venous dilation with vertical orientation.

Spectral Pattern Description

The frontal thigh surface displays a sharply demarcated hyperemissive line aligned with the medial tract. The emission follows a vertical path, uniform in intensity, and distinct from the surrounding field. The clarity of the trajectory points toward superficial venous dilation rather than diffuse circulatory stress. Its medial localization identifies the terrain as strongly consistent with the saphenous system.

Interpretive Understanding

This spectral presentation corresponds to venous dilation within the great saphenous distribution. In Biospectral Medicine, such linear medial thigh signatures indicate superficial venous overload, often related to chronic venous return strain or early varicosity development. The image provides a textbook example of localized saphenous involvement, without the diffuse collateralization seen in more advanced venous terrains.

Clinical Correlation Through Anamnesis

History refines interpretation.

- If the patient reports leg heaviness, visible varicosities, or standing-related fatigue, the medial thigh trajectory confirms symptomatic venous strain.
- In individuals with known venous insufficiency, this mapping indicates terrain-level expression of the great saphenous overload.
- If asymptomatic, the image still serves as an early-stage indicator of vascular adaptation and a strong comparative teaching plate.

Classic Value of the Image

This figure is rated ~80–85% classic because it provides a clean and specific representation of great saphenous involvement, though more localized than the full longitudinal cases. It serves as an excellent insert image to illustrate how focal venous trajectories are captured within the thigh region.

Teaching Insight

The image highlights the principle that venous terrains can be captured at both localized and systemic levels. While some cases present extended longitudinal pathways, others, like this medial thigh dilation, reveal localized venous signatures tied to specific anatomical veins. Practitioners must learn to classify both localized and extended venous terrains, appreciating the saphenous system as a central vascular axis in lower limb biospectral mapping.

Reference 32

Internal Left Leg Venous Dilation

Classic Case

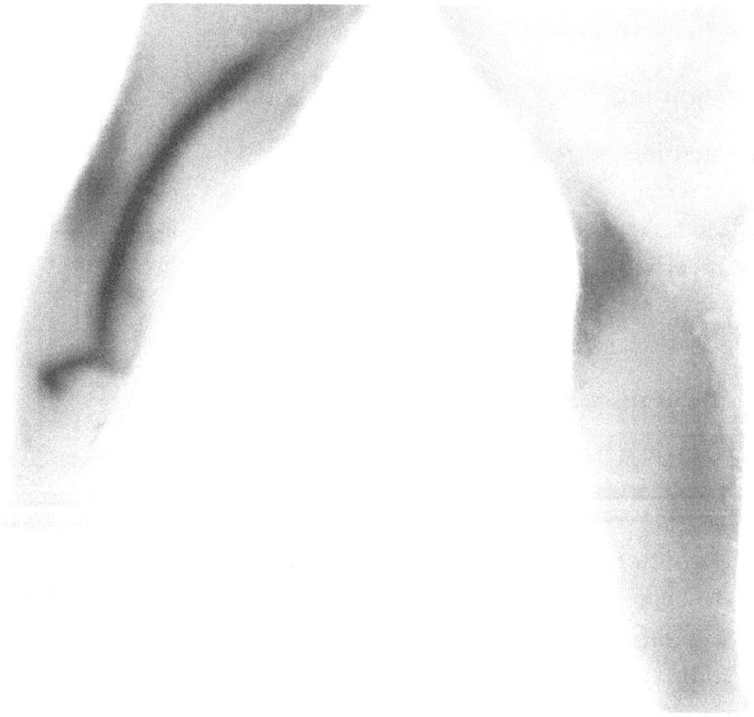

Anatomical Region & Interpretive Category

Zone 4 – Internal Left Leg

Primary Interpretive Category: Vascular / Circulatory

Spectral Pattern

A sharply defined venous hyperemission extending longitudinally along the medial aspect of the left leg, running from the thigh downward toward the calf.

Pattern Type

Unilateral venous dilation with linear medial orientation.

Spectral Pattern Description

The internal left leg surface reveals a bold venous trajectory that follows the anatomical path of the great saphenous system. The emissive signal is continuous, with slight contouring around the knee, but maintains high intensity and clear definition throughout. Unlike diffuse venous overload cases, this image emphasizes a single dominant venous line, making the pattern clean and straightforward.

Interpretive Understanding

This spectral pattern corresponds to venous dilation of the medial left leg. In Biospectral Medicine, such a presentation indicates localized superficial venous strain within the saphenous axis. The unilateral appearance differentiates it from systemic compensatory terrains, reflecting structural overload localized to the left limb. Its clarity makes it an excellent representative of focal venous adaptation.

Clinical Correlation Through Anamnesis

Patient history sharpens interpretation.

- If the patient reports localized leg heaviness, visible varicosities, or knee–calf strain, this venous dilation provides a strong correlate.
- If systemic venous insufficiency is present, the left-sided localization may represent asymmetrical collateral recruitment.
- If asymptomatic, the venous trajectory still carries didactic significance as a localized vascular terrain.

Classic Value of the Image

This figure is rated ~85% classic value. While highly didactic for showing internal left leg venous dilation, its clarity is slightly less striking than the dorsal or full longitudinal pathway cases. Nonetheless, it remains a strong teaching plate for localized venous terrains.

Teaching Insight

The image illustrates the principle that venous terrains must be assessed for both laterality and trajectory. Internal leg dilations carry particular teaching value because they map directly to the saphenous axis, yet differ in visibility and clinical emphasis from dorsal or anterior pathways. Practitioners should note that left-sided venous terrains may carry distinct associations from right-sided cases, underlining the need for comparative lateral analysis.

Reference 33

Left Axillary Mixed Venous–Lymphatic Terrain

Classic Case

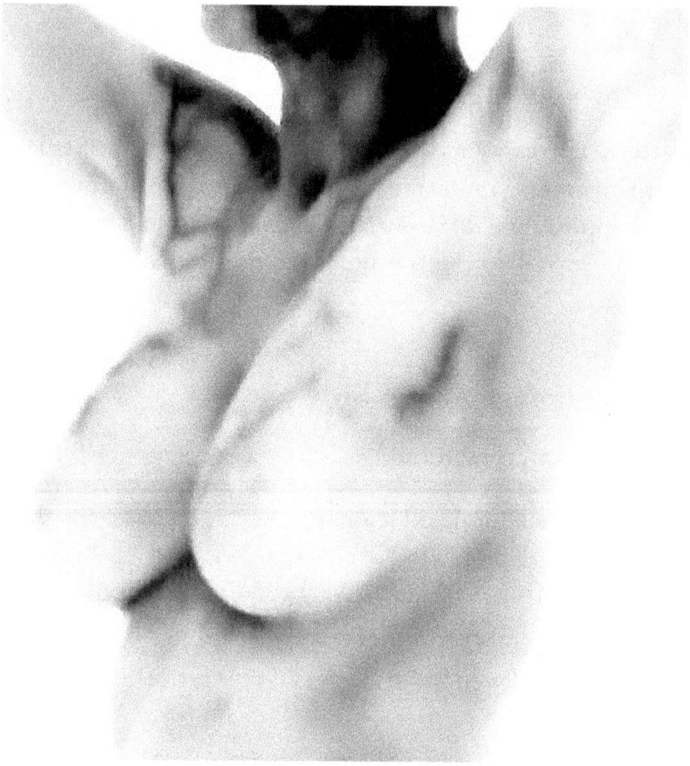

Anatomical Region & Interpretive Category

Zone 14 – Left Axillary Field

Primary Interpretive Category: Vascular / Circulatory and Lymphatic / Immune (combined involvement)

Spectral Pattern

Irregular hyperemissive branching within the left axilla, blending venous linearity with diffuse blotchy fields suggestive of lymphatic strain.

Pattern Type

Hybrid pattern: venous dilation with lymphatic–immune overlay.

Spectral Pattern Description

The oblique thoracic–axillary projection demonstrates a heterogeneous biospectral map. Linear venous hyperemission is visible along the axillary course, but it merges with patchy, irregular emissive fields that lack vascular organization. The mixed qualities of branching tracks and diffuse blotches create a dual impression, consistent with combined venous and lymphatic activity.

Interpretive Understanding

This spectral terrain reflects a mixed vascular–lymphatic involvement. In Biospectral Medicine, such hybrid signatures often suggest circulatory adaptation alongside immune or lymphatic load. The venous elements indicate superficial vascular dilation, while the blotchy irregular emissions suggest lymphatic congestion or immune system activation. The coexistence of both patterns highlights a systemic interplay within the axillary field.

Clinical Correlation Through Anamnesis

Patient history is essential for interpretation.

- If the patient reports localized swelling, axillary tenderness, or limb heaviness, the lymphatic component gains weight.
- If venous symptoms such as visible varicosities or circulatory strain are described, the vascular aspect is emphasized.
- If immune burden is part of the history (allergic reactivity, systemic fatigue, reactive states), the blotchy fields point toward immune–lymphatic contribution.

Classic Value of the Image

This figure holds ~80–85% classic value as a representative teaching plate for mixed venous–lymphatic terrains. While less "pure" than isolated vascular or lymphatic cases, its hybrid nature makes it highly instructive for demonstrating pattern overlap.

Teaching Insight

The image illustrates the interpretive principle that biospectral terrains are not always singular. Practitioners must be prepared to identify hybrid patterns, where vascular and lymphatic signals coexist within the same field. Such cases teach layered reasoning, emphasizing the need to integrate both circulatory and immune perspectives when reading axillary terrains.

Reference 34

Axillary–Breast Angiogenic Pattern

Classic Vascular Case

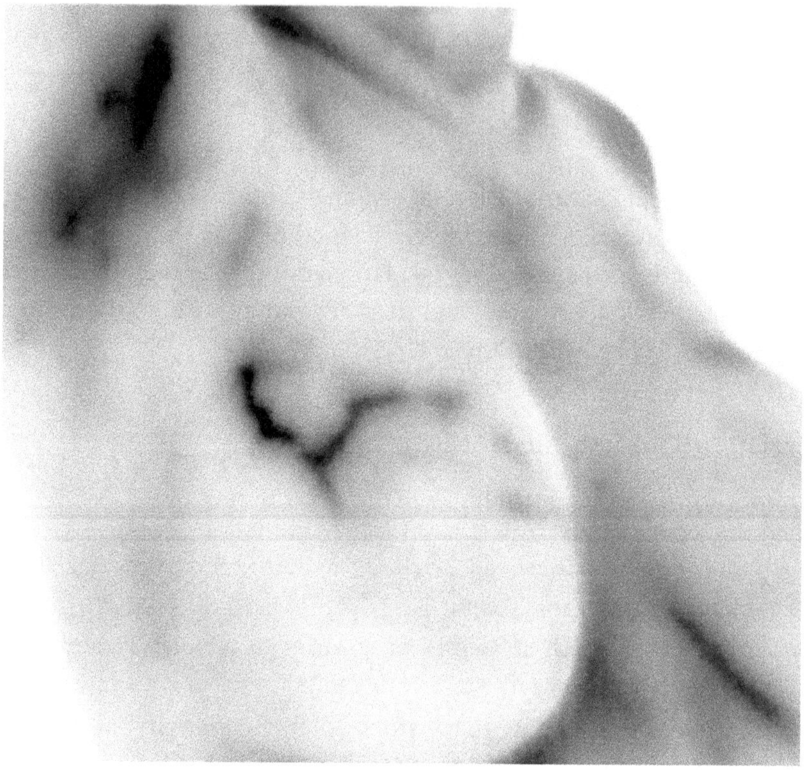

Anatomical Region & Interpretive Category

Zone **14–15: Left Axillary and Lateral Breast Projection**

Primary Interpretive Category: Vascular / Circulatory

Spectral Pattern

Curvilinear hyperemissive branching radiating within the axillary–breast field, lacking the symmetry and established pathway of typical venous drainage.

Pattern Type

Neovascular/angiogenic distribution: irregular branching not conforming to standard venous anatomy.

Spectral Pattern Description

The oblique biospectral reading shows a distinct vascular-like branching emerging from the axillary fold into the lateral breast projection. Unlike conventional venous dilations, the branches are irregular, tortuous, and lack continuity with the great saphenous or axillary venous lines. Their disorganized configuration is characteristic of angiogenic activity, the formation of new vascular networks, rather than established drainage.

Interpretive Understanding

This angiogenic spectral terrain suggests localized vascular proliferation. In Biospectral Medicine, such patterns are interpreted as terrain adaptations, often reflecting tissue demand for increased perfusion. The axillary–breast location raises interpretive questions regarding underlying regulatory signals, ranging from adaptive tissue repair to proliferative states.

Clinical Correlation Through Anamnesis

Patient context sharpens interpretation:

- In cases of recent surgery, biopsy, or trauma, angiogenic fields may indicate regenerative vascular remodelling.
- In patients with chronic breast congestion, nodular density, or hormone-driven tissue changes, these signals may reflect vascular adaptation to sustained load.
- If the history includes proliferative or neoplastic suspicion, the angiogenic field becomes a differential marker for deeper investigative correlation.

Classic Value of the Image

This case represents ~85% classic value, primarily for vascular teaching. It stands out as a differential angiogenic reference, useful for showing how neovascular activity diverges from conventional venous dilation. Its didactic strength lies in training practitioners to recognize irregular, branching patterns as distinct from symmetric, drainage-based vascular maps.

Teaching Insight

The image stress that not all vascular signals equate to venous overload. Angiogenesis represents a separate interpretive principle, requiring practitioners to distinguish between organized venous trajectories and disorganized neovascular patterns. This figure therefore provides a bridge between routine circulatory cases and more complex terrain interpretations, reinforcing the need for correlation with history and clinical context.

Reference 35

Frontal Neck Hypoemission

Classic Thyroid Hyporegulation

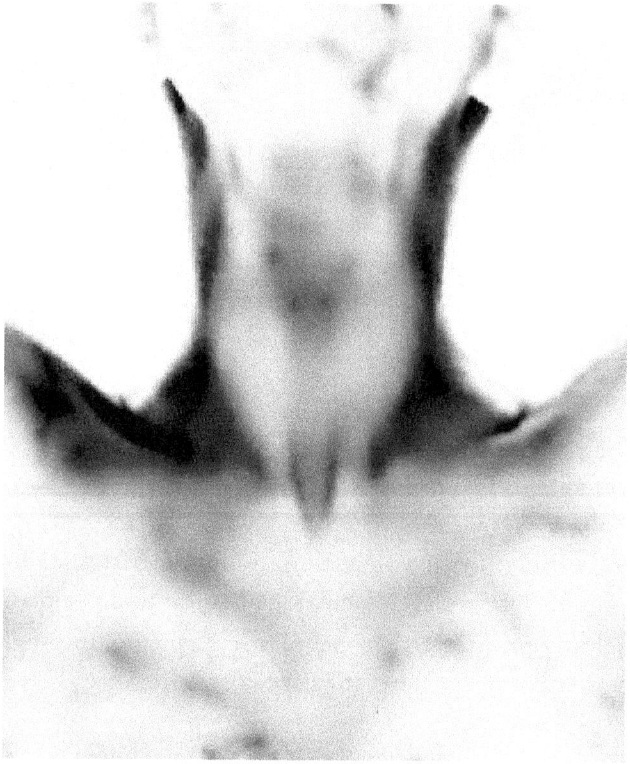

Anatomical Region & Interpretive Category

Zone 17 – Frontal Neck and Supraclavicular Region

Primary Interpretive Category: Metabolic / Endocrine

Spectral Pattern

Diffuse frontal neck hypoemission centered over the thyroid projection.

Pattern Type

Metabolic suppression signature: broad, low-signal zone indicating reduced vascular–metabolic expression.

Spectral Pattern Description

The image shows a male patient in frontal view with clear hypoemissive depression across the thyroid field. The surrounding supraclavicular and sternal zones retain normal contrast, further emphasizing the relative "cold" thyroid signature. The suppression is not patchy but rather homogeneous, delineating a clear field of reduced biospectral output in the anterior cervical zone.

Interpretive Understanding

This emissive reduction aligns with a metabolic–endocrine terrain of thyroid hyporegulation. In Biospectral Medicine, such uniform hypoemission suggests lowered perfusion, endocrine suppression, or compressive constraint within the thyroid axis. The symmetry and clarity reinforce its reading as a primary glandular terrain imbalance rather than secondary compensatory activity.

Clinical Correlation Through Anamnesis

Interpretive precision depends on case history:

- Patients reporting fatigue, metabolic slowing, or weight dysregulation may present this pattern as a direct correlate of reduced thyroid activity.
- If there is prior thyroid intervention (surgery, nodules, or autoimmune thyroiditis), the hypoemissive signature may reflect long-term suppression.
- In systemic cases with broader endocrine involvement, the thyroid hypoemission may integrate into a wider metabolic terrain imbalance.

Classic Value of the Image

This figure represents ~80% classic value as a didactic thyroid hypoemission case. Its clarity, symmetry, and homogeneous suppression make it a strong teaching reference for metabolic/endocrine hyporegulation patterns.

Teaching Insight

The case emphasizes how thyroid hypoactivity manifests spectrally not through scattered irregularity, but through diffuse and homogeneous signal loss. Practitioners must recognize this pattern as distinct from vascular or reactive presentations, situating it within the broader interpretive frame of metabolic–endocrine regulation.

Reference 36

Frontal Abdominal Hypoemission

Clasic Digestive Dysfunction Pattern

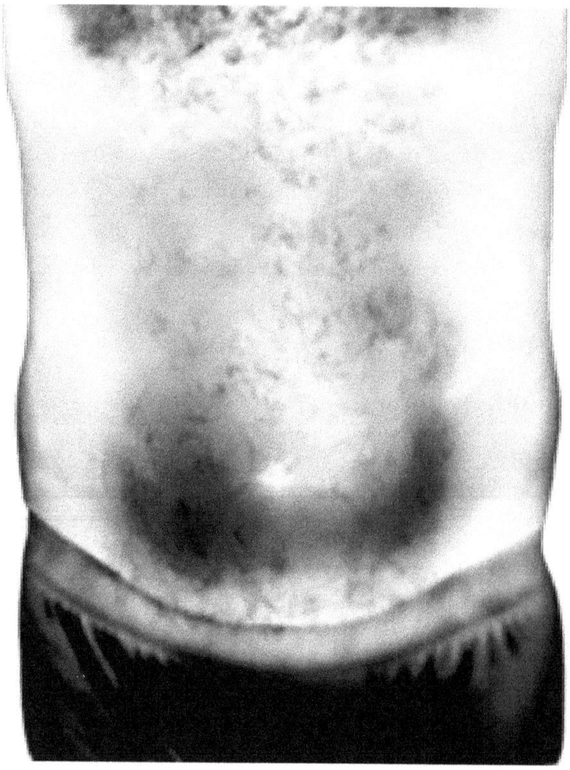

Anatomical Region & Interpretive Category

Zone 9 – Frontal Abdomen (infraumbilical region)

Primary Interpretive Category: Metabolic / Endocrine (with Digestive/Autonomic overlap)

Spectral Pattern

Localized hypoemission situated approximately four finger-breadths below the umbilicus.

Pattern Type

Focal metabolic–digestive suppression: a circumscribed low-signal field within the central abdominal projection.

Spectral Pattern Description

The image demonstrates a homogeneous hypoemissive depression clearly centered in the infraumbilical field. Its margins are well defined against surrounding abdominal zones, which retain moderate emissive activity. The uniform reduction suggests functional suppression of biospectral output in this digestive region rather than scattered or toxic–metabolic irregularity.

Interpretive Understanding

This spectral presentation aligns with digestive terrain imbalance. Two plausible mechanisms can underlie this suppression:

- Circulatory/Autonomic reduction, impaired microvascular perfusion or autonomic downregulation reducing emissive output.
- Gas insulation phenomena – digestive fermentation or enzymatic insufficiency leading to gas accumulation, insulating surface emissions and projecting as localized "cold" zones.

Clinical Correlation Through Anamnesis

Interpretive clarity emerges with history:

- Patients reporting bloating, irregular bowel movements, or postprandial heaviness may reinforce the interpretation of fermentative gas insulation.
- Reports of autonomic imbalance, stress, or pelvic–abdominal circulatory changes suggest a neurovascular regulatory component.
- If there is evidence of enzymatic insufficiency, poor absorption, or functional dysbiosis, the pattern serves as a direct biospectral correlate.

Classic Value of the Image

This case represents ~80% classic value as a digestive hyporegulation signature. Its central location and sharp hypoemissive contrast make it didactic for teaching abdominal dysfunction patterns, especially those tied to fermentation or autonomic suppression.

Teaching Insight

This figure emphasizes the principle that hypoemission in the abdominal field can arise from functional digestive terrain imbalances rather than primary organ pathology. Practitioners must be trained to distinguish focal hypoemission as a possible sign of fermentation, gas insulation, or regulatory suppression, integrating spectral findings with clinical history for accurate interpretation.

THE VALUE OF THE CLASSIC BIOSPECTRAL IMAGE

The journey through this Atlas has been guided by one central principle: that human physiology, in both health and dysfunction, leaves visible traces upon the spectral surface of the body. Across the selected images, we have traced venous overload, muscular strain, metabolic suppression, endocrine imbalance, lymphatic burden, and organ projection. Each case was chosen not merely for visual clarity but for its didactic value, offering the practitioner a reference point against which future findings may be compared.

These classic images are not ends in themselves but anchors of interpretation. They demonstrate the recurrent forms through which biospectral activity manifests, the straight linearity of a saphenous dilation, the diffuse blotching of toxic metabolic load, the focused glow of cervical strain, or the suppression of thyroidal hypoemission. By recognizing these recurring signatures, the clinician can build a framework of pattern literacy that allows the unknown to be mapped against the known.

At the same time, the Atlas has emphasized that no image stands in isolation. Each emission is part of a broader terrain, inseparable from the patient's lived experience, history, and physiology. The true power of Biospectral Medicine emerges when these patterns are not read as isolated anomalies but as integrated biosignals, pointing toward systemic states and functional dynamics. This perspective elevates emissive imaging beyond detection into interpretation, and beyond interpretation into strategy.

The final responsibility lies with the practitioner. Classic cases, while essential for learning, must never reduce clinical reasoning to mechanical recognition. Rather, they serve as reference pillars, enabling the clinician to interpret variation, asymmetry, and individuality with greater precision. The Atlas has provided a vocabulary; the art of practice is to apply this vocabulary with discernment, correlation, and care.

As the field advances, new patterns will be discovered, categories refined, and correlations expanded through research and clinical validation. Yet the images contained here will remain foundational plates, charting the beginning of a discipline that recognizes the body as an emissive field, where physiology and terrain declare themselves in visible form.

This final page affirms the mission of Biospectral Medicine; to reveal what is hidden, to teach with clarity, and to guide with purpose. The classic cases presented in this Atlas stand as a foundation for future work, supporting the growth of a science that is structured in method and centered on the human being.

Final Author's Notes

I wrote this Atlas across decades of clinical work, study, and revision. Each page reflects early mornings with datasets, long evenings refining definitions, and many hours at the bench translating observation into method.

My intention has always been simple and demanding at the same time: to make physiology legible through spectral surface reading and to give clinicians a disciplined way to apply that knowledge at the point of care. I have done my best to assemble a work that stands on scientific rigor, teaches clearly, and serves patients with precision and respect.

What you hold is a complete framework. The R-CIIM pathway sets a stepwise logic; mapped zones and fixed ROI geometry bring consistency; biospectral asymmetries receive standardized handling; the Spectrovascular Response Test (SVRT) adds a dynamic window on adaptation; the glossary and reference tables secure a unified lexicon across the nine diagnostic categories.

Acquisition standards, palette governance, overlays, and traceable metadata support reproducible practice and longitudinal tracking. These elements were built to work together, so that observation progresses to interpretation and then to action with reliability.

I invite you to engage this discipline fully. Study the definitions until they become second nature; apply the protocols exactly; document cases with overlays and clear narratives; contribute to calibration, training, and outcomes work. Share what you learn, new patterns, edge cases, refined thresholds, so the community advances while the method stays stable. Your careful practice and published results will extend the evidence base and help more clinicians use this language with confidence.

With gratitude to the patients, colleagues, mentors, and family who made this journey possible, I offer this Atlas as a foundation and an invitation. May it guide your observation, strengthen your decisions, and improve care for those you serve. If these pages help you see more clearly, act more wisely, and teach more effectively, then the years invested here achieved their purpose.

www.ingramcontent.com/pod-product-compliance
Lightning Source LLC
LaVergne TN
LVHW062040101126
852251LV00026B/338